TEXTBOOK OF PEDIATRIC INTENSIVE CARE

Dr. Beatriz Lezama

ALLIED HEALTH PRESS

Textbook of Pediatric Intensive Care

Author: **Dr. Beatriz Lezama**

Allied Health Press
4164 Lakeshore Road
Burlington ON L7L 1A4
Canada
www.alliedhealthpress.com
Email: orders@arclereducation.com

ISBN: 978-1-77956-864-9

ABOUT THE AUTHOR

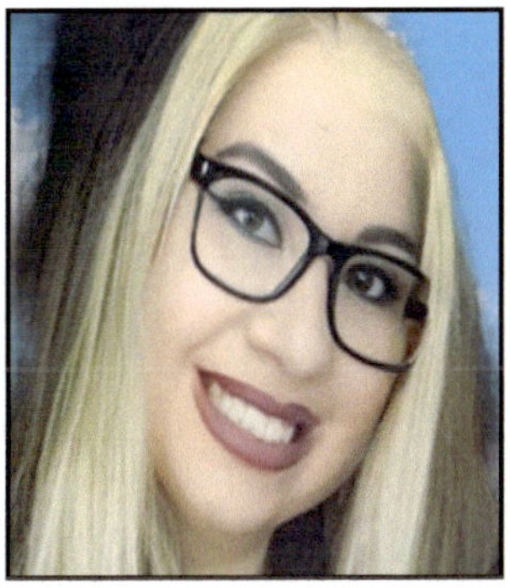

Dr. Beatriz Lezama is a pediatric specialist and fellow in neonatology, with a strong clinical foundation and a passion for early-life care. She holds certifications in general ultrasound, vascular Doppler, and maternal-fetal Doppler, enhancing her diagnostic and perinatal care skills. In addition to her clinical work, Dr. Lezama is an active health communicator and blog writer, with several health-focused articles published on LinkedIn. Her work bridges expert pediatric knowledge with accessible public education, promoting wellness and informed care for families and communities.

Brief Table of Contents

Getting Started with This Book

Chapter Openers

A list of Chapter Outline is presented providing a brief Introduction to what will be covered in the chapter.

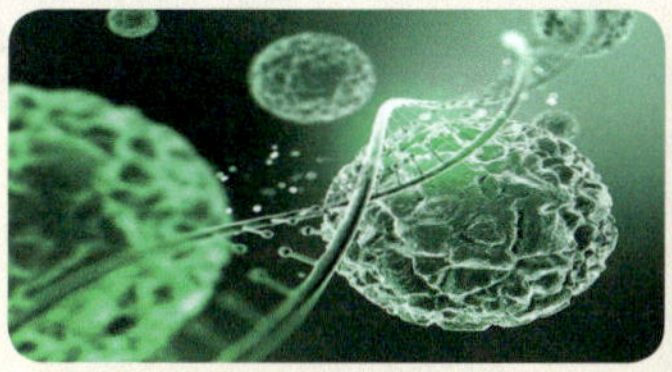

LEARNING OBJECTIVES

After studying this chapter, you will be able to:

1. Discuss the scientific method in biology;
2. Explain the cell theory;
3. Discuss the genetics and heredity;
4. Evolution and natural selection;
5. Focus on ecology and ecosystems;
6. Learn about human biology;
7. Evaluate the plant biology;
8. Explain the microbiology;
9. Focus on current trends in biology.

Introduction

Often referred to as the science of life, biology is a broad field of study aimed at comprehending the several kinds of life on Earth, from tiny creatures to sophisticated multicellular entities. Comprising several subfields, including molecular biology, ecology, and evolutionary biology, each of which advances our knowledge of living systems, this field clarifies the mechanisms controlling life events, including development, reproduction, and interaction with the surroundings, which is the central goal of biology. Moreover, biology fills in the void between the natural sciences and medicine by offering a necessary understanding of health, illness, and the interactions between organisms and their environments. Dealing with urgent global issues such as climate change, biodiversity loss, and new diseases depends on an awareness of these complex biological interactions, therefore highlighting the critical part biology plays in modern civilization. Fundamentally, biology explores and tests ideas about the living world using the scientific method. Through methodical observation and experimentation,

1.1. The Scientific Method in Biology

Learning Outcome

1. Describe the steps of the scientific method;
2. Focus on hypothesis formation;
3. Learn about experimental design.

Learning Outcomes

The beginning of each section of every chapter contains a set of Learning Outcomes that inform students of concepts they should understand. These outcomes help students understand what they should be able to do if they have mastered the material in that section.

Test Your Knowledge

Throughout each chapter, Test Your Knowledge cues you to note which topics have been covered and to self-test your understanding of the material presented.

Test Your Knowledge

1. Explain why correlation does not imply causation in scientific experiments.
2. How does the scientific method help reduce the influence of personal opinions in research?

Chapter Summary

The Summary Section appear at the end of each chapter and summarize main concepts covered throughout the chapter. These points provide key concepts in an engaging and meaningful way.

Summary

The investigation of biological principles highlights the importance of a comprehensive view of life by reflecting the intricate interactions that occur within living systems. The complexity of biology goes beyond individual species or systems, as this essay highlights; it also includes the interactions that mold ecosystems and affect biodiversity. Researchers can conduct in-depth analyses of metabolomic data using sophisticated technologies like MetaboAnalyst, which offer insights into the molecular mechanisms underlying these interactions. As demonstrated by the developments in MetaboAnalyst, for example, the integration of diverse omics data promotes a thorough understanding of metabolic pathways and helps identify important biological markers necessary for research on development and disease (Chong et al., 2018). Additionally, the phenomenon of ecological invasions is a key component of biological research and a vital field of study. The introduction of non-native species into unfamiliar habitats has significant ramifications and calls for multidisciplinary management strategies. Examining the origins and effects of these biological incursions, invasion science has become a crucial field that highlights the need to comprehend ecological dynamics and community interactions. As interest in biological invasions increases, new findings are emerging that put conventional ecological theories and practices to the test. The importance of incorporating various scientific viewpoints is shown by this developing discipline, which also highlights how invasive species shape ecosystems and advances our knowledge of ecological resilience (David et al., 2013). When taken as a whole, these discoveries from invasion science and metabolomics highlight the value of multidisciplinary biology research. Fostering cross-disciplinary collaboration and utilizing technological breakthroughs to improve our comprehension of intricate biological interactions are crucial as we look to the future of biological research. In addition to deepening our understanding of the complexities of life, this method lays the groundwork for tackling urgent environmental issues. Future studies can ensure the continued relevance of biology in a world that is constantly changing by acknowledging the interconnection of biological systems and opening the door to creative solutions that support sustainability and biodiversity conservation. We might imagine a thorough comprehension of life that serves both academia and society at large through ongoing investigation and integration of scientific knowledge.

Knowledge Assessment

The chapter includes material designed to review and reinforce each content. It includes Critical Thinking Questions to help test of your understanding of information presented in the chapter and Short answer Questions to review your understanding of the key concepts presented in the chapter.

Critical Thinking Questions

1. **Who is known as the "Father of Modern Biology"?**
   a. Aristotle
   b. Charles Darwin
   c. Gregor Mendel
   d. Louis Pasteur
2. **What is the basic unit of life?**
   a. Atom
   b. Molecule
   c. Cell
   d. Organism
3. **Which branch of biology studies the interaction of organisms with their environment?**
   a. Genetics
   b. Ecology
   c. Physiology
   d. Botany
4. **Which macromolecule is the main source of energy for living organisms?**
   a. Proteins
   b. Lipids
   c. Carbohydrates
   d. Nucleic acids
5. **DNA is primarily responsible for which function in living organisms?**
   a. Energy production
   b. Protein synthesis
   c. Storing genetic information
   d. Regulating body temperature

Short Answer Questions

1. What is biology, and why is it important to study biology?
2. What are the three main domains of life, and how are they different from one another?
3. Define homeostasis and give an example of how it works in living organisms.
4. What is the cell theory, and why is it fundamental to biology?
5. How do autotrophs and heterotrophs differ in the way they obtain energy?
6. What is the scientific method, and how is it applied in biological research?
7. Discuss how biology helps address global challenges such as climate change, disease, and food security.
8. Explain the levels of biological organization from the smallest unit to the largest. Provide examples at each level.
9. Describe the relationship between structure and function in biology, giving specific examples from cells or organs.
10. How has the discovery of genetics shaped our understanding of inheritance and variation among organisms?

Supplementary Materials

Key Terms: A list of key terms is given for quick reference

KEY TERMS FROM THIS CHAPTER

Annotation enrichment analysis	Biological structure	Cell
Cell theory	Cellular structure	Ecology
Ecosystems	Genetics	Human biology
Microbiology	Natural selection	Organism
Plant biology		

Further Resources: Recommendations for additional readings, websites, and multimedia resources.

References

1. Argelaguet, R., Velten, B., Arnol, D., Dietrich, S., Zenz, T., Marioni, J. C., Buettner, F., et al. (2018). Multi-omics factor analysis—A framework for unsupervised integration of multi-omics data sets. *Molecular Systems Biology, 14*. https://doi.org/10.15252/msb.20178124.
2. Bacher, S., Blackburn, T. M., Essl, F., & Genovesi, P. (2017). *Socio-Economic Impact Classification of Alien Taxa (SEICAT)*. https://core.ac.uk/download/286567949.pdf (accessed on 8th March 2025).
3. Barnett, R., Brace, S., Cucchi, T., & Dobney, K. (2013). *Divergent Evolutionary Processes Associated with Colonization of Offshore Islands*. https://core.ac.uk/download/20664364.pdf (accessed on 8th March 2025).

Detailed Table of Contents

CHAPTER 2

Pediatric Assessment and Monitoring 31

CHAPTER 3

Respiratory Failure and Mechanical Ventilation 59

CHAPTER 5

Neurological Emergencies 113

CHAPTER 6

Renal and Electrolyte Management 137

CHAPTER 10

Infectious Diseases and Sepsis 235

CHAPTER 11

Toxicology and Poisoning 259

CHAPTER 12

Trauma and Burns 285

CHAPTER 13

Post-Operative and Transplant Critical Care 311

LIST OF FIGURES

PREFACE

Pediatric critical care is the most demanding and high-speed of all medical specialties. It demands prompt decision-making, acute clinical acumen, and a thorough understanding of the physiological distinctions and complexities unique to infants, children, and adolescents. Since the incidence of pediatric disorders requiring intensive interventions continues to rise across the world, healthcare providers should remain updated with functional knowledge, grounded on current evidence and optimum practices. The work done in pediatric intensive care units (PICUs) is life and death, cure and disablement—hence, precision and timeliness of treatment are life-critical.

Aside from clinical responsibilities, pediatric intensive care requires empathy, toughness, and teamwork. Each case poses its own challenges—medical, emotional, and ethical. The PICU children are typically the sickest, and caring for them involves engaging families, coordinating multidisciplinary care, and planning for potential complications in various organ systems. With developing technologies and enhanced protocols, there is a demand for an orderly and readily accessible resource to assist healthcare workers in giving optimum care with assurance.

The *Textbook of Pediatric Intensive Care* has been designed to be a thorough and useful guide for clinicians, students, and nursing professionals practicing in pediatric critical care settings. Aiming to offer broad knowledge with point-of-care ease, the textbook blends clinical expertise with practical application. Whether confronted with a case of respiratory distress, with an endocrine emergency, or with ethical concerns in decisions regarding life-sustaining therapy, the book provides structured information and updated frameworks to support good clinical decision-making. With a strong focus on integration between monitoring, diagnosis, and therapeutic intervention, the book promotes an orderly and efficient process in the management of critically ill children.

Chapter 1 introduces the broad subject of pediatric intensive care, setting out the organization, function, and aim of a PICU. It defines typical indications for admission and provides an overview of the multidisciplinary composition of pediatric critical care teams. Chapter 2 is about pediatric assessment and monitoring, including age-specific interpretation of vital signs, utilization of scoring systems, and the necessity for continuing observation in early detection of deterioration.

Chapter 3 addresses respiratory failure and mechanical ventilation. Respiratory distress pathophysiology in children, causes of invasive and non-invasive ventilation, ventilator modes, and weaning strategies are addressed. Complications' identification and ventilatory support troubleshooting are also emphasized in the chapter. Chapter 4 addresses cardiovascular emergencies, with emphasis on presentation and management of shock, crises of congenital heart disease, arrhythmias, and use of vasoactive agents.

Chapter 5 deals with neurological emergencies such as altered mental status, seizures, traumatic brain injury, and elevated intracranial pressure. The importance of neuroprotection and prompt imaging is emphasized throughout. Chapter 6 deals with renal and electrolyte management. Fluid balance, acute kidney injury, electrolyte disorders, and modes of renal replacement therapy in children are all addressed.

Chapter 7 addresses endocrine and metabolic emergencies. The chapter examines diabetic ketoacidosis, adrenal insufficiency, inborn errors of metabolism, and accompanying crises that require immediate hormonal or nutritional intervention. Chapter 8 addresses gastrointestinal and hepatic disease, acute liver failure, gastrointestinal hemorrhage, pancreatitis, and nutritional supportive measures in the critically ill child.

Chapter 9 condenses hematologic and oncologic issues. It focuses on the acute care of children with febrile neutropenia, tumor lysis syndrome, coagulopathies, and transfusion treatment.

Chapter 10 covers infectious diseases and sepsis, with a focus on the identification and management of pediatric sepsis, septic shock, and multi-organ dysfunction, as well as consideration of antimicrobial stewardship and infection prevention in the PICU.

Chapter 11 covers toxicology and poisoning, including an overview of the management of typical pediatric poisonings, antidote use, decontamination, and supportive care interventions. It emphasizes initial risk stratification and decision-making when the substance is unidentified. Chapter 12 gives an overview of pediatric trauma and burn care and includes principles of stabilization, imaging, fluid resuscitation, airway management, and psychological problems with trauma recovery.

Chapter 13 addresses post-transplant and post-operative critical care. It addresses care pathways following massive surgery and organ transplant, e.g., fluid therapy, monitoring of the graft, immunosuppression, and prevention of infection. Special care considerations in liver and cardiac transplant patients are addressed. Chapter 14 addresses ethical and legal issues in pediatric critical care. Issues addressed include informed consent, end-of-life care, conflict resolution, minors' decision-making capacity, and interacting with the legal system.

Chapter 15 concludes on the topic of patient safety and quality improvement. The chapter introduces the measures of quality in PICU performance, recapitulates methods of reducing medical error, and provides tools for the success of safety interventions. How audits, feedback loops, simulation training, and family involvement contribute to quality endeavors is also addressed.

This is a book for a wide range of readers with an interest in looking after seriously ill children. Pediatricians, intensivists, residents, emergency physicians, nurses, and allied health professionals will all find it a readable overview of day-to-day clinical dilemmas. Medical and nursing students wishing to study critical care will find it helpful in its clarity of explanation and case-based approach.

INTRODUCTION TO PEDIATRIC INTENSIVE CARE

1

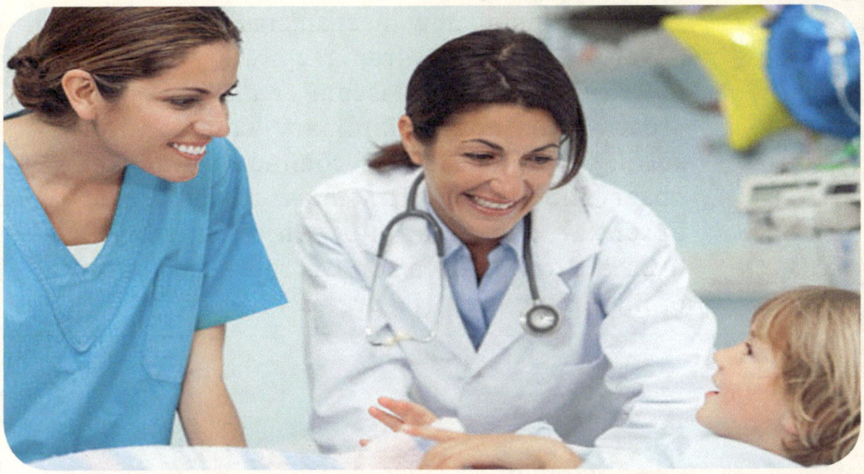

LEARNING OBJECTIVES

After studying this chapter, you will be able to:

1. Understand the structure and function of pediatric intensive care units.
2. Identify common conditions treated in pediatric intensive care.
3. Focus on psychological and emotional aspects of pediatric intensive care.
4. Discuss advances in pediatric intensive care.

Introduction

Pediatric intensive care (PIC) is a specialized subsystem of care focusing on the complexities of critically ill children. The introduction of systemic approaches to care in this setting has hugely improved patient outcomes, thus rendering the rationale for state-of-the-art practices such as centralized coordination of critical care resources unavoidable. For instance, the implementation of the Critical Care Coordination Center (C4) during the COVID-19 pandemic demonstrates that integrative management facilitates greater access to needed services for patients and enables the effective triage and transfer of critically ill children (Kelly *et al.*, 2023). Furthermore, understanding protocols about diagnostic procedures, that is, blood cultures in the PICU, is critical to maximizing care and minimizing unnecessary interventions (Charlotte *et al.*, 2023). This chapter will discuss these frameworks and practices and provide an extensive overview of the most important things that constitute good pediatric intensive care (Figure 1.1).

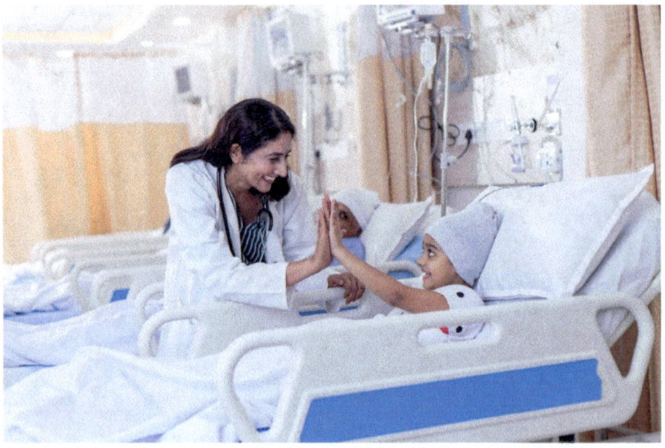

Figure 1.1. Pediatric intensive care (PIC).

Source: https://www.chop.edu/sites/default/files/styles/landscape_150_3x2_1100x733_1x/public/2024-05/Photo-ANE-PICUgetty-2624X1720-v01.jpg?itok=r6-BElG1.

1.1. Structure and Function of Pediatric Intensive Care Units

Learning Outcome

1. Understand the design and layout of PICUs.
2. Explain staffing requirements and roles.
3. Describe equipment and technology used in PICUs.
4. Focus on patient-to-nurse ratios in pediatric care.
5. Learn safety protocols and infection control measures.
6. Discuss interdisciplinary team approach in PICUs.
7. Explain family-centered care practices.
8. Focus on transitioning patients from PICU to general pediatrics.
9. Identify challenges faced by PICUs in resource allocation.

Pediatric Intensive Care Units (PICUs) are structured to provide specialized medical care to critically ill children and therefore require a delicate understanding of both their physical design and working procedures. A PICU's functioning is contingent upon its organization, like the recruitment of dedicated pediatric intensivists and adequate nursing staff, as they have a significant role in maintaining safety and patient outcomes. For instance, the development of guidelines and standards is needed in the evaluation of the risks associated with invasive interventions to enhance the overall quality of care delivered (Argent *et al.*, 2018). In addition, advances in pediatric medical care have also come a long way to streamline interventions in PICUs, providing new mechanisms to intervene in various conditions from respiratory diseases to critical care (Bernasconi *et al.*, 2019). By creating an interdisciplinary collaboration setting that focuses on communication and observation, PICUs can more easily predict potential complications, which ultimately translate to enhanced survival rates and quality of life for children (Figure 1.2).

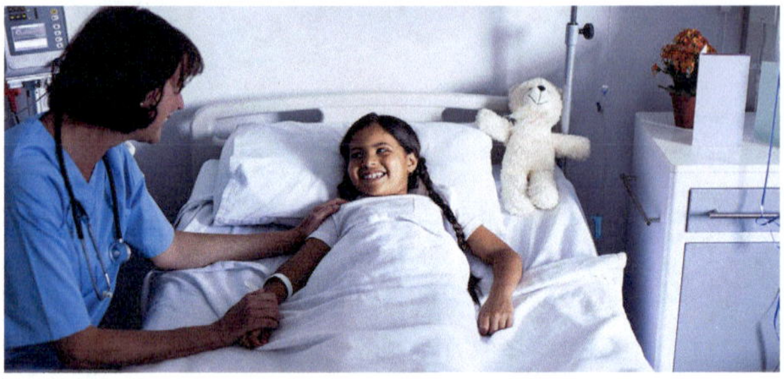

Figure 1.2. The effectiveness of a PICU hinges on its organization, which includes the appointment of dedicated pediatric intensivists and adequate nursing staffing, as these factors significantly influence safety and patient outcomes.

Source: https://cdn.prod.website-files.com/5ee7039040ea6efb80d7521c/5fe02ef510348c7dce8833c0_Inside-the-PICU-1400x700.jpg.

1.1.1. Design and Layout of PICUs

Design and planning of Pediatric Intensive Care Units (PICUs) play a significant role in enhancing patient outcomes as well as effective care in these specialized environments. Proper space arrangement can prevent the risk of infection transmission, which directly impacts the safety and recovery of susceptible pediatric patients. For instance, research has identified that the poor definition of areas of infection transmission can disrupt healthcare workers' adherence to best practices, which emphasizes the importance of a clear definition in layout (Brintnell *et al.*, 2017). In addition, the physical design must respond to the bespoke needs of young patients, which often involves the management of long-term conditions like asthma. To this end, healthcare workers are faced with complex treatment procedures and emergent therapeutic interventions unique to child development stages (Quint D *et al.*, 2014). The ideal PICU design, therefore, not only provides a healing environment but also allows for healthcare workers to deliver effective, compassionate care.

1.1.2. Staffing Requirements and Roles

In pediatric intensive care units (PICUs), staffing needs and roles are critical factors that go far in determining patient outcomes and the effectiveness of care administered. The severity of patients' conditions necessitates several disciplines of practitioners, and each member of the team has a crucial role to play in providing care for critically ill children. Research has mapped out areas of pediatric intensive care nursing priorities, such as decision-making regarding treatment options and infection prevention within healthcare, which reflect the high stakes in these roles (Latour *et al.*, 2014). And proper nurse staffing levels play a crucial role since it is directly associated with both the quality of care provided for patients and the capacity of teams to provide evidence-based practice (Latour *et al.*, 2014). As outlined in education models, nurses, teachers, and healthcare leaders work together in an attempt to maximize these staffing plans so that each child patient receives superior care and support in their most vulnerable moments (Figure 1.3).

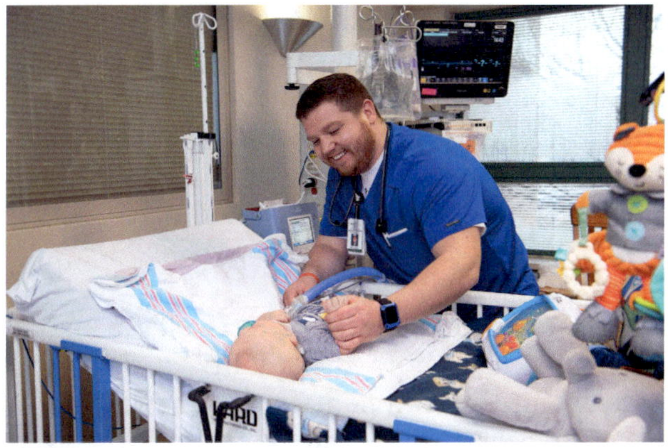

Figure 1.3. In pediatric intensive care units (PICUs), staffing requirements and roles are crucial components that significantly impact patient outcomes and the overall effectiveness of care delivery.

Source: https://www.datocms-assets.com/23576/1587664341-childrens-neuro-units-5-6.jpg.

1.1.3. Equipment and Technology Used in PICUs

The success of Pediatric Intensive Care Units (PICUs) relies heavily on a series of specialized equipment and technology for the treatment and observation of critically ill children. Such devices include ventilators that offer precise respiratory therapy, of which newer devices allow non-invasive methods of ventilation, which enhance patient outcomes and comfort significantly. Moreover, infusion pumps provide precise control of the delivery of drugs, which helps to manage complex pharmacological needs better. Advanced monitoring equipment tracks vital signs in real-time, enabling quick responses by clinicians to changes in a child's status. This group of technologies not only needs to meet the short-term clinical requirements but also be adaptable to accommodate the specific requirements of pediatric patients, particularly in low- and middle-income countries where resources are limited. Building PICUs in these settings calls for planning, equipping staff with appropriate devices, and long-term investment in healthcare staff and technology, thus creating a more effective pediatric care environment (Hervé Leleu *et al.*, 2025; Bjorklund *et al.*, 2018).

1.1.4. Patient-to-Nurse Ratios in Pediatric Care

Patient-to-nurse staffing ratio is also a major determinant of both the quality of care and patient outcomes in pediatric intensive care. A lower ratio usually facilitates more individualized care, allowing for prompt response to the extremely dependent requirements of children who are critically ill.

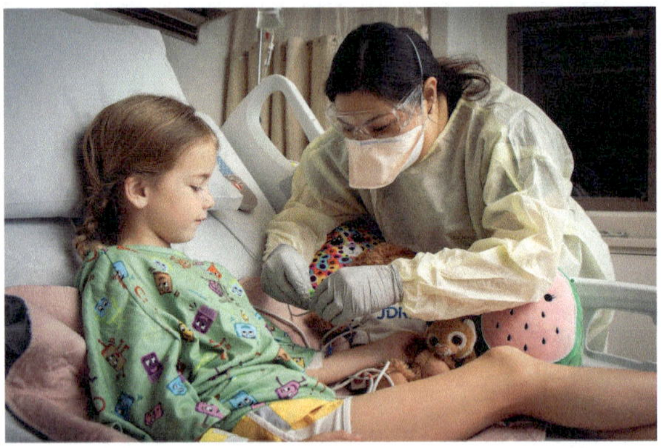

Figure 1.4. Insufficient staffing, conversely, can lead to increased morbidity and even mortality among pediatric patients, underscoring the necessity of systematic approaches to staffing in these high-pressure environments.

Source: https://media.defense.gov/2022/Mar/16/2002957357/1920/1080/0/220308-A-HZ730-9005.JPG.

Under-staffing, conversely, can contribute to increased morbidity and even death among pediatric patients, lending evidence to the demand for systematic strategies for staffing in these high-stress environments. Research has established that effective nurse staffing structures, including state-regulated nurse-to-patient ratios, can enhance patient safety and the quality of care overall through the minimization of the risk of caregiver overload. Additionally, the use of evidence-based training among nursing staff, particularly in low- and middle-income countries (LMICs), has been established to enhance the effectiveness of pediatric critical care units by empowering nurses with suitable skills and knowledge (Bjorklund *et al.*, 2018). Therefore, the nurse staffing ratio issue is vital in establishing sound pediatric intensive care systems and promoting improved health outcomes (Figure 1.4).

1.1.5. Safety Protocols and Infection Control Measures

Within Pediatric Intensive Care, the use of stringent safety measures and infection control protocols is essential for protecting vulnerable patients. Such strategies include not only the organized reporting of mistakes but also the promotion of transparency and accountability among health staff, as encouraged by the European Federation of Nurses Associations within their patient safety report (Burke *et al.*, 2008). With evidence-based protocols, such as those outlined to prevent central line-associated bloodstream infections, are necessary in this vulnerable environment. Designated teams specifically perform central line insertions and remain actively involved in monitoring infection rates, thus enhancing patient outcomes through inter-professional collaboration that facilitates optimal safety (Jennifer *et al.*, 2011). The addition of these measures is reflective of compliance with a policy of continuous improvement, the awareness that active infection control is essential in mitigating the risks involved with critically ill children who are especially susceptible to complications.

1.1.6. Interdisciplinary Team Approach in PICUs

In Pediatric Intensive Care Units (PICUs), the implementation of an interdisciplinary team approach is key to offering comprehensive and effective patient care. The approach encourages collaboration among different health professionals, including physicians, nurses, respiratory therapists, and social workers, to address the unique physical, emotional, and developmental requirements of each child holistically. Through the integration of several areas of study, the team is able to create customized care plans that not only solve the immediate healthcare concerns but also address the long-term health results and well-being of pediatric patients and their families. This approach becomes powerful when it comes to the recovery time of the patient and the satisfaction of the family, as interdisciplinary teamwork creates a more communicative and assistive environment. As has been explored in recent studies, the quality of interdisciplinary co-operation is central to building educational models in the context of health-care environments, as discussed in Boger *et al.* (2018) and School BU of Management (2002) (Figure 1.5).

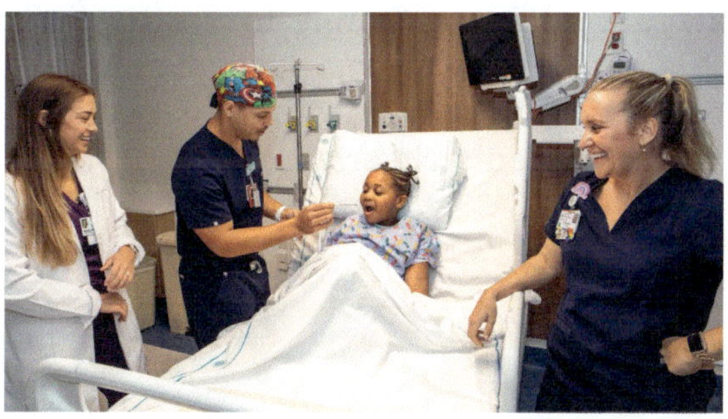

Figure 1.5. By merging expertise from various disciplines, the team can formulate tailored care plans that not only focus on the immediate medical concerns but also on the long-term health outcomes and well-being of pediatric patients and their families.

Source: https://cdn.atriumhealth.org/-/media/newsroom/featured-images/lch-picu_featured.jpg?rev=d5ffabacfc3c4a74a57cde910b2dc8c2&h=1080&w=1920&la=en&hash=81B41E3798461DCBFF4D52DFD679406A.

1.1.7. Family-Centered Care Practices

In pediatric intensive care, the implementation of family-centered care practices is crucial for optimizing patient outcomes and supporting the emotional well-being of both the child and their family members. A significant aspect of this approach is recognizing families as integral participants in the care team, particularly during medical rounds, where their presence can enhance the quality of care delivered to the child.

Evidence indicates that 85–100% of family members in intensive care settings prefer to be involved in these discussions, believing that their participation would improve their child's care (Latour *et al.*, 2015). Despite this strong desire, many pediatric intensive care units (PICUs) continue to restrict family involvement in rounds, limiting opportunities for collaboration and support. Addressing such barriers is a priority within nursing research agendas, particularly in the domain of child- and family-centered care, which remains critical for holistic treatment in PICUs (Latour *et al.*, 2014).

1.1.8. Transitioning Patients from PICU to General Pediatrics

Relocating children from the Pediatric Intensive Care Unit (PICU) to general pediatrics is a turning point in a child's health process, often plagued by emotional and practical challenges. Parents are often subjected to a dynamic emotional process during this move, having to walk through anxiety and vulnerability as they move into a new care environment, thus increasing their stress levels (Evans *et al.*, 2019).

The transition process brings significant variation in care delivery between the PICU and the regular pediatric settings, bringing with it issues of continuity and quality of care. Transfer is perceived by most families as less involvement in their child's care, and this can lead to destabilization and loss (Evans *et al.*, 2019). Moreover, studies have not been able to establish proven transition protocols, which is a practice gap that affects continuity and overall patient outcomes. Hence, targeted support from healthcare professionals is essential to counteract the issues that come with this transition (Figure 1.6).

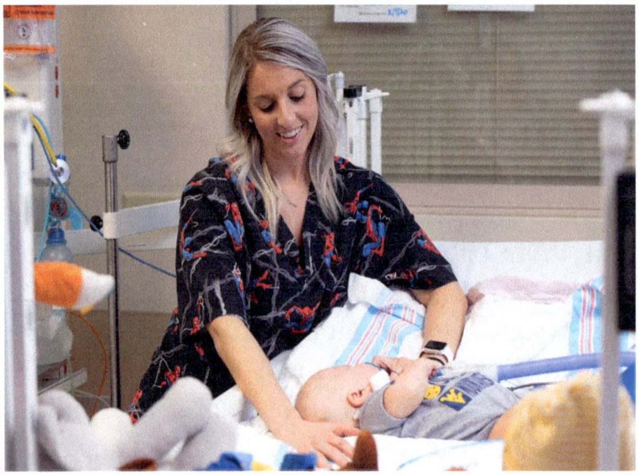

Figure 1.6. Many families report feeling less involved in their child's care upon transfer, which can lead to a sense of loss and destabilization.

Source: https://www.datocms-assets.com/23576/1584121950-childrens-neuro-units-5-5.jpg.

1.1.9. Challenges Faced by PICUs in Resource Allocation

The issues of Pediatric Intensive Care Units (PICUs) in the distribution of resources are multifaceted and involve economic constraints, high clinical load, and limited access to specialized research centers. In low- and middle-income countries (LMIC), where pediatric healthcare institutions are scarce in themselves, the issue burdens them even more. Clinician-educators in such settings report that poor funding and time-consuming requirements from their end impede the development of pediatric critical care practices, which ultimately reflects on patient outcomes (Attebery *et al.*, 2017). Additionally, specialized demands of specific populations, such as pediatric oncology patients, also make resource allocation challenging since they invariably require intensive care measures that are both costly and resource-intensive. The evidence indicates that mortality rates in PICU among such patients remain inordinately high when compared to the general pediatric population, imposing an urgent need for more strategic resource planning in PICUs (Nielsen *et al.*, 2019). Addressing such problems lies at the very core of advocating for quality and efficiency in pediatric critical care.

Test Your Knowledge

1. What types of healthcare professionals typically staff a PICU?
2. How are patients triaged and admitted to a PICU?

1.2. Common Conditions Treated in Pediatric Intensive Care

Learning Outcome

1. Focus on respiratory distress and failure.
2. Know cardiac conditions requiring intensive monitoring.
3. Discuss neurological emergencies in children.
4. Explain post-operative care for pediatric surgeries.
5. Focus on management of sepsis in children.
6. Describe trauma care in pediatric patients.
7. Learn end-of-life care and palliative options.
8. Explain chronic conditions requiring intensive management.
9. Identify infectious diseases prevalent in pediatric populations.

In the pediatric intensive care unit (PICU), clinicians are repeatedly confronted with a broad variety of conditions that reflect the individuality and high physiological demands of children. The most common illnesses are respiratory failures, typically met following a severe asthma attack or pneumonia, and must be treated with emergency and advanced respiratory care. In addition, critical care specialists treat children who have cardiovascular diseases, such as congenital heart disease or severe arrhythmias, which need strict monitoring and treatment (Bernasconi *et al.*, 2019). Conditions that are neurological in nature, such as seizures or encephalitis, are also extremely difficult, wherein an early diagnosis and treatment should be given to avoid any sequelae in the long run (Dale *et al.*, 2016). As pediatric critical care progresses, a deeper understanding of such diseases maximizes treatment methods, eventually leading to improved patient outcomes and quality of life among children who face critical health crises.

1.2.1. Respiratory Distress and Failure

Pediatric respiratory failure and distress present some of the most challenging conditions of intensive care, primarily necessitating advanced therapies. Acute lung injury (ALI) that causes impaired gas exchange and hypoxemia presents as a serious condition that has the potential to lead to increased mortality in affected children. Studies have revealed that elevated levels of PAI-1 correlate with poorer clinical outcomes because elevated plasma levels of PAI-1 are a sign of defective fibrinolysis that is detrimental during ALI episodes (Brady *et al.*, 2009).

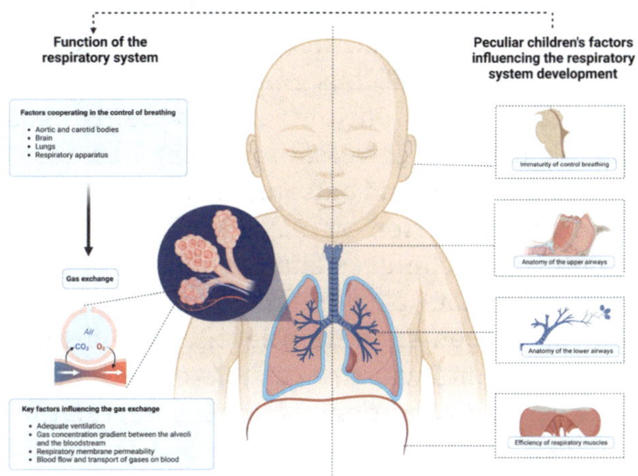

Figure 1.7. Respiratory distress and failure in pediatric patients present significant challenges in intensive care settings, often necessitating advanced therapeutic interventions.

Source: https://www.mdpi.com/children/children-11-01232/article_deploy/html/images/children-11-01232-g001.png.

For critically ill patients, extracorporeal membrane oxygenation (ECMO) has also been proposed as a potential therapy for preventing life-threatening respiratory failure, demonstrating improved outcomes when combined with protective mechanical ventilation strategies. While its application in a timely manner continues to be debated, ECMO is a rescue therapy for saving the lives of children with acute respiratory distress syndrome (Finney *et al.*, 2014). Proper treatment of respiratory distress is therefore key to optimizing the care provided in pediatric intensive units (Figure 1.7).

1.2.2. Cardiac Conditions Requiring Intensive Monitoring

In pediatric critical care, management of cardiac conditions is done under close monitoring due to the danger of immediate worsening. Congenital heart disease and acquired cardiovascular disorders have most often involved complex hemodynamics that play a significant role in the child's overall health. Specifically, the prevalence of CCHD has emphasized screening and early intervention, and evidence has established that universal screening decreases missed diagnosis and outcomes in asymptomatic newborns (Carrion *et al.*, 2014). Moreover, monitoring techniques such as pulse oximetry provide key data, allowing clinicians to critically analyze oxygen saturation levels and, in turn, identify infants who are capable of developing fatal cardiac conditions. Also, the correlation between multiple organ failure and increased mortality in cases of cardiac distress underlines the need for intensive observation in pediatric patients (Chimbira *et al.*, 2001). Hence, patient vigilance through intensive monitoring is vital to optimizing treatment and improving survival rates in this at-risk group.

1.2.3. Neurological Emergencies in Children

Neurologic emergencies in children are particularly challenging in pediatric intensive care, often needing to be immediately identified and treated to avoid subsequent effects. Seizures, stroke, or traumatic brain injury are some of the conditions that can occur abruptly and progress rapidly and, therefore, need emergency medical management. That these conditions are emergencies typically means they are harder to diagnose and manage because children present with nonspecific complaints compared to adults. For instance, increasing levels of child hypertension, as argued in Agabiti-Rosei *et al.* (2016), can be viewed as an underlying risk factor for neurological events, hence the need to track and avert these incidents. Similarly, the prevalence of Methicillin-resistant *Staphylococcus aureus* (MRSA) in critically ill patients, including children, reflects the requirement for screening and treatment of infection suspected to result in neurological complications, according to *et al.*Batra *et al.* (2008). Handling such emergencies is well accomplished by an interdisciplinary team consisting of medical and nursing personnel to provide optimal patient care (Figure 1.8).

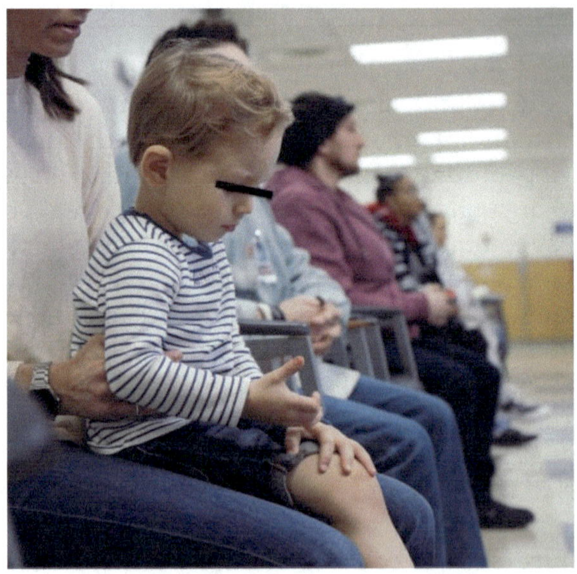

Figure 1.8. Neurological emergencies in children present unique challenges in pediatric intensive care, often demanding prompt recognition and intervention to mitigate potential long-term outcomes.

Source: https://i0.wp.com/iem-student.org/wp-content/uploads/2024/12/a-photo-of-a-4-year-old-boy.jpg?fit=500%2C500&ssl=1.

1.2.4. Post-Operative Care for Pediatric Surgeries

Pediatric post-operative management is a critical component of maximizing recovery and preventing complications in children. The care period demands careful monitoring and management, often involving particular routines that are founded on the unique physiological characteristics of children. The application of anesthesia, for instance, has made significant strides, but vigilance is necessary in light of ongoing potential for perioperative complications, including drug reaction and respiratory issues (Argo *et al.*, 2019). Proper post-operative care also involves the preservation of pain control, fluid resuscitation, and prevention of surgical site infection, all of which are of utmost importance during recovery (Antognini *et al.*, 2015). Secondly, family education and participation are essential aspects of the healing process because the family typically becomes the primary caregiver after discharge. Lastly, the goal of post-op care in pediatric settings is to provide a safe and supportive environment to maximize healing and address the physical and emotional needs of the child and family.

1.2.5. Management of Sepsis in Children

Sepsis treatment in children requires a multidimensional approach with an emphasis on early diagnosis and timely intervention to lead to improved outcomes. Central to this is the identification of prognostic indicators that determine the extent of the condition and potential mortality risk. A recent study highlighted that those children with a modified Sequential Organ Failure assessment (mSOFA) score of more than 12 showed a sensitivity of 92% and specificity of 96%, demonstrating its validity to anticipate mortality in pediatric sepsis (Youssry *et al.*, 2024). In addition, some special considerations must be taken into account when caring for children with congenital heart disease (CHD), as the unique cardiovascular pathophysiology may obfuscate traditional sepsis guidelines (Babu *et al.*, 2023). Thus, the inclusion of traditional scoring systems, e.g., PRISM, and laboratory findings like reticulocyte distribution width can enhance predictive validity and eventually facilitate timely referral to the Pediatric Intensive Care Unit, where therapeutic interventions can significantly reduce mortality (Figure 1.9).

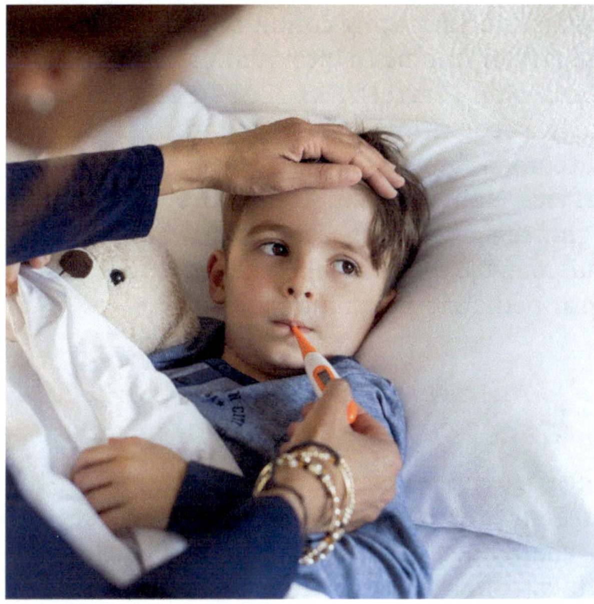

Figure 1.9. The management of sepsis in children requires a multifaceted approach that prioritizes early diagnosis and timely intervention to improve outcomes.

Source: https://ysm-res.cloudinary.com/image/upload/ar_1:1,c_fill,dpr_3.0,f_auto,g_faces:auto,q_auto:eco,w_500/v1/yms/prod/5564139d-5345-484a-bf79-97171f34e2bf.

1.2.6. Trauma Care in Pediatric Patients

Effective management of trauma in children is a critical component of pediatric intensive care, demanding specially targeted approaches due to the typical physiological and psychological responses of children. Early detection and treatment are given priority in a pediatric intensive care unit (PICU), particularly considering the fact that trauma can lead to complex complications like brain death, which was seen in 14 patients in a population studied, where asphyxia and drowning were the leading causes (Sucu *et al.*, 2018). Implementation of systems like Pediatric Early Warning systems (PEWs) has been shown to enhance clinical outcomes by assisting in taking timely action against deteriorating conditions, thus reducing the risk of traumatic interventions like invasive ventilation (Carrol *et al.*, 2014). This focus on early recognition not only improves patient outcomes but also reinforces overall PICU service delivery, and it mirrors the serious significance of specialized trauma care protocols that manage the particular challenges associated with pediatric populations.

1.2.7. End-of-Life Care and Palliative Options

The provision of palliative and end-of-life care in the pediatric intensive care setting is challenged with particular difficulties and ethical dilemmas. As these are addressed by healthcare professionals, however, the ethical precept of beneficence remains predominant, guiding decision-making for the child's and family's best interests (Diana Špoljar *et al.*, 2025). It is the central premise that underscores the relevance of interdisciplinary care in pediatric palliative medicine, particularly in cases where life-sustaining interventions are no longer commensurate with the quality of life of the child. Pediatric palliative transport (PPT) steps in as a vital option, which allows for the transport of critically ill children from intensive care to hospice or home environments, facilitating a more compassionate terminal process (Swasey *et al.*, 2024). The integration of PPT into palliative care practices is not merely aligned with family-centered care but also provides critical support to families when they are under extreme emotional duress, further confirming the value of continued investment in the development and formalization of such interventions (Figure 1.10).

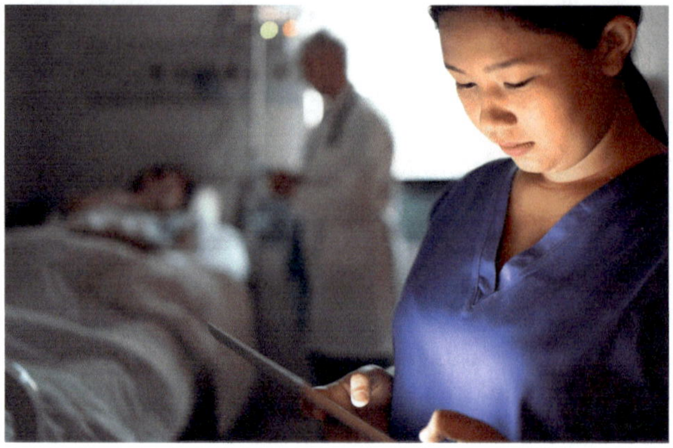

Figure 1.10. The provision of end-of-life care and palliative options within pediatric intensive care settings presents unique challenges and ethical dilemmas.

Source: https://assets.contenthub.wolterskluwer.com/api/public/content/5169dbb0c1b540b295f6c0de583bab53?v=4171ea1c.

1.2.8. Chronic Conditions Requiring Intensive Management

Long-term illnesses requiring intense management in children present unique challenges to health professionals and families alike. Illnesses such as chronic respiratory failure, seizure disorders, chronic kidney disease, and nutritional dependencies typically arise or worsen in children after critical illness, most notably sepsis. A large study highlighted that approximately 19.4% of critically ill survivors of sepsis developed worsening or new chronic conditions in six months following hospital discharge, indicating an immediate need for systematized follow-up care (Carlton *et al.*, 2022). The nurses' role in the group management of these chronic diseases is of particular significance, as evidenced by the existence of studies that noted a high positive relationship between perceived nursing staff support and successful disease management strategies among parents (Akbulut *et al.*, 2022). Of importance, therefore, is comprehension of group complexity in chronic conditions within a pediatric intensive care context in order to improve long-term health outcomes and provide holistic care to children involved.

1.2.9. Common Infectious Diseases of Pediatric Populations

Infectious illnesses are among the prominent issues among pediatric patients, often needing intensive care owing to their severity. Of these, viral infections, such as SARS-CoV-2, are of significant concern as many of them have the possibility of changing from mild to serious over a short duration, with hospitalization and, in some cases, mortality among children, even when cases are normally lower than in adults. Recent research points to the need to identify the risk determinants for severe COVID-19 to enhance focused interventions for optimizing the response to treatment among children (Zachary *et al.*, 2024). Besides, illnesses such as sepsis and myocarditis have turned into severe complications of multifocal infectious processes, demonstrating the need for more efficient diagnostic tools such as targeted echocardiography, which is totally indispensable in the intensive care setting to assess cardiovascular dysfunction due to infectious disease (Ermolenko *et al.*, 2025). Thus, understanding these dynamics is necessary to improve pediatric intensive care interventions and patient outcomes.

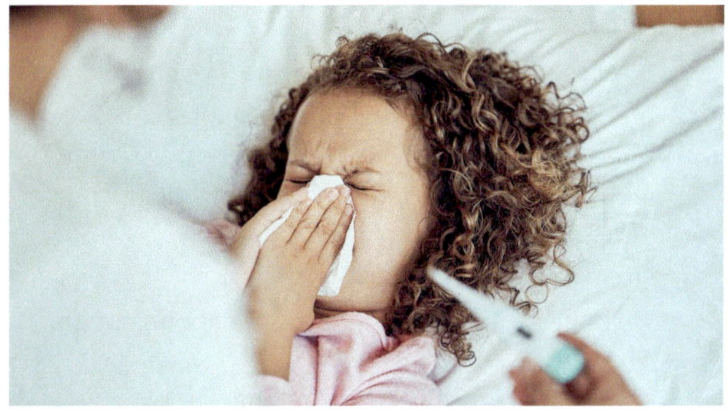

Figure 1.11. Viral infections, such as SARS-CoV-2, represent a critical concern, as many cases can escalate from mild to severe, culminating in hospitalization and even fatal outcomes in children despite a generally lower incidence compared to adults.

Source: https://www.childrenscolorado.org/globalassets/parenting-advice/articles/cold-vs-flu-article-image_1280x720.jpeg?v=4a556a.

Test Your Knowledge

1. What are common post-operative complications that lead to PICU admission?
2. How are congenital heart defects managed in the PICU setting?

1.3. Psychological and Emotional Aspects of Pediatric Intensive Care

Learning Outcome

1. Know the impact of hospitalization on children.
2. Focus on coping mechanisms for pediatric patients.
3. Discuss psychological support for families.
4. Discuss the role of child life specialists in PICUs.
5. Address anxiety and fear in young patients.
6. Understand long-term psychological effects of intensive care.
7. Describe strategies for effective communication with children.
8. Know the importance of play therapy in recovery.
9. List resources for mental health support in PICUs.

Pediatric intensive care units (PICUs) present a rare intersection of psychological and emotional challenges, not only for children in the hospital but also for their families and the caregivers. The experience of critical illness can trigger significant emotional distress, anxiety, and uncertainty among patients as well as families, making it essential that there are integrated psychological support systems in PICUs. Parents tend to feel helpless and fearful, whereas nurses, due to their direct role in the care process, understand the critical role played by parents in the care and recovery of the child. This mutualistic relationship emphasizes the need for healthcare providers to bridge the gap between medical staff and parents to alleviate emotional distress and improve outcomes of patient care (Toscano *et al.*, 2016). Evidence-based strategies for monitoring and improving patient and family experiences further alleviate these challenges, ultimately generating a supportive healing environment (Hays *et al.*, 2020).

1.3.1. Impact of Hospitalization on Children

Hospitalization poses serious consequences for children in terms of their physical status, emotional condition, and developmental progress. Stress due to being in the medical environment, undergoing appropriate therapies, or facing uncertainties can elicit anxiety and post-traumatic stress responses among pediatric patients. Research has revealed that respiratory syncytial virus (RSV) is among the leading causes of significant pediatric admissions, where a large number of cases require intensive care unit (ICU) admission, thereby establishing the vulnerability of infants and young children in these situations (Bourdeau *et al.*, 2023).

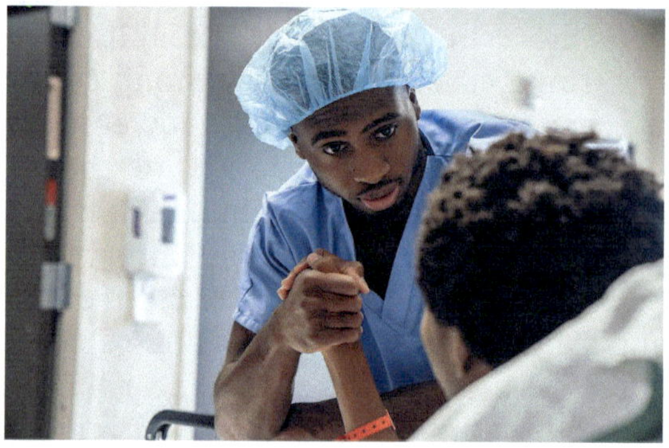

Figure 1.12. Hospitalization can have profound effects on children, influencing their physical health, emotional well-being, and developmental progress.

Source: https://www.mcw.edu/-/media/MCW/Image-Library/Stock-Photography/Stock-Clinical/GettyImages-925542218.jpg?anchor=middlecenter&scale=both&m ode=crop&hash=7BF98E624933EEB13BE98011E2EC5002.

In addition, during the COVID-19 pandemic, there were significant declines in pediatric emergency department utilization for conditions such as asthma, which implies that decreased exposure to usual seasonal triggers may decrease hospitalization rates. But this also raises questions about children's access to obligatory medical attention, which could result in increased exacerbation severity in the future (William *et al.*, 2021). Substantiating this knowledge is important for optimizing pediatric healthcare plans (Figure 1.12).

1.3.2. Coping Mechanisms for Pediatric Patients

Pediatric intensive care unit patients' coping mechanisms are necessary to decrease stress and anxiety, which are often present during hospital stays. Coping mechanisms are intricate and may include psychological, social, and environmental changes. Effective interventions may include play therapy, through which children are able to express their fears and emotions in a safe environment, and family-centered care, with an emphasis on parent participation in medical management and daily care, to bring a sense of control and reassurance. Empirical research indicates that a transfer from a pediatric intensive care unit to a general ward can possibly cause an increase in emotional distress in patients and their families, as was noted in studies examining parents' experiences during such a critical stage (Evans *et al.*, 2019). Furthermore, awareness among healthcare workers regarding how they manage is important in maintaining a supportive atmosphere for families, thereby improving the overall quality of care (Bagatell *et al.*, 2016). Lastly, the above strategies are crucial in enhancing the well-being of pediatric patients and their families within intensive care units.

1.3.3. Psychological Support to Families

Psychological support for the families is an essential part of care for pediatric intensive care unit (PICU) cases. When a child is faced with an acute health crisis that merits admission to the PICU, the family usually suffers from heightened stress, anxiety, and psychological distress. Evidence implies that, upon discharge, the majority of families still encounter physical, functional, and emotional challenges, emphasizing the need for coordinated psychological care (Coad *et al.*, 2020). Effective interventions can include family-based therapies that treat not just the child but also enhance family coping mechanisms. For instance, the integration of group therapy with peer support has been found to improve psychosocial functioning and quality of life for parents and youth living with chronic conditions like Type 1 diabetes mellitus (Alemzadeh *et al.*, 2013). Thus, including psychological support in the care model fosters resilience and prevents long-term psychological impacts of PICU experience for families (Figure 1.13).

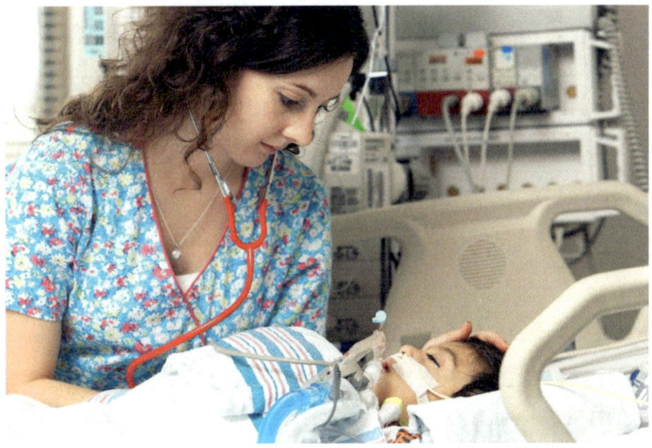

Figure 1.13. When a child faces a severe health crisis that necessitates PICU admission, the entire family often experiences heightened levels of stress, anxiety, and emotional turmoil.

Source: https://dam.northwell.edu/m/4859e26a49ea4eda/Drupal-Web_GettyImages-76131994.jpg.

1.3.4. Role of Child Life Specialists in PICUs

In the stressful environment of Pediatric Intensive Care Units (PICUs), child life specialists play the important role of alleviating the emotional and developmental challenges of hospitalized children and their families.

Specifically trained to provide psychological care, child life specialists help young patients navigate complex medical interventions and cope with hospital anxiety. By employing the intervention of therapeutic play, education, and emotional support, child life specialists prepare children to express their feelings, thereby inducing resilience during periods of importance. Additionally, they work extremely closely with medical teams to implement interventions that are tailored to individual children's special developmental needs. Such collaborative practices are particularly relevant to families confronting end-of-life care decisions, as documented by research emphasizing the amount of difference supportive staff make towards emotional well-being as well as care quality in pediatric patients (Behee-Semler *et al.*, 1990; Bagatell *et al.*, 2016). The general value of child life specialists is that they assist in making the medical environment more sympathetic and supportive within PICUs.

1.3.5. Dealing with Fear and Anxiety in Pediatric Patients

Anxiety and fear management in pediatric intensive care in children is vital to both psychological well-being and recovery. Children will experience enhanced distress due to being in a new setting, unpleasant procedures, and separation from family members, heightening their anxiety. Health care professionals should therefore emphasize effective communication and establish settings that facilitate feeling expression since children's rights to be heard are accorded paramount importance in clinical settings. Such measures not only reduce fear but also enhance the trusting patient-physician relationship. Despite this, available evidence indicates a disturbing trend in the use of restraint during clinical interventions that can precipitate experiences of moral distress in caregivers and, in the worst case, harm the therapeutic relationship with young patients (Alderson *et al.*, 2014). In addition, a lack of prescribed transition programs for young patients receiving palliative care also prevents care continuity, typically resulting in emotional concerns inadequately addressed (Adi *et al.*, 2009) (Figure 1.14).

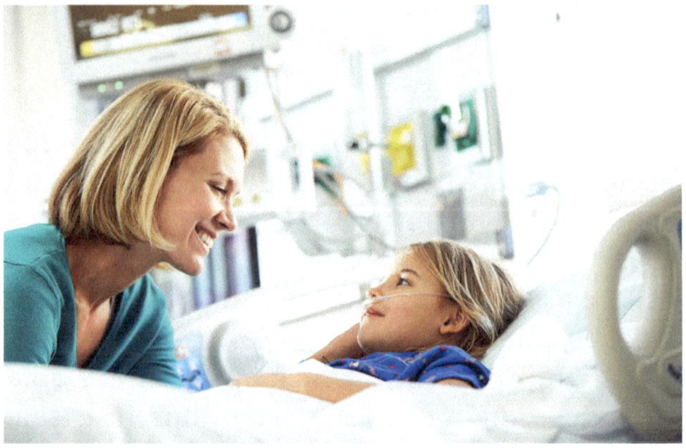

Figure 1.14. Addressing anxiety and fear in young patients within the context of pediatric intensive care is essential for promoting both psychological well-being and overall recovery.

Source: https://img.lb.wbmdstatic.com/vim/live/webmd/consumer_assets/site_images/article_thumbnails/SEEDs/picu-pediatric-intensive-care-unit-seeds/1800x1200-picu-pediatric-intensive-care-unit-seed.jpg.

1.3.6. Long-Term Psychological Effects of Intensive Care

The long-term psychological effects of intensive care on children are strong and multifaceted, continuing far longer than the short-term acute medical crisis. Most children, following hospitalization in a pediatric intensive care unit (PICU), experience significant emotional and cognitive problems, which present as post-traumatic stress, anxiety, and depression. A study on pediatric non-accidental trauma consequences shows that hospital survivors often require ongoing psychological care to cope with emotional and behavioral issues resulting from their exposure (Bassili *et al.*, 2020). In addition, a UK study indicates that the impact of surviving a PICU admission may create emotional problems not only for the child but also for his or her parents and siblings, evidencing the family aspect of this problem (Coad *et al.*, 2020). The requirement to acknowledge and satisfy such enduring psychological needs is of prime importance in designing certain interventions that support healing and enhance the lives of pediatric survivors.

1.3.7. Effective Communication Strategies with Children

Good communication in the pediatric intensive care environment is a key to the delivery of an amiable environment that enhances improved comprehension and coping mechanisms of the children. Simple, child-friendly language and effective narration skills can do much to bridge communication gaps between the clinicians and child patients.

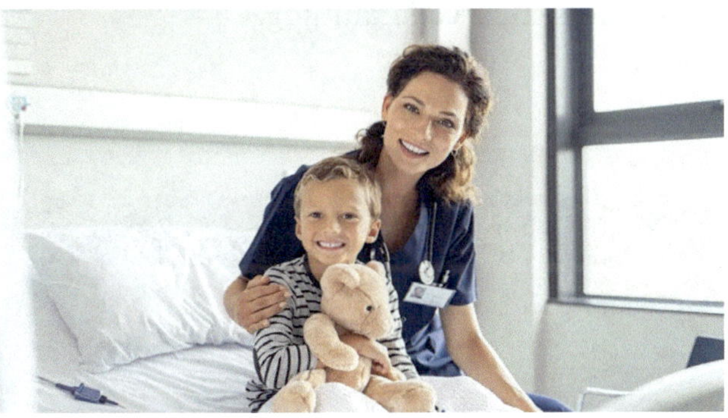

Figure 1.15. Utilizing child-friendly language and engaging storytelling techniques can significantly aid in bridging the communication gap between healthcare professionals and young patients.

Source: https://cdn.prod.website-files.com/63a1cbc81b0e903002cf9cec/669149e4818b42a8fc7031cf_Nursa%20PICU%20Specialty%20Post.webp.

Caregivers have to adapt their style of communication based on the stage of development of each child, since it might influence their comprehension and emotional response. Secondly, incorporation of family-centered methods, such as rounds that are family-centered, has been found to enhance patterns of communication, facilitating effective communication in the care team and the family of the child (Utami *et al.*, 2012). By prioritizing these strategies, healthcare professionals are able to optimize the child's experience, as well as family resiliency, so that there is an alignment of decisions in critical care with shared values and meaning (Latour *et al.*, 2014). Successful communication, then, becomes a platform for delivering patient-focused pediatric care (Figure 1.15).

1.3.8. Importance of Play Therapy in Recovery

In pediatric intensive care, play therapy is a critical intervention that facilitates recovery, most notably in children who are faced with the emotional and psychological trauma that accompanies life-threatening conditions. Play therapy enables children to express their fears, worries, and feelings within a safe environment, aiding in emotional regulation and coping mechanisms. Studies point to the fact that integrating play in treatment both promotes normalcy and enhances healthcare team and child patient communication, and thus increases adherence to treatment. Besides, just like a therapist's personality is crucial in the rehabilitation of patients undertaking physical therapy, according to a patient-therapist rapport study by Richmond *et al.* (2019), the relational aspect of play therapy is key in establishing comfort and trust. Therefore, the proper implementation of play therapy in the pediatric intensive care unit can play a vital role in integral healing as well as better overall outcomes among vulnerable children (Aebi *et al.*, 2017).

1.3.9. Mental Health Resources in PICUs

Inclusive of pediatric intensive care units (PICUs), satisfying mental health care needs both for the patients and their families is vital in mitigating the psychological impact of critical illness. Mental health services in these settings have evolved, with the inclusion of pediatric psychologists as a primary strategy. These practitioners provide critical support, particularly as it has been found that a significant percentage of families experience clinical levels of distress, including depression and anxiety, during the process of hospitalization (Balistreri *et al.*, 2024). Implementation of structured programs, like the Skin Champion program for preventing pressure injury, also demands prioritization of in-depth care practices that promote psychological flourishing as well as physical health (Gordon *et al.*, 2018). Through the establishment of a multi-disciplinary practice incorporating dedicated psychological support within the PICU, healthcare centers can enhance resilience among families, give mental wellness a high priority, and ultimately enhance the overall trajectory of patient care for these high-stress units (Figure 1.16).

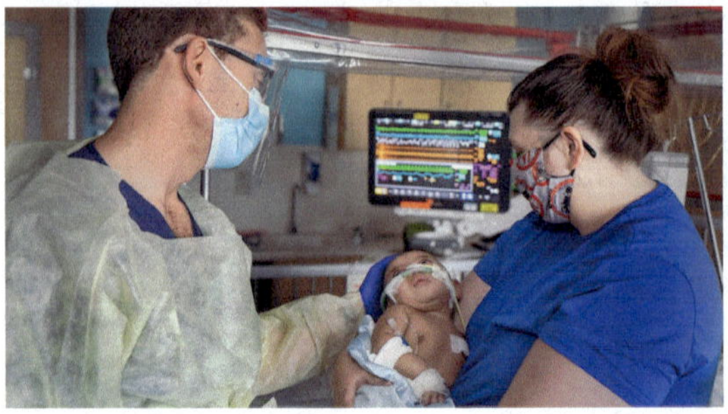

Figure 1.16. Resources for mental health in these settings have evolved, with the integration of pediatric psychologists emerging as a key strategy.

Source: https://www.hopkinsmedicine.org/-/media/youtube-video-thumbnails/critical-care-medicine-fellowships/critical-care-medicine-fellowships-maxresdefault.jpg.

Test Your Knowledge

1. What support systems are available for families during a PICU admission?
2. How are end-of-life decisions and palliative care handled in a PICU?

1.4. Advances in Pediatric Intensive Care

Learning Outcome

1. Understand innovations in medical technology.
2. Explain research and clinical trials in pediatric care.
3. Focus on telemedicine in pediatric intensive care.
4. 1Discuss evidence-based practices in PICUs.
5. Focus on training and education for PICU staff.
6. Describe the role of simulation training in improving outcomes.
7. Know future trends in pediatric intensive care.
8. Analyze global perspectives on pediatric intensive care.
9. Discuss collaborations between institutions for better care.

The appearance of pediatric intensive care has undergone significant change with advancements in sedation protocols and respiratory care, thereby enhancing patient outcomes. One of them is the comparison between intermittent bolus (IB) and continuous infusion (CI) of propofol for deep procedural sedation for procedures such as Auditory Brainstem Response tests. Evidence shows that while both methods of sedation are adequate, the CG technique comes with quicker recovery and discharge times despite a prolonged procedure duration and a greater total propofol dose (Ahmed *et al.*, 2017). Further developments, like the reclassification of disorders like bronchopulmonary dysplasia (BPD), have produced a broader patient care mandate allowing for individualized therapeutic intervention (Bancalari *et al.*, 2018). Together, these innovations reflect the dynamic and evolving nature of pediatric intensive care, with an emphasis on a continued focus on enhancing the safety and effectiveness of treatments within this critical care area.

1.4.1. Medical Technology Innovations

In the past few years, technological progress has profoundly influenced pediatric intensive care, as patient outcomes and the quality of care have both been enhanced considerably. New technologies, like advanced monitoring equipment, telemedicine, and minimally invasive procedures, have become a vital component of intensive care practices. These technologies enable clinicians to provide instant analysis of information and favor multidisciplinary approaches to managing patients. Interestingly, bibliometric analysis highlights the significance of cross-disciplinary work in this domain as critical care's seminal papers are mostly multi-author, which points towards a collaborative effort in refining knowledge and practices (Esmaeilzadeh *et al.*, 2019). In addition, case studies across various health care institutions reveal impactful innovations that have significantly improved patient safety and care delivery (Blumenthal *et al.*, 2006).

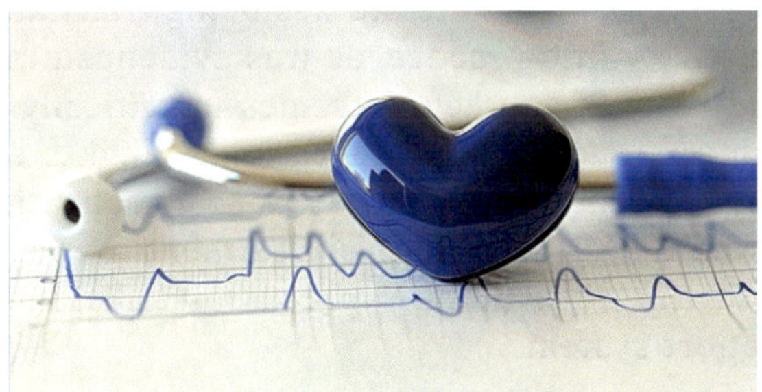

Figure 1.17. Cutting-edge developments, such as advanced monitoring systems, telemedicine capabilities, and minimally invasive surgical techniques, have become integral to intensive care practices.

Source: https://www.apexhospitals.com/_next/image?url=https%3A%2F%2Fbed.apexhospitals.com%2Fuploads%2Ftele_icu2_79f213a029.jpg&w=1920&q=75.

Thus, ongoing innovation in medical technology continues to shape pediatric intensive care, with medical professionals becoming increasingly better equipped to address the unique needs of critically ill children (Figure 1.17).

1.4.2. Research and Clinical Trials in Pediatric Care

Research and clinical trials are highly relevant in formulating pediatric care, particularly in pediatric intensive care units (PICUs), where children's needs can be subtle and varied. They not only assess the efficacy of interventions but also emphasize the significance of psychiatric care of parents during their children's hospitalization, particularly in congenital heart disease (CHD) (Kan *et al.*, 2019). It has been proven that therapeutic interventions can significantly reduce maternal anxiety and improve infant-parent attachment, but more high-quality trials need to be undertaken in order to back these findings (Kan *et al.*, 2019). In addition, the selection of outcomes that are relevant and of clinical importance is necessary to facilitate studies being translated effectively into practice, as was evidenced in a study identifying key outcomes in critically ill children. Such focused research highlights the ever-existent demand for rigorous investigation in the arena of pediatric treatment in order to fortify both therapy processes and family support systems.

1.4.3. Telemedicine in Pediatric Intensive Care

In the rapidly evolving age of pediatric intensive care, telemedicine seems to be a revolutionary step that escalates the level of diagnosis and treatment. With the use of real-time video conferencing technology and remote monitoring, healthcare providers are able to provide complicated care to critically ill children regardless of where they are located. For instance, studies indicate the efficacy of the use of tele-ultrasound technologies in enabling experts to remotely guide less qualified practitioners in conducting complex studies from miles away, hence avoiding delayed and accurate diagnoses of cardiac and respiratory ailments (Austin *et al.*, 2019). Additionally, telecardiology services have proven that remote consultations can reduce the demand for physical visits and provide acceptable clinical outcomes and costs, as demonstrated by a cohort study between teleconsultation and face-to-face visits (Dowie *et al.*, 2008). Such advances prove that telemedicine does not merely enhance access to required pediatric services but optimizes the use of resources under the circumstances of pediatric intensive care (Figure 1.18).

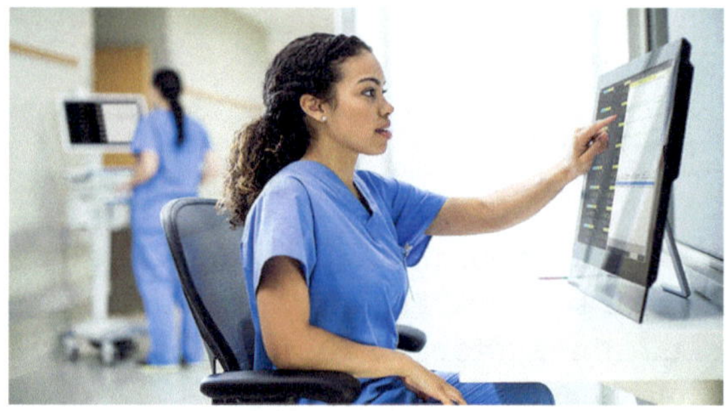

Figure 1.18. By integrating real-time video conferencing and remote monitoring technologies, healthcare providers can offer specialized care to critically ill children, regardless of their geographical location.

Source: https://www.philips.com/c-dam/corporate/innovation-and-you/global/june-2023/masthead-patient-monitoring-thumbnail.jpg.

1.4.4. Evidence-Based Practices in PICUs

In pediatric intensive care units (PICUs), the incorporation of evidence-based practice is essential in enhancing patient outcomes and guaranteeing the delivery of high-quality care. One excellent example is the implementation of the evidence-based liberation bundle, which is empirically proven to improve the management of critically ill children by maximizing care approaches and encouraging interdisciplinary teamwork among healthcare team members (Ali *et al.*, 2025). In addition, correcting fields already identified, like oral care, can also improve the quality of care being provided overall. Research has established that pediatric critical care nurses possess different levels of knowledge and practice regarding necessary guidelines, further emphasizing the relevance of standardized education and training in closing gaps (Moustafa *et al.*, 2024). By providing nurses with hands-on skills and ensuring adherence to evidence-based guidelines, PICUs can significantly reduce complications, shorten hospital stays, and ultimately improve the long-term health outcomes for their pediatric patients.

1.4.5. PICU Staff Training and Education

Effective staff education and training in the Pediatric Intensive Care Unit (PICU) are vital if high-quality patient care is to be delivered, particularly in specialist areas such as pressure ulcer prevention and burn care. Execution of a special training program for PICU nurses to carry out burn dressing changes significantly improved their skill and confidence levels so that they could provide care focusing on the complexities of pediatric burn victims (Carr *et al.*, 2025). Furthermore, ongoing education regarding pressure ulcer prevention was found to reduce the prevalence of pressure ulcers and enhance patient outcomes. Research identified that in the face of challenges such as personnel gaps, long-term practicing nurses with professional training exhibited a greater likelihood of embracing preventive measures (Mostafa *et al.*, 2024). Such targeted training programs are central to equipping PICU staff to become well-informed and capable enough to address the intricate needs of critical children's care, thus delivering better patient outcomes (Figure 1.19).

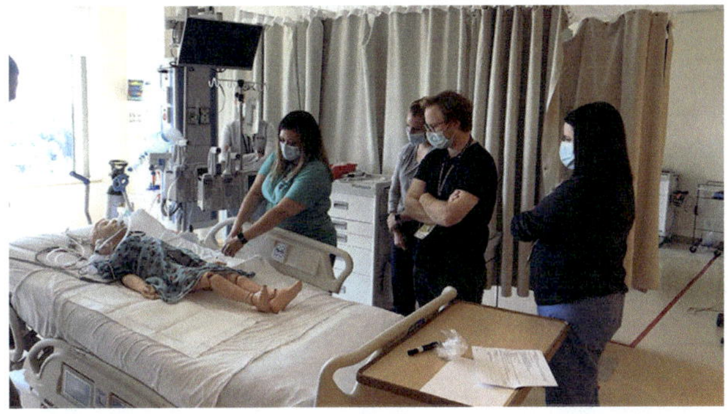

Figure 1.19. Effective training and education for staff in the Pediatric Intensive Care Unit (PICU) are crucial for delivering high-quality patient care, particularly in specialized areas such as burn treatment and pressure ulcer prevention.

Source: https://medicine.umich.edu/sites/default/files/styles/large_gallery_16x9/public/gallery/PCC-Research-Gallery1.jpg?itok=K_ae_w05.

1.4.6. Role of Simulation Training in Improving Outcomes

Simulation training integration in pediatric intensive care units (PICUs) enhances clinical skills to a tremendous extent as well as patient care outcomes. Simulation training subjects healthcare personnel to the practice of high-stakes conditions in a simulated environment, thereby instilling teamwork and communication skills required for handling complex pediatric cases. Through the use of simulators, the ability to mimic such critical incidents as rapid response and code blue events is possible, in which timely intervention can dramatically alter patient trajectories. There is evidence to suggest that if telemedicine is supplemented with simulation, as has been determined in the rapid response team telemedicine model, the quality and reliability of critical care interventions may be enhanced dramatically, with results comparable to proven face-to-face models (Berrens *et al.*, 2019). Further, case studies reveal that these innovations enhance procedural knowledge as well as promote a culture of teamwork and safety among pediatric healthcare teams (Blumenthal *et al.*, 2006) (Figure 1.20).

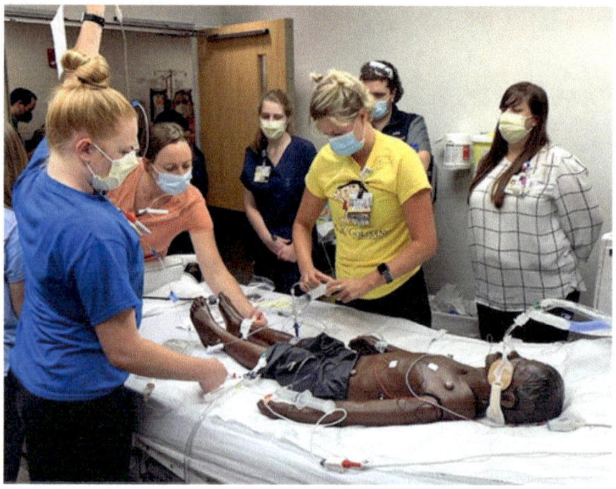

Figure 1.20. Incorporating simulation training into pediatric intensive care units (PICUs) significantly enhances clinical competencies and improves patient outcomes.

Source: https://www.urmc.rochester.edu/MediaLibraries/URMCMedia/childrens-hospital/critical-care/images/picu-simulation-crop-sq.jpg.

1.4.7. Future Trends in Pediatric Intensive Care

With pediatric intensive care evolving, several trends suggest an innovative future focusing on technical advancement and patient-centered practice. One of the key trends is the integration of mental health screening and intervention for children, particularly those aged below five, as seen through the ongoing efforts in states like Colorado and Massachusetts. These attempts, as discussed in Lyman *et al.* (2010), highlight the importance of early mental health identification as an integrated part of pediatric practice. Furthermore, innovation in clinical partnerships and patient safety is central to enhancing comprehensive quality of care within intensive care units. Case studies in Blumenthal *et al.* (2006) demonstrate how pediatric intensive care units have utilized innovative practice to not only improve patient outcomes but also establish a learning culture and safety. Overall, these trends indicate a future where pediatric intensive care deals with physical and psychological health problems in efficient manners.

1.4.8. Global Views on Pediatric Intensive Care

The understanding of global perceptions of pediatric intensive care employs a mosaic of diverse practices, cultural environments, and provision of health. It has experienced problems such as identification and management of deteriorating children and the safe interhospital transfer of critically ill children in nations like Ireland, which provide common challenges for child healthcare practitioners (Adshead *et al.*, 2014).

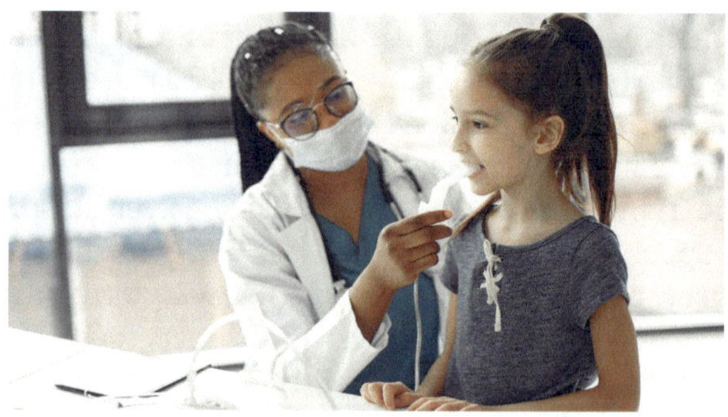

Figure 1.21. Understanding global perspectives on pediatric intensive care reveals a diverse landscape shaped by varying practices, cultural norms, and healthcare systems.

Source: https://medicalnewsbulletin.com/wp-content/uploads/2025/01/Untitled-design-2.jpg.

The issues are indicative of broader concerns regarding the quality of care and highlight research priorities within children's nursing. In addition, the Pediatric Self-Management Model illustrates the role of behavioral elements in having a significant impact upon the outcomes of health, particularly for disorders such as type 1 diabetes, and highlights the importance of adapting care methods to respond to different patient needs (Kaugars *et al.*, 2012). Through an examination of these global contexts, pediatric intensive care specialists can develop a more holistic conceptualization of pediatric intensive care, enabling intervention design that is tailored to the specific concerns faced within various cultural and systems environments (Figure 1.21).

1.4.9. Collaborations Between Institutions for Better Care

With the evolving times of pediatric intensive care, institution collaborations are the cornerstones of improvement in quality and outcomes of care for critically ill children. Such collaborations facilitate the sharing of knowledge, resources, and best practices, which can significantly offset the issues in lower- and middle-income countries (LMIC). For instance, a recent study noted that LMIC clinician-researchers enumerated lack of sufficient funding and support as major barriers to the conduct of successful pediatric critical care research, stressing the need for collaborative efforts to establish mutual guidelines and standardized care protocols (Attebery *et al.*, 2017). Furthermore, case studies show that learning collaborations involving health-care organizations have succeeded in applying innovations aimed at improving patient safety and overall quality of care (Blumenthal *et al.*, 2006). Pooling the strengths of several institutions, these collaborations can potentially develop an environment conducive to improving the provision of health-care services to critically ill children, ultimately reducing mortality rates and enhancing patient outcomes.

Test Your Knowledge

1. What are the recent advancements in mechanical ventilation techniques in pediatric intensive care?
2. How is point-of-care testing (POCT) influencing decision-making in the PICU?

SUMMARY

The very nature of the complexities in pediatric intensive care demands a multidimensional approach to both the educational and clinical competency of managing patients. By acknowledging the imperatively required effective interventions, such as the Skin Champion program that saw an incredible 85% reduction in severe harm caused by pressure injury, healthcare providers can enhance the quality of care offered to vulnerable pediatric patients (Gordon *et al.*, 2018). Also, the problem of tackling nurses' difficulties with teaching medication underscores the need to reconcile educational strategies with discharge outcome improvement. As the descriptive qualitative study discovered, a wide range of structural and process-related barriers negatively affect the successful transfer of knowledge to caregivers, indicating the need for a system shift to establish a culture of safety and high-quality care in pediatrics. Therefore, ongoing activities in nurse education and program planning are very important in ensuring best practices are not just established but also sustained in the long term.

In examining the complexities of pediatric intensive care, a series of prominent observations stand out that demonstrate the need for this medical specialty. Firstly, the setting of intensive care is troubled with challenges, specifically the added risk of preventable medical errors, which bear consequences for patient outcomes and safety. It has been established that these kinds of mistakes are most prevalent in high-pressure situations such as the ICU, where physicians have lower situational awareness during resuscitative efforts, thereby needing mental aids such as Visual TASK to enhance teamwork and decision-making (Calhoun *et al.*, 2016). Additionally, the unique pharmacokinetic differences that accompany therapies, that is, extracorporeal membrane oxygenation (ECMO), contribute to the complicating factors in medication management because the safety and efficacy of drug therapy may be severely affected in the pediatric intensive care population (Aebi *et al.*, 2017). At a broader level, these complications indicate the high-level complexity of pediatric intensive care and the ongoing necessity for innovation and practice enhancement.

KEY TERMS FROM THIS CHAPTER

- Care
- COVID-19 pandemic
- Services
- Protocols
- Blood cultures
- Specialized medical care
- Organization
- Nursing staff
- Guidelines
- Quality of care
- Communication
- Children
- Management
- Patients
- Diagnostic procedures
- Pediatric intensive care
- Contingent
- Recruitment
- Safety
- Standards
- Interdisciplinary collaboration
- Observation

CRITICAL THINKING QUESTIONS

1. **What is the primary goal of a Pediatric Intensive Care Unit (PICU)?**
   a. To provide long-term residential care for children
   b. To perform surgical procedures for pediatric patients
   c. To provide intensive monitoring and treatment for critically ill children
   d. To offer outpatient pediatric services
2. **Which of the following is NOT typically a part of the PICU team?**
   a. Pediatric intensivist
   b. Respiratory therapist
   c. Oncologist
   d. Child life specialist
3. **What is a common reason for admission to a pediatric intensive care unit?**
   a. Mild asthma
   b. Upper respiratory infection
   c. Respiratory failure
   d. Routine vaccination
4. **Which of the following best describes a key difference between a PICU and a general pediatric ward?**
   a. PICUs have fewer staff members
   b. Patients in the PICU are generally healthier
   c. PICUs provide intensive monitoring and life support equipment
   d. General pediatric wards use more advanced technology
5. **What is the ideal nurse-to-patient ratio in most PICUs?**
   a. 1:4
   b. 1:3
   c. 1:2 or 1:1
   d. 1:6

Short Answer Questions

1. What is the primary function of a Pediatric Intensive Care Unit (PICU)?
2. How does the structure of a PICU differ from an adult ICU or general pediatric ward?
3. What are the most common reasons for admission to a PICU?
4. How is respiratory failure managed in pediatric patients?
5. What are common emotional reactions of children in intensive care settings?
6. How does a PICU stay affect the mental health of parents and siblings?

Answers to Critical Thinking Questions

1. (c) 2. (c) 3. (c) 4. (c) 5. (c)

REFERENCES

1. Adi, Y., Carter, Y., Doug, M., *et al.* (2009). Transition to adult services for children and young people with palliative care needs: A systematic review. https://core.ac.uk/download/44454.pdf (accessed on 30th June 2025).
2. Adshead, A., Aherne, A., Ajizian, A., Association for Children with Life-Threatening or Terminal Conditions and Their Families (ACT), & Royal College of Pediatrics and Child Health (RCPCH), Azize, B., Coughlan, B., *et al.* (2014). Research priorities for children's nursing in Ireland: A Delphi study. https://core.ac.uk/download/30733090.pdf (accessed on 30th June 2025).
3. Aebi, A., Shah, A. G., Anderson, A., Arlt, B., Barr, B., Barthelemy, B., *et al.* (2017). Medication complications in extracorporeal membrane oxygenation. https://core.ac.uk/download/129191716.pdf (accessed on 30th June 2025).
4. Agabiti-Rosei, E., Cruickshank, J. K., Dominiczak, A., *et al.* (2016). 2016 European Society of Hypertension guidelines for the management of high blood pressure in children and adolescents. https://core.ac.uk/download/46165193.pdf (accessed on 30th June 2025).
5. Ahmed, S. S., Hicks, S., Nitu, M., *et al.* (2017). Intermittent bolus versus continuous infusion of propofol for deep sedation during ABR/nuclear medicine studies. https://core.ac.uk/download/227054213.pdf (accessed on 30th June 2025).
6. Akbulut, H., & Uysal, G. (2022). Determination of the relationship between disease managements and the perception of nursing support of parents whose children are monitored in an intensive care unit. *The Journal of Pediatric Research.* https://www.semanticscholar.org/paper/21f565bab5aa6fe7eada42ad557b94d6af3e74e1 (accessed on 30th June 2025).
7. Alderson, A., Bigwood, B., Bradlyn, B., Brenner, B., Bricher, B., *et al.* (2014). Holding and restraining children for clinical procedures within an acute care setting: An ethical consideration of the evidence. https://core.ac.uk/download/42137676.pdf (accessed on 30th June 2025).
8. Alemzadeh, R., Kaugars, A. S., Kichler, J. C., *et al.* (2013). Effectiveness of groups for adolescents with Type 1 diabetes mellitus and their parents. https://core.ac.uk/download/213076442.pdf (accessed on 30th June 2025).
9. Ali, R. M. S., Mosbeh, A. N., & Hafez, M. M. (2025). Effect of educational program on nurses' performance regarding application of liberation bundle in pediatric intensive care unit. *BMC Nursing, 24.* https://www.semanticscholar.org/paper/82bf7c2cf3994b56c999a57bc90a15dc2beb6d81 (accessed on 30th June 2025).
10. Nielsen Angaard, J. S., Brierley, J., Dohna-Schwake, C., *et al.* (2019). PICU mortality of children with cancer admitted to pediatric intensive care unit: A systematic review and meta-analysis. https://core.ac.uk/download/227040533.pdf (accessed on 30th June 2025).
11. Antognini, J. F., Antognini, J. M., O'Brien, K., & Khatri, V. (2015). How many operating rooms are needed to manage non-elective surgical cases? A Monte Carlo simulation study. https://core.ac.uk/download/323071788.pdf (accessed on 30th June 2025).
12. Argent, A., & Frey, B. (2018). Safe pediatric intensive care: Part 2: Workplace organization, critical incident monitoring and guidelines. https://core.ac.uk/download/159154992.pdf (accessed on 30th June 2025).

13. Argo, A., Buscemi, R., Karch, S. B., Lanzarone, A., Roccuzzo, R., & Zerbo, S. (2019). Perioperative and anesthetic deaths: Toxicological and medico legal aspects. https://core.ac.uk/download/224993621.pdf (accessed on 30th June 2025).

14. Attebery, J., Fink, E. L., Kissoon, N., *et al.* (2017). Challenges and priorities for pediatric critical care clinician-researchers in low- and middle-income countries. https://core.ac.uk/download/212859289.pdf (accessed on 30th June 2025).

15. Austin, B., Davis, W., Le, D. Q., *et al.* (2019). Feasibility evaluation of commercially available video conferencing devices to technically direct untrained nonmedical personnel to perform a rapid trauma ultrasound examination. https://core.ac.uk/download/323310769.pdf (accessed on 30th June 2025).

16. Babu, S., Sreedhar, R., Munaf, M., & Gadhinglajkar, S. (2023). Sepsis in the pediatric cardiac intensive care unit: An updated review. *Journal of Cardiothoracic and Vascular Anesthesia*. https://www.semanticscholar.org/paper/f9935652100cf6dc40d513f960a9ea19886190f2 (accessed on 30th June 2025).

17. Bagatell, R., Bloomer, M., Bryson, A., Scott, D., Davies, B., Doka, K. J., Downey, V., *et al.* (2016). Healthcare staff's experience in providing end-of-life care to children: A mixed-method review. https://core.ac.uk/download/74204640.pdf (accessed on 30th June 2025).

18. Balistreri, K. A. (2024). Description and critical evaluation of models of psychology practice in the pediatric intensive care unit. https://core.ac.uk/download/619714983.pdf (accessed on 30th June 2025).

19. Bancalari, E., Clyman, R. I., Collaco, J. M., *et al.* (2018). Bronchopulmonary dysplasia: Executive summary of a workshop. https://core.ac.uk/download/227054384.pdf (accessed on 30th June 2025).

20. Bassili, M. (2020). Non-accidental trauma: Nature of subsequent encounters and related outcomes. https://core.ac.uk/download/477681284.pdf (accessed on 30th June 2025).

21. Batra, R., Edgeworth, J., Eziefula, A. C., *et al.* (2008). Throat and rectal swabs may have an important role in MRSA screening of critically ill patients.

22. Behee-Semler, B. J., Fox, R. A., & Ragatz, S. C. (1990). Implications of a NICU perinatal follow through program for the primary care physician. https://core.ac.uk/download/213084301.pdf (accessed on 30th June 2025).

23. Bernasconi, S., Borrelli, M., Caffarelli, C., Corsello, G., Di Pinto, R., Gaeta, V., Iovane, B., *et al.* (2019). Report on advances for pediatricians in 2018: Allergy, cardiology, critical care, endocrinology, hereditary metabolic diseases, gastroenterology, infectious diseases, neonatology, nutrition, respiratory tract disorders and surgery. https://core.ac.uk/download/286528671.pdf (accessed on 30th June 2025).

24. Berrens, Z. J., Brady, P. W., Gosdin, C. H., *et al.* (2019). Efficacy and safety of pediatric critical care physician telemedicine involvement in rapid response team and code response in a satellite facility. https://core.ac.uk/download/299809011.pdf (accessed on 30th June 2025).

25. Bjorklund, A. R., Day, L. T., Hagen, S. A., Johannsen, E., *et al.* (2018). Pediatric critical care in resource-limited settings—Overview and lessons learned. https://core.ac.uk/download/154430985.pdf (accessed on 30th June 2025).

26. Blumenthal, D., & McCarthy, D. (2006). *Committed to Safety: Ten Case Studies on Reducing Harm to Patients*. https://core.ac.uk/download/71350251.pdf (accessed on 30th June 2025).
27. Boger, K. D., Bozzone, D., Cook, S. E., Donohue, K., *et al.* (2018). *The Journal of the Center for Interdisciplinary Teaching and Learning*. https://open.bu.edu/bitstream/2144/29602/1/WINTER-2018-IMPACT.pdf (accessed on 30th June 2025).
28. Bonica, M., Students of Health Management 721.01, University of New Hampshire. (2017). *Healthcare Management Primer*. https://core.ac.uk/download/215509297.pdf (accessed on 30th June 2025).
29. Boston University School of Management. (2002). *Research Highlights*. https://open.bu.edu/bitstream/2144/32996/1/research_highlights_Summer2002_web.pdf (accessed on 30th June 2025).
30. Bourdeau, M., Vadlamudi, N. K., Bastien, N., Embreé, J., Halperin, S. A., Jadavji, T., Kazmi, K., *et al.* (2023). Pediatric RSV-associated hospitalizations before and during the COVID-19 pandemic. *JAMA Network Open, 6*, e2336863–e2336863. https://doi.org/10.1001/jamanetworkopen.2023.36863 (accessed on 30th June 2025).
31. Brady, S., Curley, M. A. Q., Flori, H., Matthay, M. A., *et al.* (2009). Elevated PAI-1 is associated with poor clinical outcomes in pediatric patients with acute lung injury. https://core.ac.uk/download/323078706.pdf (accessed on 30th June 2025).
32. Brintnell, J., Cobb, S., Mitchell, A., Momtahan, K., *et al.* (2017). Human factors considerations in designing for infection prevention and control in neonatal care–Findings from a pre-design inquiry. https://core.ac.uk/download/84636920.pdf (accessed on 30th June 2025).
33. Burke, J., Smith, L. N., Sveinsdóttir, H., Willman, A., *et al.* (2008). Patient safety in Europe: Medication errors and hospital-acquired infections. https://core.ac.uk/download/90014.pdf (accessed on 30th June 2025).
34. Calhoun, A. W., Gonzales, M. J., Henry, J. M., Riek, L. D., *et al.* (2016). Visual TASK: A collaborative cognitive aid for acute care resuscitation. http://arxiv.org/abs/1605.05224 (accessed on 30th June 2025).
35. Carlton, E., Gebremariam, A., Maddux, A., McNamara, N. A., Barbaro, R., Cornell, T. T., Iwashyna, T. J., *et al.* (2022). New and progressive medical conditions after pediatric sepsis hospitalization requiring critical care. *JAMA Pediatrics*. https://www.semanticscholar.org/paper/02d8ea8a45a055382f4e70833a4dff7887726a45 (accessed on 30th June 2025).
36. Carr, C., Beck, P., Kazlauskas, K., & Moody, A. (2025). 922 igniting a change: Development of a PICU burn program. *Journal of Burn Care & Research: Official Publication of the American Burn Association, 46*, S342–S342. https://www.semanticscholar.org/paper/c24135f8284f8d776045646c3d13f50cc856cf18 (accessed on 30th June 2025).
37. Carrion, V., Lakshminrusimha, S., Manja, V., Mathew, B., *et al.* (2014). Critical congenital heart disease screening by pulse oximetry in a neonatal intensive care unit. https://core.ac.uk/download/323069960.pdf (accessed on 30th June 2025).
38. Carrol, E. D., Lane, S., Lisboa, P. J. G., McGrath, M., *et al.* (2014). What impact did a pediatric early warning system have on emergency admissions to the pediatric intensive care unit? An observational cohort studies. https://core.ac.uk/download/42136646.pdf (accessed on 30th June 2025).

39. Chimbira, W., Crawford, H., Gupta, S., Legg, J. P., *et al.* (2001). Acute lung injury in pediatric intensive care: Course and outcome. https://core.ac.uk/download/pdf/8715345.pdf (accessed on 30th June 2025).

40. Coad, J., Colville, G., Curley, M. A. Q., Draper, E. S., *et al.* (2020). Study protocol for a multicenter longitudinal mixed methods study to explore the outcomes of children and families in the first year after pediatric intensive care: The OCEANIC study. https://core.ac.uk/download/323385694.pdf (accessed on 30th June 2025).

41. Dale, R. C., Nosadini, M., & Lim, M. (2016). Therapeutic decision making in autoimmune and inflammatory disorders of the central nervous system in children. https://core.ac.uk/download/154325209.pdf (accessed on 30th June 2025).

42. Dowie, R., Franklin, R. C., Mistry, H., Rigby, M. J., *et al.* (2008). A pediatric telecardiology service for district hospitals in south-east England: An observational study. https://core.ac.uk/download/337059.pdf (accessed on 30th June 2025).

43. Edwards, J. N., & Silow-Carroll, S. (2011). Eliminating central line infections and spreading success at high-performing hospitals. https://core.ac.uk/download/71358071.pdf (accessed on 30th June 2025).

44. Ermolenko, K., Pshenisnov, K. V., Aleksandrovich, Y., Aleksandrovich, I. V., & Konev, A. I. (2025). Focused echocardiography as a tool for differential diagnosis of cardiovascular dysfunction in children with infections: Case reports. *Russian Journal of Pediatric Surgery, Anesthesia and Intensive Care.* https://www.semanticscholar.org/paper/95747f91a4e21176b1e5295226202ef70218b482 (accessed on 30th June 2025).

45. Esmaeilzadeh, M., Mahdiyoun, S. A., & Mokhtari, H. (2019). Classic papers in critical care: A bibliometric analysis. https://core.ac.uk/download/286730461.pdf (accessed on 30th June 2025).

46. Evans, C., Manning, J. C., & Suleman, Z. (2019). Parents' and careers' experiences of transition and aftercare following a child's discharge from a pediatric intensive care unit to an in-patient ward setting: A qualitative systematic review. https://core.ac.uk/download/228155955.pdf (accessed on 30th June 2025).

47. Finney, S. J. (2014). Extracorporeal support for patients with acute respiratory distress syndrome. https://core.ac.uk/download/77004032.pdf (accessed on 30th June 2025).

48. Gordon, M. D., Hagan, J., *et al.* (2018). Evidence-based skin champion program reduces pressure injuries in a pediatric hospital. https://core.ac.uk/download/212897182.pdf (accessed on 30th June 2025).

49. Hays, R. D., Lerner, C., Palimaru, A., Quigley, L., *et al.* (2020). A review of best practices for monitoring and improving inpatient pediatric patient experiences. https://core.ac.uk/download/287622168.pdf (accessed on 30th June 2025).

50. Kan, J. M., Kasparian, N. A., Newburger, J. W., Pincus, H. A., *et al.* (2019). Mental health care for parents of babies with congenital heart disease during intensive care unit admission: Systematic review and statement of best practice. https://core.ac.uk/download/323195256.pdf (accessed on 30th June 2025).

51. Kaugars, A. S., Kichler, J. C., & Moss, A. (2012). Behavioral factors influencing health outcomes in youth with Type 1 diabetes. https://core.ac.uk/download/213084246.pdf (accessed on 30th June 2025).

52. Kelly, M., Pinet-Peralta, L. M., Roque, T., Scalea, T., Delbridge, T., & Galvagno, S. M. (2023). The Maryland (USA) Critical Care Coordination Center (C4): From pandemic to permanence. *Prehospital and Disaster Medicine, 38*, 311–318. https://www.semanticscholar.org/paper/add6a9890cf116810669fe9542ba07253bba7eea (accessed on 30th June 2025).

53. Latour, J. M., & Tume, L. N. (2015). Family involvement in PICU rounds: Reality or rhetoric? https://core.ac.uk/download/74390205.pdf (accessed on 30th June 2025).

54. Latour, J. M., Tume, L. N., van den Hoogen, A., Wielenga, J., *et al.* (2014). An electronic Delphi study to establish pediatric intensive care nursing research priorities in twenty European countries. https://core.ac.uk/download/42136644.pdf (accessed on 30th June 2025).

55. Leleu, H., Moises, J., & Valdmanis, V. (2025). Optimal productive size of hospital's intensive care units. https://core.ac.uk/download/pdf/6218470.pdf (accessed on 30th June 2025).

56. Lyman, D. R., Dougherty, R. H., & Holt, W. (2010). State case studies of infant and early childhood mental health systems: Strategies for change. https://core.ac.uk/download/71355034.pdf (accessed on 30th June 2025).

57. Mostafa, O. E., Zakari, N., & Al Salem, M. (2024). Evaluation of nurses' attitudes, behaviors, and barriers toward pressure ulcer prevention in neonatal and pediatric intensive care units. *Frontiers in Pediatrics, 12*. https://www.semanticscholar.org/paper/6cca50b328edb48bcccd8525786087d6c676659e (accessed on 30th June 2025).

58. Quint, D., Berman, J., McDaniel, M., Barahona, P., Saxena, P., Teach, S. J., & Popkin, S. J. (2014). Helping low-income families manage childhood asthma: Solutions for healthcare & beyond. https://core.ac.uk/download/75777733.pdf (accessed on 30th June 2025).

59. Richmond, A. A. (2019). The links between motivational techniques, successful physical therapists, and successful rehab clinics. https://core.ac.uk/download/213463605.pdf (accessed on 30th June 2025).

60. Sheehan, W. J., Patel, S. J., Margolis, R., Fox, E., Shelef, D. Q., Kachroo, N., Pillai, D. K., *et al.* (2021). Pediatric asthma exacerbations during the COVID-19 pandemic: Absence of the typical fall seasonal spike in Washington, DC. *The Journal of Allergy and Clinical Immunology: In Practice, 9*, 2073–2076. https://doi.org/10.1016/j.jaip.2021.02.008 (accessed on 30th June 2025).

61. Špoljar, D., Jankovic, S., Vrkic, D., McNamara, G., Curkovic, M., Novak, M., Filipović-Grčić, B., *et al.* (2025). Ethics and end-of-life in pediatric and neonatal ICUs: A systematic review of recommendations. *BMC Palliative Care, 24*. https://www.semanticscholar.org/paper/64fe485ea2ddec1716e6b9d80678a36c38ba67bf (accessed on 30th June 2025).

62. Sucu, A., Kahveci, B., Celiloğlu, C., Tolunay, O., Çelik, T., Özdemir, U., & Çelik, Ü. (2018). Evaluation of patients diagnosed with brain death in pediatric critical care. https://core.ac.uk/download/201499296.pdf (accessed on 30th June 2025).

63. Swasey, H., Morrill, D., Mott, S., Engstrand, S., & Connor, J. A. (2024). Perceptions of interprofessional practitioners regarding pediatric palliative transports. *American Journal of Critical Care: An Official Publication, American Association of Critical-Care Nurses, 33*(2), 133–139. https://www.semanticscholar.org/paper/a0ee5f7f03c6d367222a9445b68c563dcac88f21 (accessed on 30th June 2025).

64. Toscano, N. (2016). Nurses' perceptions of parents staying during chronically ill child's hospitalization: Learning to speak the same language. https://core.ac.uk/download/56327896.pdf (accessed on 30th June 2025).

65. Utami, R. S. (2012). The challenges and strategies to improve family-centered round: A literature review. https://media.neliti.com/media/publications/154611-EN-the-challenges-and-strategies-to-improve.pdf (accessed on 30th June 2025).

66. Willis, Z. I., Oliveira, C. R., Abzug, M., Anosike, B. I., Ardura, M., Bio, L. L., Boguniewicz, J., *et al.* (2024). Guidance for prevention and management of COVID-19 in children and adolescents: A consensus statement from the Pediatric Infectious Diseases Society Pediatric COVID-19 Therapies Taskforce. *Journal of the Pediatric Infectious Diseases Society*. https://www.semanticscholar.org/paper/32a4e9f3be75cdd58c2859e73c4c0c397eb7783e (accessed on 30th June 2025).

67. Woods-Hill, C. Z., Nelson, M. N., Eriksen, W., Rendle, K. A., Beidas, R. S., Bonafide, C. P., Brajcich, M. R., *et al.* (2023). Determinants of blood culture use in critically ill children: A multicenter qualitative study. *Pediatric Quality & Safety, 8*. https://www.semanticscholar.org/paper/bedbb7d474bf5b1bf089e204ea185117a4d76b58 (accessed on 30th June 2025).

68. Youssry, I., Zarea, H., Rady, H., & Khedr, D. (2024). Improving prediction of severity of sepsis in children: A single center trial. *Pediatric Sciences Journal*. https://www.semanticscholar.org/paper/b81e39e5871900b74cdc4ff70278392010ef0346 (accessed on 30th June 2025).

PEDIATRIC ASSESSMENT AND MONITORING

2

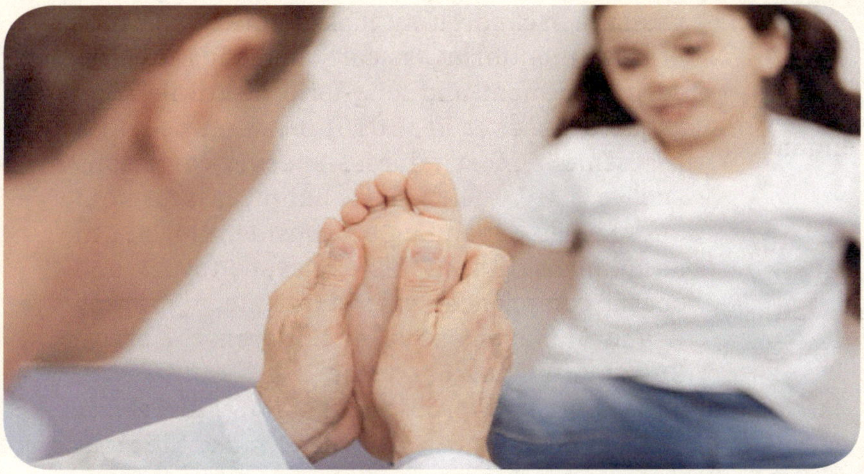

LEARNING OBJECTIVES

After studying this chapter, you will be able to:

1. Understand growth and development assessment.
2. Explain health history and physical examination.
3. Identify diagnostic tools and techniques.
4. Perform monitoring and follow-up care.

Introduction

Pediatric monitoring and assessment cannot be overstressed, as they form the cornerstones on which effective healthcare delivery for children is founded. Effective assessments enable health professionals to effectively identify a child's unique health status, growth, and developmental milestones, so that interventions, which can significantly enhance long-term health outcomes, are instituted in a timely manner. Recently, it has been observed that there is an urgent need to implement behaviorally individualized elements in pediatric practice, particularly in managing childhood obesity and associated health conditions (Sahota *et al.*, 2010). Furthermore, considerations of special populations, such as children with autism spectrum disorder, call for advanced methods for identifying and managing challenging behaviors effectively (Johnson *et al.*, 2013). With the evolving healthcare situation, in-depth knowledge of pediatric monitoring and assessment will not only ensure the provision of better care but also offer the means for framing effective interventions as per the varying needs of children from diverse backgrounds (Figure 2.1).

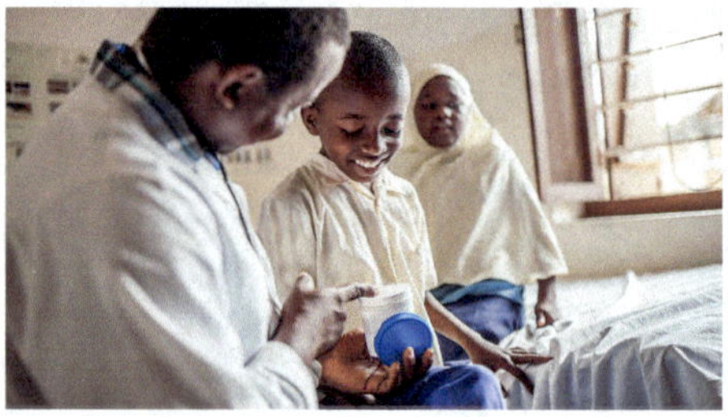

Figure 2.1. Accurate assessments enable healthcare providers to identify a child's unique health status, growth patterns, and developmental milestones, leading to timely interventions that can significantly enhance long-term health outcomes.

Source: https://www.philips.com/c-dam/corporate/newscenter/global/standard/resources/healthcare/2024/transform-health-fund/header-transform-health-fund-getty-images-1189735296.jpg.

2.1. Growth and Development Assessment

Learning Outcome

1. Understand stages of growth in children.
2. Know developmental milestones.
3. Explain physical growth measurements.
4. Focus on cognitive development assessments.
5. Discuss social and emotional development indicators.
6. Learn language and communication skills evaluation.
7. Understand the importance of growth charts.
8. Identify factors affecting growth and development.
9. Understand the role of parents in monitoring development.

Children's growth and development assessment lies at the heart of identifying potential health issues and guaranteeing interventions. The assessment is not just a measurement of physical values such as height and weight, but also a measurement of development milestones in order to assess the intellectual, emotional, and social progress of the child. Through the integration of growth charts and developmental screening tests, healthcare providers can have better information on whether a child's development is within expected expectations. For example, the importance of increasing blood pressure in children emphasizes the significance of close monitoring, as early detection leads to early treatment and long-term health benefits (Agabiti-Rosei *et al.*, 2016). Besides, pediatric assessment must address specific conditions such as HIV, which have unique assessment approaches depending on considerations such as immunologic markers relevant to age and special compliance issues in treatment (Therapy A and Management M of Children H-I *et al.*, 2003). Last but not least, a general growth and development assessment allows caregivers and healthcare professionals to make the right decisions, enhancing pediatric health outcomes.

2.1.1. Stages of Growth in Children

Understanding the stages of growth in children is essential in pediatric assessment and monitoring, as the stages of growth reflect important physical, intellectual, and emotional developments. During early childhood, height and weight undergo a profound transformation with a significant reliance on nutritious intake and health care interventions to promote healthy growth patterns. For instance, adherence to growth hormone (GH) therapy has been linked with improved clinical outcomes such as increased linear growth and overall quality of life in children (Carlo *et al.*, 2017). Surveillance of developmental milestones becomes essential during the transition from infancy to school age. Programs like the BRIDGE program recognize the requirement for home support for at-risk newborns to ensure a smooth transition from neonatal care to home (Patel *et al.*, 2015). Through intervention in the various stages of development, healthcare providers can intervene with targeted interventions that optimize the health and developmental status of children through their early years (Figure 2.2).

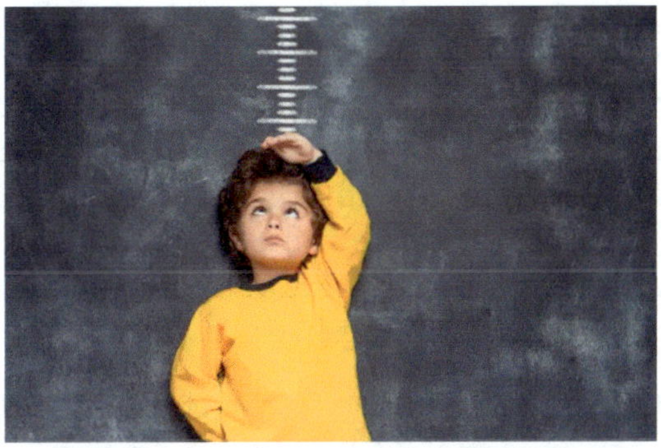

Figure 2.2. Understanding the stages of growth in children is essential for effective pediatric assessment and monitoring, as these stages encompass significant physical, cognitive, and emotional developments.

Source: https://www.carehospitals.com/ckfinder/userfiles/images/understanding_the_stages_of_child_growth_and_development_i_.webps.

2.1.2. Developmental Milestones

Developmental milestones in child monitoring and evaluation are primary markers that medical professionals utilize to determine a child's growth and potential developmental delays.

These consist of a number of areas of development, such as motor skills, language, cognitive abilities, and social-emotional growth, that are milestones of the child's overall well-being. Regular monitoring of these milestones allows the early identification of any abnormalities, which is essential in carrying out early interventions that significantly influence a child's developmental trajectory. As highlighted in recent studies, constant monitoring of growth, like weight, length, and head circumference, is important in identifying at-risk infants who can experience growth faltering or undernutrition, particularly in preterm populations (Haiden *et al.*, 2025). Further, incorporation of developmental milestones assessment into propaedeutics not only supports accurate diagnosis but also enhances planning for prevention, with consequent optimal health outcomes in pediatric patients (Mukhamattairovna, 2024). Incorporation of developmental milestones into routine monitoring is, therefore, still an important aspect of quality pediatrics.

2.1.3. Physical Growth Measurements

An integral component of pediatric monitoring and assessment is the precise measurement of physical growth indexes, that is, height, weight, and body mass index (BMI). Measurement of these values is not only a monitoring tool for nutritional status but also a key to the screening of possible health issues in children and adolescents.

For instance, inappropriate growth patterns may indicate conditions like obesity or undernutrition, both with significant long-term health implications. With the rise in the prevalence of diseases like hypertension among young individuals, the necessity for accurate monitoring grows ever more imperative (Agabiti-Rosei *et al.*, 2016). Additional intervention through growth measurement can enhance outcomes, such as efforts to combat obesity in children, particularly those with special needs like autism spectrum disorder (Boutelle *et al.*, 2019). Hence, regular physical growth assessments are necessary to form an overall impression of a child's well-being and development progression (Figure 2.3).

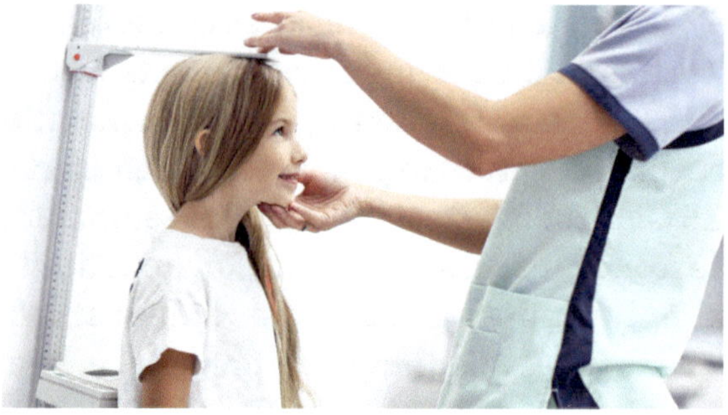

Figure 2.3. An essential component of pediatric assessment and monitoring involves the precise evaluation of physical growth measurements, which include height, weight, and body mass index (BMI).

Source: https://www.healthdigest.com/img/gallery/bmi-everything-you-need-to-know/or-to-children-or-teens-1612381041.jpg.

2.1.4. Cognitive Development Assessments

Cognitive developmental testing is also an important aspect of pediatric assessment and follow-up, as it provides precious information about the intellectual development of a child and the risk for developmental delay. Early detection of cognitive delays is thus extremely valuable as it allows for early intervention, which may drastically alter a child's course of development. Research has demonstrated that primary care professionals tend to overestimate such delays, and thus the requirement for increased monitoring and screening activity (Sices, 2007). Secondly, techniques adopted in cognitive assessments must be strictly tested for uniformity and reliability (Cordingley *et al.*, 2017). Standard reporting and administration procedures do not exist, and thus, heterogeneity across studies exists, rendering such assessments futile. Therefore, establishing comprehensive rules and boosting training for healthcare professionals will not only provide accurate evaluations but also foster enhanced long-term outcomes for children's mental growth.

2.1.5. Indicators for Social and Emotional Development

The assessment of social and emotional development indicators in pediatric populations is essential for ensuring holistic growth and well-being. These indicators provide valuable insights into a child's mental health and cognitive functions, which are crucial during formative years. Research indicates significant connections between mental health and child development, noting that preschoolers are particularly susceptible to mental health conditions that can disrupt social-emotional functioning (Suryaningsih *et al.*, 2025).

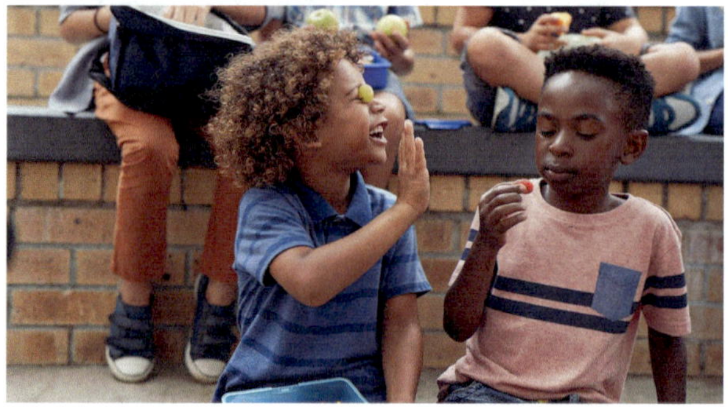

Figure 2.4. The assessment of social and emotional development indicators in pediatric populations is essential for ensuring holistic growth and well-being.

Source: https://i0.wp.com/post.healthline.com/wp-content/uploads/2019/12/Male_Children_Playing_1296x728-header-1296x728.jpg?w=1155&h=1528.

Utilizing standardized instruments like the Strengths and Difficulties Questionnaire (SDQ) in pediatric assessment, practitioners can effectively monitor these indicators. Besides, an understanding of how external stimuli, such as local conditions influencing community moods, are manifested in children's emotional landscape can enable targeted interventions (Serkina *et al.*, 2025). This integrated process not only optimizes early identification of delays in development but also informs evidence-based policy and intervention measures to optimize outcomes among children with varying developmental backgrounds (Figure 2.4).

2.1.6. Language and Communication Skills Evaluation

Effective language and communication skills are essential components of pediatric monitoring and assessment because they directly influence a child's ability to interact with and perceive the world around them. Measurement of these skills includes various areas, for example, receptive and expressive language, articulation, and social communication. The measurement of these skills allows clinicians to ascertain potential developmental delay and tailor interventions accordingly. For instance, implementation of a theory-based conversation guide has been enacted to ensure the optimal preparation of parents for discharge and nurses' home-based self-management competency (Gralton *et al.*, 2017). Secondly, the integration of model practices in education and related services, particularly in adherence to the Individuals with Disabilities Education Act (IDEA), attempts to ensure a supportive environment for children with communicative challenges (Dennis *et al.*, 1999). Consequently, early detection and intervention for language and communication abilities are crucial in forming effective caregiver-child relationships and providing overall developmental success.

2.1.7. Importance of Growth Charts

Growth charts are invaluable tools in pediatric assessment and follow-up, providing critical data regarding a child's growth pattern vis-a-vis accepted norms. Growth charts enable medical professionals to identify deviations in growth patterns that may signal attendant health issues, such as malnutrition or growth abnormalities. For instance, a child's head circumference is a vital auxological parameter; deviations from the norm can indicate conditions such as microcephaly or macrocephaly, with significant developmental implications (Corsello *et al.*, 2019). Systematic follow-up with the aid of growth charts facilitates early identification and intervention, which is crucial in managing impending health problems. Also, the detailed information provided by growth charts informs policymakers and healthcare providers of the general health status of child populations, guiding resource allocation and health policy (McCarthy *et al.*, 2004). Hence, growth charts are quantitative values but so much more than just a number and an integral component of anticipatory pediatric care facilitating better health outcomes through close monitoring (Figure 2.5).

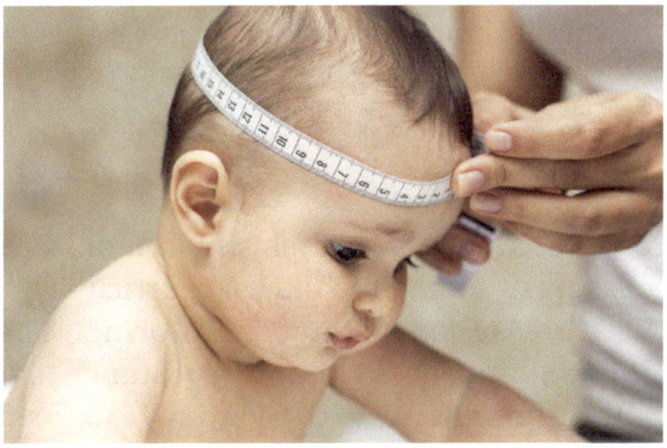

Figure 2.5. Growth charts serve as essential tools in pediatric assessment and monitoring, providing critical insights into a child's growth trajectory relative to established norms.

Source: https://emh5334n65w.exactdn.com/wp-content/uploads/2022/06/iStock-481561138.jpg?strip=all&lossy=1&ssl=1.

2.1.8. Factors Affecting Growth and Development

Being aware of what contributes to children's growth and development is a component of good assessment and monitoring. A number of factors, such as nutritional status, a chronic illness, and family functioning, are significant.

For instance, vitamin D deficiency would result in growth retardation and skeletal deformity, particularly in children with a family history of atopy, where chronic inflammation would also enhance growth impairments (Ardiaria *et al.*, 2024). Additionally, the influence of preterm birth on developmental outcomes highlights the role of family interactions and parental stress in modeling child behavior in early years. Preterm children often remain under the care of families with adversity that can impede the quality of mother-father-child relations, thereby decelerating their optimal growth and development (Gatta *et al.*, 2017). Pediatric assessment processes can be enhanced by healthcare professionals through addressing these issues, thus ensuring the monitoring of developmental milestones in a more comprehensive manner.

2.1.9. Parents' Role in Monitoring Development

Parents must take a pivotal role in monitoring the progress of their children, particularly in pediatric assessment and monitoring. Their role is significant in that they stand to be the first persons to recognize any abnormal development, and their observations would be of great value to clinical assessment. Parents can, for instance, provide useful information regarding their child's psychosocial adjustment and intrafamilial dynamics, which are significant factors to consider in relation to understanding the development of the child against the backdrop of the family. As emphasized in the biopsychosocial model, mental and social determinants play a role in child disease and its management (Maartje de Wit *et al.*, 2022). Moreover, if parents are actively engaged in taking care of the child, their emotional status and coping ability can directly affect the behavior of the child and compliance with treatment. Thus, it is essential to create a fruitful collaboration between parents, healthcare professionals, and the interdisciplinary team in order to achieve successful surveillance and positive developmental results, as described in the context of mental health assistance (Marilyn *et al.*, 2022) (Figure 2.6).

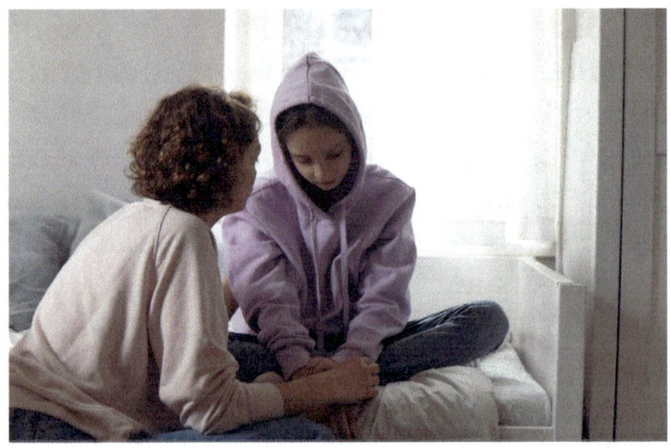

Figure 2.6. Parents play a pivotal role in monitoring their children's development, particularly in the context of pediatric assessment and monitoring.

Source: https://www.news-medical.net/images/news/ImageForNews_747363_16832732061856822.jpg.

Test Your Knowledge

1. How do PICU providers monitor growth in children with prolonged ICU stays?
2. Why is age-appropriate developmental assessment important in the PICU setting?

2.2. Health History and Physical Examination

Learning Outcome

1. Understand the importance of a comprehensive health history.
2. Identify components of a pediatric health history.
3. Know techniques for effective physical examination.
4. Focus on vital signs assessment in children.
5. Perform screening for common pediatric conditions.
6. Explain immunization history and its relevance.
7. Discuss family history and genetic considerations.
8. Describe cultural and social factors in health history.
9. Explain documentation and communication of findings.

A full physical examination and health history are integral components of pediatric assessment and monitoring upon which successful diagnosis and management are founded. During health history taking, practitioners must consider a sequence of factors, including family medical histories that can illuminate potential genetic susceptibility as well as lifestyle factors that can influence outcomes.

Pediatric patients are particularly vulnerable to conditions such as hypertension; the growing prevalence of hypertension among children underscores the necessity for caution on the part of the practitioner during examination, with the guidelines emphasizing the importance of clinical evaluation and out-of-office blood pressure assessment (Agabiti-Rosei *et al.*, 2016). Pediatricians need to remain vigilant regarding conditions such as obstructive sleep apnea syndrome (OSAS), which can potentially affect the health of children. The interplay of the risk factors, such as hyperadenoidal tissue, further complicates diagnosis, highlighting the need for comprehensive evaluations in order to create efficient management plans (Bellini *et al.*, 2019).

2.2.1. Importance of Comprehensive Health History

Comprehensive health history is at the forefront of pediatric monitoring and evaluation since it encompasses a wide variety of factors essential in the evaluation of a child's overall health and growth. In gathering complete medical, family, and social histories, health practitioners are able to identify risk factors, background conditions, and developmental milestones that are essential to the child's well-being.

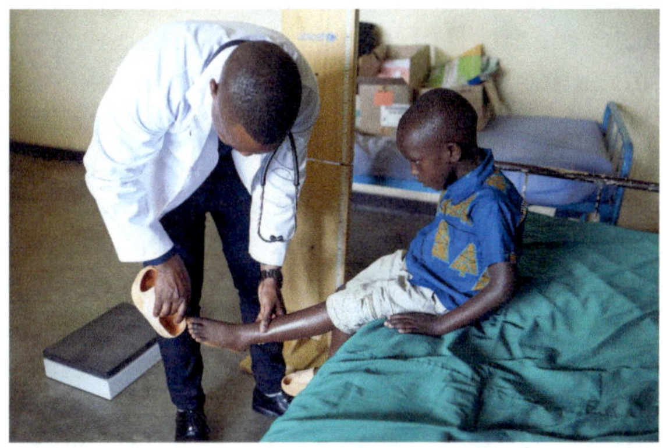

Figure 2.7. Collecting detailed medical, familial, and social histories enables healthcare providers to identify potential risks, underlying conditions, and developmental milestones critical to the child's well-being.

Source: https://www.compassion.com/Images/effects-of-poverty-img3-0125.jpg.

This is particularly significant for CYSHCN, as managed care plans are increasingly looking to serve this at-risk population well. For instance, California, Massachusetts, and Michigan have developed individualized processes for the identification and assessment of CYSHCN in their Medicaid programs and are looking to meet federal requirements. Also, implementing national preventive care standards and enhancing health providers' training can improve the quality of such assessments in such settings (Stevens *et al.*, 2005; Jee *et al.*, 2014). Hence, a thorough health history is essential for individualized care and care integration in children (Figure 2.7).

2.2.2. Components of a Pediatric Health History

An adequate pediatric health history is essential to effective assessment and surveillance, enabling health professionals to become aware of the unique requirements of children. A pediatric health history involves several key factors, including developmental and birth milestones, immunizations, and significant family medical history. It also encompasses information regarding eating patterns, exercise, and social determinants of health that are most likely to impact the child's health. Above all else, transition from pediatric to adult care is best described by the need for individualized health histories; successful models of transition incorporate interprofessional collaboration and include the incorporation of developmentally appropriate education for adolescents and families (Bagnall *et al.*, 2013). Furthermore, implementing evidence-based pathways within healthcare settings has also been shown to increase quality of care by integrating interdisciplinary care, although challenges such as reshaping electronic health records can hinder implementation of the pathways (Cabana *et al.*, 2021). Overall, these elements introduce a formalized framework for the delivery of the best pediatric care.

2.2.3. Efficient Physical Examination Methods

An effective pediatric physical examination requires a mixture of formal approaches and sensitivity. Physicians must create a comfortable atmosphere in order to calm patients early enough, typically by talking with them in their own realm, both physically and psychologically. Proper communication techniques that match the child's age ensure more cooperation from the child, enabling an extensive checkup. Moreover, using standardized evaluation measures can reduce the process to its essentials and allow for thorough assessment of developmental milestones as well as physical health. As described in several promising practices, including those highlighted in the context of related services in special education, the importance of prioritizing individual needs and making corresponding adjustments in techniques cannot be overstated (Dennis *et al.*, 1999). Secondly, the appreciation for the necessity of routine screening and routine monitoring assists practitioners in identifying any emergent health matters, thereby allowing for timely interventions that are consistent with the goals of IDEAs and pediatric standards of care (Figure 2.8).

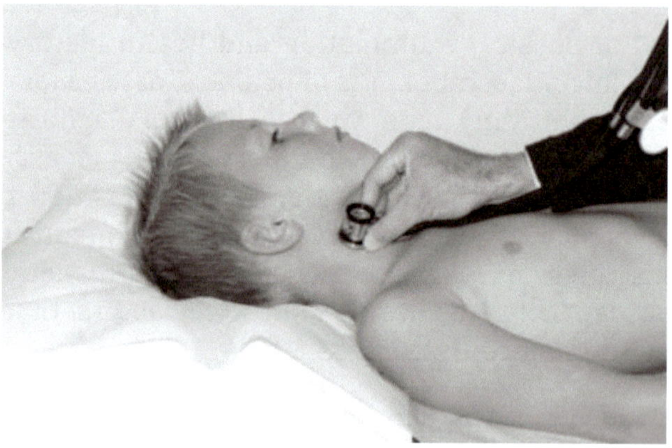

Figure 2.8. Conducting an effective physical examination in pediatric assessment requires a blend of systematic techniques and a compassionate approach.

Source: https://i0.wp.com/clinicalgate.com/wp-content/uploads/2015/06/B9781437713978000101_f10-17-9781437713978.jpg?fit=376%2C250&ssl=1.

2.2.4. Vital Signs Assessment in Children

Child vital signs assessment is a critical component of pediatric practice as it provides useful information regarding their physiological status and overall well-being. The evaluation of vital signs, including respiratory rate, heart rate, blood pressure, and temperature, allows health practitioners to detect impending deterioration or distress. Such an innovation is the innovation of contactless devices for accurate monitoring of respiratory rate, which has been recognized as a key triage factor in clinical assessment (Burke *et al.*, 2020). Further, Pediatric Early Warning Score (PEWS) has been found to be an effective model for pediatric monitoring, particularly in high-risk populations such as those undergoing hematopoietic cell transplant. Studies demonstrate that higher PEWS significantly predict the need for intensive care intervention, and the model's success in identifying patients at risk (Cater *et al.*, 2018). Through vigilant monitoring of vital signs, health workers are able to enhance outcomes and provide timely intervention in the care of children.

2.2.5. Screening for Common Pediatric Conditions

Accurate screening for common childhood disorders is crucial in the optimization of child health outcomes and allows early diagnosis of potential disorders. Routine checks may identify various disorders such as developmental delay, obesity, and malnutrition, which otherwise may lead to significant long-term consequences. For instance, research highlighted that ongoing weight loss and poor energy intake were of most significance as indicators of disease-associated malnutrition among children, with emphasis on regular nutritional screening in practice (Bian *et al.*, 2018). Furthermore, evidence-based clinical practice recommendations, including those authored by the American Diabetes Association, suggest regular screenings for chronic diseases, like type 1 diabetes, to boost compliance as well as timely intervention (Bartz *et al.*, 2019). By applying standardized screening methods, clinicians are not only able to enhance the detection of common childhood disorders but also to start selective interventions that lead to better health trajectories in children (Figure 2.9).

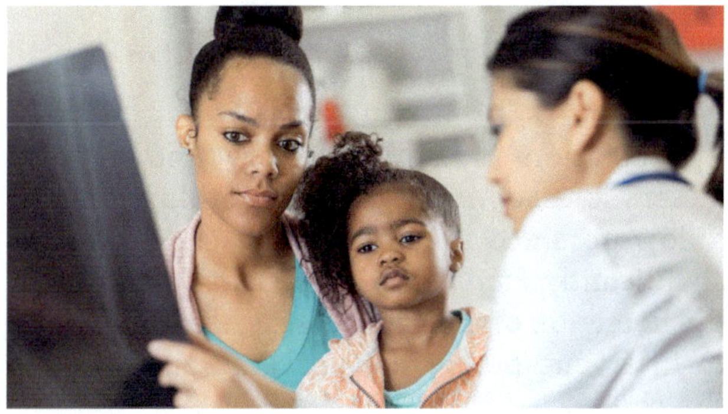

Figure 2.9. Effective screening for common pediatric conditions is critical in optimizing child health outcomes and ensuring early detection of potential issues.

Source: https://www.fda.gov/files/pediatric%20xray_drupal.jpg.

2.2.6. Immunization History and Its Relevance

Understanding a child's vaccination history is central to pediatric monitoring and assessment because it provides an immediate picture of their overall state of health and vulnerability to being contaminated by vaccine-preventable diseases. Comprehensive immunization history not only assures compliance with vaccination schedules but also assists providers in identifying and closing gaps in protection proactively. For instance, the use of allergen immunotherapy has emphasized the importance of complete immunization histories when managing allergies in children, especially considering their susceptibility to anaphylactic reactions (Montserrat Álvaro-Lozano *et al.*, 2020). The

American Diabetes Association also points out the role of preventive services like vaccinations in long-term health outcomes among pediatric patients with chronic diseases (Nuha *et al.*, 2022). Lastly, having correct immunization records is significant for encouraging immunologic assessments and care planning on an individual basis, thereby enhancing pediatric health interventions.

2.2.7. Family History and Genetic Considerations

Appreciation of family history and genetic factors is essential in pediatric evaluation and follow-up since it can impact a child's health significantly. Family history is usually the key to the detection of inherited diseases early enough to intervene before they become an issue for the child.

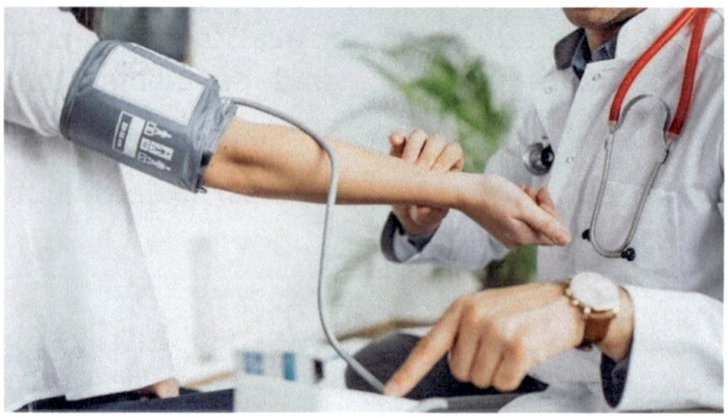

Figure 2.10. Family history often plays an instrumental role in the early identification of hereditary conditions, allowing for timely interventions that can mitigate risks associated with diseases such as hypertension and immunodeficiency.

Source: https://www.hindustantimes.com/ht-img/img/2024/03/07/1600x900/hypertension_1705661357154_1709801154625.jpg.

Interventions in such conditions are sure to reduce disease-related risks like immunodeficiency and hypertension. For instance, the increasing prevalence of hypertension in children emphasizes the necessity to assess family health patterns that can be employed to guide clinical practices based on patient risk profiles (Agabiti-Rosei *et al.*, 2016). Similarly, conditions like HIV necessitate careful consideration of genetic background, particularly in perinatal transmission risks and varying clinical presentations among various populations of pediatric patients (Therapy A and Management M of Children H-I *et al.*, 2003). By integrating genetic information and family history into regular assessments, clinicians may develop tailored care plans maximizing preventive measures and treatment efficacy, resulting in enhanced health outcomes for children (Figure 2.10).

2.2.8. Cultural and Social Factors in Health History

The connection between social and cultural factors significantly affects health histories, particularly in pediatric visits. These consist of numerous influences from socioeconomic status to cultural notions about illness and health that can significantly impact children's health outcomes. For instance, social determinants of health (SDOH) and childhood adverse experiences (ACEs) have been discovered to have short-term as well as long-term effects on children's health, necessitating their identification in primary care (Corvini *et al.*, 2018). In addition, parental perceptions and fears, as can be witnessed in long-term condition-managing families such as Type 1 Diabetes, can also yield conflict that undermines treatment adherence and blood sugar control among pediatric patients (Bonichini *et al.*, 2017). By being able to recognize such complex cultural and social factors, healthcare professionals are better able to develop more effective, tailored interventions that better support families and result in healthier child outcomes.

2.2.9. Documentation and Communication of Findings

Good documentation and reporting of results are essential elements in pediatric examination and monitoring to guarantee that health professionals are able to provide high-quality care that matches the individual needs of children. Good documentation allows for easy transfer of patient data among multi-disciplinary teams, which enables sound clinical decision-making and fosters continuity of care.

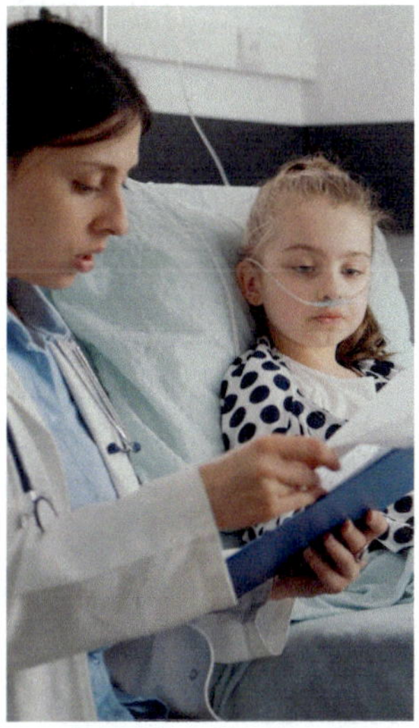

Figure 2.11. Effective documentation and communication of findings are critical components in the pediatric assessment and monitoring process, ensuring that healthcare providers can deliver high-quality care tailored to the unique needs of children.

Source: https://img.freepik.com/free-photo/sick-child-patient-wearing-oxygen-nasal-tube-resting-bed-recovering-after-breathing-sickness-surgery-medical-consultation-physician-woman-doctor-analyzing-disease-expertise-hospital-ward_482257-9355.jpg?semt=ais_hybrid&w=740.

Particularly, following evidence-based guidelines, for example, those that are issued by professional organizations, ensures that practitioners remain current with evidence-based practice, reducing variability in care and improving patient outcomes (Stout *et al.*, 2018). Additionally, engaging families in documentation facilitates inter-professional collaboration that can assist in clarifying the child's state and treatment options (Judy *et al.*, 2016). Because pediatric practice largely involves complex interactions among various stakeholders, effective communication not only aids informed clinical choices but also empowers families by engaging them as responsible stakeholders in their child's healthcare process.

Test Your Knowledge

1. Why is birth history particularly important in assessing critically ill infants?
2. What are red flags in a pediatric history that may indicate underlying metabolic or genetic conditions?

2.3. Diagnostic Tools and Techniques

Learning Outcome

1. Identify laboratory tests commonly used in pediatrics.
2. Explain imaging studies and their applications.
3. Describe developmental screening tools.
4. Focus on behavioral assessments and questionnaires.
5. Know the use of technology in pediatric assessments.
6. Discuss the importance of accurate interpretation of results.
7. Understand ethical considerations in diagnostic testing.
8. Describe collaboration with specialists for complex cases.

In the field of pediatric assessment and monitoring, the application of an array of diagnostic tools and techniques plays a vital role in maximizing the health condition of children. They range from growth charts to advanced imaging systems, each of which is integral for precise assessment and intervention. For instance, observation through the application of growth hormone (GH) therapy has been highlighted as key in the case of children with growth deficiency. Low compliance with GH therapy can have the ability to induce negative clinical outcomes, reinforcing the significance of comprehensive evaluation approaches that integrate multi-disciplinary therapies. Secondly, new technology in electronic technology applied in injection devices is improving patient compliance by automating the recording of injection data, thus maximizing treatment compliance rates. Lastly, proper use of these methods of diagnosis not only informs pediatric practice but also facilitates an empowering environment that is conducive to the child's long-term health and development.

2.3.1. Laboratory Tests Routinely Used in Pediatrics

Effective pediatric monitoring and evaluation are greatly reliant on an array of laboratory tests tailored to the unique physiological and developmental requirements of children. Among the tests required are complete blood counts, which provide information on nutritional status, in addition to detecting infections, and blood chemistry panels assessing metabolic function and organ function. Significantly, recognition of hypertension in childhood has emerged as a significant field, with the increasing prevalence of the disorder among children and adolescents highlighting the demand for proper protocols of diagnosis as described in new guidelines (Agabiti-Rosei *et al.*, 2016).

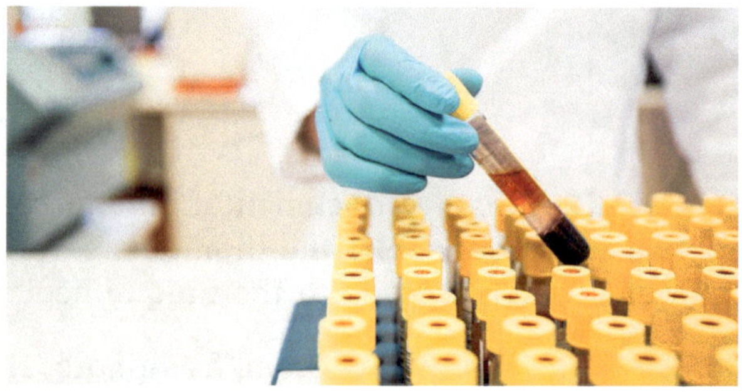

Figure 2.12. Essential tests include complete blood counts, which provide insights into nutritional status and detect infections, along with blood chemistry panels that assess metabolic function and organ health.

Source: https://media.post.rvohealth.io/wp-content/uploads/2022/02/blood-test-1200x628-facebook-1200x628.jpg.

Also, laboratory evaluation of hyperbilirubinemia plays a critical role in newborn health, particularly with respect to the risk of bilirubin-induced neurologic dysfunction and its potential long-term complications if not properly managed (Boo *et al.*, 2015). Such incorporation of these laboratory measurements into standard pediatric practice, therefore, enables early intervention and ensures improved health status with avoidance of associated risks in this group of vulnerable individuals (Figure 2.12).

2.3.2. Imaging Studies and Their Applications

Imaging studies are a core part of pediatric evaluation and follow-up, which allow for early diagnosis and treatment of several conditions. Employing tools such as ultrasound, magnetic resonance imaging (MRI), and computed tomography (CT) is core in the evaluation of developmental anomalies, gastrointestinal diseases, and neurological disorders. For instance, the increasing prevalence of nonalcoholic fatty liver disease (NAFLD) among children underscores the need for effective imaging technology to monitor liver health and inform therapy protocols (Miriam *et al.*, 2016). Additionally, imaging is instrumental in conditions such as disorders of sex development (DSDs), where comprehensive clinical evaluation relies significantly on accurate imaging to inform management decisions (Peter *et al.*, 2016). These breakthroughs not only enhance diagnostic precision but also help in targeted interventions, resulting in better health outcomes. As imaging technology continues to advance, its applications in pediatric medicine will increasingly lead to improved monitoring and interventions, giving way to the best developmental trajectories for the children involved.

2.3.3. Developmental Screening Tools

Developmental screening tools play a critical role in children's evaluation and surveillance, leading to early detection of potential delays and disabilities. The tools are required for early intervention to avoid untoward effects on a child's development and health. Detailed examination reveals extensive variation in the validity and usefulness of these tools, particularly with reference to cultural issues and genetic influences on children's development. Studies have identified various screening instruments, with the Ages and Stages Questionnaire (ASQ) and Battelle Developmental Inventory (BDI) being especially noted as useful instruments, but most lack cultural sensitivity (Kurbatfinski *et al.*, 2024). Moreover, the advancement of technology has also come with possibilities and challenges, most importantly, app-based screening instruments. The issue of compatibility, usability, and confidentiality must be addressed so that such technology tools can enhance clinical outcomes without compromising the validity of assessments (Waugh, 2023) (Figure 2.13).

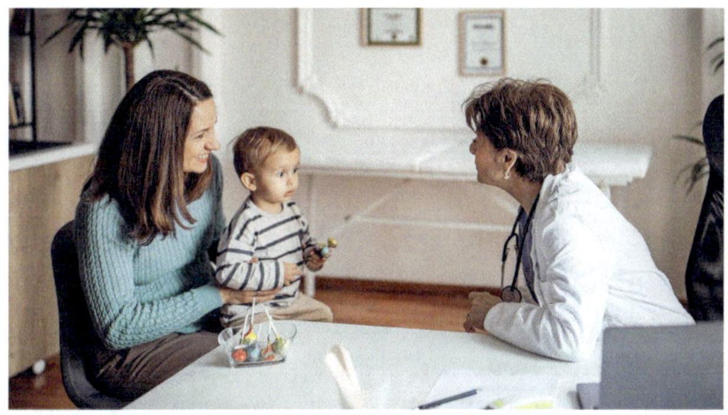

Figure 2.13. Developmental screening tools play a crucial role in the assessment and monitoring of pediatric populations, enabling early identification of potential delays and disabilities.

Source: https://media.post.rvohealth.io/wp-content/uploads/2023/10/mom-son-with-pediatrician-1296-728-header.jpg.

2.3.4. Behavioral Assessments and Questionnaires

Under pediatric monitoring and assessment, behavioral measures and questionnaires are significant for the evaluation of the psychosocial status of children and adolescents. The tools enable physicians to identify mental illnesses, behavior, and coping mechanisms systematically among young people, especially youths with chronic illnesses like diabetes. Questionnaires that have been validated can reveal vital information regarding emotional states, resilience, and family functioning that are critical in developing interventions to support children's adaptation and coping (Maartje de Wit *et al.*, 2022). Finally, the emergence of post-acute sequelae of SARS-CoV-2 infection (PASC) underscores the value of sound screening instruments to address the psychological impact of illness and isolation (Laura *et al.*, 2022). By implementing routine psychosocial screenings, healthcare teams can promote active care, allowing for early referrals and promoting team-based approaches to coordinating the physical and emotional well-being of pediatric patients.

2.3.5. Use of Technology in Pediatric Assessment

The integration of technology into pediatric testing is quickly transforming the landscape of clinical testing and monitoring. Advanced devices such as cardiopulmonary exercise testing (CPET) and near-infrared spectroscopy (NIRS) demonstrate this trend, offering noninvasive measurements of complex physiological responses in children. CPET challenges the integrative function of the pulmonary, cardiovascular, and skeletal muscle systems, yet it has been hampered in the past by the need for patient compliance. However, with the incorporation of two-site NIRS monitoring in their arsenal, clinicians can now noninvasively estimate anaerobic thresholds and make exercise testing in children more effective (Danduran *et al.*, 2012). It not only provides real-time regional tissue oxygenation monitoring but also supports clinical outcomes by providing patient-specific, individualized interventions. Thus, the use of technological innovation in pediatric assessment is promoting more patient-centered and holistic care, which in turn leads to better health outcomes in children (Figure 2.14).

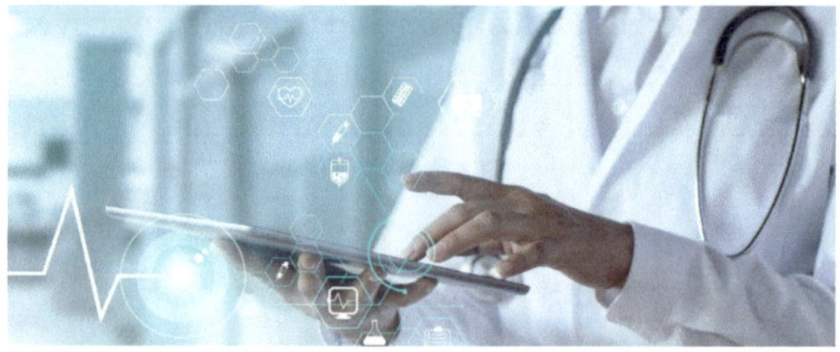

Figure 2.14. The integration of technology in pediatric assessments is rapidly transforming the landscape of clinical evaluations and monitoring.

Source: https://res.cloudinary.com/dlpitjizv/image/upload/v1688671479/impact/Examples_of_Smart_Technology_in_Healthcare_Hero_D_e7d99fb4a0.jpg.

2.3.6. Importance of Accurate Interpretation of Results

Proper interpretation of pediatric monitoring and assessment findings plays a crucial role in guaranteeing optimal health outcomes among children. Misinterpretation will lead to non-representative clinical decisions, which may have adverse effects on a child's treatment regimen. This is particularly evident in cases such as Type 1 Diabetes Mellitus (T1DM), where aggressive SMBG is required. Evidence demonstrates that major HbA1c improvement can be achieved only if children are educated to control their glucose level effectively (Formosa *et al.*, 2013). Similarly, the availability of high-resolution HLA typing has transformed our understanding regarding the compatibility of donor and recipient in solid organ transplantation, highlighting the requirement for proper assessment of antibody profiles to minimize post-transplant complications (Dinh *et al.*, 2019). Hence, prolonged training and prolonged analysis of results are part of pediatric practice, ensuring interventions are timely and appropriate, ultimately ensuring the protection of children's health and development.

2.3.7. Ethical Considerations in Diagnostic Testing

In pediatric monitoring and evaluation, ethical considerations of diagnostic testing come into focus. With advances in technology, particularly with next-generation sequencing (NGS), where genetic material can be rapidly evaluated, health implications in children become complex. Parents may be faced with difficult decisions on the extent of genetic testing, particularly in the context of a potential for discovering surprises, such as vulnerabilities to serious conditions. Engagement in informed consent processes is crucial, where parents are informed about the significance of test results and their medical and emotional impacts that they may entail (Paepe *et al.*, 2013).

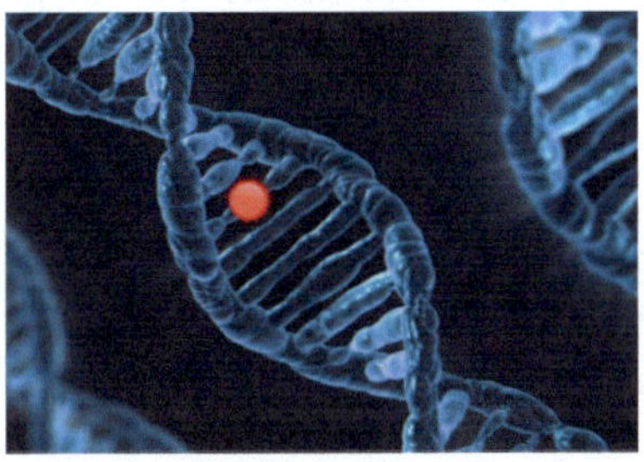

Figure 2.15. As advances in technology, particularly next-generation sequencing (NGS), facilitate the rapid analysis of genetic material, the implications for children's health become increasingly complex.

Source: https://cdn.prod.website-files.com/65b10cf2a9c7f9d23b4bb47d/65b10cf2a9c7f9d23b4bb4db_what-is-ngs-testing-unveiling-the-essentials-of-next-generation-sequencing.jpg.

Even newer technologies like liquid biopsy, while promising in the non-invasive monitoring of cancer in children, pose challenges to the validity and ethical use of such data towards treatment planning (Astrahantseff *et al.*, 2020). As professionals confront these issues, they need to place transparency and advocacy of pediatric patients' best interests foremost among their concerns (Figure 2.15).

2.3.8. Collaboration with Specialists for Complex Cases

In pediatric assessment and monitoring, the intensity of the cases of children with special health care needs emphasizes the vital necessity of collaboration with experts. Partnerships ensure an integrated image of each child's unique difficulties, and this is particularly relevant in managing intricate medical and educational necessities. Experts like pediatricians, psychologists, and therapists bring their knowledge that enhances the one-to-one assessment process and informs individualized interventions. The inclusion of ancillary services, as noted in models of education, is aimed at the significance of inter-disciplinary coordination in establishing effective Individualized Education Programs (IEPs) that are specifically for students with disability, between the ages of 3 and 21 years (Dennis *et al.*, 1999). Along with this, management of care delivery systems relies more and more on the identification and assessment of children and youth with special healthcare needs (CYSHCN) in order to maintain state policies consistent with optimal management best practices (Jee *et al.*, 2014). Ultimately, this collaboration leads to improved outcomes and facilitates comprehensive development in pediatric populations.

Test Your Knowledge

1. What are the indications for arterial blood gas analysis in children?
2. How is continuous EEG monitoring used in the management of seizures or encephalopathy?

2.4. Monitoring and Follow-Up Care

Learning Outcome

1. Know the importance of regular follow-up visits.
2. Track developmental progress over time.
3. Adjust care plans based on assessments.
4. Discuss the role of multidisciplinary teams in monitoring.
5. Focus on parental involvement in follow-up care.
6. Address concerns and questions from families.
7. Explain transitioning care as children grow.
8. Describe long-term monitoring for chronic conditions.
9. Evaluate the effectiveness of interventions.

Ideal monitoring and follow-up care are integral components in guaranteeing that pediatric patients are provided with the optimum management during their developmental phases. Given the unique physiological and psychological characteristics of children, health professionals ought to be vigilant in their observation and interventions. For instance, monitoring of chronic conditions such as HIV calls for an understanding of age-specific immunological markers and personal pharmacokinetics in drug metabolism in children, as emphasized in Therapy A and Management M of Children H-I *et al.* (2003). Integrated care, including, for instance, health care and education, is necessary for overall care in pediatrics. A pediatric care coordination framework suggested highlights how essential it is that these domains are brought together in the form of an end-to-end support system for children and families, which identifies the difference that proper follow-up care can make to health outcomes and welfare, as stated in Jeanne *et al.* (2009). Thus, routine monitoring and coordinating follow-up is necessary in the management of pediatric health.

2.4.1. Importance of Regular Follow-up Clinic Visits

Regular follow-up visits are a crucial aspect of pediatric monitoring and evaluation, with an invaluable opportunity to evaluate a child's development level and address any emerging health problems. The regular visits offer a chance to identify early on any health, developmental, or behavioral issues so that prompt interventions that can make a significant difference in a child's course towards better health can be initiated. Besides, the inclusion of prevention services, including dental care in well-child check-ups, underscores the requirement for a broader approach to child health. Services that integrate oral and general pediatrics can promote increased access to needed services and bridge socioeconomic as well as geographic barriers to care (Krol *et al.*, 2013).

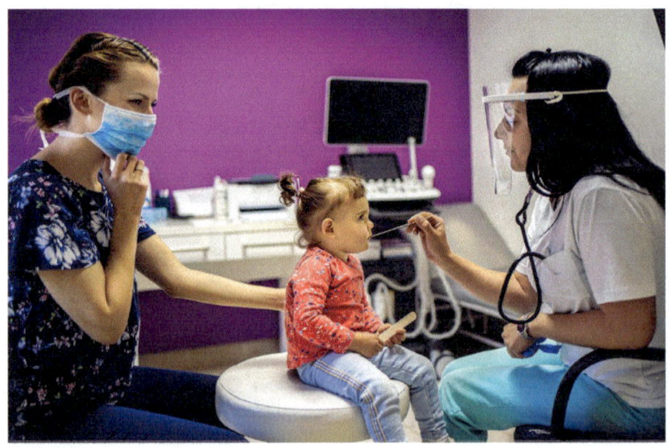

Figure 2.16. Regular follow-up visits play a crucial role in pediatric assessment and monitoring, serving as vital opportunities to gauge a child's developmental progress and address any emerging health concerns.

Source: https://insights.ibx.com/wp-content/uploads/2021/06/toddler-checkup.jpg.

Further, attending follow-up appointments on a regular basis is crucial in maintaining active engagement and up-to-date information from the families, considering that policies for additional enrollment in health programs like

Medicaid and Well-Child Visits have a direct impact on children's health and development (Genevieve *et al.*, 2010) (Figure 2.16).

2.4.2. Tracking Developmental Progress Over Time

Monitoring children's developmental progress over the long term is a significant aspect of pediatric assessment, giving information regarding physical, cognitive, and emotional development. Effective monitoring strategies enable early detection of developmental delay or concern and timely intervention that can significantly alter outcomes. Applying systematic checklists and continuous assessment supports a systematic approach to monitor developmental milestones and keep pediatric care workers vigilant and responsive to changing needs among children. For instance, the application of evidence-based checklists in pediatric endocrinology not only facilitates streamlined evaluation but also encourages clinician engagement and satisfaction with the care program (Legierse *et al.*, 2022). Further, monitoring platforms for developmental progress can capitalize on technology to track growth and learning patterns, similar to how e-learning platforms have in healthcare training (Maimon *et al.*, 2025). The combined method of monitoring is thus essential to ensure maximal pediatric health and seamless transitions to adulthood.

2.4.3. Adjustment of Care Plans Based on Assessments

Amending care plans on the basis of ongoing assessment is a critical part of successful pediatric monitoring and assessment. Ongoing assessment makes it possible to adjust treatment methods in a timely manner to suit the specific needs of pediatric patients. For instance, as has been emphasized in recent applications of Measurement-Based Care (MBC), the application of widely accepted Patient-Reported Outcome Measures (PROMs) improves the precision of care interventions, particularly in identifying new ongoing mental health problems among children (Kapila *et al.*, 2025). Such assessments enable medical care professionals to improve care plans collectively so that they are not only updated but also effective in the long term. In addition, transfer of care in such complex conditions as Osteogenesis Imperfecta (OI) suggests the requirement to modify treatment plans as patients transition to adulthood (Celli *et al.*, 2024). With evidence-based data and real-time information incorporated into the care planning, health professionals can optimize patient outcomes, hence bringing out the dynamic nature of pediatric care (Figure 2.17).

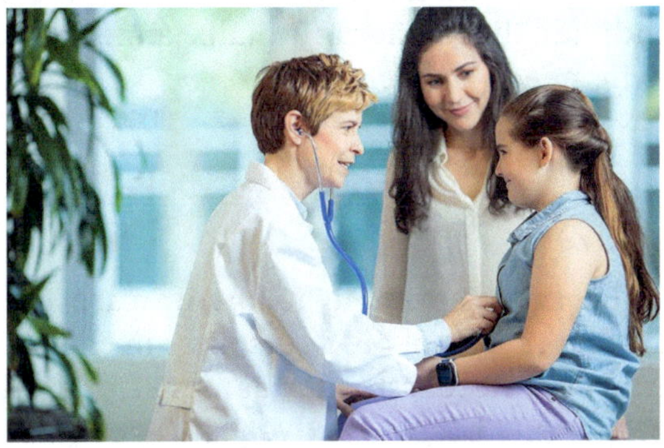

Figure 2.17. Adjusting care plans based on ongoing assessments is a critical component of effective pediatric assessment and monitoring.

Source: https://i0.wp.com/www.usa.edu/wp-content/uploads/2021/04/nurse-interventions-hero.jpg?resize=1000%2C666&quality=89&ssl=1.

2.4.4. Role of Multidisciplinary Teams in Monitoring

The efficacy of pediatric monitoring and evaluation is significantly supported by the intervention of multidisciplinary groups that bring together a range of skills necessary in addressing children's illness complexities. The standard ingredients of such teams include pediatricians, nurses, anesthesiologists, and allied healthcare providers who collaborate to offer a holistic care approach. For instance, in child anesthesia, a structured approach enables effective preoperative evaluation and meticulous planning to minimize perioperative danger and enhance patient experiences, as presented in Kamlesh *et al.* (2025). In addition, in the differentiation of such illnesses as bone infection and sarcomas, it is a collaboration between oncologists, pathologists, and radiologists that comes up with timely and adequate diagnoses, which are essential for optimal outcomes in children, as emphasized in Main *et al.* (2025). Not only does collaboration produce ongoing surveillance, but it also facilitates effective communication, which finally leads to individualized therapy plans aimed at the specific needs of each child.

2.4.5. Parent Involvement in Follow-up Care

Parental involvement in follow-up care is key to the facilitation of best outcomes in children's healthcare. Research has demonstrated that when parents become actively engaged in their child's follow-up care, there are significant increases in compliance with treatment and overall well-being. For instance, a review by NHS Health Scotland emphasizes the efficacy of strong behavioral aspects within child health schemes, best delivered with excellent parental involvement (Sahota *et al.*, 2010). This involvement is particularly crucial in the management of chronic disease, where ongoing management is essential. In addition, a parent-child study of Type 1 diabetic children reveals parental conflict and worry can negatively affect the child's glycemic control, illustrating the importance of supportive interaction in follow-up care (Bonichini *et al.*, 2017). Thus, strengthening parental roles benefits health monitoring, but also allows for an understanding of the emotional dynamics that accompany managing chronic disease in pediatric patients (Figure 2.18).

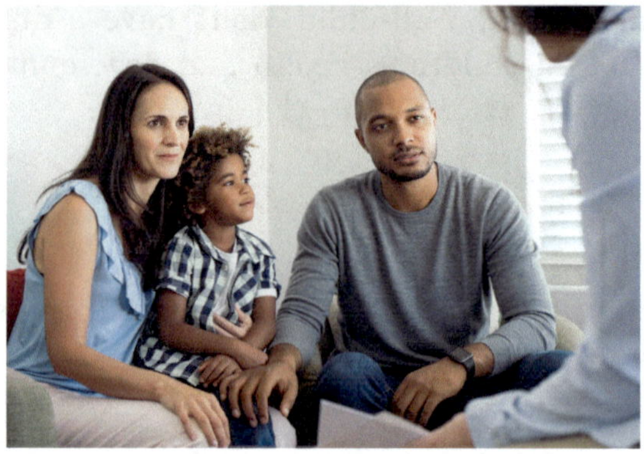

Figure 2.18. The role of parental involvement in follow-up care is pivotal in fostering optimal outcomes in pediatric health management.

Source: https://nam.edu/wp-content/uploads/2020/07/PFEC-Paper-graphics-1.png.

2.4.6. Addressing Concerns and Questions from Families

In pediatric practice, adequate reaction to the family's concerns and questions is critical in establishing trust and offering comprehensive care. Parents are typically wrestling with fears regarding their child's developmental milestones, screenings, and the whole pediatrics process itself. Through the utilization of tools such as the American Academy of Pediatrics Bright Futures guidelines, these interactions can be significantly eased, enhancing provider adherence to well-child visits and answering questions from parents more consistently (Davis *et al.*, 2016). Furthermore, studies have indicated that children's nurses perceive health promotion with families to be a complex conversation due to sensitivities regarding issues like obesity, which can dissuade honest discussion (Greenwood *et al.*, 2015). Hence, it is essential that healthcare practitioners actively listen and create a conducive atmosphere where families feel comfortable expressing their concerns. Such bidirectional communication not only empowers parents but also improves the pediatric monitoring and assessment process and fosters care collaboration relationships.

2.4.7. Transitioning Care as Children Grow

Since children are undergoing several developmental stages, the transference of care is increasingly essential in offering them physical and psychological well-being. The process is characterized by the need for age-related checks and checking systems that adapt and evolve together with the developing child, addressing problems specific to each age.

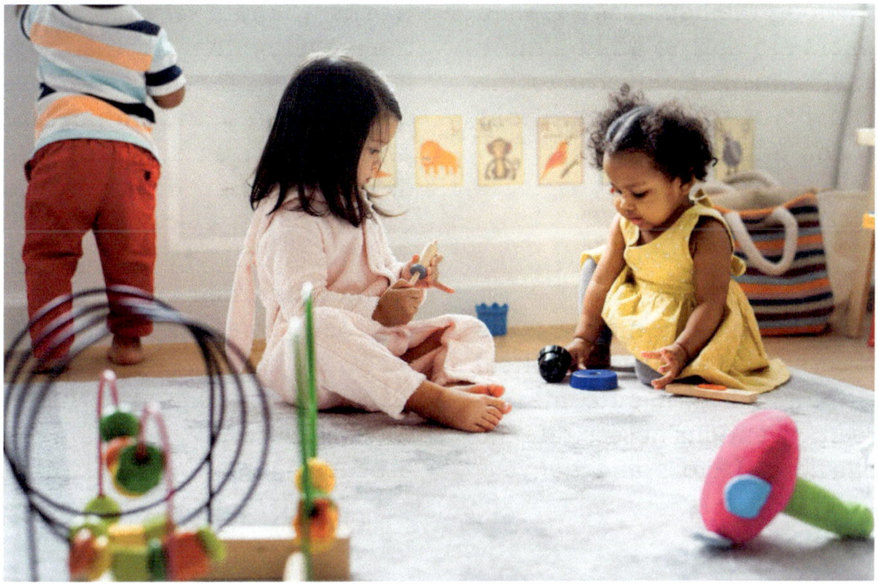

Figure 2.19. As children progress through various developmental stages, the transitioning of care becomes increasingly crucial in ensuring their physical and psychological well-being.

Source: https://kidscareclub.com/wp-content/uploads/2014/01/iStock-1074135186.jpg.

For instance, the use of devices like the ACTi graph and activPAL to monitor physical activity in children underscores the need for precise measurement of levels of physical activity among children, with research evidence showing that the two devices are equally valid at a group level (Dall *et al.*, 2011). Additionally, the enactment of inclusive state policies with an emphasis on improving primary care and chronic care provision is central to ensuring this transition. By focusing on leadership, payment incentives, and support for infrastructure, the guidelines enable practitioners to maximize the capacity to adapt to changing needs in the health of children (Anne *et al.*, 2010). Finally, an effective transition of care maximizes health outcomes as children grow up (Figure 2.19).

2.4.8. Long-Term Monitoring for Chronic Conditions

Follow-up of chronic diseases in children for the long term is necessary for the provision of the best health outcomes and prevention of disease progression complications. Recent focus has been on a concerning rise in hypertension (HTN) among children and youth, which calls for the immediate application of routine monitoring and control regimes (Agabiti-Rosei *et al.*, 2016). Effective monitoring not only allows early detection of complications but also allows interventions in a timely fashion that can avoid long-term cardiovascular hazards. Moreover, the transition of young patients with chronic illness, such as Type 1 diabetes, from pediatric to adult care is associated with certain challenges that need ongoing monitoring (Bagnall *et al.*, 2013). By making prioritization of structured monitoring techniques that are focused on patient care, family involvement, and mutual practices among the healthcare team a priority, practitioners are able to build a more compassionate environment conducive to the effective management of chronic conditions throughout childhood into adulthood.

2.4.9. Evaluating the Impact of Interventions

In pediatric assessment and monitoring, the evaluation of intervention effects is critical to realizing the optimal health outcomes in children. Effective interventions necessitate the evaluation of behavioral factors and delivery formats, particularly in interventions to treat obesity in children. The need to include models of behavior change in such programs has been stressed by the literature review undertaken by NHS Health Scotland, voicing the absence of knowledge around which technique best works (Sahota *et al.*, 2010). Additionally, the development of theory-based discharge interventions for children's hospitalized parents demonstrates the importance of parents' preparation for self-care following hospital discharge based on models for best-practice care (Gralton *et al.*, 2017). Through critical analysis of such interventions, clinicians are able to maximize their approaches, incorporating an approach where pediatric healthcare not only meets the immediate requirements of health but also promotes long-term healthy behaviors. Over time, these evaluations inform deeper clinical practice and policy frameworks in child health.

Test Your Knowledge

1. What are the parameters for weaning children off ventilators?
2. What long-term complications should be monitored after PICU discharge?

SUMMARY

Optimal health outcomes require effective monitoring and evaluation of pediatric patients. As seen through initiatives like the Skin Champion initiative, which decreased hospital-acquired pressure wounds by a significant percentage, the introduction of evidence-based care into practice among pediatric patients is imperative. Not only do these programs assist frontline healthcare providers, but they also ensure that quality of care is provided in an even manner across all settings. The pediatric care coordination framework also points out the need to connect healthcare, education, and family support, which is important for overall pediatric evaluation (Jeanne *et al.*, 2009). Lastly, an integrated approach with novel methods and interdisciplinarity can enhance the quality of care in pediatrics and safeguard the health of young vulnerable patients, ensuring they receive the categorical care they deserve at pivotal development stages (Gordon *et al.*, 2018).

In summary, the discussion about pediatric monitoring and evaluation brings to the fore the critical need to measure patient and family experience with the aim of enhancing the quality of care. The central theme that emerges is the necessity for hospitals to employ evidence-based practices that facilitate effective communication of care performance, which is important in developing staff and ensuring leadership accountability. The integration of patient survey data becomes a revolutionary strategy for introducing quality improvement (QI) interventions and, subsequently, decision-making based on immediate effects on care. Of special interest is maintaining continuous feedback loops, particularly at points of major decision, such as discharge. Additionally, homology between adult inpatient and neonatal care highlights universal principles of culture change and multidisciplinary collaboration to facilitate a robust QI infrastructure. These strategies not only yield improved pediatric care outcomes but also yield continuous enhancements in patient experience (Murphy *et al.*, 2008; Hays *et al.*, 2020).

KEY TERMS FROM THIS CHAPTER

- Monitoring
- Health professionals
- Growth
- Childhood obesity
- Provision
- Height
- Growth charts
- Assessment
- Health status
- Developmental milestones
- Autism spectrum disorder
- Diverse backgrounds
- Weight
- Developmental screening tests

CRITICAL THINKING QUESTIONS

1. **What is the primary purpose of continuous cardiorespiratory monitoring in the PICU?**
   a. To track growth patterns
   b. To detect early signs of clinical deterioration
   c. To reduce the need for nursing staff
   d. To replace physical examination
2. **Which of the following is the most appropriate method for monitoring oxygen saturation in a PICU patient?**
   a. Blood pressure cuff
   b. ECG monitor
   c. Pulse oximetry
   d. Capnography
3. **Capnography in pediatric intensive care primarily monitors:**
   a. Oxygen saturation
   b. Blood glucose levels
   c. Exhaled carbon dioxide
   d. Intracranial pressure
4. **Which of the following scoring systems is commonly used to assess the severity of illness in pediatric ICU patients?**
   a. APGAR
   b. GCS
   c. PEWS (Pediatric Early Warning Score)
   d. PRISM (Pediatric Risk of Mortality)
5. **Which vital sign is the most sensitive indicator of clinical deterioration in a child?**
   a. Blood pressure
   b. Temperature
   c. Heart rate
   d. Respiratory rate

Short Answer Questions

1. How does critical illness impact physical growth and development in pediatric patients?
2. What tools are used to assess developmental milestones in critically ill children?
3. What elements of a child's health history are most critical during PICU admission?
4. How is the physical exam adapted for intubated or sedated pediatric patients?
5. What laboratory investigations are routinely ordered upon PICU admission?
6. How is bedside ultrasound used in pediatric intensive care?
7. What vital signs are continuously monitored in the PICU and why?
8. How is fluid balance monitored and managed in critically ill children?

Answers to Critical Thinking Questions

1. (b) 2. (c) 3. (c) 4. (d) 5. (d)

REFERENCES

1. Acerini, C. L., Lehwalder, D., Wac, K., & Bang, P. (2017). Optimizing patient management and adherence for children receiving growth hormone. https://core.ac.uk/download/146491367.pdf (accessed on 30th June 2025).
2. Agabiti-Rosei, E., Cruickshank, J. K., Dominiczak, A., Erdine, S., *et al.* (2016). *2016 European Society of Hypertension Guidelines for the Management of High Blood Pressure in Children and Adolescents.* https://core.ac.uk/download/46165193.pdf (accessed on 30th June 2025).
3. Álvaro-Lozano, M., Akdiş, C. A., Akdiş, M., Alviani, C., Angier, E., Arasi, S., Arzt-Gradwohl, L., *et al.* (2020). Allergen immunotherapy in children user's guide. *Pediatric Allergy and Immunology, 31,* 1–101. https://doi.org/10.1111/pai.13189 (accessed on 30th June 2025).
4. Antiretroviral Therapy and Medical Management of HIV-Infected Children (ATMMHC), Health Resources and Services Administration (HRSA), National Institutes of Health (NIH), National Pediatric and Family HIV Resource Center, *et al.* (2003). *Guidelines for the Use of Antiretroviral Agents in Pediatric HIV Infection.* https://core.ac.uk/download/pdf/11307015.pdf (accessed on 30th June 2025).
5. Ardiaria, M., Hardaningsih, G., Pratiwi, R., Putra, R., *et al.* (2024). The relationship between 25-hydroxyvitamin (OH) D levels and nutritional status in children with family history of atopy. https://core.ac.uk/download/636476407.pdf (accessed on 30th June 2025).
6. Astrahantseff, K., Chaali-Vlug, R., De Preter, K., De Wilde, S., *et al.* (2020). The pitfalls and promise of liquid biopsies for diagnosing and treating solid tumors in children: A review. https://core.ac.uk/download/286549310.pdf (accessed on 30th June 2025).
7. Bagnall, A., Day, R., & Kime, N. H. (2013). *Systematic Review of Transition Models for Young People with Long-Term Conditions: A Report for NHS Diabetes.* https://core.ac.uk/download/29018738.pdf (accessed on 30th June 2025).
8. Bakhavadinova, Z. M. (2024). Propaedeutics of childhood diseases. *International Journal of Medical Sciences and Clinical Research.* https://www.semanticscholar.org/paper/ecb0531625794b11ccb76e880695736f16fe8145 (accessed on 30th June 2025).
9. Bartz, S. K., DeSalvo, D., Mockler, B., Sonabend, R., *et al.* (2019). Use of best practice alerts to improve adherence to evidence-based screening in pediatric diabetes care. https://core.ac.uk/download/212903935.pdf (accessed on 30th June 2025).
10. Bellini, C., Cammaroto, G., Colizza, A., de Vincentiis, M., *et al.* (2019). Risk factors for obstructive sleep apnea syndrome in children: State of the art. https://core.ac.uk/download/231747914.pdf (accessed on 30th June 2025).
11. Bian, F., Galera-Martinez, R., Gerasimidis, K., Hulst, J., *et al.* (2018). Opinions and practices of healthcare professionals on assessment of disease-associated malnutrition in children: Results from an international survey. https://core.ac.uk/download/pdf/296205775.pdf (accessed on 30th June 2025).
12. Bonichini, S., Mazzoldi, M. A., Pastore, N., Piovan, R., *et al.* (2017). Psychological well-being in parents of pediatric patients with TD1: Role of family conflict and parental fear of children's self-injecting on their glycemic control and psychological well-being. https://core.ac.uk/download/80154835.pdf (accessed on 30th June 2025).

13. Boo, N. Y., de Almeida, M. F. B., Iskander, I. F., Kumar, S., *et al.* (2015). Management of late-preterm and term infants with hyperbilirubinemia in resource-constrained settings. https://core.ac.uk/download/323066114.pdf (accessed on 30th June 2025).

14. Boutelle, K. N., Drahota, A., & Matheson, B. E. (2019). A pilot study investigating the feasibility and acceptability of a parent-only behavioral weight-loss treatment for children with autism spectrum disorder. https://core.ac.uk/download/323308512.pdf (accessed on 30th June 2025).

15. Bull, M. J., Trotter, T. L., Santoro, S. L., Christensen, C. K., & Grout, R. W. (2022). Health supervision for children and adolescents with Down syndrome. *Pediatrics, 149*. https://doi.org/10.1542/peds.2022-057010 (accessed on 30th June 2025).

16. Burke, D., Daw, W., Elphick, H. E., Evans, R., *et al.* (2020). A novel, contactless, portable "spot-check" device accurately measures respiratory rate. https://core.ac.uk/download/322489452.pdf (accessed on 30th June 2025).

17. Cabana, M. D., Cattamanchi, A., Gupta, N., Jennings, S., *et al.* (2021). Implementing pediatric inpatient asthma pathways. https://core.ac.uk/download/323082497.pdf (accessed on 30th June 2025).

18. Cater, D. T., Moser, E. A. S., Rowan, C. M., Tori, S., *et al.* (2018). Modification and assessment of the Bedside Pediatric Early Warning Score in the pediatric allogeneic hematopoietic cell transplant population. https://core.ac.uk/download/227054287.pdf (accessed on 30th June 2025).

19. Celli, L., Garrelfs, M. R., Sakkers, R. J. B., Elting, M., Celli, M., Bökenkamp, A., Smits, C., *et al.* (2024). Adapting to adulthood: A review of transition strategies for osteogenesis imperfecta. *Calcified Tissue International, 115*, 960–975. https://www.semanticscholar.org/paper/6a0cb736dc7ab868dd3b484c2f74701e65785dcc (accessed on 30th June 2025).

20. Cordingley, L., Ghio, D., Lee, R. R., Rashid, A., *et al.* (2017). Chronic pain assessments in children and adolescents: A systematic literature review of the selection, administration, interpretation, and reporting of unidimensional pain intensity scales. https://core.ac.uk/download/288395031.pdf (accessed on 30th June 2025).

21. Corsello, G., Mancuso, G., Martorana, C., Montante, C., Notarbartolo, V., Piro, E., Schierz, I. A. M., *et al.* (2019). Microcephaly and macrocephaly: A study on anthropometric and clinical data from 308 subjects. https://core.ac.uk/download/287859205.pdf (accessed on 30th June 2025).

22. Corvini, M., Cox, K., O'Neil, M., Ryer, R., *et al.* (2018). Addressing childhood adversity and social determinants in pediatric primary care: Recommendations for New Hampshire. https://core.ac.uk/download/215540986.pdf (accessed on 30th June 2025).

23. Dall, P., Granat, M., Martin, A., McNeil, J., *et al.* (2011). Objective measurement of habitual sedentary behavior in pre-school children: Comparison of activPAL with actigraph monitors. https://core.ac.uk/download/110646.pdf (accessed on 30th June 2025).

24. Danduran, M. J., Dixon, J. E., Hoffman, G. M., Loomba, R., *et al.* (2012). Near infrared spectroscopic monitoring during cardiopulmonary exercise testing detects anaerobic threshold. https://core.ac.uk/download/213086413.pdf (accessed on 30th June 2025).

25. Davidson, J. E., Aslakson, R. A., Long, A. C., Puntillo, K., Kross, E. K., Hart, J. L., Cox, C. E., *et al.* (2016). Guidelines for family-centered care in the neonatal, pediatric, and adult ICU. *Critical*

Care Medicine, 45, 103–128. https://doi.org/10.1097/ccm.0000000000002169 (accessed on 30th June 2025).

26. Davis, J. L. (2016). Quality improvement for well child care. https://core.ac.uk/download/162578549.pdf (accessed on 30th June 2025).
27. De Paepe, A., & Vanakker, O. (2013). Pharmacogenomics in children: Advantages and challenges of next generation sequencing applications. https://core.ac.uk/download/55848729.pdf (accessed on 30th June 2025).
28. de Wit, M., Gajewska, K. A., Goethals, E. R., McDarby, V., Zhao, X., Hapunda, G., Delamater, A. M., *et al.* (2022). ISPAD Clinical Practice Consensus Guidelines 2022: Psychological care of children, adolescents and young adults with diabetes. *Pediatric Diabetes, 23*, 1373–1389. https://doi.org/10.1111/pedi.13428 (accessed on 30th June 2025).
29. Dennis, R. E., Edelman, S. W., Giangreco, M. F., *et al.* (1999). Related services for Vermont's students with disabilities. https://core.ac.uk/download/51067326.pdf (accessed on 30th June 2025).
30. Dinh, A., Duke, J. L., Ferriola, D., Frackelton, R., *et al.* (2019). Assessing the utilization of high-resolution 2-field HLA typing in solid organ transplantation. https://core.ac.uk/download/213445234.pdf (accessed on 30th June 2025).
31. ElSayed, N. A., Aleppo, G., Aroda, V. R., Bannuru, R. R., Brown, F. M., Bruemmer, D., Collins, B. S., *et al.* (2022). 4. Comprehensive medical evaluation and assessment of comorbidities: Standards of care in diabetes—2023. *Diabetes Care, 46*, S49–S67.2. https://doi.org/10.2337/dc23-s004 (accessed on 30th June 2025).
32. Formosa, N. (2013). Blood glucose monitoring in children and adolescents with Type 1 Diabetes Mellitus. https://core.ac.uk/download/46602350.pdf (accessed on 30th June 2025).
33. Gatta, M., Miscioscia, M., Peraro, C., Simonelli, A., *et al.* (2017). A psychological perspective on preterm children: The influence of contextual factors on quality of family interactions. https://core.ac.uk/download/129592820.pdf (accessed on 30th June 2025).
34. Gauthier, A. K., Sims-Kastelein, K., Takach, M., & Kaye, N. (2010). *Strengthening Primary and Chronic Care: State Innovations to Transform and Link Small Practices.* https://core.ac.uk/download/71355266.pdf (accessed on 30th June 2025).
35. Gordon, M. D., Hagan, J., *et al.* (2018). Evidence-based skin champion program reduces pressure injuries in a pediatric hospital. https://core.ac.uk/download/212897182.pdf (accessed on 30th June 2025).
36. Gralton, K., Johnson, N. L., Kaul, M., Klingbeil, H., *et al.* (2017). Development of a self-management theory-guided discharge intervention for parents of hospitalized children. https://core.ac.uk/download/213087168.pdf (accessed on 30th June 2025).
37. Greenwood, N., & Lewis, K. (2015). Opportunistic health promotion among overweight children. https://core.ac.uk/download/30731293.pdf (accessed on 30th June 2025).
38. Haiden, N., Luque, V., Domellöf, M., Hill, S., Kivelä, L., de Koning, B. D., Köglmeier, J., *et al.* (2025). Assessment of growth status and nutritional management of prematurely born infants after hospital discharge: A position paper of the ESPGHAN Nutrition Committee. *Journal of Pediatric Gastroenterology and Nutrition*. https://www.semanticscholar.org/paper/1686726aa1f89da5bc3b3b1ee91d35cc39d1afc1 (accessed on 30th June 2025).

39. Hays, R. D., Lerner, C., Palimaru, A., Quigley, D., *et al.* (2020). A review of best practices for monitoring and improving inpatient pediatric patient experiences. https://core.ac.uk/download/287622168.pdf (accessed on 30th June 2025).

40. Jee, J., & Nagarajan, J. (2014). Identification and assessment of children and youth with special health care needs in Medicaid managed care: Approaches from three states. https://core.ac.uk/download/71365115.pdf (accessed on 30th June 2025).

41. Johnson, N. L., & Rodriguez, D. (2013). Children with autism spectrum disorder at a pediatric hospital: A systematic review of the literature. https://core.ac.uk/download/213081757.pdf (accessed on 30th June 2025).

42. Kamlesh, K., & Prajapati, H. (2025). Optimizing preoperative assessment and preparation for safe pediatric anesthesia. *International Journal of Anesthesiology Sciences.* https://www.semanticscholar.org/paper/4d9bc49ea5edc8d503ea095bb773f935556b5937 (accessed on 30th June 2025).

43. Kapila, S., Saunders, N., Anthony, S., Pol, S. J., Paz-Soldan, M., Samardzic, T., & Monga, S. (2025). Advancements in pediatric mental healthcare through implementation and evaluation of measurement-based care in a hospital setting. *International Journal of Integrated Care.* https://www.semanticscholar.org/paper/d5e306ef7c8d0a057df08d505edb26d7ad7998ea (accessed on 30th June 2025).

44. Kenney, G. M., & Pelletier, J. E. (2010). Improving the lives of young children: The role of developmental screenings in Medicaid and CHIP. https://core.ac.uk/download/71347983.pdf (accessed on 30th June 2025).

45. Krol, D., Cheung, K., Cruz, K., Carver, L., & Revels, M. (2013). Providing preventive oral health care to infants and young children in Women, Infants, and Children (WIC), Early Head Start, and primary care settings. https://core.ac.uk/download/71362896.pdf (accessed on 30th June 2025).

46. Kurbatfinski, S., Komanchuk, J., Dosani, A., & Letourneau, N. (2024). Validity, reliability, accessibility, and applicability of young children's developmental screening and assessment tools across different demographics: A realist review. *Children, 11.* https://www.semanticscholar.org/paper/a6c5851cdd3c18afaa13c05185167fba03d076b5 (accessed on 30th June 2025).

47. Lee, P. A., Nordenström, A., Houk, C. P., Ahmed, S. F., Auchus, R. J., Baratz, A. B., Dalke, K. B., *et al.* (2016). Global disorders of sex development update since 2006: Perceptions, approach and care. *Hormone Research in Pediatrics, 85*, 158–180. https://doi.org/10.1159/000442975 (accessed on 30th June 2025).

48. Legierse, J., González, G., Marvicsin, D., & Anderson, C. J. (2022). Using age-specific checklists to help transition adolescents with Type 1 diabetes to adult care. *ADCES in Practice, 11*, 8–18. https://www.semanticscholar.org/paper/26fe39ec7b84d666c8282efe48bf9664e0f1d92b (accessed on 30th June 2025).

49. Maimon, Y., & Traiber, G. (2025). TCM Academy–Online platform for acupuncture and traditional Chinese medicine education: Advancing global standards. *Medical Acupuncture, 37*(2), 96–99. https://www.semanticscholar.org/paper/03a2b2285abe02ae69931899cedd927b3b639db1 (accessed on 30th June 2025).

50. Malone, L. A., Morrow, A. K., Chen, Y., Curtis, D., de Ferranti, S. D., Desai, M., Fleming, T. K., *et al.* (2022). Multi-disciplinary collaborative consensus guidance statement on the assessment and

treatment of post-acute sequelae of SARS-CoV-2 infection (PASC) in children and adolescents. *PM&R, 14*, 1241–1269. https://doi.org/10.1002/pmrj.12890 (accessed on 30th June 2025).

51. McAllister, J. W., Popp, J., & Antonelli, R. (2009). Making care coordination a critical component of the pediatric health system: A multidisciplinary framework. https://core.ac.uk/download/71352885.pdf (accessed on 30th June 2025).

52. McCarthy, D., & Leatherman, S. (2004). Quality of health care for children and adolescents: A chartbook. https://core.ac.uk/download/71354153.pdf (accessed on 30th June 2025).

53. Murphy, C. G., Alendy, C., Cooper, J., & Simpson, L. (2008). Childhood obesity: The role of health policy. https://core.ac.uk/download/71342400.pdf (accessed on 30th June 2025).

54. Patel, R. (2015). Pediatric nurse practitioner home visitation is associated with a decrease in home care and healthcare utilization errors in high-risk infants. https://core.ac.uk/download/129532636.pdf (accessed on 30th June 2025).

55. Saberi Main, S., Naghizadeh, H., & Khabiri, S. S. (2025). Diagnostic challenges and multidisciplinary approaches in differentiating pediatric bone infections from sarcomas: A narrative review. *International Journal of Cancer Management*. https://www.semanticscholar.org/paper/085cc84d95443a130cadcce3dc8de2583fe9be93 (accessed on 30th June 2025).

56. Sahota, P., Woodward, J., & Wordley, J. (2010). Literature review–Health behavior changes models and approaches for families and young people to support HEAT 3: Child healthy weight programmers. https://core.ac.uk/download/29018931.pdf (accessed on 30th June 2025).

57. Serkina, Y., Pshenichnaya, N. N., & Velikikh, P. K. (2025). The transformation of the life of the population of the border region in the conditions of a special military operation: A sociological analysis. *Proceedings of the Southwest State University. Series: Economics. Sociology. Management*. https://www.semanticscholar.org/paper/5cb9cd26dd03a14b44d34fc50e5841 3368bb19fb (accessed on 30th June 2025).

58. Sices, L. (2007). Developmental screening in primary care: The effectiveness of current practice and recommendations for improvement. https://core.ac.uk/download/71350769.pdf (accessed on 30th June 2025).

59. Stevens, G., Abrams, M. K., Inkelas, M., & Halfon, N. (2005). Quality of preventive health care for young children: Strategies for improvement. https://core.ac.uk/download/71354158.pdf (accessed on 30th June 2025).

60. Stout, K., Daniels, C. J., Aboulhosn, J., Bozkurt, B., Broberg, C. S., Colman, J. M., Crumb, S. R., *et al.* (2018). 2018 AHA/ACC guideline for the management of adults with congenital heart disease: A report of the American College of Cardiology/American Heart Association Task Force on Clinical Practice Guidelines. *Circulation, 139*. https://doi.org/10.1161/cir.0000000000000603 (accessed on 30th June 2025).

61. Suryaningsih, C., Adiviso, F., Estiva, E. A., Aliswag, E., Aggari, M., & Santos, M. (2025). The association between mental health, social-emotional health, and child development in preschool children: A structural equation modelling approach. *Gema Lingkungan Kesehatan*. https://www.semanticscholar.org/paper/fcbce6abda16bfafb5197229708f7bc18222540f (accessed on 30th June 2025).

62. Vos, M. B., Abrams, S. H., Barlow, S. E., Caprio, S., Daniels, S. R., Kohli, R., Mouzaki, M., *et al.* (2016). NASPGHAN clinical practice guideline for the diagnosis and treatment of nonalcoholic

fatty liver disease in children. *Journal of Pediatric Gastroenterology and Nutrition, 64*, 319–334. https://doi.org/10.1097/mpg.0000000000001482 (accessed on 30th June 2025).

63. Waugh, J. (2023). Functional symptoms in children may be much more common than previously believed. *Developmental Medicine & Child Neurology, 65.* https://www.semanticscholar.org/paper/128a13a89565b188da5693b0933c44d52e57322e (accessed on 30th June 2025).

RESPIRATORY FAILURE AND MECHANICAL VENTILATION

3

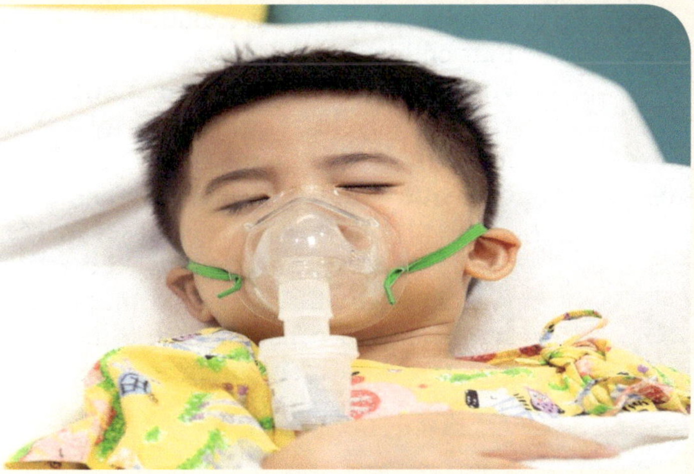

Introduction

Pediatric respiratory failure is a matter of utmost concern in intensive care, with the complexities of dealing with young, delicate systems demanding expert handling. Acute lung injury and acute respiratory distress syndrome are severe presentations of respiratory dysfunction, with non-cardiogenic pulmonary edema and refractory hypoxemia, and mortality ranging between 10 to 90% depending on a number of factors (Chimbira *et al.*, 2001). Most importantly, particularly in pediatrics, the high incidence of infections like bronchiolitis underscores the necessity of more sophisticated interventions, as this illness is the leading cause of non-elective admissions to the pediatric ICU. Understanding the pathophysiologic mechanism of the illness and therapeutic options, including mechanical ventilation, plays a key role in predicting outcomes. Since pediatric patients exhibit typical physiological responses that are distinct from those of adults, certain approaches are necessary in order to achieve better survival rates and reduce long-term consequences of respiratory failure (Figure 3.1).

LEARNING OBJECTIVES

After studying this chapter, you will be able to:

1. Understand Causes of Respiratory Failure in Children.
2. Explain the Assessment and Diagnosis of Respiratory Failure.
3. Describe Mechanical Ventilation Techniques.

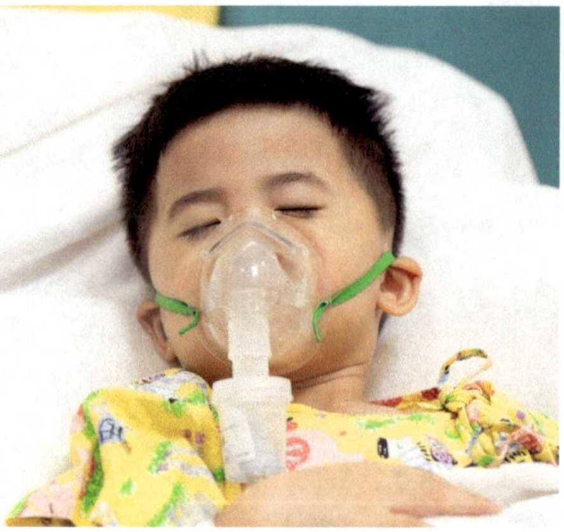

Figure 3.1. Respiratory failure in pediatric patients.

Source: https://careoptionsforkids.com/wp-content/uploads/2025/04/respiratory-distress-vs-failure-1.jpg.

3.1. Causes of Respiratory Failure in Children

Learning Outcome

1. Understand acute respiratory distress syndrome (ARDS).
2. Explain pneumonia and its impact on respiratory function.
3. Describe asthma exacerbations in pediatric patients.
4. Focus on congenital anomalies affecting the respiratory system.
5. Identify neuromuscular disorders leading to respiratory failure.
6. Explain infections and their role in respiratory compromise.
7. Focus on environmental factors contributing to respiratory issues.
8. Identify trauma and its effects on respiratory health.
9. Understand chronic conditions leading to acute respiratory failure.

Respiratory failure in children can be due to numerous complicated causes, the majority of which are related to basic medical conditions and environmental conditions. Pneumonia, asthma, and bronchitis are important considerations since they have a tendency to severely compromise lung function and gas exchange, leading to hypoxia and hypercapnia. Neuromuscular diseases, such as spinal muscular atrophy, can also compromise respiratory muscle function further, adding to the susceptibility for respiratory failure. The recent coronavirus disease 2019 (COVID-19) epidemic introduced novel factors in this calculation; there are reports that children are afflicted with a syndrome of virus-linked fever and inflammation (Whittaker *et al.*, 2020). In addition, obesity has also been identified as a significant risk factor, with one study finding a high correlation between elevated body mass index and severe respiratory disease necessitating intensive care treatment (Sattar *et al.*, 2020). All of these reasons are significant to consider in the development of effective treatment interventions in pediatric intensive care units.

3.1.1. Acute Respiratory Distress Syndrome (ARDS)

Acute respiratory distress syndrome (ARDS) is a critical illness that poses gigantic challenges in pediatric intensive care, particularly due to its acute presentation and variable aetiology. ARDS pathophysiology represents a complex interaction of systemic inflammation and compromised pulmonary function, which justifies therapeutic interventions directed to alleviate its severity. Long-term glucocorticoid treatment has been a vital intervention, with a marked correlation with patient outcomes, as measured by the decrease in inflammation, thus enhancing pulmonary recovery and hospital survival rates. Specifically, the therapy has been associated with an increase in mechanical ventilation-free days, which is a factor of critical significance in treating pediatric patients with ARDS (Meduri *et al.*, 2016). Also, extracorporeal membrane oxygenation (ECMO) has become a rescue therapy for severe disease, offering a means of delivering high-quality lung-protective ventilation—essential in the management of this challenging syndrome (Finney *et al.*, 2014). The widespread adoption of these therapies in practice shows that there is ongoing intention to refine care in children with the syndrome (Figure 3.2).

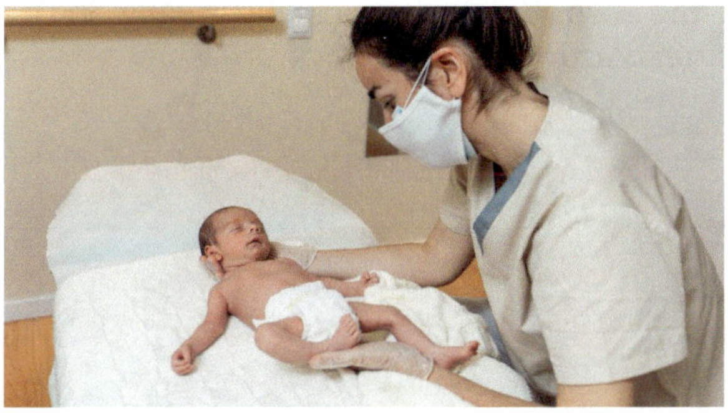

Figure 3.2. Acute respiratory distress syndrome (ARDS) is a critical condition that poses significant challenges in pediatric intensive care, particularly due to its rapid onset and variable etiology.

Source: https://i0.wp.com/airwayjedi.com/wp-content/uploads/2022/12/baby-w-RN_AdobeStock_475081802.jpeg?resize=778%2C438&ssl=1.

3.1.2. Pneumonia and Its Impact on Respiratory Function

Pneumonia has a serious impact on respiratory function, particularly in children, with the consequences being devastating. Pneumonia induces alveolar inflammation and consolidation, which ultimately compromises gas exchange and encourages hypoxemia. Severe pneumonia may precipitate acute respiratory distress syndrome (ARDS), with diffuse pulmonary inflammation and compromised lung compliance. Systemic inflammatory response due to cytokine release worsens the respiratory failure further, and the condition requires interventions such as mechanical ventilation in order to boost the breathing capacity of the child. Evidence suggests that anti-inflammatory strategies such as glucocorticoid therapy recover pulmonary function and improve clinical outcomes among patients with ARDS (Meduri *et al.*, 2016). Additionally, prolonged immobilization with mechanical ventilation is also risky for intensive care unit-acquired weakness (ICUAW), complicating recovery (Hermans *et al.*, 2016). Therefore, the management of pneumonia requires an integrated approach considering respiratory and overall neuromuscular well-being in pediatric patients with critical illness.

3.1.3. Asthma Exacerbations in Pediatric Patients

Exacerbations of asthma are a serious problem in children, often needing intensive therapy. Exacerbation may lead to respiratory failure and, therefore, needs careful monitoring and management in pediatric intensive care. Pathophysiologic mechanisms of asthma should be understood because inflammation and airway hyperresponsiveness are the main factors in exacerbation severity. Pharmacologic management, including bronchodilators and corticosteroids, is typically aimed at reducing inflammation in the airway and increasing airflow. The Infectious Diseases Society of America has developed guidelines proposing evidence-based practice management concepts that emphasize the multidimensionality of respiratory conditions such as asthma during periods of heightened respiratory distress (Bhimraj *et al.*, 2020). The guidelines also emphasize the need for immediate intervention among critically ill children because early interventions can significantly improve the outcomes (Timothy *et al.*, 2018). Here, the relationship between early medical intervention and elaborate care planning is vital in the prevention of recurrent exacerbations and patient stabilization (Figure 3.3).

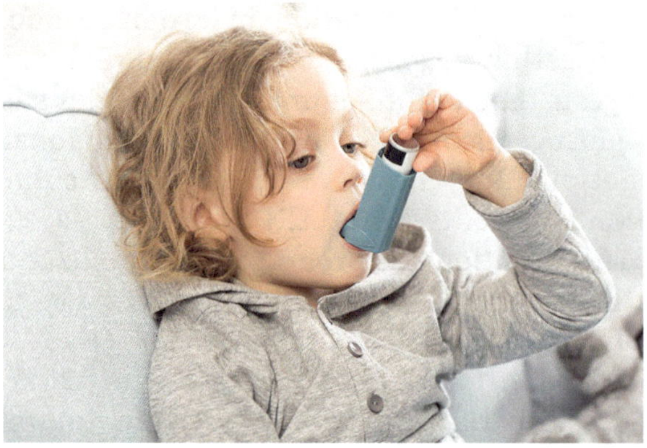

Figure 3.3. Asthma exacerbations represent a significant concern in pediatric patients, often necessitating intensive medical intervention.

Source: https://hospitalpharmacyeurope.com/wp-content/uploads/2002/06/HPE-asthma.jpg.

3.1.4. Congenital Anomalies Affecting the Respiratory System

Congenital respiratory malformations are a serious problem in pediatric critical care and often cause respiratory failure that necessitates mechanical ventilation. These malformations, which can range from congenital diaphragmatic hernia to tracheoesophageal fistula, often disrupt normal respiratory function, causing compromised oxygenation and ventilation. The complexity of such cases is underscored by the need for careful monitoring and assessment, as indicated by the Vasoactive-Ventilation-Renal score, which has been established as a reliable predictor of postoperative situations in neonates with congenital cardiac abnormalities (Cashen *et al.*, 2018). Furthermore, studies show that some of the physiological indicators, such as hypothermia and excess oxygen demand at presentation, are strongly associated with mortality risk in ventilated neonates, thus making the treatment of congenital respiratory anomalies difficult (Chudasama *et al.*, 2009). Such crucial interdependencies need to be known when improving care measures in the pediatric intensive care unit.

3.1.5. Neuromuscular Disorders Leading to Respiratory Failure

Neuromuscular disorders (NMD) are one of the leading causes of respiratory failure among children, hence the use of mechanical ventilation as a leading intervention. These disorders, which affect the neuromuscular junction or muscle function, lead to inadequate strength of the respiratory muscles, eventually leading to ventilatory insufficiency.

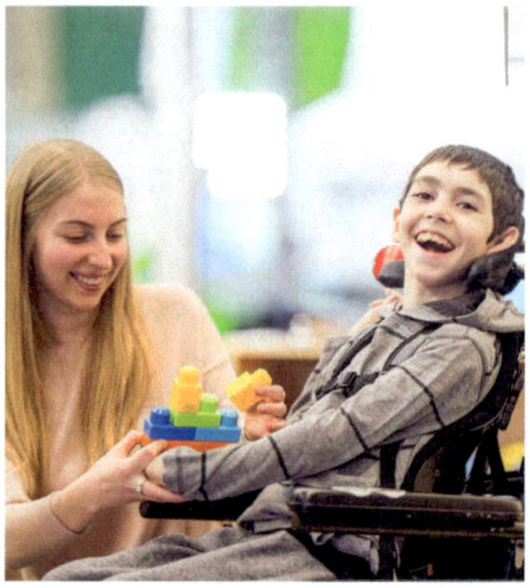

Figure 3.4. Neuromuscular disorders (NMD) are a significant contributor to respiratory failure in pediatric patients, necessitating the consideration of mechanical ventilation as a critical intervention.

Source: https://wp04-media.cdn.ihealthspot.com/wp-content/uploads/sites/122/2021/03/content-img-neuromuscular.jpg.

Since children with NMD experience stressful respiratory dynamics, the likelihood of complications like respiratory infection and atelectasis is considerably amplified. Besides, airway clearance technique (ACT) evolution has fostered management strategies among this population as described in the systematic review of adult and pediatric neuromuscular disorder cases (Chatwin *et al.*, 2018). The severity of the care required highlights the need for proper monitoring and early intervention, as respiratory failure would progress rapidly if not addressed early. Thus, it is essential to understand the effects of NMD on respiratory health in the pediatric intensive care unit (Inoue *et al.*, 2019) (Figure 3.4).

3.1.6. Infections and Their Role in Respiratory Compromise

In pediatric patients, infection is a frequent etiology of respiratory dysfunction, contributing significantly to the need for mechanical ventilation in the intensive care unit. Respiratory infections such as pneumonia and viral infections can potentially cause severe hypoxemia and respiratory failure within a short period, necessitating early intervention. Such infections in the majority are caused by the inflammatory process leading to airway obstruction and compromised gas exchange, and thus early effective management is vital. It is necessary, in the treatment of such infections, to consider gender disparities in outcomes since evidence in the form of data shows male patients developing more serious disease than female patients in COVID-19 and SARS, with increased mortality reported among males (Jin *et al.*, 2020). In addition, complications due to infection, including cytokine release syndrome, add an additional level of complexity, and the necessity for meticulous monitoring and therapeutic maneuvering in critically ill children is highlighted (Shimabukuro *et al.*, 2018).

3.1.7. Environmental Causes Resulting in Respiratory Complications

Environmental determinants of relevance significantly influence the severity and scope of respiratory illness in children, particularly in terms of respiratory failure and mechanical ventilation in pediatric intensive care patients. Among them is the high prevalence of viral infections such as the respiratory syncytial virus (RSV), which is disproportionately prevalent in children under five years, particularly those with compromised immunity or comorbid conditions (Kaler *et al.*, 2023). The transmission of RSV through respiratory droplets indicates environmental cleanliness as well as infection control policies. Moreover, the exposure to environmental toxins, allergens, and other irritants exacerbates respiratory illnesses among vulnerable populations. The application of lung ultrasound (LUS) in clinical practice has elucidated the impact of such environmental determinants on lung function, guiding interventions aimed at the alleviation of respiratory distress (Demi *et al.*, 2022). Hence, the tackling of these environmental factors is necessary to enhance children's outcomes in intensive care (Figure 3.5).

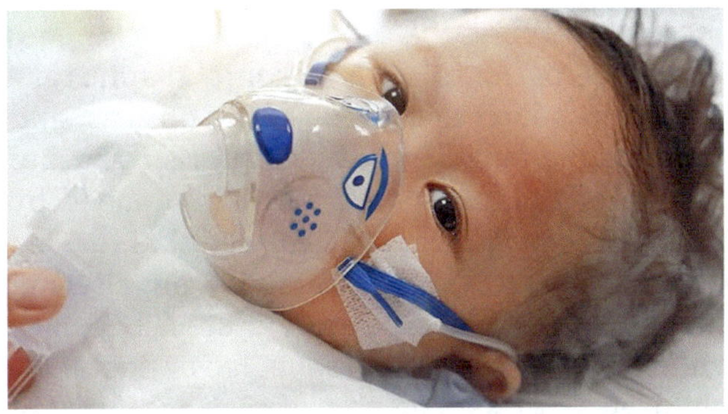

Figure 3.5. Respiratory syncytial virus (RSV).

Source: https://asm.org/ASM/media/Article-Images/2022/December/RSV-Feature-879x492.jpg?ext=.jpg.

3.1.8. Trauma and Its Effects on Respiratory Health

Trauma's impact on respiratory status is profoundly significant, particularly in pediatric patients who have sustained significant injuries. Trauma reliably leads to respiratory failure, for which mechanical ventilation can be instituted as a supportive measure of life. Trauma-induced inflammation can lead to an elevated metabolic rate with increased breakdown of nutrients and, therefore, malnutrition, which is very prevalent in PICU patients (Somani *et al.*, 2025). This nutritional deficiency can further exacerbate respiratory complications, contributing to a higher risk of mechanical ventilation and longer hospital stays. In addition, mechanical ventilation complications such as ventilator-associated pneumonia and atelectasis can also enhance risks in already compromised children (Shawn *et al.*, 2023). Thus, fulfilling the nutritional needs of such patients while being able to manage respiratory conditions effectively is critical in order to improve outcomes in PICU, highlighting the sophisticated interconnection among trauma, malnutrition, and acute respiratory failure in children.

3.1.9. Chronic Conditions Leading to Acute Respiratory Failure

Pediatric patients with chronic respiratory conditions, such as asthma, cystic fibrosis, and congenital anomalies, have a high risk of acute respiratory failure, which can be managed by interventions like mechanical ventilation. The chronic disease can progressively impair lung function, and the respiratory system becomes vulnerable to acute worsening. For instance, children with asthma can experience forceful bronchospasm, causing respiratory distress and compromising acute lung injury (ALI) or acute respiratory distress syndrome (ARDS), two conditions characterized by severe hypoxemia and respiratory failure (Chimbira *et al.*, 2001). Furthermore, the presence of multiple organ failure is frequently observed in patients with chronic respiratory complications, increasing the risk of mortality and making it difficult to treat (Kazuyoshi *et al.*, 2018). Identification and early management of these chronic respiratory disorders prevent acute occurrences and improve outcomes in pediatric intensive care units (Figure 3.6).

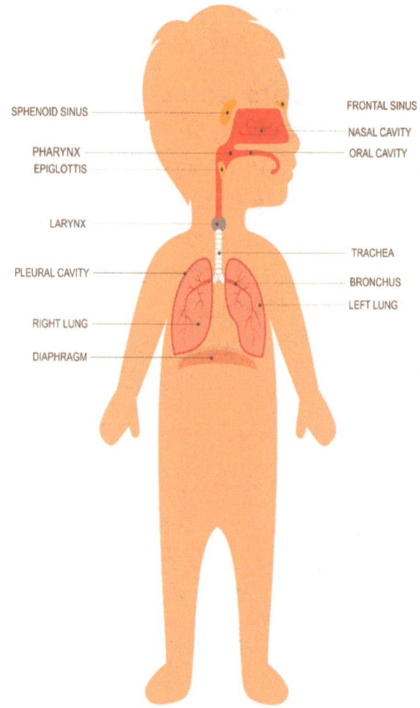

Figure 3.6. Chronic respiratory conditions in pediatric patients, such as asthma, cystic fibrosis, and congenital abnormalities, significantly increase the risk of acute respiratory failure, necessitating advanced interventions like mechanical ventilation.

Source: https://ceufast.com/imgs/image-1--pediatric-respiratory-tract_800px.jpg.

Test Your Knowledge

1. What role do neuromuscular diseases play in causing hypoventilation in children?
2. How can congenital heart disease lead to respiratory failure?

3.2. Assessment and Diagnosis of Respiratory Failure

Learning Outcome

1. Identify clinical signs and symptoms of respiratory failure.
2. Know the importance of patient history in diagnosis.
3. Learn physical examination techniques.
4. Perform diagnostic imaging methods.
5. Focus on laboratory tests and their relevance.
6. Monitor vital signs and oxygen saturation.
7. Discuss use of arterial blood gases (ABGs).
8. Explain the role of pulse oximetry in assessment.
9. Focus on differential diagnosis considerations.

Respiratory failure in children is diagnosed and evaluated with a multidimensional system, involving both clinical evaluation and higher-level diagnostic approaches. Initially, a complete history of the child's complaint and any comorbid disease is essential since respiratory failure can present differently based on age and comorbid disease. These tools, including the Lung Injury Score and the Pediatric Sequential Organ Failure Assessment (pSOFA), play a critical role in quantifying the level of severity of respiratory disease as well as predicting the prognosis of patients, especially in acute hypoxemic respiratory failure (AHRF) (Damps *et al.*, 2023). Interestingly, according to studies, SARS-CoV-2-induced hypoxemic respiratory failure is typically linked with children having higher oxygenation levels compared to their non-COVID peers, calling for timely and proper assessment (Yolanda *et al.*, 2021). It is critical that there be a proper diagnosis since it forms the foundation of an effective management plan, which includes potential mechanical ventilation, typically necessary for serious cases.

3.2.1. Clinical Signs and Symptoms of Respiratory Failure

Recognition of clinical signs and symptoms of respiratory failure is critical in the pediatric intensive care setting since prompt diagnosis will greatly impact the outcome of the patient. Tachypnea, retractions, and cyanosis are typical presentations, indicative of compromised oxygenation and ventilation. Altered mental status or exhaustion may be due to the children's failure to maintain adequate respiratory function. Monitoring heart rate and respiratory rate is valuable since persistently abnormal readings may indicate impending deterioration.

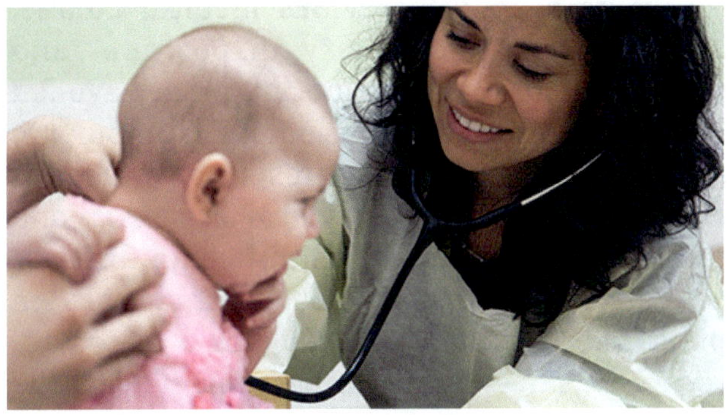

Figure 3.7. Identifying clinical signs and symptoms of respiratory failure is crucial in pediatric intensive care, as early recognition can significantly impact patient outcomes.

Source: https://www.mottchildren.org/sites/default/files/styles/full_size_image/public/mottchildren%20-%20pulm%20overview%20spotlight%20graphic.png?itok=gkmr6Mt3.

The significance of non-invasive therapy modalities, such as High Flow Nasal Cannula (HFNC) therapy, is underscored through evidence of its capacity to prevent further deterioration of respiratory status in infants with conditions such as bronchiolitis (Schibler *et al.*, 2015). Furthermore, advances in diagnostic technologies, including the application of critical care ultrasound, enhance clinicians' ability to investigate underlying pathologies, thereby informing the use of focused management for respiratory failure (Chong *et al.*, 2020). In all, a thorough understanding of these clinical indicators is imperative in optimizing treatment effectiveness in pediatric patients who experience respiratory difficulties (Figure 3.7).

3.2.2. Importance of Patient History in Diagnosis

Patient history in the intricate life of pediatric intensive care cannot be overstated, particularly in the diagnosis of respiratory failure. A good patient history provides valuable information regarding a child's previous medical course, any suspected hereditary disposition, and certain environmental exposures that have led to their illness. This information is important in distinguishing between respiratory distress caused by sepsis, as is typical in sepsis, and other etiologies such as chronic lung diseases or congenital malformations. As a case in point, the fact that the child has a history of recurrent infections is in agreement with the need to assess primary immune deficiencies, which may complicate the development of sepsis (McCulloh *et al.*, 2014). In addressing conditions like respiratory failure, where time is of the essence, patient history is utilized by clinicians to successfully individualize mechanical ventilation therapy, ensuring that treatment is aligned with the specific pediatric patient requirements (Kazuyoshi *et al.*, 2018). Thus, careful patient history forms the foundation for accurate diagnosis and optimal practice treatment planning.

3.2.3. Physical Examination Techniques

Good physical examination techniques are important for early diagnosis and appropriate treatment of pediatric respiratory failure. Clinicians must systematically assess respiratory effort, auscultate lung sounds, and observe for distress, such as retractions or nasal flaring. Physical examination can provide critical information about the patient's condition, including acute lung injury or the need for mechanical ventilation. For instance, familiarization with the nuances of expected patterns of respiration can guide the selection of non-invasive methods for support, e.g., High Flow Nasal Cannula therapy, which has been reported to be useful in optimizing outcomes in conditions like bronchiolitis (Schibler *et al.*, 2015). Secondly, competent physical examination is also included in monitoring patient response to interventions like High Frequency Oscillation Ventilation, especially in populations with acute respiratory distress syndrome (Chimbira *et al.*, 2001). Using systematic methods, healthcare providers can enhance the quality of care in children's intensive care settings (Figure 3.8).

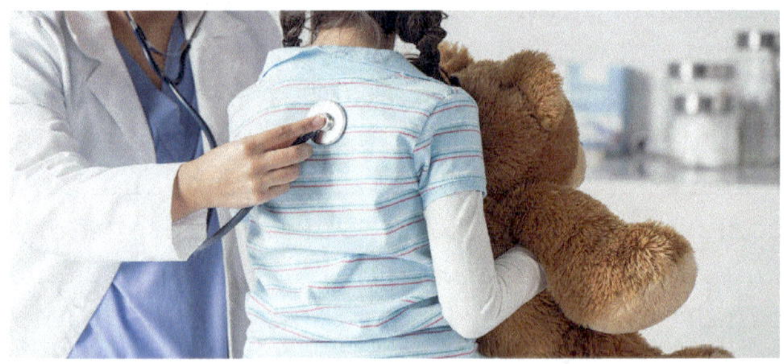

Figure 3.8. Clinicians must systematically assess respiratory effort, auscultate lung sounds, and observe for signs of distress, such as retractions or nasal flaring.

Source: https://s3-us-west-2.amazonaws.com/utsw-patientcare-web-production/original_images/pediatric-respiratory-medicine-1600x732.jpg.

3.2.4. Diagnostic Imaging Methods (e.g., X-rays, CT scans)

Imaging modalities such as X-rays and CT scans play a critical role in the diagnosis and treatment of children's respiratory failure in intensive care units. These imaging modalities provide invaluable information regarding the structure and function of the respiratory tract that enables clinicians to diagnose various conditions such as pneumonia, bronchopulmonary dysplasia, and structural abnormalities. X-rays are often employed as an initial imaging strategy since they can be completed rapidly and are widely accessible, allowing for instantaneous evaluation of the airways and lungs. The CT scan provides more advanced cross-sectional views, defining fine pathology not visible on X-ray and facilitating targeted therapeutic intervention. Their importance is echoed by their integration in clinical practice, allowing clinicians to utilize the most recent standards of diagnostic imaging, maximizing patient outcomes for pediatric respiratory distress (Kazuyoshi *et al.*, 2018; Bancalari *et al.*, 2018).

3.2.5. Laboratory Tests and Their Relevance

In pediatric intensive care, laboratory investigations have a pivotal role in the diagnosis and management of respiratory failure, therapeutic decision-making, and assessment of the efficacy of mechanical ventilation. Laboratory investigations like arterial blood gas analysis, complete blood counts, and electrolyte panels provide precious information regarding a patient's physiological status. For instance, arterial blood gases (ABGs) help in assessing oxygenation and acid-base status, which is crucial in patients with respiratory failure. Secondly, measurements of markers such as hemoglobin levels can inform clinicians about transfusions, especially when anemia underlying the respiratory illness is a complicating factor. Most importantly, the accuracy of these tests enhances clinical decision-making so that personalized strategies for ventilation can be created to suit each child patient's individual requirements (Docking *et al.*, 2012). Also, routine laboratory examinations can identify potential complications and follow the overall response to treatment, so that the mechanical ventilation settings can be manipulated in a timely fashion as necessary (Balázs *et al.*, 2018) (Figure 3.9).

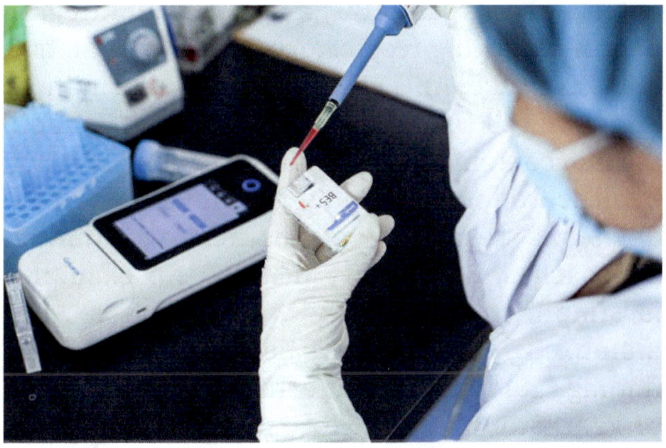

Figure 3.9. Laboratory tests, including arterial blood gas analysis, complete blood counts, and electrolyte panels, provide essential insights into a patient's physiological status.

Source: https://en.seamaty.com/Uploads/2024-05-24/6650369ae6a61.jpg.

3.2.6. Monitoring Vital Signs and Oxygen Saturation

In pediatric intensive care, observation of oxygenation and vital signs is critical, particularly for patients who are experiencing respiratory failure. Real-time and precise monitoring of the same enables clinicians to track the earliest signs of clinical deterioration and intervene in time. For instance, the Pediatric Early Warning Score (PEWS) has been proven to be a good instrument in this regard, where an eight or higher score has been found to correlate highly with intensive interventions, including mechanical ventilation (Cater *et al.*, 2018). Its application not only facilitates ease of respiratory status monitoring but also aids in patient detection who are at higher risk for PICU admission (Argent *et al.*, 2017). Early intervention is critical in bridging improvements in patient outcomes, particularly in a field where every second counts in respiratory emergency situations.

3.2.7. Use of Arterial Blood Gases (ABGs)

Arterial blood gas (ABG) analysis is an integral part of managing respiratory failure in pediatric intensive care. ABG gives essential information regarding a patient's oxygenation, carbon dioxide content, and acid-base balance, allowing healthcare professionals to make informed decisions regarding mechanical ventilation approaches. Respiratory distress, for example, is simplified to identify with repeated ABG monitoring once they have been established, the findings guiding the readjustment of parameters of ventilatory support to optimize respiratory function.

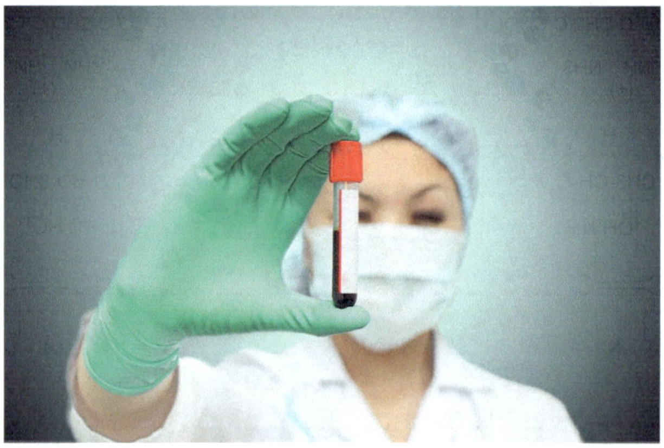

Figure 3.10. The analysis of arterial blood gases (ABGs) is a critical component in the management of respiratory failure within pediatric intensive care settings.

Source: https://respiratory-therapy.com/wp-content/uploads/2019/12/testing-blood-vial-2k1.jpg.

Most crucially, inclusion of newer monitoring techniques into the debate in more recent literature demonstrates that including ABG analysis in combination with other noninvasive measures must be done to optimize clinical outcome in critically ill children (Trivedi *et al.*, 2015). Through extensive monitoring, clinicians are able to effectively tailor interventions, improving patient safety and reducing risks from prolonged mechanical ventilation (Karakitsos *et al.*, 2014). Hence, ABGs remain a vital tool in the management of pediatric respiratory failure (Figure 3.10).

3.2.8. Role of Pulse Oximetry in Assessment

In pediatric intensive care, pulse oximetry is a critical tool in assessing and managing respiratory failure. Pulse oximetry is a minimally invasive technique that continuously monitors peripheral oxygen saturation, providing critical information regarding the patient's respiratory status in real time. With timely intervention, pulse oximetry enhances the capacity of health professionals to make unambiguous decisions regarding mechanical ventilation and other interventions. Notably, pediatric critical care has resulted in improved outcomes among children who are critically ill, but overreliance on high-technology diagnostics can obscure the importance of conventional examination and clinical acumen, a matter noted in controversy over the evolving nature of pediatric care (Argent *et al.*, 2018). Consequently, while pulse oximetry is an important tool, it must be embedded within a broader strategy of measurement that includes interdisciplinary interventions that enhance practitioner competency and patient safety (Huffer *et al.*, 2017).

3.2.9. Differential Diagnosis Considerations

In pediatric respiratory failure, differential diagnosis is key to appropriate care in the intensive care unit. Therapists and other healthcare providers need to evaluate a broad spectrum of potential underlying diseases, ranging from infectious processes through structural abnormalities, that may result in respiratory insufficiency. Of particular significance, the onset of severe acute respiratory syndrome coronavirus 2 (SARS-CoV-2) has added some complexity, since children can also present with multisystem inflammatory syndrome (MIS-C) due to post-infectious immune dysregulation, a condition that adds complexity to the clinical profile and requires close monitoring (Nakra *et al.*, 2020). Moreover, respiratory failure also has a correlation with myocarditis symptomatology by virtue of direct viral injury and immune-mediated damage to the heart, which is additionally responsible for the respiratory impairment (Siripanthong *et al.*, 2020). For this reason, a multi-modal diagnostic workup incorporating clinical evaluation, imaging, and laboratory testing is appropriate in order to determine the specific etiology and appropriately direct therapeutic interventions.

Test Your Knowledge

1. What vital signs are most sensitive to changes in respiratory function in pediatric patients?
2. How is arterial blood gas (ABG) interpretation used to diagnose respiratory failure?

3.3. Mechanical Ventilation Techniques

Learning Outcome

1. Understand the overview of mechanical ventilation modes.
2. Learn indications for initiating mechanical ventilation.
3. Explain non-invasive ventilation options.
4. Focus on invasive ventilation techniques.
5. Discuss settings and parameters in mechanical ventilation.
6. Focus on monitoring and adjusting ventilator settings.
7. Know complications associated with mechanical ventilation.
8. Understand weaning protocols from mechanical ventilation.
9. Discuss the role of multidisciplinary teams in ventilation management.

In pediatric intensive care, the application of mechanical ventilation strategies plays a pivotal role in managing respiratory failure, particularly in children with acute respiratory distress syndrome (ARDS). Of the various methods applied, Extracorporeal Membrane Oxygenation (ECMO) is a significant intervention in cases of severe hypoxemia or hypercapnia. Current developments also emphasize the interplay between ECMO and lung protective strategies as critical in strengthening patient outcomes and avoiding complications of mechanical ventilation (Finney *et al.*, 2014).

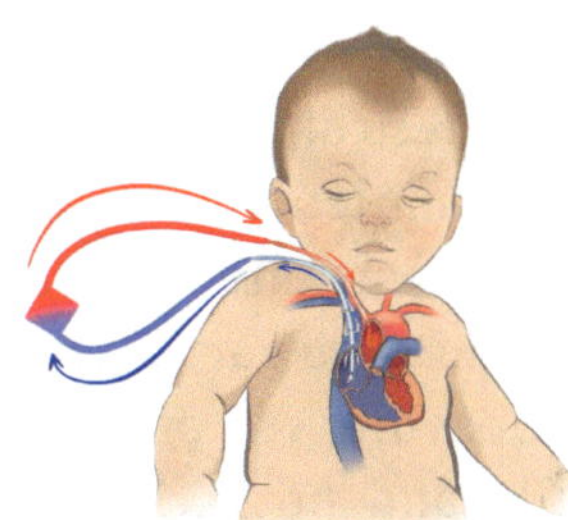

Figure 3.11. Extracorporeal membrane oxygenation (ECMO) has emerged as a significant intervention, especially for cases of severe hypoxemia or hypercapnia.

Source: https://www.mdpi.com/jcm/jcm-12-06661/article_deploy/html/images/jcm-12-06661-g004.png.

In addition, High Flow Nasal Therapy (HFNT) is a breakthrough non-invasive therapy that offers efficient respiratory support using heated and humidified air with variable oxygenation levels, a practice greatly beneficial in the management of acute and chronic respiratory conditions (Cortegiani *et al.*, 2019).

Medical practitioners can significantly improve survival rates and quality of care in pediatric patients with respiratory failure through the addition of these new approaches (Figure 3.11).

3.3.1. Overview of Mechanical Ventilation Modes

It is essential to understand various modes of mechanical ventilation in pediatric intensive care to manage respiratory failure effectively. These have primarily been divided into assist-control, pressure support, and synchronized intermittent mandatory ventilation, each of which has specific patient needs. Assist-control mode allows inspirations initiated by the patient with a fixed tidal volume to provide respiratory support as well as weaning.

Conversely, pressure support ventilation supports patient-breathed efforts with a fixed pressure, thus promoting spontaneity and comfort in the process of ventilation. In addition, synchronized intermittent mandatory ventilation combines spontaneous and mandatory breaths and promotes patients to participate in their own respiratory endeavors. All of the modes have specific benefits and potential complications, such as ventilator-associated pneumonia and airway trauma, which reflect the importance of judicious choice on the basis of individual patient profile and clinical status (Shawn *et al.*, 2023). Steady progress in mechanical ventilation not only enhances acute care but also enables long-term therapies, such as home mechanical ventilation (Kwak, 2022).

3.3.2. Indications for Initiating Mechanical Ventilation

In pediatric intensive care, initiation of mechanical ventilation is a life-sustaining intervention determined by the severity of respiratory failure as well as underlying pathophysiology. The main indications for mechanical ventilation are the existence of insufficient respiratory effort, severe hypoxemia, and uncorrectable hypercapnia. In addition, illnesses like severe acute respiratory distress syndrome (ARDS) in children typically need this procedure, especially if other forms of treatment are not able to facilitate adequate gas exchange. Even modern treatment emphasizes the timing of mechanical ventilation initiation, as timely treatment is beneficial in hereditary neuromuscular disorders, which have high respiratory morbidity if left untreated (as reflected by elevated pre-HMV respiratory morbidity in pre-diagnosis patients) (Han *et al.*, 2015). Further, novel evidence emphasizes the need for critical evaluation of new ventilation strategies, such as high-frequency oscillatory ventilation, with variable results in children (Bateman *et al.*, 2016) (Figure 3.12).

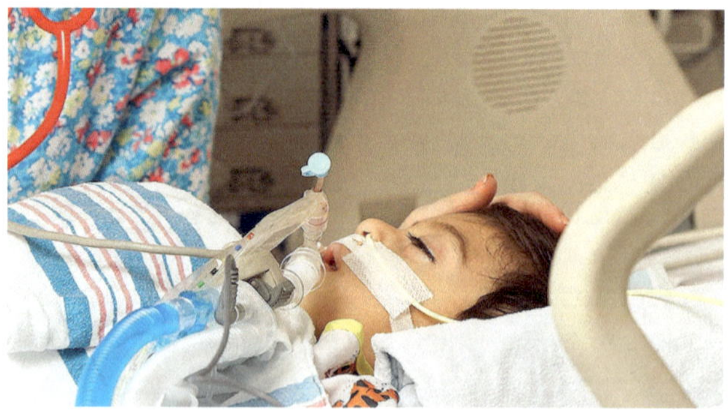

Figure 3.12. In pediatric intensive care, the decision to initiate mechanical ventilation is a critical intervention dictated by the severity of respiratory failure and the underlying pathology.

Source: https://img.medscape.com/thumbnail_library/gty_220301_child_ventilator_icu_800x450.jpg.

3.3.3. Non-Invasive Ventilation Options

For pediatric intensive care, non-invasive ventilation (NIV) modalities have a significant function to play in the management of respiratory failure, especially when it is acute hypercapnic in nature. With the development of technology and improved understanding, NIV has become a mode of support of choice because it can decrease the necessity for endotracheal intubation, which carries greater risks of morbidity and mortality. Research has shown that early intervention with NIV has the potential to improve significantly, as shown by the HACOR score, which predicts NIV failure and helps make decisions about intubation in a timely manner (Saha *et al.*, 2024). Also, while high-flow nasal cannula oxygen (HFNC) has been shown to have its own merits in respiratory support, it was not non-inferior to NIV for acute exacerbations of chronic obstructive pulmonary disease, highlighting the ongoing relevance of proper selection and use of respiratory support methods (Tan *et al.*, 2024).

3.3.4. Invasive Ventilation Techniques

Invasive ventilation techniques are pivotal to the management of pediatric respiratory failure in intensive care, particularly in conditions where patients have severe conditions such as adenovirus infection. Invasive techniques become vital when non-invasive strategies fail because they contribute to oxygenation and ventilation directly, effectively preventing further complications arising from prolonged hypoxemia. Critical factors have been determined through research, like acute respiratory distress syndrome, which warrant the transition to invasive mechanical ventilation in a bid to deliver adequate respiratory assistance (Tao *et al.*, 2025). Also, risk factor assessment with the aid of machine learning models has improved the decision-making process clinically, allowing clinicians to determine the need for invasive support with precision. These predictions enhance the treatment of critical children, enabling interventions that can reduce mortality rates by quite a lot (Chiaruttini *et al.*, 2024). Lastly, understanding the indications for invasive ventilation is vital to optimizing patient outcomes in the pediatric intensive care unit (Figure 3.13).

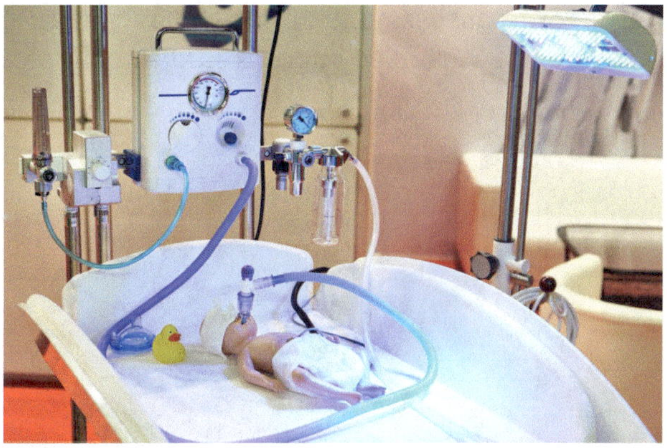

Figure 3.13. Invasive ventilation techniques in pediatric intensive care settings.

Source: https://medanta.s3.ap-south-1.amazonaws.com/blogs/April2024/9tgBZKV3eiFELROUhiHhX0V3B17qvW-metaMjVBLmpwZw==-.jpg.

3.3.5. Settings and Parameters in Mechanical Ventilation

In pediatric intensive care, respiratory failure, mechanical ventilator parameters, and settings are instrumental in enhancing patient outcomes. Individualization of ventilator modes and settings is essential due to the unique physiological demands of children who are likely to have dissimilar pathophysiologic conditions from those of adults. Adjustment of the ventilator settings—e.g., tidal volume, respiratory rate, and positive end-expiratory pressure—is necessary to address individualized needs and optimize alveolar ventilation while minimizing lung injury. Also, parameters such as adequate humidity and circuit configurations must be properly set to ensure comfort and efficient gas exchange. Caregiver and healthcare provider educational interventions on these parameters are central to the effective application of home mechanical ventilation (HMV) therapies, and recent studies indicate that best-practice HMV protocols can exponentially decrease respiratory morbidity in children (Kwak, 2022) and increase overall long-term outcomes in such populations (Sattar *et al.*, 2020).

3.3.6. Monitoring and Adjusting Ventilator Settings

Ventilator setting titration and monitoring are necessary in pediatric intensive care to optimize respiratory support in infants with respiratory failure. A successful ventilation can be achieved by the ongoing assessment of patient oxygenation and ventilation status, which may be governed by a number of variables such as lung mechanics and synchrony with the patient.

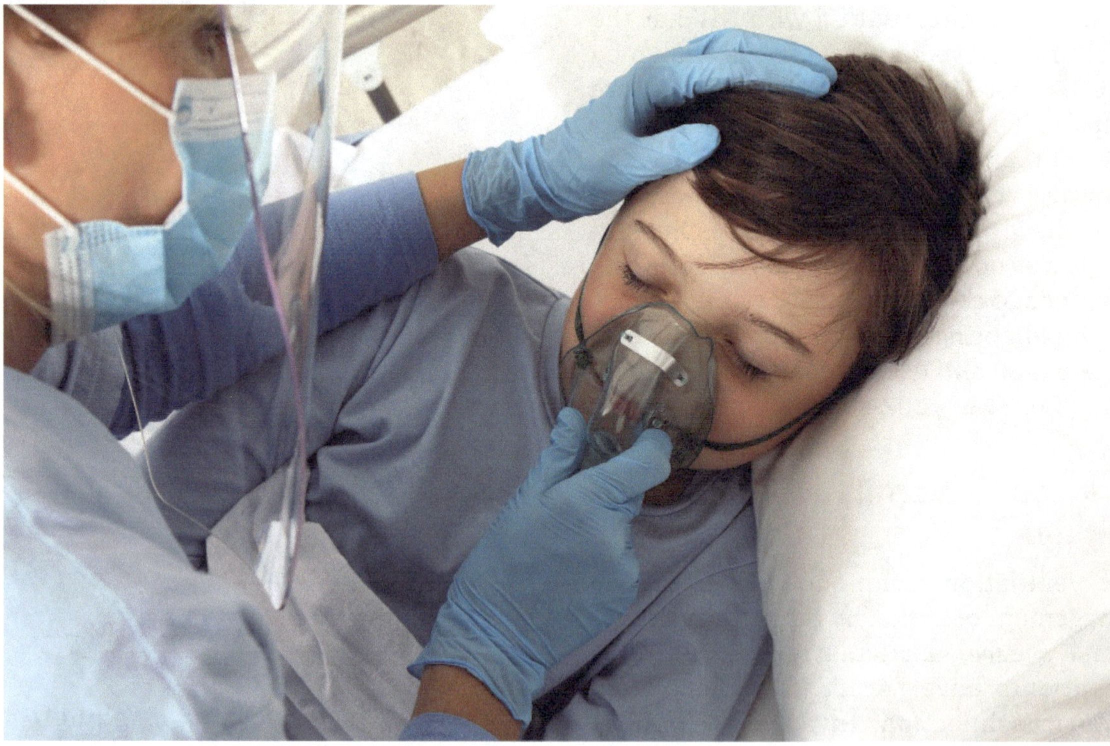

Figure 3.14. Effective ventilation management necessitates a continuous assessment of the patient's oxygenation and ventilation status, which can be influenced by various factors such as lung mechanics and patient-ventilator synchrony.

Source: https://respiratory-therapy.com/wp-content/uploads/2023/04/oxygen-mask-pediatric-2k.jpg.

Modification of ventilator settings, including tidal volume, respiratory rate, and inspiratory pressure, decreases the probability of developing complications like ventilator-induced lung injury. Stepwise introduction of new technology, such as high-flow nasal cannula (HFNC), has resulted in a significant decrease in mechanical ventilation length of stay, especially among patients who are on long-term respiratory support or post-operative support (Choi *et al.*, 2024). Furthermore, it has been demonstrated through research that time delays in intervention algorithms, such as post-extubation nebulization, are responsible for increased rates of extubation failure, necessitating the highest level of vigilance in monitoring and timely modification of ventilatory management (Belayhun *et al.*, 2025) (Figure 3.14).

3.3.7. Complications Associated with Mechanical Ventilation

Mechanical ventilation in pediatric intensive care units, while critical to the treatment of respiratory failure, may cause many serious complications. Among these, ventilator-associated pneumonia (VAP) is frequent and may prolong hospitalization, leading to high morbidity and mortality rates. Barotrauma and volutrauma, resulting from inappropriately set pressures and tidal volumes, are other complications and may lead to lung injury. Further, prolonged mechanical ventilation makes patients vulnerable to muscle weakening and atrophy of the diaphragm due to disuse. Being aware of the balance that is present in providing adequate respiratory support with minimal risk of these complications is essential. The incorporation of advanced techniques, such as extracorporeal membrane oxygenation (ECMO), has been shown to be promising in complementing lung protective ventilation tactics, ultimately influencing patient outcomes (Finney *et al.*, 2014). Recent studies of high-frequency oscillatory ventilation (HFOV) further imply that it can be employed safely with satisfactory survival rates in pediatric acute hypoxemic respiratory failure patients, yet randomized trials must be conducted to affirm its efficacy unambiguously (Babbitt *et al.*, 2012).

3.3.8. Protocols for Weaning from Mechanical Ventilation

Implementation of weaning algorithms from mechanical ventilation is a crucial part of intensive care in children, particularly in those with respiratory failure. There is widespread variation in current practice, typically determined more by the individual preference of the clinician than by explicit criteria, leading to inconsistent patient management approaches.

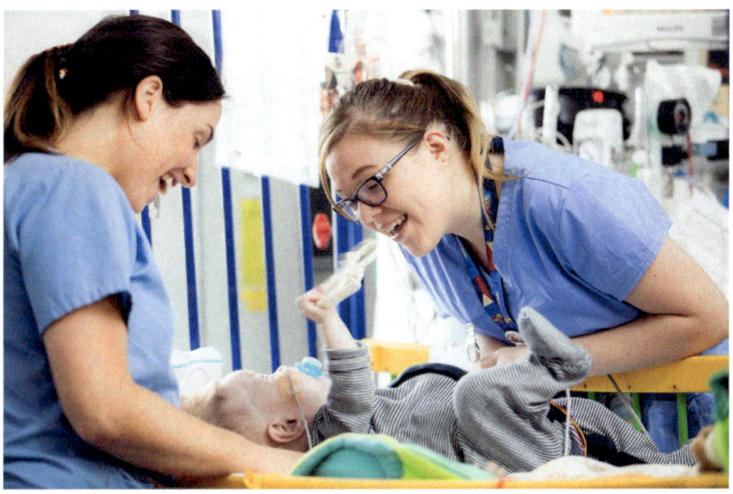

Figure 3.15. The implementation of weaning protocols from mechanical ventilation is a critical aspect of pediatric intensive care, particularly for patients experiencing respiratory failure.

Source: https://www.qub.ac.uk/research-centres/media/Media,920706,smxx-1600x1066.jpg.

For instance, studies indicated that only 9% of pediatric intensive care units (PICUs) had formal weaning programs, and the majority relied on physician decisions without evidence-based consideration of patient readiness to be extubated, for instance, spontaneous breathing trials (Ambuel *et al.*, 2015). This lack of formalized protocols can compromise patient outcomes, particularly since evidence has been shown for the benefits of weaning protocols involving reductions in days of ventilation and improvements in survival rates (Meduri *et al.*, 2016). Thus, developing and adhering to evidence-based weaning protocols may make care provided in PICUs higher in quality regarding more consistent practice that tends to improve clinical outcomes in seriously ill children (Figure 3.15).

3.3.9. Role of Multidisciplinary Teams in Ventilation Management

Pediatric intensive care unit ventilation management involves teamwork with special emphasis on the importance of multidisciplinary teams. The teams, such as physicians, nurses, respiratory therapists, and allied health professionals, collaborate to formulate personalized ventilation plans that address every patient's complex needs. By calling upon the diverse knowledge of its members, such teams are more able to utilize interventions, such as weaning protocols and sedation regimens, that are critical in caring for patients with respiratory failure. Evidence indicates that the implementation of a multidisciplinary package of interventions, including early mobility and the control of delirium, has the ability to reduce the length of mechanical ventilation in critically ill children (Curley *et al.*, 2015). Moreover, the inclusion of routine training and communication among team members makes care delivered more effective, thus enhancing outcomes in pediatric patients needing mechanical ventilation (Ambrosino *et al.*, 2008). Last but not least, a well-coordinated multidisciplinary team is central to enhancing ventilation management to a maximum level and promoting recovery in this vulnerable population.

Test Your Knowledge

1. How is non-invasive ventilation (NIV) used in pediatric respiratory support?
2. What are the advantages and risks of high-frequency oscillatory ventilation (HFOV) in pediatric patients?

SUMMARY

Management of pediatric respiratory failure needs multidimensionality, particularly when mechanical ventilation is a part of it. Complexity in the weaning process of patients from mechanical breathing to spontaneous breathing demands a good understanding of patient-related factors along with a step-by-step implementation of clinical guidelines. Successful weaning from ventilation is not only crucial for the patient's short-term recovery but also marks his return to his normal life, thus making successful weaning methods all the more paramount. The given case study follows suit with the need for pulmonary mechanics assessment and implementation of muscle conditioning regimens to increase the outcome. Further, clinical practice guidelines, for example, those provided by the Korean Society of Critical Care Medicine, provide evidence-based interventions to guide clinicians regarding effective weaning regimens, emphasizing the central role of multidisciplinary practice in achieving optimal care for these vulnerable patients (Hariyanto *et al.*, 2025; Ha *et al.*, 2024).

In discussing the intricate relationship between mechanical ventilation and respiratory failure in pediatric intensive care, certain crucial facts are recognized. The increasing prevalence of obesity and other concomitant conditions has been seen to exacerbate the severity of respiratory disease, elevating hospitalization risk and the need for intensive care management, particularly where COVID-19 is the case and obesity significantly elevates the risk for invasive mechanical ventilation (Huang *et al.*, 2020). Further, new pediatric illnesses, such as multisystem inflammatory syndrome in children (MIS-C), also require heightened sensitization and specific management in pediatric patients presenting with respiratory failure. There is a need to differentiate between MIS-C and atypical presentations of COVID-19 in order to provide appropriate treatment (Diorio *et al.*, 2020). These discussions confirm the need for therapy tailored to pediatric respiratory failure, emphasizing the need for ongoing study and clinical vigilance in the treatment of high-risk populations in the intensive care setting.

KEY TERMS FROM THIS CHAPTER

- Respiratory failure
- Acute lung injury
- Respiratory dysfunction
- Refractory hypoxemia
- Mechanical ventilation
- Pneumonia
- Bronchitis
- Hypoxia
- Spinal muscular atrophy
- Intensive care
- Acute respiratory distress
- Non-cardiogenic pulmonary edema
- Non-elective admissions
- Survival rates
- Asthma
- Gas exchange
- Hypercapnia
- Fever

CRITICAL THINKING QUESTIONS

1. **Which of the following is the most common cause of respiratory failure in children?**
    a. Chronic obstructive pulmonary disease (COPD)
    b. Bronchiolitis
    c. Myocardial infarction
    d. Stroke
2. **What is the primary goal of mechanical ventilation in pediatric patients?**
    a. To sedate the child completely
    b. To cure underlying infections
    c. To support oxygenation and ventilation
    d. To increase blood pressure
3. **Which type of respiratory failure is characterized by low oxygen levels with normal or low carbon dioxide levels?**
    a. Type I (Hypoxemic) respiratory failure
    b. Type II (Hypercapnic) respiratory failure
    c. Mixed respiratory failure
    d. Metabolic acidosis
4. **Which of the following parameters is most commonly used to initiate mechanical ventilation in a child?**
    a. Serum sodium
    b. Glasgow Coma Scale (GCS)
    c. Arterial blood gases (ABG)
    d. Hematocrit levels
5. **What is the best initial ventilator mode for a child with acute respiratory distress?**
    a. CPAP
    b. Pressure-controlled ventilation (PCV)
    c. High-frequency oscillatory ventilation (HFOV)
    d. SIMV or Assist-Control (A/C)

Short Answer Questions

1. What are the most common causes of acute respiratory failure in infants and young children?
2. How do upper versus lower airway obstructions contribute to pediatric respiratory failure?
3. What are the early clinical signs of respiratory distress in children?
4. How does the Pediatric Assessment Triangle (PAT) aid in identifying respiratory compromise?
5. What are the primary indications for initiating mechanical ventilation in children?
6. What is the difference between pressure-controlled and volume-controlled ventilation modes?
7. What are the short-term outcomes for children requiring mechanical ventilation in the PICU?
8. What factors predict poor prognosis in pediatric respiratory failure?

Answers to Critical Thinking Questions

1. (b) 2. (c) 3. (a) 4. (c) 5. (d)

REFERENCES

1. Ambrosino, N., & Goldstein, R. (2008). Ventilatory support for chronic respiratory failure. https://www.semanticscholar.org/paper/01546e76e3cd1e7bec620ea13d1e19575c903318 (accessed on 30th June 2025).
2. Ambuel, B., Blackwood, B., Maloney, C., *et al.* (2015). The implausibility of 'usual care' in an open system: Sedation and weaning practices in pediatric Intensive Care Units (PICUs) in the United Kingdom (UK). https://core.ac.uk/download/42138145.pdf (accessed on 30th June 2025).
3. Aoyama, K., Azuhata, T., Doi, K., Doi, M., Egi, M., Fujimura, N., Fujishima, S., *et al.* (2018). The Japanese clinical practice guidelines for management of sepsis and septic shock 2016 (J-SSCG 2016). https://core.ac.uk/download/154950014.pdf (accessed on 30th June 2025).
4. Argent, A., & Frey, B. (2018). Safe pediatric intensive care: Part 1: Does more medical care lead to improved outcome? https://core.ac.uk/download/159151916.pdf (accessed on 30th June 2025).
5. Argent, A., Festa, M., Lacroix, J., Leteurtre, S., *et al.* (2017). The intensive care medicine clinical research agenda in pediatrics. https://core.ac.uk/download/158171535.pdf (accessed on 30th June 2025).
6. Babbitt, C. J., Cooper, M. C., Levine, G. K., Liao, J., *et al.* (2012). High-frequency oscillatory ventilation in pediatric acute hypoxemic respiratory failure: Disease-specific morbidity survival analysis. https://core.ac.uk/download/323075275.pdf (accessed on 30th June 2025).
7. Balázs, G., Dahlem, P., Elek, N., Szima, B., *et al.* (2018). Pediatric sepsis: Clinical considerations. https://core.ac.uk/download/161060610.pdf (accessed on 30th June 2025).
8. Bancalari, E., Clyman, R. I., Collaco, J. M., Davis, S. D., *et al.* (2018). Bronchopulmonary dysplasia: Executive summary of a workshop. https://core.ac.uk/download/227054384.pdf (accessed on 30th June 2025).
9. Bateman, S., Borasino, S., Asaro, L., Cheifetz, I., Diane, S., Wypij, D., & Curley, M. (2016). Reply: Do we really know how to use high-frequency oscillatory ventilation in critically ill children? *American Journal of Respiratory and Critical Care Medicine, 193*(9), 1068–1069. https://www.semanticscholar.org/paper/60876e0e42bce01deb2eeecec9dcafc5e7097e3f (accessed on 30th June 2025).
10. Belayhun, Y., Ambachew, S., & Damite, A. (2025). Prevalence of extubating failure and associated factors among pediatric patients admitted to the Pediatric Intensive Care Unit at Tikor Anbessa Specialized Hospital, Ethiopia. *Ethiopian Journal of Pediatrics and Child Health.* https://www.semanticscholar.org/paper/67b4859a83b892ba001f05897a48b95fc239a0db (accessed on 30th June 2025).
11. Bhimraj, A., Morgan, R. L., Shumaker, A. H., Lavergne, V., Baden, L. R., Cheng, V. C. C., Edwards, K. M., *et al.* (2020). Infectious Diseases Society of America guidelines on the treatment and management of patients with COVID-19 (April 2020). *Clinical Infectious Diseases, 78*, e83–e102. https://doi.org/10.1093/cid/ciaa478 (accessed on 30th June 2025).
12. Cashen, K., Costello, J. M., Gowda, K. M. N., Grimaldi, M., *et al.* (2018). Multicenter validation of the vasoactive-ventilation-renal score as a predictor of prolonged mechanical ventilation after neonatal cardiac surgery. https://core.ac.uk/download/227054193.pdf (accessed on 30th June 2025).

13. Cater, D. T., Moser, E. A. S., Rowan, C. M., Tori, S., *et al.* (2018). Modification and assessment of the Bedside Pediatric Early Warning Score in the pediatric allogeneic hematopoietic cell transplant population. https://core.ac.uk/download/227054287.pdf (accessed on 30th June 2025).

14. Chatwin, M., Toussaint, M., Gonçalves, M., Sheers, N., Mellies, U., Gonzales-Bermejo, J., Sancho, J., *et al.* (2018). Airway clearance techniques in neuromuscular disorders: A state of the art review. *Respiratory Medicine, 136*, 98–110. https://doi.org/10.1016/j.rmed.2018.01.012 (accessed on 30th June 2025).

15. Chiaruttini, M. V., Lorenzoni, G., Daverio, M., Marchetto, L., Izzo, F., Chidini, G., Picconi, E., *et al.* (2024). Non-invasive ventilation failure in pediatric ICU: A machine learning driven prediction. *Diagnostics, 14*. https://www.semanticscholar.org/paper/25dfbd91d7c146460962a9e367ddf599d6b769af (accessed on 30th June 2025).

16. Chimbira, W., Crawford, H., Gupta, S., Legg, J., *et al.* (2001). Acute lung injury in pediatric intensive care: Course and outcome. https://core.ac.uk/download/pdf/8715345.pdf (accessed on 30th June 2025).

17. Choi, J., Park, E., Park, H., Kang, D., Yang, J. H., Kim, H., Cho, J., *et al.* (2024). Effect of high-flow nasal cannula therapy on mechanical ventilation duration in the pediatric intensive care unit. *PLOS One, 19*. https://www.semanticscholar.org/paper/e999edaeb8cce23ca7e6cd18d9251ae3f6d326b9 (accessed on 30th June 2025).

18. Chong, W., Hai, M. D., Liu, Y., *et al.* (2020). Critical care ultrasonography and its application for COVID-19. https://core.ac.uk/download/322850187.pdf (accessed on 30th June 2025).

19. Chudasama, R. K., Srivastava, A., & Trivedi, S. S. (2009). Study of early predictors of fatality in mechanically ventilated neonates in NICU. https://core.ac.uk/download/pdf/87413.pdf (accessed on 30th June 2025).

20. Colleti Junior, J., Prata-Barbosa, A., & Tonial, C. (2024). Ventilation liberation in Ibero-American pediatric intensive care units. *Critical Care Science, 36*. https://www.semanticscholar.org/paper/5dddfb76b6c3ff98b4960024b6dcc8582aefdba4 (accessed on 30th June 2025).

21. Cortegiani, A., Gregoretti, C., & Spoletini, G. (2019). Physio pathological rationale of using high-flow nasal therapy in the acute and chronic setting: A narrative review. https://core.ac.uk/download/224993362.pdf (accessed on 30th June 2025).

22. Curley, M., Wypij, D., & Matthay, M. (2015). Sedation protocol for critically ill pediatric patients—reply. *JAMA, 313*(17), 1754–1755. https://www.semanticscholar.org/paper/182d42316f3ac787943686dbdb26a15394bf70e0 (accessed on 30th June 2025).

23. Damps, M., Byrska-Maciejasz, E., Kowalska, M., Rosada-Kurasińska, J., Rybojad, B., Sordyl, J., Zielińska, M., *et al.* (2023). COVID-19 in pediatric intensive care units in Poland, PAPITCO-19 study (Polish analysis of PICU trends during COVID-19). *Journal of Clinical Medicine, 12*. https://www.semanticscholar.org/paper/fa7339b6d6ec11d8bf9d6b4ed1a75832d60cb3ac (accessed on 30th June 2025).

24. Demi, L., Wolfram, F., Klersy, C., De Silvestri, A., Ferretti, V. V., Müller, M., Miller, D. L., *et al.* (2022). New international guidelines and consensus on the use of lung ultrasound. *Journal of Ultrasound in Medicine, 42*, 309–344. https://doi.org/10.1002/jum.16088 (accessed on 30th June 2025).

25. Diniz-Silva, F., Pinheiro, B. V., Reyes, L., Cavalcanti, A. B., Figueredo, B., Rios, F., Machado, F. R., *et al.* (2024). Adherence to low tidal volume in the transition to spontaneous ventilation in patients with acute respiratory failure in intensive care units in Latin America (SPIRAL): A study protocol. *Critical Care Science, 36*. https://www.semanticscholar.org/paper/add48332d3652f5bccab9e59e4aa5624c2535ac0 (accessed on 30th June 2025).

26. Diorio, C., Henrickson, S. E., Vella, L. A., McNerney, K. O., Chase, J., Burudpakdee, C., Lee, J. H., *et al.* (2020). Multisystem inflammatory syndrome in children and COVID-19 are distinct presentations of SARS–CoV-2. *Journal of Clinical Investigation, 130*, 5967–5975. https://doi.org/10.1172/jci140970 (accessed on 30th June 2025).

27. Docking, R., Kinsella, J., Moss, L., Sim, R., *et al.* (2012). An investigation into the effects of commencing hemodialysis in the critically ill. https://core.ac.uk/download/1439066.pdf (accessed on 30th June 2025).

28. Finney, S. J. (2014). Extracorporeal support for patients with acute respiratory distress syndrome. https://core.ac.uk/download/77004032.pdf (accessed on 30th June 2025).

29. Gao, Y., Ding, M., Dong, X., Zhang, J., Azkur, A. K., Azkur, D., Gan, H., *et al.* (2020). Risk factors for severe and critically ill COVID-19 patients: A review. *Allergy, 76*, 428–455. https://doi.org/10.1111/all.14657 (accessed on 30th June 2025).

30. Ha, T. S., Oh, D., Lee, H. J., Chang, Y., Jeong, I., Sim, Y., Hong, S. K., *et al.* (2024). Liberation from mechanical ventilation in critically ill patients: Korean Society of Critical Care Medicine Clinical Practice Guidelines. *Acute and Critical Care, 39*, 1–23. https://www.semanticscholar.org/paper/b467d2621c7e870e90f12c2f0af4ba462374e486 (accessed on 30th June 2025).

31. Han, Y. J., Park, J. D., Lee, B., Choi, Y. H., Suh, D., Lim, B., & Chae, J. (2015). Home mechanical ventilation in childhood-onset hereditary neuromuscular diseases: 13 years' experience at a single center in Korea. *PLoS ONE, 10*. https://www.semanticscholar.org/paper/e53e400df10ea18d861a717bbe09fad0d7627de0 (accessed on 30th June 2025).

32. Hariyanto, H., Yahya, C. Q., & Sangia, A. A. T. (2025). Mechanical ventilation in acute respiratory distress syndrome and severe scoliosis: A case report. *Journal of Comprehensive Pediatrics*. https://www.semanticscholar.org/paper/b9e90c25d5bd39f24575f30daf443dd0757ddbee (accessed on 30th June 2025).

33. Harris, J., Harris, J., Ista, E., Ista, S., *et al.* (2016). Clinical recommendations for pain, sedation, withdrawal and delirium assessment in critically ill infants and children: An ESPNIC position statement for healthcare professionals. https://core.ac.uk/download/46665888.pdf (accessed on 30th June 2025).

34. Hermans, G., Meduri, G. U., & Schwingshackl, A. (2016). Prolonged glucocorticoid treatment in ARDS: Impact on intensive care unit-acquired weakness. https://core.ac.uk/download/323077025.pdf (accessed on 30th June 2025).

35. Huang, Y., Lu, Y., Huang, Y., Wang, M., Ling, W., Sui, Y., & Zhao, H. L. (2020). Obesity in patients with COVID-19: A systematic review and meta-analysis. *Metabolism, 113*, 154378. https://doi.org/10.1016/j.metabol.2020.154378 (accessed on 30th June 2025).

36. Huffer, K. (2017). Improving new graduate critical care nurse practitioner knowledge and retention using a dedicated orientation and mentoring program. https://core.ac.uk/download/217321337.pdf (accessed on 30th June 2025).

37. Inoue, S., Hatakeyama, J., Kondo, Y., Hifumi, T., Sakuramoto, H., Kawasaki, T., Taito, S., *et al.* (2019). Post-intensive care syndrome: Its pathophysiology, prevention, and future directions. *Acute Medicine & Surgery, 6*, 233–246. https://doi.org/10.1002/ams2.415 (accessed on 30th June 2025).

38. Jin, J., Bai, P., He, W., Wu, F., Liu, X., Han, D., Liu, S., *et al.* (2020). Gender differences in patients with COVID-19: Focus on severity and mortality. *Frontiers in Public Health, 8.* https://doi.org/10.3389/fpubh.2020.00152 (accessed on 30th June 2025).

39. Kaler, J., Hussain, A., Patel, K., Hernández, T., & Ray, S. D. (2023). Respiratory syncytial virus: A comprehensive review of transmission, pathophysiology, and manifestation. *Cureus.* https://doi.org/10.7759/cureus.36342 (accessed on 30th June 2025).

40. Karakitsos, D., El Barbary, M., Gillman, L., Papalois, A., & Shiloh, A. (2014). Critical care and perioperative monitoring. *The Scientific World Journal, 2014.* https://www.semanticscholar.org/paper/5d1bf6b3597952064d302be7ef8ebdd129cd985a (accessed on 30th June 2025).

41. Kwak, S. (2022). Home mechanical ventilation in children with chronic respiratory failure: A narrative review. *Journal of Yeungnam Medical Science, 40*, 123–135. https://doi.org/10.12701/jyms.2022.00227 (accessed on 30th June 2025).

42. Lee, S. Y., Huh, J. W., Hong, S. B., Lim, C., & Ahn, J. H. (2024). Short-term and long-term outcomes of critically ill patients with solid malignancy: A retrospective cohort study. *The Korean Journal of Internal Medicine, 39*, 957–966. https://www.semanticscholar.org/paper/5ce03fc36e232a45156ea12178a6a30ff1d19531 (accessed on 30th June 2025).

43. López-Fernández, Y. M., Martínez-de-Azagra, A., González-Gómez, J. M., Pérez-Caballero Macarrón, C., García-González, M., Parrilla-Parrilla, J., Miñambres-Rodríguez, M., *et al.* (2021). Acute hypoxemic respiratory failure in children at the start of COVID-19 outbreak: A nationwide experience. *Journal of Clinical Medicine, 10.* https://www.semanticscholar.org/paper/78cee09ba7c45aa9c90a5930efbea0fe5936d8d5 (accessed on 30th June 2025).

44. McCulloh, R. J., & Randolph, A. G. (2014). Pediatric sepsis: Important considerations for diagnosing and managing severe infections in infants, children, and adolescents. https://core.ac.uk/download/28948161.pdf (accessed on 30th June 2025).

45. Meduri, G. U., & Schwingshackl, A. (2016). Rationale for prolonged glucocorticoid use in pediatric ARDS: What the adults can teach us. https://core.ac.uk/download/323079960.pdf (accessed on 30th June 2025).

46. Nakra, N., Blumberg, D. A., Herrera-Guerra, A., & Lakshminrusimha, S. (2020). Multi-system inflammatory syndrome in children (MIS-C) following SARS-CoV-2 infection: Review of clinical presentation, hypothetical pathogenesis, and proposed management. *Children, 7*, 69–69. https://doi.org/10.3390/children7070069 (accessed on 30th June 2025).

47. Ragab, D., Salah Eldin, H., Taeimah, M., Khattab, R., & Salem, R. (2020). The COVID-19 cytokine storm; What we know so far. *Frontiers in Immunology, 11.* https://doi.org/10.3389/fimmu.2020.01446 (accessed on 30th June 2025).

48. Rooney, S., Donohue, J. E., Bush, L., Zhang, W., Banerjee, M., Pasquali, S. K., & Gaies, M. (2019). Extubating failure rates after pediatric cardiac surgery vary across hospitals. *Pediatric Critical Care Medicine, 20*, 450–456. https://doi.org/10.1097/pcc.0000000000001877 (accessed on 30th June 2025).

49. Saha, P., & Agrawal, R. (2024). Prediction of success of non-invasive ventilation in type II respiratory failure in intensive care unit using HACOR score. *Indian Journal of Critical Care Medicine: Peer-reviewed, Official Publication of Indian Society of Critical Care Medicine, 28*, S253–S255. https://www.semanticscholar.org/paper/3be7c79adcbc30b42220e775df12bb8b4290cfc7 (accessed on 30th June 2025).

50. Sattar, N., McInnes, I. B., & McMurray, J. J. V. (2020). Obesity is a risk factor for severe COVID-19 infection. *Circulation, 142*, 4–6. https://doi.org/10.1161/circulationaha.120.047659 (accessed on 30th June 2025).

51. Schibler, A., Franklin, D., Oakley, E., Babl, F. E., Whitty, J. A., Furyk, J. S., Neutze, J., *et al.* (2015). Early high flow nasal cannula therapy in bronchiolitis, a prospective randomized control trial (protocol): A Pediatric Acute Respiratory Intervention Study (PARIS). https://core.ac.uk/download/41993892.pdf (accessed on 30th June 2025).

52. Seol, K. H., Lee, B. S., Yoo, K., Roh, J. H., Lee, J. M., Kwak, J. I., Kim, T. G., *et al.* (2025). Brain injury and short-term neurodevelopmental outcomes in neonates treated with respiratory extracorporeal membrane oxygenation: A single-center experience. *Neonatal Medicine*. https://www.semanticscholar.org/paper/fdae0d2748b17c832c9601c9b57afa8416ccd0fc (accessed on 30th June 2025).

53. Shekerdemian, L. S., Mahmood, N., Wolfe, K. K., Riggs, B. J., Ross, C. E., McKiernan, C., Heidemann, S. M., *et al.* (2020). Characteristics and outcomes of children with coronavirus disease 2019 (COVID-19) infection admitted to US and Canadian pediatric intensive care units. *JAMA Pediatrics, 174*, 868–868. https://doi.org/10.1001/jamapediatrics.2020.1948 (accessed on 30th June 2025).

54. Shimabukuro-Vornhagen, A., Gödel, P., Subklewe, M., Stemmler, H. J., Schlößer, H., Schlaak, M., Kochanek, M., *et al.* (2018). Cytokine release syndrome. *Journal for Immunotherapy of Cancer, 6*. https://doi.org/10.1186/s40425-018-0343-9 (accessed on 30th June 2025).

55. Siripanthong, B., Nazarian, S., Muser, D., Deo, R., Santangeli, P., Khanji, M. Y., Cooper, L. T., *et al.* (2020). Recognizing COVID-19–related myocarditis: The possible pathophysiology and proposed guideline for diagnosis and management. *Heart Rhythm, 17*, 1463–1471. https://doi.org/10.1016/j.hrthm.2020.05.001 (accessed on 30th June 2025).

56. Somani, N., Batth, N. K., Beri, N., Jindal, P., & Kansal, M. (2025). Evaluating the impact of enteral nutrition on pediatric outcomes in PICU patients: A study of morbidity and mortality effects. *National Board of Examinations Journal of Medical Sciences*. https://www.semanticscholar.org/paper/06891e16a9b1f62267e161116a93c836020e8878 (accessed on 30th June 2025).

57. Sood, S. B., Ganatra, H. A., Perez Marques, F., & Langner, T. (2023). Complications during mechanical ventilation—A pediatric intensive care perspective. *Frontiers in Medicine, 10*. https://www.semanticscholar.org/paper/06ccbe5ac28e0f36973f80b92286e90debe0905e (accessed on 30th June 2025).

58. Tan, D., Wang, B., Cao, P., Wang, Y., Sun, J., Geng, P., Walline, J., *et al.* (2024). High flow nasal cannula oxygen therapy versus non-invasive ventilation for acute exacerbations of chronic obstructive pulmonary disease with acute-moderate hypercapnic respiratory failure: A randomized controlled non-inferiority trial. *Critical Care, 28*. https://www.semanticscholar.org/paper/d1e77a4d400cae67f23af656fb826cf38f39533c (accessed on 30th June 2025).

59. Tao, X., & Ye, S. (2025). Risk factors for invasive mechanical ventilation, extracorporeal membrane oxygenation, and mortality in children with severe adenovirus infection in the pediatric intensive care unit: A retrospective study. *BMC Pediatrics, 25.* https://www.semanticscholar.org/paper/5e1f69512840f6226e221696f0fa8e8c22370f46 (accessed on 30th June 2025).

60. Trivedi, S., Tibrewala, N., & Balsara, K. (2015). Anesthetic management of a patient with amyotrophic lateral sclerosis undergoing laparoscopic diaphragmatic pacing. *Indian Journal of Anesthesia, 59*, 683–685. https://www.semanticscholar.org/paper/e1dc66cda6ad7e7e97ad22dee4e5fc948ea91858 (accessed on 30th June 2025).

61. Uyeki, T. M., Bernstein, H. H., Bradley, J. S., Englund, J. A., File, T. M., Fry, A. M., Gravenstein, S., *et al.* (2018). Clinical practice guidelines by the Infectious Diseases Society of America: 2018 update on diagnosis, treatment, chemoprophylaxis, and institutional outbreak management of seasonal influenza. *Clinical Infectious Diseases, 68*, e1–e47. https://doi.org/10.1093/cid/ciy866 (accessed on 30th June 2025).

62. Whittaker, E., Bamford, A., Kenny, J., Kaforou, M., Jones, C. E., Shah, P., Ramnarayan, P., *et al.* (2020). Clinical characteristics of 58 children with a pediatric inflammatory multisystem syndrome temporally associated with SARS-CoV-2. *JAMA, 324*, 259–259. https://doi.org/10.1001/jama.2020.10369 (accessed on 30th June 2025).

CARDIOVASCULAR EMERGENCIES

4

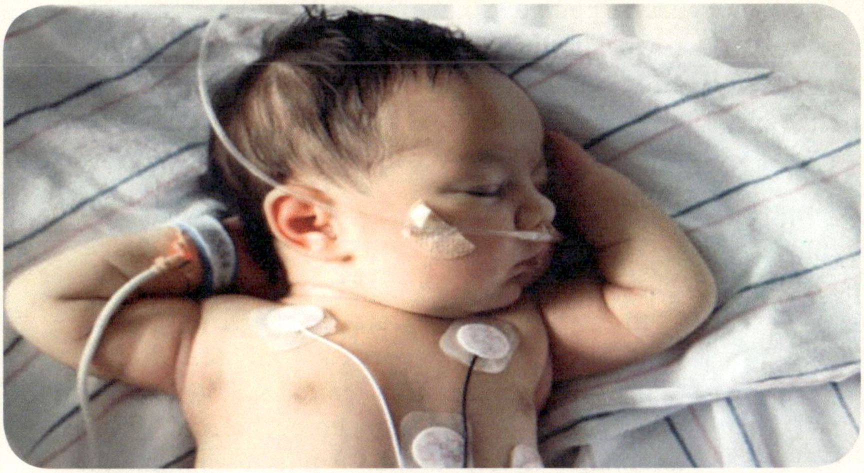

LEARNING OBJECTIVES

After studying this chapter, you will be able to:

1. Understand Common Cardiovascular Emergencies in Pediatrics.
2. Explain Assessment and Diagnosis.
3. Describe Management and Treatment Strategies.
4. Focus on Challenges and Considerations in Pediatric Intensive Care.

Introduction

Pediatric cardiovascular emergencies are a serious and rapidly growing area of pediatric intensive care, demanding immediate diagnosis and treatment to avoid potential morbidity and mortality. New modalities for the changing face of pediatric practice include the use of point-of-care ultrasound (POCUS), which is growing in popularity for acute use. A study quotes that 100% of pediatric intensive care units (PICUs) are applying POCUS for cardiovascular assessment, pointing towards its role in rendering prompt diagnosis and interventions in situations of emergencies (Şık *et al.*, 2024). Complications such as those of hematopoietic cell transplantation (HCT) also point towards the relevance of prompt cardiovascular management of critically ill children. Recent articles indicate infection and associated cardiovascular complications significantly predict death in children undergoing HCT in the PICU, and close surveillance and intentional treatment are recommended (Rubén *et al.*, 2024). Collectively, these data attest to the importance of cardiovascular emergency management to the general pediatric intensive care scenario (Figure 4.1).

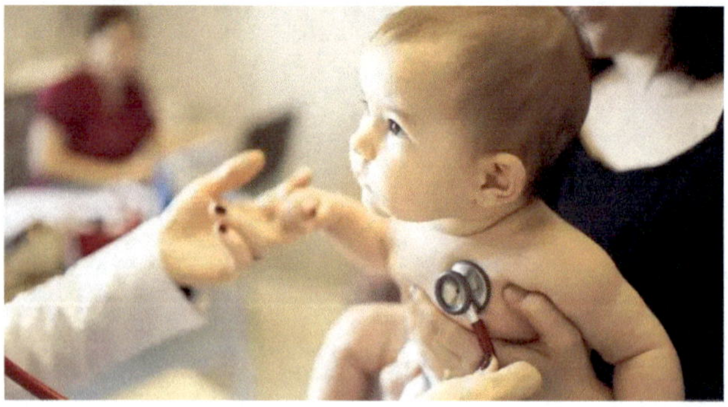

Figure 4.1. Cardiovascular emergencies in pediatric patients.

Source: https://stgaccinwbsdevlrs01.blob.core.windows.net/newcorporatewbsite/blogs/February2024/AZIQ1gjEtSecpTQaOmMM.webp.

4.1. Common Cardiovascular Emergencies in Pediatrics

Learning Outcome

1. Understand congenital heart defects.
2. Explain myocarditis and pericarditis.
3. Focus on arrhythmias in children.
4. Describe cardiogenic shock.
5. Know hypertensive emergencies.
6. Focus on pulmonary embolism.
7. Explain aortic dissection.
8. Describe heart failure in pediatric patients.
9. Understand cardiac arrest in children.

Pediatric cardiovascular emergencies also have unique challenges that need to be identified and treated early. The most prevalent of these are arrhythmias, which can lead to acute cardiac arrest in children and adolescents, often accompanied by intrinsic conditions such as congenital heart defects. *Mycoplasma pneumoniae* infection has been reported to be a significant cause of these emergencies, particularly in immunocompromised pediatric patients, with hypoxemia being a critical indicator of severity (Espeleta-Fox *et al.*, 2025). Moreover, intensified asthma may complicate the clinical presentation because respiratory distress may inadvertently induce cardiovascular distress, putting even more stress on the pediatric patient's already weakened system (Selmano Ağlu *et al.*, 2025).

It is important for medical staff to critically assess pediatric patients' cardiovascular stability since early intervention averts long-term effects and enhances survival rates. Understanding how respiratory and cardiovascular functions interact is important in order to manage these emergencies effectively.

4.1.1. Congenital Heart Defects

Congenital heart defects (CHDs) are a significant issue in pediatric medicine, often demanding prompt intervention and meticulous postoperative care. The defects, from trivial anomalies to critical malformations, impair the structure and function of the heart, leading to severe complications such as impaired blood flow and oxygenation.

For instance, blocked total anomalous pulmonary venous return (TAPVR) affects 7–9 per 100,000 infants and is a high-risk factor for morbidity and mortality, particularly with preoperative obstruction. In diagnostics, echocardiography is now routine in the diagnosis of these defects, as advances in techniques permit precise anatomical descriptions and functional assessments (Thomas, 1999). The incorporation of such diagnostic equipment not only enhances hemodynamics of the patients but also aids the clinicians in making appropriate judgments, ultimately leading to better results in high-risk environments such as pediatric intensive care units (Figure 4.2).

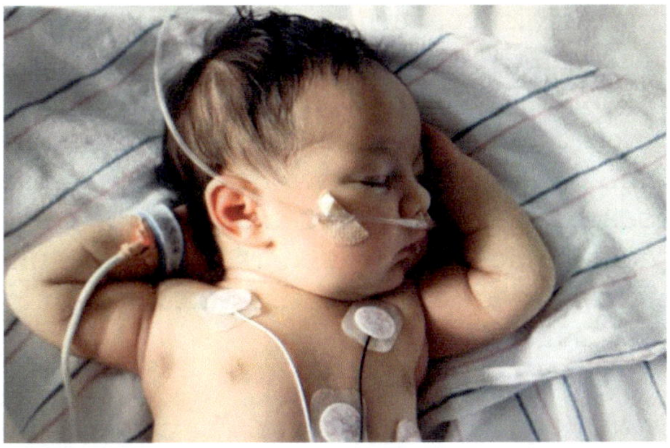

Figure 4.2. Congenital heart defects (CHDs) represent a significant challenge in pediatric medicine, often necessitating urgent intervention and meticulous postoperative care.

Source: https://www.heart.org/-/media/Images/Health-Topics/Congenital-Heart-Defects/Survivor-photos/Sloan-in-hospital.jpg?h=533&w=800&sc_lang=en.

4.1.2. Myocarditis and Pericarditis

Myocarditis and pericarditis are conditions that pose a severe problem in terms of cardiovascular emergencies in pediatric critical care, particularly following some precipitants like viral infections and, very recently, vaccinations. The occurrence of these conditions can result in severe complications like heart failure and arrhythmias, which are very serious in children whose cardiovascular system is still in its immature state. Research revealed that the majority of myocarditis cases in individuals younger than 21 were after mRNA COVID-19 vaccines, with a high prevalence of chest pain and increased cardiac biomarkers in the affected (Dongngan *et al.*, 2021). Although most cases presented a benign clinical course, the prevalence of abnormal cardiac MRI scans indicates the relevance of monitoring for long-term effects (Bryan *et al.*, 2021). Early diagnosis and effective management are also important in avoiding the dangers of these conditions, emphasizing their importance in the care of children in pediatric cardiology.

4.1.3. Child Arrhythmias

The manifestation of arrhythmias in children represents a daunting challenge in pediatric cardiovascular emergencies, with a requirement for early detection and intervention. The cardiac rhythm alterations may be brought about by a myriad of underlying etiologies varying from congenital heart anomalies to acquired conditions such as electrolyte abnormalities or infection. Identification of the particular etiology is vital since the clinical implications often dictate the need for urgent treatment interventions. For instance, studies have demonstrated that arrhythmias can complicate postoperative recovery in congenital conditions, such as total anomalous pulmonary venous return, where about 52% of patients develop postoperative arrhythmias, testifying to the need for close monitoring. Further, having conditions such as low cardiac output syndrome also raises the risk of arrhythmias, testifying to the interaction of several cardiovascular challenges in this compromised population (Kuok *et al.*, 2022). Thus, a comprehensive management style is needed to optimize the outcomes for pediatric patients with arrhythmias (Figure 4.3).

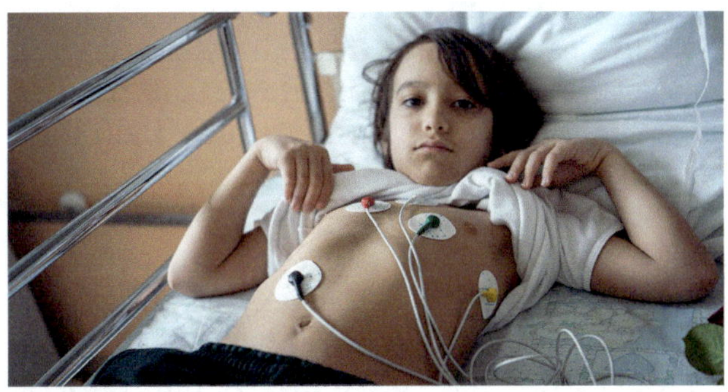

Figure 4.3. Arrhythmias.

Source: https://media.post.rvohealth.io/wp-content/uploads/2023/06/boy-hospital-heart-cardiac-arrhythmia-medical-exam-1200x628-facebook-1200x628.jpg.

4.1.4. Cardiogenic Shock

Cardiogenic shock is a critical emergency condition in pediatric intensive care characterized by the failure of the heart to establish adequate blood circulation to meet the body's demands. This process normally ensues as an aftermath of underlying heart dysfunction, especially acute decompensated heart failure, whose incidence has increased dramatically in recent years, which calls for current treatment practices that consider its multifactorial pathophysiology (Colombo *et al.*, 2024). Interestingly, sex differences in cardiogenic shock treatment have been noted, and those concerned with cases of heart failure are such that females present with lower intensive care unit stays but higher in-hospital mortality compared to their male counterparts (Lori *et al.*, 2024). The absence of good-standardized treatment protocols within most critical care settings adds to the complexity of management strategies, emphasizing the need for more refined diagnostic and therapeutic approaches aimed at improving outcomes in pediatric patients faced with this malignant disease (Colombo *et al.*, 2024).

4.1.5. Hypertensive Emergencies

Hypertensive emergencies constitute a critical subgroup of cardiovascular emergencies that call for urgent intervention within pediatric intensive care settings. They are characterized by a severe elevation in blood pressure coupled with acute end-organ damage, including neurological impairment, cardiac arrest, or renal dysfunction. Given the specific physiological and developmental factors of the pediatric cohort, recognition and management of the condition are of the greatest priority. Effective treatment strategies often involve the stepwise reduction of blood pressure using intravenous antihypertensives under tight monitoring of the patient to prevent complications such as ischemic events or stroke. Failure in the management of hypertensive emergencies in children will lead to much worse outcomes, and this is concerning because it is also exacerbated by the higher rates of mortality with inappropriate management strategies in critical care, as reflected in intensive care unit admission analysis for various cardiovascular diseases (Kuwabara *et al.*, 2025). These dynamics need to be understood in seeking improved pediatric care and outcomes (Yuriy *et al.*, 2025) (Figure 4.4).

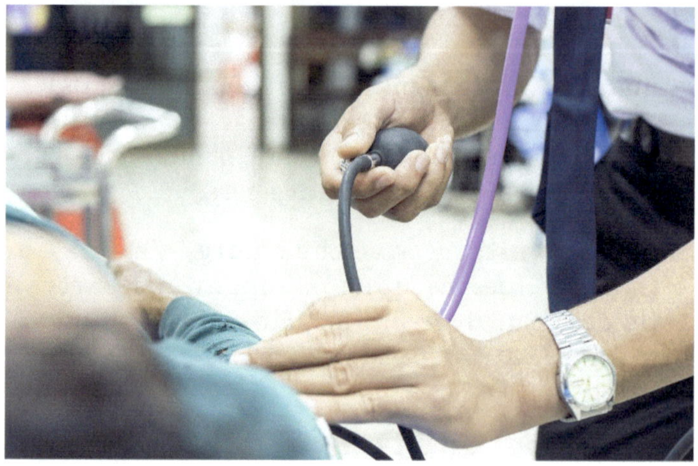

Figure 4.4. Hypertensive emergencies represent a critical subset of cardiovascular crises that necessitate prompt intervention within pediatric intensive care settings.

Source: https://www.myamericannurse.com/wp-content/uploads/2012/03/shutterstock_572920273-scaled.jpg.

4.1.6. Pulmonary Embolism

Pulmonary embolism (PE) is a severe cardiovascular emergency, particularly in the pediatric intensive care unit, where early detection and management are critical. Although PE is not as common in children compared to adults, when it is present, it can lead to severe complications, including respiratory failure and hemodynamic instability, and thus needs close monitoring and management. Based on reports, pediatric patients undergoing hematopoietic cell transplantation are more likely to require PICU treatment for pulmonary complications and meet the need for advanced treatment in cases of PE (Amanda *et al.*, 2024). Moreover, outcomes differ substantially with the clinical setting; studies indicate that patients treated in general wards have perilously high mortality rates and therefore the imperative for early ICU admission in PE, just like in acute myocardial infarction and other aortic emergencies (Kuwabara *et al.*, 2025). Thus, the understanding of the nuances of PE in pediatrics is vital to optimizing treatment and improving survival.

4.1.7. Aortic Dissection

Aortic dissection, while more prevalent in adults, is dangerous in children because of anatomical variations and developmental factors.

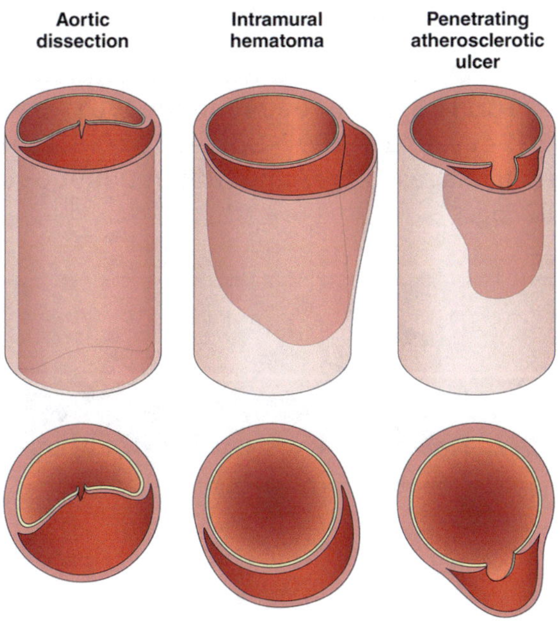

Figure 4.5. Aortic dissection, while more common in adults, poses significant risks in the pediatric population due to anatomical differences and developmental considerations.

Source: https://www.jtcvs.org/cms/10.1016/j.jtcvs.2023.04.023/asset/a1d398ca-7960-4630-a2b5-97fa3e23c114/main.assets/gr7_lrg.jpg.

The cardiovascular crisis involves a tear in the intimal layer of the aorta with blood tracking between layers, with a potential for calamitous consequences if not immediately treated. Early diagnosis and treatment are crucial, especially in the pediatric setting, where the symptoms may be atypical or misdiagnosed. The 2022 ACC/AHA Guideline for the Diagnosis and Management of Aortic Disease also underscores the necessity of a child-specific systematic approach to diagnosis and intervention, which ranges from medical therapy to surgery (Eric *et al.*, 2022). In addition, as was emphasized during the COVID-19 pandemic, hospitals must have preparedness plans in place to manage such high-acuity cases effectively, establishing resource readiness and patient and healthcare worker safety (Christopher *et al.*, 2020) (Figure 4.5).

4.1.8. Heart Failure in Pediatric Patients

Pediatric heart failure is a complicated issue in the realm of cardiovascular emergencies, particularly in the pediatric intensive care setting. The novel addition of multisystem inflammatory syndrome in children (MIS-C) linked to SARS-CoV-2 has placed the critical juncture of viral infection and acute cardiac failure into the limelight. It is reported that children with MIS-C typically present with severe inflammatory conditions, which result in cardiogenic shock and left ventricular dysfunction; approximately one-third of patients initially present with a left ventricular ejection fraction of below 30% (Belhadjer *et al.*, 2020). Furthermore, a case report in an 11-year-old girl presented with acute worsening to cardiac failure, underlining the necessity of diagnosis and heart failure management in such individuals (Dolhnikoff *et al.*, 2020). Prompt recognition and management, including intravenous immunoglobulin and inotropic therapy, are required to minimize the risk of long-term cardiac sequelae and improve the prognosis of these vulnerable patients.

4.1.9. Cardiac Arrest in Children

Cardiac arrest in a child is an emergent condition that is life-threatening and needs immediate and expert medical management to prevent long-term morbidity or death. Underlying etiologies of cardiac arrest in a child can be entirely different from those in adults, usually consisting of respiratory issues or critical illness rather than primary cardiovascular diseases. A recent study demonstrated that the modified Pediatric Sequential Organ Failure Assessment (mpSOFA) score could predict survival outcomes following in-hospital cardiac arrest (IHCA) among pediatric patients, making it relevant in post-arrest treatment planning in a cardiac intensive care unit (CICU) (Haar *et al.*, 2024). Additionally, ongoing research conducted by the International Liaison Committee on Resuscitation emphasizes the need to implement evidence-based practice and continuous improvement in resuscitation sciences among children and to bridge knowledge gaps to enhance overall outcomes during such crises (Berg *et al.*, 2023). The dynamics of these factors are crucial in optimizing pediatric resuscitation and care protocols in emergencies (Figure 4.6).

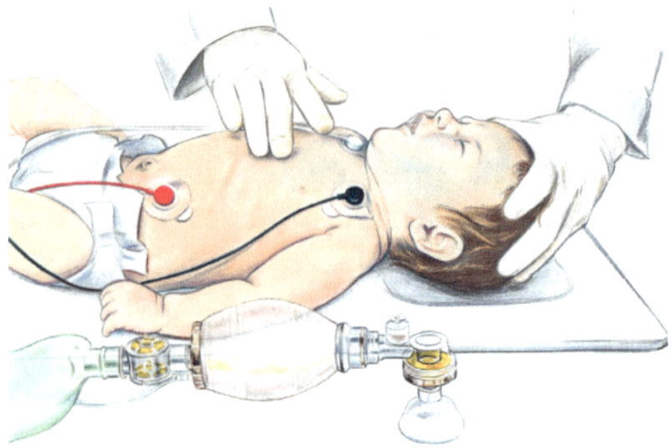

Figure 4.6. Cardiac arrest in children represents a critical event that necessitates immediate and specialized medical intervention to prevent long-term morbidity or mortality.

Source: https://www.ahajournals.org/cms/10.1161/CIR.0000000000000901/asset/d32354c9-941b-4d97-866f-2567f48fac03/assets/images/large/cir.0000000000000901.fig02.jpg.

Test Your Knowledge

1. What congenital heart conditions may result in early cardiovascular emergencies in neonates?
2. How does myocarditis commonly present in a pediatric patient in the PICU?

4.2. Assessment and Diagnosis

Learning Outcome

1. Understand clinical presentation of cardiovascular emergencies.
2. Know the importance of history taking.
3. Focus on physical examination techniques.
4. Learn diagnostic imaging modalities.
5. Discuss laboratory tests and biomarkers.
6. Explain electrocardiogram (ECG) interpretation.
7. Describe echocardiography in pediatric patients.
8. Discuss the role of telemetry monitoring.
9. Understand differential diagnosis considerations.

Accurate assessment and diagnosis are crucial in the management of cardiovascular emergencies in the pediatric intensive care unit. Pediatric physiology demands a systematic approach with appropriate clinical assessment and diagnostic investigations to accommodate the peculiar needs of younger patients.

Most importantly, pre-sedation assessments should be closely done by clinicians to identify any pre-existing medical conditions that enhance procedural risk (Charles *et al.*, 2019). Further, increasing dependence on electronic health records (EHRs) can impact clinician effectiveness and patient safety since it has been proven that the heavy workload associated with the use of EHRs is a reason for clinician burnout and shapes overall care delivery (Downing *et al.*, 2018). Thus, all of these elements are significant in ensuring accurate diagnosis and timely interventions and, ultimately, better outcomes for children under cardiovascular emergencies. By integrating both clinical assessments and technological tools thoughtfully, healthcare providers can maximize the effectiveness of their diagnoses in critical pediatric situations.

4.2.1. Clinical Presentation of Cardiovascular Emergencies

In pediatric intensive care, presentation of cardiovascular emergencies can be very unpredictable and typically presents with acute presentations that necessitate immediate medical intervention. Children may present with tachycardia, hypotension, and altered mental status, which may be presentations of critical conditions like cardiogenic shock or acute heart failure. Recent literature has pointed out alarming patterns in which kids have been presenting with symptoms of multisystem inflammatory syndrome in children (MIS-C), typically in the aftermath of SARS-CoV-2 infection, characterized by fulminant inflammatory syndromes that can lead to severe left ventricular dysfunction and raised inflammatory markers like interleukin-6 and D-dimer levels (Belhadjer *et al.*, 2020). Recognition of such presentations is important, as timely treatment with intravenous immunoglobulin and other measures has been associated with good outcomes, that is, restoration of ventricular function in the affected patients (Paul *et al.*, 2017). Early and appropriate diagnosis is therefore essential in the management of these life-threatening cardiovascular emergencies (Figure 4.7).

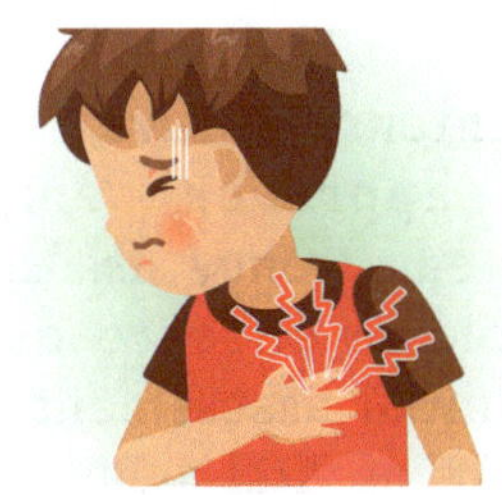

Figure 4.7. Children may exhibit signs such as tachycardia, hypotension, and altered mental status, which can indicate severe underlying conditions like cardiogenic shock or acute heart failure.

Source: https://sachkhandhospital.in/wp-content/uploads/2024/05/Untitled-design-11.png.

4.2.2. Importance of History Taking

In pediatric critical care, the importance of careful history taking cannot be overestimated, particularly in cardiovascular emergencies. Careful history provides healthcare providers with insight into a child's basic health status, comorbid conditions, and possible precipitating causes for cardiovascular emergencies. This information is crucial for early diagnosis and tailored treatment, as the same manifestation of cardiovascular distress can have multiple etiologies, e.g., congenital cardiac defects or acquired conditions such as myocarditis. The American Heart Association and the American College of Cardiology emphasize that systemically incorporated evidence-based guidelines defining the protocols of therapy for cardiovascular disease form part of organized patient history (Paul *et al.*, 2017). In addition, making it clear to talk to families during history taking builds trust and can provide valuable information about the child's health, which is most likely neglected in emergency situations. Thus, effective history taking becomes a bulwark of good care in the management of cardiovascular emergencies in children.

4.2.3. Physical Examination Techniques

In pediatric intensive care, the physical examination approach employed in cardiovascular emergency assessment plays an essential role in effective diagnosis and management. Initial assessment begins with close observation of vital signs such as heart rate, blood pressure, and respiratory rate, which are important indicators of hemodynamic stability. Accurate peripheral pulse palpation and auscultation of heart sounds also contribute to the assessment of cardiac function in suspected cardiogenic shock or myocarditis, which is common in febrile children with sepsis-like severe inflammatory disease caused by SARS-CoV-2 infection (Belhadjer *et al.*, 2020). In addition, careful monitoring for respiratory distress and fluid overload, as indicated by increased work of breathing or peripheral edema, is paramount. That combination of these testing modalities not only makes real-time clinical decision-making possible, but it also creates a baseline upon which ongoing follow-up may be based, thus allowing timely intervention in critically ill children (Charles *et al.*, 2019) (Figure 4.8).

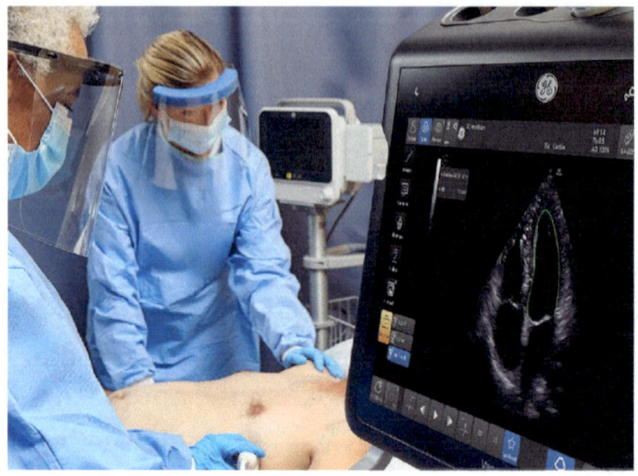

Figure 4.8. In pediatric intensive care, the physical examination techniques employed during the evaluation of cardiovascular emergencies are critical for accurate diagnosis and management.

Source: https://images-cdn.welcomesoftware.com/Zz02ZGM3M2VlZTUzYjAxMWVkYjkyYmRlODhjZWY2OTFkOQ==/real-time-desktop.webp.

4.2.4. Diagnostic Imaging Modalities

Diagnostic imaging modalities in pediatric intensive care have a vital role in the early detection and management of cardiovascular emergencies. Imaging methods such as echocardiography, computed tomography (CT), and magnetic resonance imaging (MRI) enable complete evaluations of cardiac structure and function in children. Echocardiography, in particular, is critical because it is transportable and does not use ionizing radiation, thus being appropriate for continuously monitored critically ill children. Advanced imaging modalities also make it possible to diagnose conditions such as aortic disease, which, as the recent guidelines have stressed, needs to be treated early to prevent complications (Eric *et al.*, 2022). Additionally, the current reflections on shielding both patients and healthcare providers while undergoing imaging procedures bring to the forefront the importance of modifying protocols for echocardiography, particularly during the COVID-19 outbreak, ensuring effective and safe provision of care in a challenging clinical environment (Barker *et al.*, 2020).

4.2.5. Laboratory Tests and Biomarkers

In pediatric intensive care cardiovascular emergencies, laboratory evaluation and biomarkers play a crucial role in early diagnosis and treatment management. Laboratory investigations provide valuable information about liver conditions, such as pneumonia, with a direct bearing on the cardiovascular status of children.

For instance, with research, biomarkers like C-reactive protein (CRP) and lactate levels have been found to be helpful in predicting clinical severity and mortality risk among intensive care unit (ICU) admission pediatric pneumonia patients (Ar Mı *et al.*, 2025). Further, the identification of numerous other lab markers like white blood cell (WBC) count and absolute lymphocyte counts has been associated with prognostic outcomes in critically ill children (Jia *et al.*, 2025). By applying these patterns of biomarkers, clinicians can not only assess the acute physiological status of children but also tailor interventions in a timely manner, improving overall survival in cardiovascular emergencies (Figure 4.9).

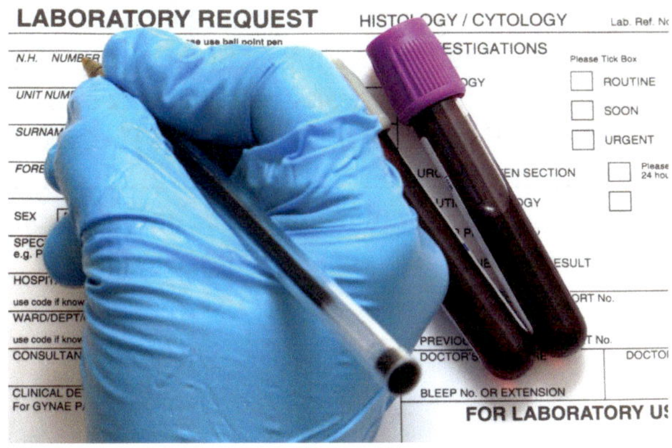

Figure 4.9. The identification of various other laboratory indicators, such as white blood cell (WBC) counts and absolute lymphocyte counts, has been associated with prognostic outcomes in critically ill children.

Source: https://cdn-prod.medicalnewstoday.com/content/images/articles/322/322289/differential-blood-test-paperwork-from-lab-being-filled-out-by-gloved-hand-next-to-blood-sample-vials.jpg.

4.2.6. Electrocardiogram (ECG) Interpretation

In pediatric intensive care, cardiovascular emergencies, and electrocardiogram (ECG) reading are among the most critical skills that directly influence a patient's outcome. Accurate ECG reading enables practitioners to quickly identify arrhythmias, ischemia, and other cardiac abnormalities, particularly pertinent given the unique physiological differences between children and adults. The interpretation process entails identifying age-dependent norms of heart rate as well as common states of the child's heart, such as congenital heart defects and myocarditis. Evidence from available literature promotes the application of point-of-care ultrasound (POCUS) in conjunction with ECGs in pediatric settings, with wide clinical benefits such as expedited diagnosis and reduced complications in intervention (Şık *et al.*, 2024). Moreover, diagnosis of acute cerebrovascular accidents among children primarily relies on ECG findings, hence the importance of rigorous training of pediatric intensive care unit staff in interpreting ECG (Bykov *et al.*, 2024). Therefore, a robust mechanism for ECG evaluation is crucial for effective emergency treatment among vulnerable children.

4.2.7. Pediatric Patients and Echocardiography

Echocardiography plays a pivotal role in the evaluation and management of pediatric patients with cardiac emergencies, particularly in the pediatric intensive care unit (PICU). The non-invasive imaging technique allows for the timely assessment of cardiac form and function, allowing clinicians to detect abnormalities like congenital heart disease, myocardial dysfunction, and pericardial effusion.

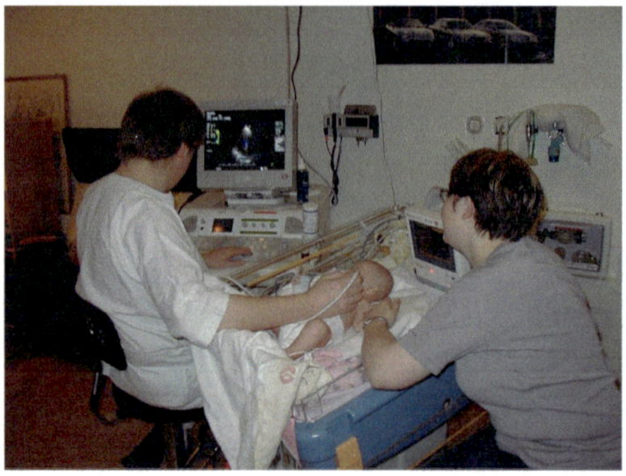

Figure 4.10. Echocardiography plays a pivotal role in the evaluation and management of pediatric patients experiencing cardiovascular emergencies, particularly within the pediatric intensive care unit (PICU).

Source: https://dmhca.in/wp-content/uploads/2024/09/Sonographer_doing_pediatric_echocardiography.jpg.

For example, for patients who present with septic shock or acute respiratory distress, echocardiography can help to identify underlying cardiac etiology that can either worsen these conditions. Its use has been emphasized in recent studies in monitoring patients who are related to COVID-19, wherein some develop multisystem inflammatory syndrome affecting cardiac conditions. Incorporating echocardiography into routine screening in the PICU not only enhances diagnostic accuracy but also directs proper management protocols, stressing the need to adhere to guidelines set for cardiology management in pediatrics (Eric *et al.*, 2022). Moreover, visualization of immediate cardiovascular variations underscores its critical function in managing pediatric patients within the context of acute care (Dallan *et al.*, 2020) (Figure 4.10).

4.2.8. Role of Telemetry Monitoring

Telemetry monitoring is a crucial element of timely evaluation and management of critically ill patients in pediatric intensive care cardiovascular emergencies. Monitoring is dynamic feedback of vital signs and can detect hemodynamic changes and arrhythmias, enabling timely intervention whenever necessary.

Moreover, combining telemetry with advanced neuromonitoring techniques such as electroencephalography makes the detection of concurrent neurological activity more sensitive in the presence of metabolic crises while improving outcomes for patients. Studies demonstrate a substantial rate of subclinical and clinical seizure occurrence among patients with inborn errors of metabolism, making careful monitoring in the PICU justified (Sen *et al.*, 2024). In addition, advances in point-of-care ultrasound enable telemetry effectiveness through rapid diagnostics and clinical decision-making for cardiovascular testing (Şık *et al.*, 2024). Overall, comprehensive telemetry monitoring is crucial to ensuring proper care and avoiding risks from life-threatening cardiovascular diseases in children.

4.2.9. Differential Diagnosis Considerations

In pediatric intensive care cardiovascular emergencies, strict differential diagnosis considerations are instrumental in the effective management of patients. The subtle nature of the presentations in children will often demand immediate assessment tools such as focused echocardiography, which has been extremely helpful in enabling the detection of underlying cardiovascular dysfunction in a timely manner. (Ermolenko *et al.*, 2025)

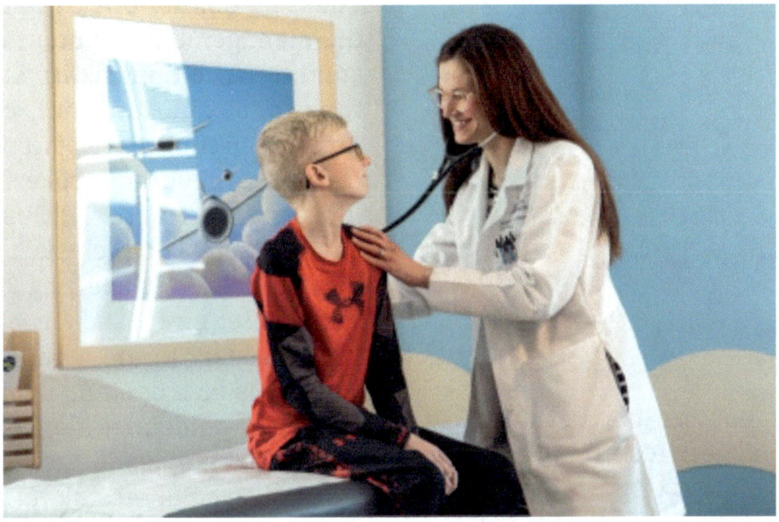

Figure 4.11. The complexity of pediatric presentations often demands immediate assessment techniques such as focused echocardiography, which has proven invaluable in identifying underlying cardiovascular dysfunction rapidly.

Source: https://www.childrensdayton.org/sites/default/files/styles/400px_wide/public/20171227Dayton_ml-4067.jpg?itok=JjRt_MOW.

This non-invasive method not only enables precise diagnostics but also enables timely interventions, which are vital in the prevention of severe complications like sepsis or cardiogenic shock. Further, the inclusion of point-of-care ultrasound (POCUS) has become more trending among pediatric emergency departments, enhancing diagnostic capability and procedural precision. (Şık *et al.*, 2024) Without its limitations, obstacles like limited equipment, staff, and training have hindered its wide implementation. Resolving these issues will make clinicians capable of conducting differential diagnoses efficiently, and in the long run, this will lead to better outcomes for critically ill children experiencing cardiovascular emergencies in intensive care unit environments.

Test Your Knowledge

1. How is blood pressure interpreted in neonates versus older children in the context of shock?
2. What are the ECG findings in pediatric patients with SVT, VT, or heart block?

4.3. Management and Treatment Strategies

Learning Outcome

1. Understand initial stabilization protocols.
2. Focus on pharmacological interventions.
3. Discuss advanced cardiac life support (ACLS).
4. Explain surgical interventions for congenital defects.
5. Know the role of interventional cardiology.
6. Describe fluid management in emergencies.
7. Know the use of mechanical support devices.
8. Discuss family-centered care during emergencies.
9. Focus on transitioning to long-term care.

Effective management and treatment of cardiovascular emergencies in pediatric intensive care are the most important ways of improving patient outcomes. The multifaceted nature of these emergencies requires an extensive response with the integration of aggressive clinical monitoring and advanced therapeutic maneuvers. For instance, in drug carrying complications of medication, such as drug transport-related complications like those resulting from clandestine drug carrying methods, such as body packing, careful imaging, particularly a CT scan, is required for cardiovascular and gastrointestinal effects assessment to inform treatment decision-making (Aitelkhadir *et al.*, 2025). In addition, the development of opportunistic pathogens, such as *Ralstonia pickettii* in vulnerable pediatric patients, further highlights the need for personalized therapeutic treatment regimens, including the delivery of broad-spectrum antibiotics and careful observation for systemic infection signs (Nabih *et al.*, 2025). These treatment interventions should include multi-disciplinary integration to implement immediate interventions and enable recovery among critically ill children, ultimately reducing cardiovascular crisis mortality rates.

4.3.1. Initial Stabilization Protocols

In pediatric cardiovascular emergency care, initial stabilization guidelines are important in minimizing the risk of morbidity and mortality. These guidelines offer a structured approach to the management of potentially life-threatening conditions, emphasizing stabilization of vital functions and optimal cerebral perfusion pressure in children experiencing life-threatening processes such as stroke or sepsis. Pediatric intensive care units (PICUs) provide the ideal environment in which such protocols would be best delivered, including those interventions that are required, such as airway management, fluid resuscitation, and monitoring of vital signs. The lack of standardized pediatric stroke treatment guidelines highlights the necessity for tailored strategies to the management of acute cerebrovascular accidents in children, as the majority of practices now take a cue from adult guidelines with doubtful direct applicability (Bykov *et al.*, 2024). In addition, there is a need to understand the nuances of sepsis in children since current definitions are inadequate, hence compromising early treatment (Schwalbach *et al.*, 2018) (Figure 4.12).

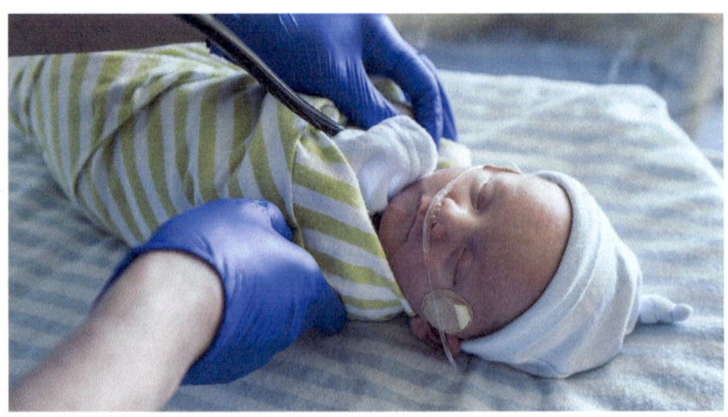

Figure 4.12. Initial stabilization protocols.

Source: https://www.childrenscolorado.org/contentassets/2b6b74c1ae5c4eed9c6d82ddd66a3034/ecmo.jpeg?v=4a6502.

4.3.2. Pharmacological Interventions

Pharmaceutical treatment plays a critical role in pediatric intensive care in dealing with cardiovascular emergencies because it enables rapid hemodynamic stabilization of acutely ill children. Specific medications, e.g., inotropes and vasopressors, are routinely used to boost myocardial contractility and optimize systemic vascular resistance, thereby improving perfusion during shock states. For instance, medications like epinephrine and dopamine can prove pivotal in therapeutic intervention in a child with imminent cardiac failure or septic shock. Further, careful monitoring of sedation, particularly against the backdrop of potential airway complications that can arise in emergency procedures, is necessary. As highlighted in current recommendations, a systematic approach to safe sedation—such as precautions for pre-sedation assessment and adequate monitoring—provides effective analgesia and patient safety during procedures (Charles *et al.*, 2019). Application of these pharmacologic strategies is required to decrease morbidity and improve outcomes in this high-risk population (James *et al.*, 2020).

4.3.3. Advanced Cardiac Life Support (ACLS)

Advanced Cardiac Life Support (ACLS) is one of the most important models of care in pediatric intensive care that has been used to enhance the management of children with cardiovascular emergencies. This protocol, which emphasizes early recognition of cardiac arrest and prompt activation of resuscitative measures, was designed to increase survival and neurological quality of life for children. Significantly, recent research places greater value on incorporating evidence-based practices in practice and training protocols of ACLS. For instance, the 2023 American Heart Association Focused Update on Adult Advanced Cardiovascular Life Support places greater emphasis on the growing knowledge of drug therapy and interventions applicable to resuscitation in heterogeneous populations, stressing the need for a tailored approach in pediatric populations (Sarah *et al.*, 2023). Furthermore, the requirement for formal training programs within healthcare teams, according to the 2020 International Consensus on Cardiopulmonary Resuscitation, supplements the call for continuous education to enable efficient implementation of critical care guidelines (Greif *et al.*, 2020) (Figure 4.13).

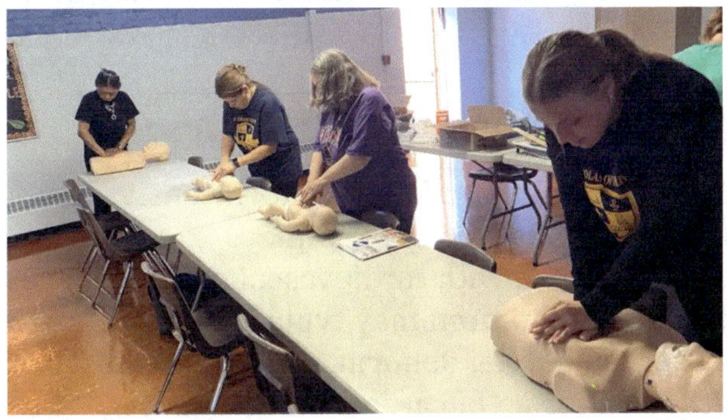

Figure 4.13. Advanced cardiac life support (ACLS) is a critical framework designed to enhance the management of cardiovascular emergencies in children.

Source: https://illinoissafety.com/wp-content/uploads/2024/05/ACLS-training.webp.

4.3.4. Surgical Interventions for Congenital Defects

Surgical corrections of congenital defects are very important procedures that have a great impact on the long-term health and quality of life for children's patients, particularly those with critical congenital heart disease, CCHD. Prompt corrective surgery is frequently necessary to repair structural abnormalities that will seriously decline if left untreated. The subtleties of pediatric cardiac surgery extend beyond technical competency, as the involved sophisticated physiology demands intimate familiarity with the individualized physiological adaptations present in neonates and infants.

Furthermore, literature indicates that children with severe chronic illness exhibit substantially increased healthcare utilization, requiring multiple surgeries, and thus underscores the importance of individualized care plans. Notably, quality pediatric palliative care can prolong decision-making for families with high-risk surgical options, potentially improving their experience and outcomes (Talwar *et al.*, 2025). A multidisciplinary intervention is thus warranted to address the issues that congenital defects create in pediatric intensive care (Talwar *et al.*, 2025).

4.3.5. Interventional Cardiology Role

In the domains of pediatric intensive care, interventional cardiology plays a significant role in dealing with cardiovascular emergencies effectively. Children may typically present with either congenital abnormalities of the heart or acquired forms of cardiac disease that must be addressed at the earliest to avoid complications that may be perilous in nature.

Techniques such as balloon angioplasty, stent placements, and catheter-based intracardiac shunt closures have proved to be very useful in restoring hemodynamic stability in seriously ill children. The ability to perform these interventions on a minimally invasive scale reduces recuperation time and reduces trauma in young patients, particularly in the delicate children population. Advances in imaging technologies, namely echocardiography and fluoroscopy, have enhanced the precision of such interventions as well as allowed for more desirable results on complex cases (Acar *et al.*, 2016). With evolving interventional techniques, they are still part of the multidisciplinary intervention needed for the successful treatment of cardiovascular emergencies in children within the intensive care unit (Karon, 2004) (Figure 4.14).

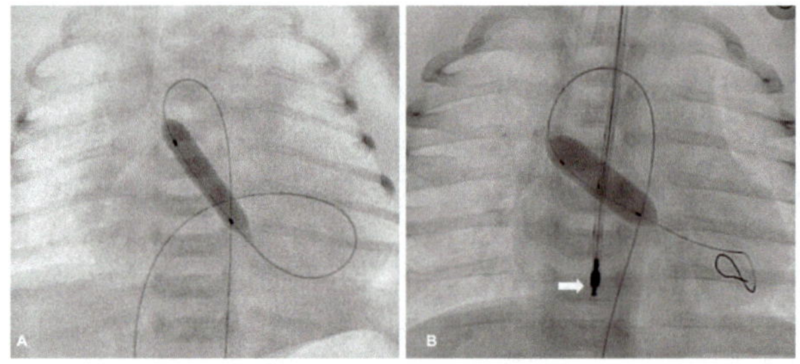

Figure 4.14. Procedures such as balloon angioplasty, stent placements, and catheter-based closures of intracardiac shunts have proven invaluable in restoring hemodynamic stability in critically ill pediatric patients.

Source: https://www.mdpi.com/diagnostics/diagnostics-13-02673/article_deploy/html/images/diagnostics-13-02673-g002.png.

4.3.6. Fluid Management in Emergencies

Fluid management in emergency situations, particularly pediatric intensive care, plays a crucial role in outcome determination for cardiovascular emergencies. Restoration of circulation and support of blood pressure are dependent on the timely administration of intravenous fluids, particularly in shock or sepsis. New forms of modalities have been established to support fluid resuscitation, and great stress has been put on how an individualized approach must be adjusted to the unique condition of each patient. To illustrate, recent sepsis definitions emphasize the importance of rapidly instituting organ dysfunction to direct fluid therapy, which profoundly influences mortality (Singer *et al.*, 2016). Furthermore, evidence-based guidelines developed by the ACC and AHA highlight the importance of systematic evaluation in fluid management, attempting to harmonize clinical evaluation with pharmacological treatments for optimal therapy (Paul *et al.*, 2017). Thus, efficient fluid management, in addition to minimizing morbidity, also improves recovery patterns in critically ill children.

4.3.7. Application of Mechanical Support Devices

In the context of pediatric intensive care, mechanical support devices have emerged as a significant intervention for several cardiovascular emergencies. These devices, like ventricular assist devices (VAD) and intra-aortic balloon pumps (IABP), are utilized to stabilize the hemodynamics of children who are at risk of severe circulatory failure or cardiogenic shock. Use of these devices requires careful consideration of many factors, such as the child's physiological and anatomical constitution, which can greatly differ from that of adults. Moreover, as a result of the sophisticated support technologies, clinicians are expected to adhere to guidelines so that they may achieve maximal outcomes.

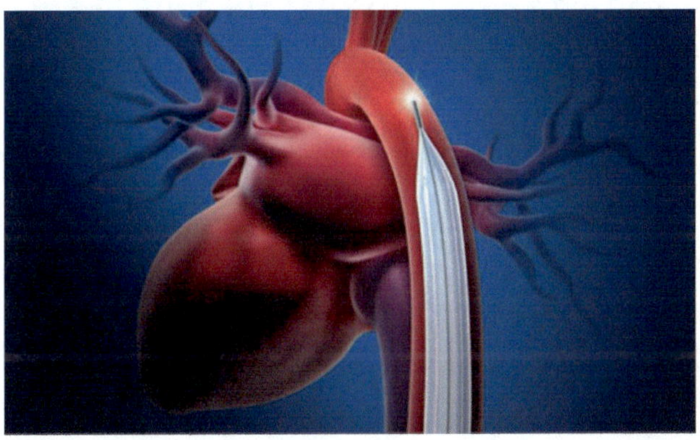

Figure 4.15. Intra-aortic balloon pumps (IABPs) serve to stabilize hemodynamics in children facing severe circulatory failure or cardiogenic shock.

Source: https://www.dicardiology.com/sites/default/files/styles/content_feed_large/public/field/image/Maquet%20IABP%20invivo.jpg?itok=63-Jotrv.

American College of Cardiology and American Heart Association guidelines point out multidisciplinary care in the management of cardiovascular emergencies through the integration of pharmaceutical and procedural interventions with mechanical support modalities to ensure recovery of the child (Charles *et al.*, 2019; Paul *et al.*, 2017). Lastly, mechanical support devices are a critical component in the comprehensive care of pediatric patients with severe cardiovascular issues (Figure 4.15).

4.3.8. Family-Centered Care During Emergencies

Family-centered care deployment in pediatric critical care is crucial in ensuring the physical and emotional well-being of young cardiovascular emergency patients. The strategy aims at the inclusion of family members in the process of decision-making in order to foster an environment of support that is crucial during high-stress situations. Communication and interprofessional care strategies can enhance trust and understanding between families and healthcare providers. For instance, in cases where the assignment of resources like extracorporeal membrane oxygenation (ECMO) is going on amidst crises, families must be well-informed about the risks and benefits of treatment to promote shared decision-making (Matthew *et al.*, 2020). Further, ensuring families are given adequate sedation guidelines for their children, particularly in the course of emergency procedures, might avoid fear and improve recovery outcomes (Charles *et al.*, 2019). Lastly, the involvement of families in care procedures not only enhances patient satisfaction but also strengthens therapeutic alliances, which are essential in critical care settings.

4.3.9. Transition to Long-Term Care

The transition to long-term care of children following cardiovascular emergencies is a critical turning point that requires organization and planning. As the intensive care measures are weaned off, during which patients are supported with life-sustaining interventions such as extracorporeal membrane oxygenation, ongoing rehabilitation and care of such individuals becomes focal. This is particularly important for children, who may experience differential outcomes based on the unique challenges of managing congenital heart diseases and recovery complications in the long term. Evidence indicates that ineffective management during this process has serious implications, including high hospital readmission rates due to inadequate follow-up care or inadequate patient education for post-discharge care (Sim Aões Moizés *et al.*, 2016).

Also, the requirement of uninterrupted monitoring of cardiovascular function post-discharge is also pointed out by evidence of a high incidence of new cerebral infarcts after carotid artery reconstruction in children (Chau *et al.*, 2025). A smooth transition to long-term care not only assists in reducing readmissions but also plays an important role in maximizing long-term outcomes and quality of life for these vulnerable patients (Figure 4.16).

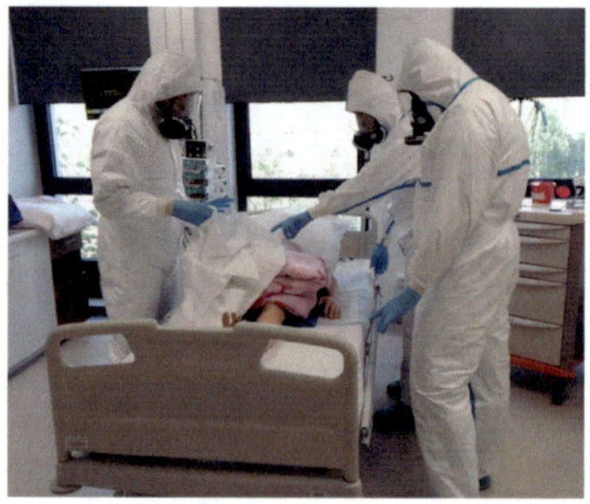

Figure 4.16. As patients emerge from intensive care, where they have received life-saving interventions such as extracorporeal membrane oxygenation, the focus shifts to their ongoing rehabilitation and health management.

Source: https://media.springernature.com/lw685/springer-static/image/art%3A10.1186%2Fs12912-021-00736-7/MediaObjects/12912_2021_736_Fig1_HTML.png.

Test Your Knowledge

1. How are fluids managed differently in hypovolemic versus cardiogenic shock in children?
2. How is acute heart failure managed in the PICU setting?

4.4. Challenges and Considerations in Pediatric Intensive Care

Learning Outcome

1. Understand age-specific physiological differences.
2. Explain ethical considerations in treatment decisions.
3. Identify communication barriers with families.
4. Focus on resource limitations in pediatric ICUs.
5. Describe training and education for healthcare providers.
6. Know the psychological impact on patients and families.
7. Focus on a multidisciplinary team approach.
8. Explain cultural considerations in care.
9. Discuss future directions in pediatric cardiovascular care.

More in cardiovascular emergencies, in pediatric intensive care, clinicians are faced with numerous complexities that complicate patient management. The challenges include the inherent physiological diversities in pediatric patients that necessitate special diagnostic and therapeutic management. For instance, disorders like patent ductus arteriosus and pulmonary hypertension can present with characteristic hemodynamic instabilities that necessitate precise interventions to stabilize the vulnerable cardiovascular status of such patients (Sehgal *et al.*, 2025). Further, the need for emergent procedures such as bedside endoscopy during critical situations introduces additional complexities where hemodynamic instability and coagulopathy are complications that must be managed cautiously (Jagirdhar *et al.*, 2024). These complications combined create the necessity for careful selection of patients and multidisciplinary treatment, a significant requirement for the pediatric ICU setting, which ultimately strives to optimize outcomes while maintaining corresponding risks at their lowest within this vulnerable population. Correcting these concerns not only improves existing care but also serves as guidance for future research priorities in pediatric cardiology.

4.4.1. Age-Specific Physiological Differences

Understanding physiological variation with age is crucial in the treatment of cardiovascular emergencies in the pediatric intensive care unit. Infants and children possess distinct anatomical and physiological characteristics in comparison to adults, particularly in cardiovascular physiology. The infant's heart rate is significantly higher, necessitating diversified interventions in cardiac emergencies.

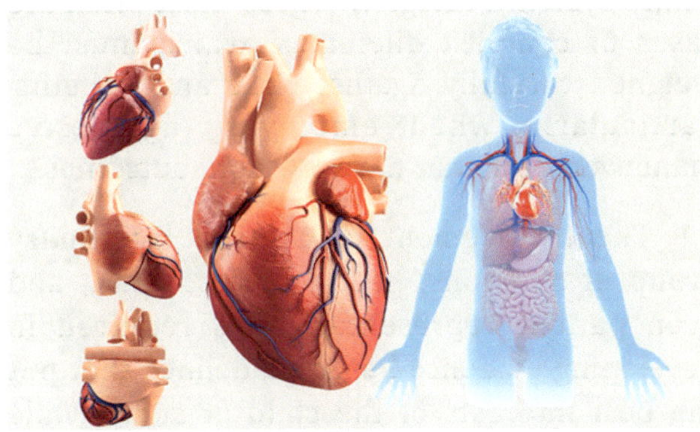

Figure 4.17. Infants and children exhibit distinct anatomical and functional characteristics compared to adults, particularly in cardiovascular physiology.

Source: https://dm3omg1n1n7zx.cloudfront.net/rcni/static/journals/ncyp/aop/ncyp.2020.e1245/tile/ncyp.2020.e1245_abs.jpg.

Children also possess a higher fraction of total body water, influencing fluid management strategy during acute heart failure or shock. This physiological background is particularly relevant in conditions like multisystem inflammatory syndrome in children, where acute cardiac impairment can occur after

SARS-CoV-2 infection (Belhadjer *et al.*, 2020). In accordance with evolving guidelines in the management of cardiovascular disease, it is crucial to make changes accordingly to facilitate these differences, as established by the ACC and AHA (Paul *et al.*, 2017). Inadequate recognition of these differences yields inappropriate management and bad outcomes, which justifies the employment of individualized strategies in pediatric intensive care.

4.4.2. Ethical Considerations in Treatment Decisions

In the case of cardiovascular emergencies in pediatric intensive care, ethical considerations in planning treatment are significant in safeguarding the child's welfare as well as the health system's integrity. These most often are cases of complex dilemmas, which must be weighed carefully against risks and benefits, particularly when employing aggressive maneuvers that can have variable outcomes.

The involvement of a multidisciplinary group of surgeons, health professionals, and even patient representatives is required in developing evidence-based guidelines that put the best interests of the child at stake while remaining up to speed with ethical standards. In addition, as treatment conditions evolve—usually governed by novel data and long-term outcomes—healthcare providers must remain responsive and change recommendations accordingly, particularly when confronting unforeseen challenges such as the impact of pandemics on patient treatment (Lorenzo *et al.*, 2020; Oren *et al.*, 2020).

With open communication and decision-sharing, ethical frameworks can help clinicians navigate through these intricate clinical settings effectively.

4.4.3. Communication Barriers with Families

Effective communication among pediatric intensive care unit (PICU) health care providers and families is critical, particularly with regard to cardiovascular emergencies. However, a number of barriers usually interfere with this process, including cultural differences as well as language barriers, which can have a remarkable impact on family involvement in care decision-making. The presence of language minority groups within ICUs necessitates targeted communication strategies aimed at promoting the understanding of treatment options and their meanings to the families.

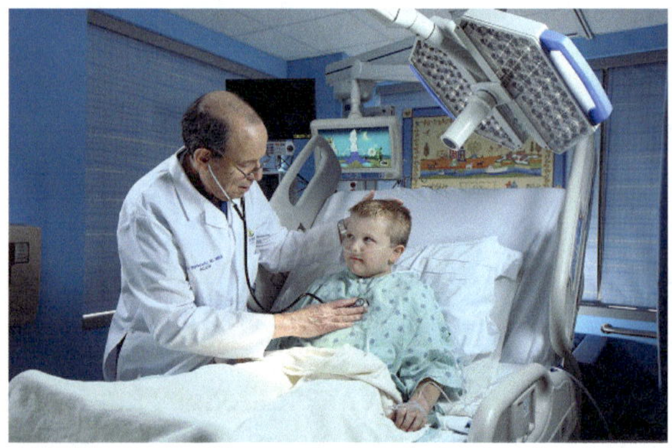

Figure 4.18. Effective communication between healthcare providers and families in pediatric intensive care units (PICUs) is critical, particularly during cardiovascular emergencies.

Source: https://anesthesiology.hopkinsmedicine.org/wp-content/uploads/2022/09/PICUStethescopeBoy.06082016-2.jpg.

For instance, recent studies show that online resources like Google Translate do not necessarily deal with the complexities of medical terms, and it is imperative that specialized translation tools be developed. Developing an artificial intelligence-driven translation tool for PICUs could possibly transmit timely and efficient communication, thereby enhancing family involvement and understanding (Bahrami *et al.*, 2025). Additionally, barriers such as poor training in the application of point-of-care ultrasound technology also disrupt quality communication in such points of crisis, casting the need for ongoing education in pediatric emergency care (Şık *et al.*, 2024) (Figure 4.18).

4.4.4. Resource Limitations in Pediatric ICUs

Resource limitation is a critical concern in pediatric intensive care units (PICUs), particularly in crisis situations such as pandemics or natural disasters. The limitations most commonly manifest as shortfalls in basic equipment, including mechanical ventilators and advanced monitoring devices, required for the management of cardiovascular emergencies in children. For instance, the application of extracorporeal membrane oxygenation (ECMO) as a rescue therapy is not merely technology-dependent but also depends on skilled personnel who might not be present in sufficient numbers to address high demand. The uneven allocation of resources, which is sustained by an uneven distribution of expertise, underscores the need for an active model for optimizing outcomes of critically ill children. Research calls for developing strategies for equitable distribution of resources, particularly in times of crisis, in a manner that ensures proper care to vulnerable populations without compromising it (Matthew *et al.*, 2020; James *et al.*, 2020). Implementation of these strategies is required to ensure pediatric critical care systems are strengthened.

4.4.5. Training and Education for Healthcare Providers

In the context of cardiovascular emergencies in pediatric intensive care, training and education of healthcare professionals are key. Appropriate management of such life-threatening conditions hinges on a proper understanding of existing resuscitation techniques and how to make optimal use of advanced technology such as echocardiography. Ongoing education classes should focus on identification and management of conditions that lead to heart arrest, including the use of critical interventions like defibrillators and intraosseous infusions, as noted in Raina *et al.* (2020). The special precautions, like the use of personal protective equipment during examinations, pose challenges that need persistent training in the clinical setting. Prioritization measures and echocardiographic service adjustment in the event of public health crises provide focus on preparedness and response for clinicians, so that healthcare professionals can still provide optimal care in spite of altered circumstances, as guided by recommendations of the ASE and other specialized organizations (James *et al.*, 2020) (Figure 4.19).

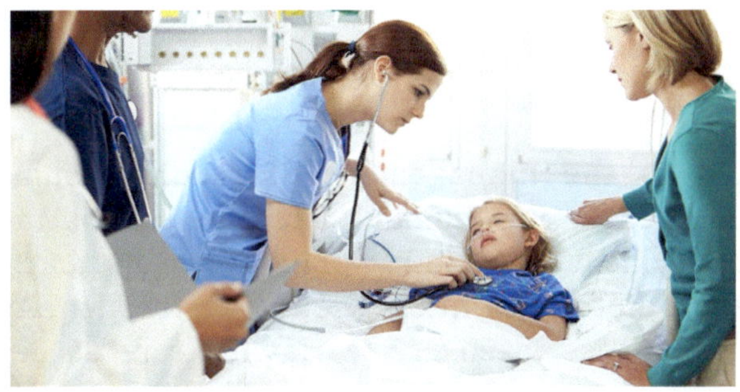

Figure 4.19. Effective response to such critical situations requires a comprehensive understanding of the latest resuscitation techniques and the appropriate use of advanced technologies such as echocardiography.

Source: https://www.kkcth.org/Blog/1748327737_1723181241_Untitled%20design%20(49).webp.

4.4.6. Psychological Impact on Patients and Families

The psychological impact of cardiovascular emergencies on the patient and family is widespread and complicated, particularly in the pediatric intensive care unit. Relatives are usually under acute stress, anxiety, and uncertainty while experiencing their child's life-threatening illness, which adds to helplessness and fear. There is evidence that effective communication from health professionals in such moments is crucial in reducing psychological distress and fostering an optimistic atmosphere. In some countries, there are structured programs for addressing the emotional needs of surviving patients and family members of non-survivors that are highly recommended for comprehensive care. These programs should aim at enhancing the emotional well-being of the surviving patients as well as their family members. These considerations emphasize the necessity of a description of the psychological aspects of pediatric critical care, as outlined in guidelines for improving the quality and outcomes of healthcare (Paul *et al.*, 2023; Kleinpell *et al.*, 2021).

4.4.7. Multidisciplinary Team Approach

Key to the management of cardiovascular emergencies in pediatric intensive care is the deployment of a multidisciplinary team approach. It promotes the integration of heterogeneity of expertise to ensure worldwide care as per the unique needs of critically ill children. For instance, with the emergence of Multisystem Inflammatory Syndrome in Children (MIS-C), a coalition of experts, including infectious disease experts, cardiologists, and intensivists, enabled effective management through clinical guideline development and conducting multidisciplinary rounds. Such a collaborative framework not only improved patient outcomes via standardized care but also facilitated seamless communication between clinical settings (Gillen *et al.*, 2023). Similarly, the response to treating patients with advanced pathogens like viral hemorrhagic fevers required proceduralized processes that involved interdepartmental coordination between multiple hospital departments to enhance readiness and response capacity (Brewer *et al.*, 2024). Lastly, the integration of various professional disciplines becomes imperative in pediatric cardiovascular emergencies management, reinforcing the importance of multidisciplinary collaboration within intensive care units (Figure 4.20).

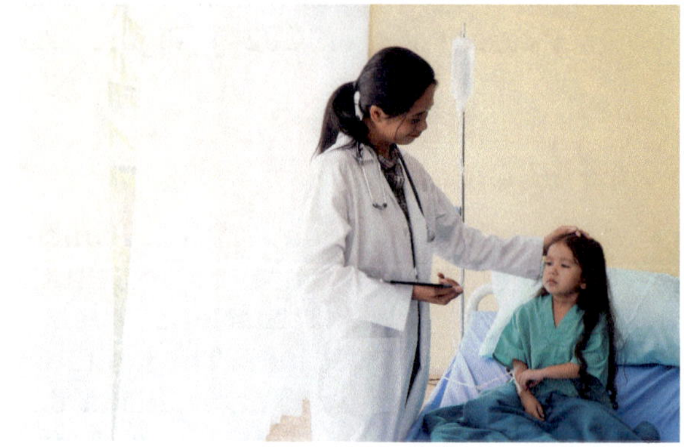

Figure 4.20. The implementation of a multidisciplinary team approach is pivotal in addressing cardiovascular emergencies in pediatric intensive care.

Source: https://medanta.s3.ap-south-1.amazonaws.com/blogs/December2024/DuBoDUM6l09JpzbJttQiXToGGzKRFc-metaUGFlZGlhdHJpYyBjYXJkaW9sb2d5LmpwZw==-.jpg.

4.4.8. Cultural Considerations in Care

Cultural considerations form the core of the management of pediatric patients who come to the intensive care unit with cardiovascular emergencies. Understanding the heterogeneity of the patients is enough to influence treatment outcome and delivery of care. For instance, cultural beliefs about healthcare procedures may determine parental preferences for treatment and compliance. Good communication in this case is important as the medical practitioners need to fill any gaps in trust and understanding. The example of the use of point-of-care ultrasound (POCUS) in pediatric emergency medicine is a good one; it has been proven to have clinical benefits like rapid diagnosis and treatment, but is hindered by cultural beliefs and training deficits among the staff members (Şık *et al.*, 2024). Besides, concerns regarding the child and family's psychosocial needs, shaped by their own cultural paradigms, can impact recovery and emotional well-being. Therefore, culturally responsive care must be prioritized in order to optimize patient outcomes in such situation-critical cases (Amanda *et al.*, 2024).

4.4.9. Future Directions in Pediatric Cardiovascular Care

With pediatric cardiovascular treatment continuously evolving, future directions are likely to be centered on new approaches that enhance the management of cardiovascular emergencies in the pediatric intensive care unit. Emphasis should also be placed on education and simulation training for medical professionals, enabling them to properly manage complicated cases typically posed by tracheostomy-dependent children who are at risk of heightened dangers during emergencies (Erin *et al.*, 2020). Such integration of advanced technologies, like telemedicine and wearable technology, is also likely to play a crucial role in early diagnosis and timely intervention, improving the outcomes of patients in acute conditions. Immunoscore-based data regarding pediatric patients, especially those under immune checkpoint therapies, will also further simplify the treatment pathways of associated cardiovascular events by acknowledging the specificity of the concern in such patients (Bryan *et al.*, 2021). These advancements altogether are anticipated to develop a more holistic and responsive pediatric cardiovascular treatment system in intensive care environments.

Test Your Knowledge

1. Why is hypotension a late and ominous sign in pediatric shock?
2. What are the key considerations when titrating inotropes in children?

SUMMARY

Pediatric intensive care cardiovascular emergency management is an emerging and complex field of study that necessitates sincere preparedness and compensatory action. As evidenced by recent cases following natural disasters, where surgical disaster response teams were mobilized to address extremity injuries, it is imperative to ensure that the medical fraternity is well prepared to address the multidimensional situation presented by pediatric cardiovascular accidents (Ümit Özdemir *et al.*, 2025). Furthermore, the increasing numbers of pediatric patients who receive ventricular assist devices further underscore the requirement for specialty training for critical care physicians because the majority of them have encounters with no validated resuscitation protocols for this specialist population (Ivie *et al.*, 2023). The integration of comprehensive disaster preparedness programs and well-structured emergency response teams, with ongoing training and education, will eventually enhance patient outcomes and streamline care delivery in pediatric intensive care units, ensuring caregivers are best positioned to deal with the intricacies of cardiovascular emergencies.

In pediatric intensive care cardiovascular emergencies, the importance of efficient guidelines and planning for resource strategies cannot be exaggerated. Evidence suggests that advance planning is required, particularly during crisis situations, to ensure equitable distribution of advanced care modalities such as extracorporeal membrane oxygenation (ECMO) when there is surge demand, such as during the COVID-19 pandemic (Matthew *et al.*, 2020). The American Diabetes Association emphasizes standardization of condition management and, with it, the necessity for continuous updates to clinical practice that can act on new challenges in patient care. Targeted decision-making processes centered on patient outcomes and resource availability are still necessary. Lastly, such methods aim to balance ethical considerations with clinical effectiveness, providing pediatric patients with timely and efficient interventions within acute cardiovascular events in order to enhance survival rates and outcomes.

KEY TERMS FROM THIS CHAPTER

- Cardiovascular emergencies
- Treatment
- Point-of-care ultrasound (POCUS)
- Pediatric intensive care units (picus)
- Cardiovascular emergency management
- Medical staff
- Echocardiography
- Hemodynamics
- Arrhythmias
- Diagnosis
- Morbidity
- Total anomalous pulmonary venous return
- Hematopoietic cell transplantation (HCT)
- Stress
- Congenital heart defects (CHDs)
- Cardiogenic shock
- Viral infections
- Myocarditis

CRITICAL THINKING QUESTIONS

1. **What is the most common cause of shock in pediatric patients?**
   a. Cardiogenic shock
   b. Distributive shock
   c. Obstructive shock
   d. Hypovolemic shock
2. **Which of the following signs is LEAST likely to be seen in a child with compensated shock?**
   a. Tachycardia
   b. Cool extremities
   c. Hypotension
   d. Delayed capillary refill
3. **Which medication is typically used as a first-line inotropic agent in pediatric cardiogenic shock?**
   a. Epinephrine
   b. Amiodarone
   c. Atropine
   d. Lidocaine
4. **In pediatric cardiac arrest, what is the most common initial rhythm?**
   a. Ventricular fibrillation (VF)
   b. Pulseless electrical activity (PEA)
   c. Asystole
   d. Supraventricular tachycardia (SVT)
5. **Which of the following findings suggests cardiac tamponade in a child?**
   a. Bradycardia, bounding pulses, increased BP
   b. Muffled heart sounds, distended neck veins, hypotension
   c. Rales, crackles, hypertension
   d. Loud S1, cyanosis, widened pulse pressure

Short Answer Questions

1. What are the most frequently encountered cardiovascular emergencies in the PICU?
2. How does the presentation of shock differ between hypovolemic, cardiogenic, and distributive types in children?
3. What are the key components of cardiovascular assessment in critically ill pediatric patients?
4. How is the Pediatric Assessment Triangle (PAT) used to identify hemodynamic instability?
5. What is the first-line treatment for pediatric supraventricular tachycardia (SVT)?
6. When is synchronized cardioversion indicated in pediatric arrhythmias?
7. How do age and developmental stage affect the presentation of cardiovascular emergencies?
8. What are the challenges in recognizing compensated shock in children?

Answers to Critical Thinking Questions

1. (d) 2. (c) 3. (a) 4. (b) 5. (b)

REFERENCES

1. Acar, Y., Tezel, O., Salman, N., Çevik, E., Algaba-Montes, M., Oviedo-García, A., Patricio-Bordomás, M., *et al.* (2016). 12th WINFOCUS World Congress on ultrasound in emergency and critical care. *Critical Ultrasound Journal, 8.* https://www.semanticscholar.org/paper/85b5046ad234e5fb11c7048192c0dcbc34cb13d5 (accessed on 30th June 2025).
2. Aitelkhadir, M., Khaleq, K., Bouhouri, M. A., Ettaoussi, A., & Hattabi, K. (2025). Body packing and surgical intensive care: Analysis of complications and management strategies. *International Journal of Advanced Research.* https://www.semanticscholar.org/paper/dae74a02b27995ddb418d7c09a216066a22dff2f (accessed on 30th June 2025).
3. Arı, M., Arı, H., & Cengiz, H. (2025). Advanced biomarkers for prognostic evaluation of pneumonia severity in pediatric intensive care: Focus on novel inflammatory and hematological ratios. *Italian Journal of Pediatrics, 51.* https://www.semanticscholar.org/paper/e41e28c8cca66fe94765d4288e23dda480021945 (accessed on 30th June 2025).
4. Bahrami, S., & Rubulotta, F. (2025). Artificial intelligence-driven translation tools in intensive care units for enhancing communication and research. *International Journal of Environmental Research and Public Health, 22.* https://www.semanticscholar.org/paper/481bc3c0d381da52322efa8f310bcb74e9016310 (accessed on 30th June 2025).
5. Barker, P., Lewin, M., Donofrio, M. T., Altman, C. A., Ensing, G. J., Arya, B., & Swaminathan, M. (2020). Specific considerations for pediatric, fetal, and congenital heart disease patients and echocardiography service providers during the 2019 novel coronavirus outbreak: Council on Pediatric and Congenital Heart Disease supplement to the statement of the American Society of Echocardiography. *Journal of the American Society of Echocardiography, 33*, 658–665. https://doi.org/10.1016/j.echo.2020.04.005 (accessed on 30th June 2025).
6. Belhadjer, Z., Méot, M., Bajolle, F., Khraiche, D., Legendre, A., Abakka, S., Auriau, J., *et al.* (2020). Acute heart failure in multisystem inflammatory syndrome in children in the context of global SARS-CoV-2 pandemic. *Circulation, 142*, 429–436. https://doi.org/10.1161/circulationaha.120.048360 (accessed on 30th June 2025).
7. Berg, K., Bray, J. E., Ng, K. C., Liley, H., Greif, R., Carlson, J., Morley, P. T., *et al.* (2023). 2023 international consensus on cardiopulmonary resuscitation and emergency cardiovascular care science with treatment recommendations: Summary from the Basic Life Support; Advanced Life Support; Pediatric Life Support; Neonatal Life Support; Education, Implementation, and Teams; and First Aid Task. *Circulation, 148*, e187–e280. https://www.semanticscholar.org/paper/428dbe6e859cec59a5f9cc6d786eabe4f68ba929 (accessed on 30th June 2025).
8. Brewer, B., Schnell, N. A., Sickbert-Bennett Vavalle, E., Weber, D., Wohl, D., & Fischer, W. A. (2024). Building a special pathogen response center from the ground up. *Antimicrobial Stewardship & Healthcare Epidemiology: ASHE, 4*, s95. https://www.semanticscholar.org/paper/741a4681f40d93dbbe5bb27922a130b4db58b82b (accessed on 30th June 2025).
9. Bykov, Y. V., Obedin, A. N., Muravyova, A., & Zinchenko, O. (2025). Intensive care management of pediatric status asthmaticus. *Innovative Medicine of Kuban.* https://www.semanticscholar.org/paper/21dd5c93619de27aed5b345d5dfc53e8dcb7cf08 (accessed on 30th June 2025).
10. Bykov, Y., Obedin, A. N., Fischer, V., Volkov, E., Zinchenko, O., Muravyova, A., & Yatsuk, I. (2024). Acute cerebrovascular accident in children: Clinical presentation and intensive

care management. *Avicenna Bulletin.* https://www.semanticscholar.org/paper/e4257342f5ce88f417442d1a734b301f9ecd17f9 (accessed on 30th June 2025).

11. Chan, P. S., Greif, R., Anderson, T. D., Atiq, H., Couto, T. B., Considine, J., de Caen, A. R., *et al.* (2023). Ten steps toward improving in-hospital cardiac arrest quality of care and outcomes. *Resuscitation, 193*, 109996. https://doi.org/10.1016/j.resuscitation.2023.109996 (accessed on 30th June 2025).

12. Chau, A., Maskatia, S., Albuliwi, B., Martin, E., & Ryan, K. (2025). Favorable vessel patency following carotid artery reconstruction during extracorporeal membrane oxygenation decannulation in children with congenital heart disease. *World Journal for Pediatric & Congenital Heart Surgery.* https://www.semanticscholar.org/paper/0e794ad93a537e11919f5bb6e78fdfa2a0979af7 (accessed on 30th June 2025).

13. Colombo, C. N., Tavazzi, G., Zanetti, M., Dore, F., & Finazzi, S. (2024). Cardiogenic shock diagnosis and management in general intensive care: A nationwide survey. *Minerva Anesthesiologic.* https://www.semanticscholar.org/paper/8d045e5deff543a2b92bb4f613c22ec6b69305ff (accessed on 30th June 2025).

14. Coté, C. J., & Wilson, S. (2019). Guidelines for monitoring and management of pediatric patients before, during, and after sedation for diagnostic and therapeutic procedures. *Pediatrics, 143.* https://doi.org/10.1542/peds.2019-1000 (accessed on 30th June 2025).

15. Dallan, C., Romano, F., Siebert, J. N., Politi, S., Lacroix, L., & Sahyoun, C. (2020). Septic shock presentation in adolescents with COVID-19. *The Lancet Child & Adolescent Health, 4*, e21–e23. https://doi.org/10.1016/s2352-4642(20)30164-4 (accessed on 30th June 2025).

16. Daniels, L. B., Phreaner, N., Berg, D. D., Bohula, E., Chaudhry, S., Fordyce, C. B., Goldfarb, M. J., *et al.* (2024). Sex differences in characteristics, resource utilization, and outcomes of cardiogenic shock: Data from the Critical Care Cardiology Trials Network (CCCTN) Registry. *Circulation: Cardiovascular Quality and Outcomes, 17*, e010614. https://www.semanticscholar.org/paper/cce33bce71049a882e5f62466651c716de161006 (accessed on 30th June 2025).

17. Di Lorenzo, N., Antoniou, S. A., Batterham, R. L., Busetto, L., Godoroja, D., Iossa, A., Carrano, F. M., *et al.* (2020). Clinical practice guidelines of the European Association for Endoscopic Surgery (EAES) on bariatric surgery: Update 2020 endorsed by IFSO-EC, EASO and ESPCOP. *Surgical Endoscopy, 34*, 2332–2358. https://doi.org/10.1007/s00464-020-07555-y (accessed on 30th June 2025).

18. Dolhnikoff, M., Ferranti, J. F., Monteiro, R. A. A., Duarte-Neto, A. N., Gomes-Gouvêa, M. S., Degaspare, N. V., Delgado, A. F., *et al.* (2020). SARS-CoV-2 in cardiac tissue of a child with COVID-19-related multisystem inflammatory syndrome. *The Lancet Child & Adolescent Health, 4*, 790–794. https://doi.org/10.1016/s2352-4642(20)30257-1 (accessed on 30th June 2025).

19. Downing, N. L., Bates, D. W., & Longhurst, C. (2018). Physician burnout in the electronic health record era: Are we ignoring the real cause? *Annals of Internal Medicine, 169*, 50–50. https://doi.org/10.7326/m18-0139 (accessed on 30th June 2025).

20. Ellis, D., Hall, M., Blume, E., Wolfe, J., Snaman, J., & Berry, J. (2024). Abstract 4139570: A hard start: Early, intensive healthcare utilization for children with critical congenital heart disease. *Circulation.* https://www.semanticscholar.org/paper/1a845792d15803bbd7bb1bdb4951daff0dbe1a88 (accessed on 30th June 2025).

21. Ermolenko, K., Pshenisnov, K. V., Aleksandrovich, Y., Aleksandrovich, I. V., & Konev, A. I. (2025). Focused echocardiography as a tool for differential diagnosis of cardiovascular dysfunction in children with infections: Case reports. *Russian Journal of Pediatric Surgery, Anesthesia and Intensive Care.* https://www.semanticscholar.org/paper/95747f91a4e21176b1e5295226202ef70218b482 (accessed on 30th June 2025).

22. Esangbedo, I. D., Yu, P., Choudhury, T. A., Tume, S., & Lasa, J. (2023). Ventricular assist device training and emergency management among pediatric cardiac intensive care physicians–Multicenter cross-sectional survey. *World Journal for Pediatric and Congenital Heart Surgery, 15*, 202–208. https://www.semanticscholar.org/paper/1e384b680e8542b315eac0ce65e798f09f9aa126 (accessed on 30th June 2025).

23. Espeleta-Fox, A., García-Salido, A., de Unzueta-Roch, J. L., de Lama Caro-Patón, G., Moral-Larraz, A., Toledano-Revenga, J., Leoz-Gordillo, I., *et al.* (2025). Severe *Mycoplasma pneumoniae* infections during the 2023–2024 outbreak: A single-center descriptive study in a pediatric intensive care. *The Pediatric Infectious Disease Journal, 44*, e225–e228. https://www.semanticscholar.org/paper/9baae64a97eb020fa74a9ca2d37dbb6e897a6d86 (accessed on 30th June 2025).

24. Fix, O. K., Hameed, B., Fontana, R. J., Kwok, R. M., McGuire, B. M., Mulligan, D. C., Pratt, D. S., *et al.* (2020). Clinical best practice advice for hepatology and liver transplant providers during the COVID-19 pandemic: AASLD expert panel consensus statement. *Hepatology, 72*, 287–304. https://doi.org/10.1002/hep.31281 (accessed on 30th June 2025).

25. Gillen, S., Knutson, S., Strutt, J., Fischer, G., Sharon, B., Boucher, A. A., Steiner, M. E., *et al.* (2023). 402. Multidisciplinary management model for multisystem inflammatory syndrome in children: A comprehensive approach for improved patient outcomes. *Open Forum Infectious Diseases, 10.* https://www.semanticscholar.org/paper/20ddc2f36d59e1e20c70e388e1c897c0d23e091d (accessed on 30th June 2025).

26. Greif, R., Bhanji, F., Bigham, B. L., Bray, J., Breckwoldt, J., Cheng, A., Duff, J. P., *et al.* (2020). Education, implementation, and teams: 2020 international consensus on cardiopulmonary resuscitation and emergency cardiovascular care science with treatment recommendations. *Circulation, 142.* https://doi.org/10.1161/cir.0000000000000896 (accessed on 30th June 2025).

27. Isselbacher, E. M., Preventza, O., Black, J. H., Augoustides, J., Beck, A. W., Bolen, M. A., Braverman, A. C., *et al.* (2022). 2022 ACC/AHA guideline for the diagnosis and management of aortic disease: A report of the American Heart Association/American College of Cardiology Joint Committee on Clinical Practice Guidelines. *Circulation, 146.* https://doi.org/10.1161/cir.0000000000001106 (accessed on 30th June 2025).

28. Jagirdhar, G., Elmati, P., Pattnaik, H., Shah, M., & Surani, S. (2024). Navigating gastrointestinal endoscopy challenges in the intensive care unit: A mini review. *World Journal of Critical Care Medicine, 13.* https://www.semanticscholar.org/paper/95325115fd5ddba4df4b3d84f4f356c4611e60fc (accessed on 30th June 2025).

29. Jia, M., Hu, X., Ji, L., Lin, J., Liu, J., & Wang, Y. (2025). Predictive for patients with pneumonia in pediatric intensive care unit. *Frontiers in Pediatrics.* https://www.semanticscholar.org/paper/4835f9d8d7ef9260e68d384d0e215eff8c9d1721 (accessed on 30th June 2025).

30. Johnson, A. K., Cornea, S., Goldfarb, S., Cao, Q., Heneghan, J., & Gupta, A. O. (2024). Risk factors predicting need for the pediatric intensive care unit (PICU) post-hematopoietic cell transplant, PICU utilization, and outcomes following HCT: A single center retrospective analysis. *Frontiers in Pediatrics, 12*, 1385153. https://www.semanticscholar.org/paper/28f23aaee89ca3c07e2109289b45706377bf9ca8 (accessed on 30th June 2025).

31. Karon, B. L. (2004). Practical cardiology: Evaluation and treatment of common cardiovascular disorders. *79*, 716. https://www.semanticscholar.org/paper/40485e565b41ba190adc208f9acda19df01f9cb0 (accessed on 30th June 2025).

32. Khan, E. K., Lockspeiser, T. M., Liptzin, D. R., Meier, M., & Baker, C. D. (2020). "When in doubt, change it out": A case-based simulation for pediatric residents caring for hospitalized tracheostomy-dependent children. *MedEdPORTAL*. https://doi.org/10.15766/mep_2374-8265.10994 (accessed on 30th June 2025).

33. Kiall, T. R. (1999). Online quantification of cardiovascular function in children. *Echocardiography, 16*(1), 77–84. https://www.semanticscholar.org/paper/9bcff82b9c332e969c05a57a3d1509895c6f0f56 (accessed on 30th June 2025).

34. Kirkpatrick, J. N., Mitchell, C., Taub, C., Kort, S., Hung, J., & Swaminathan, M. (2020). ASE statement on protection of patients and echocardiography service providers during the 2019 novel coronavirus outbreak: Endorsed by the American College of Cardiology. *Journal of the American Society of Echocardiography, 33*, 648–653. https://doi.org/10.1016/j.echo.2020.04.001 (accessed on 30th June 2025).

35. Kleinpell, R., Grabenkort, W. R., Boyle, W. A., Vines, D., & Olsen, K. M. (2021). The Society of Critical Care Medicine at 50 years: Interprofessional practice in critical care: Looking back and forging ahead. *Critical Care Medicine, 49*, 2017–2032. https://doi.org/10.1097/ccm.0000000000005276 (accessed on 30th June 2025).

36. Kuok, C., & Chan, W. (2022). Motor vehicle collision and acute kidney injury in children. *Pediatric Emergency Care, 38*, 545–549. https://www.semanticscholar.org/paper/7dec0d0dc465b4291182683b2c12b1dbfdb32280 (accessed on 30th June 2025).

37. Kuwabara, M., Yamamoto, T., Tahara, Y., Kikuchi, M., Imamura, H., Takeuchi, I., Sato, N., *et al.* (2025). Utilization of intensive care units and outcomes based on admission wards in cardiovascular emergencies. *Circulation Journal: Official Journal of the Japanese Circulation Society.* https://www.semanticscholar.org/paper/a7308e34e3f098f3d886e36fce642d368178f57e (accessed on 30th June 2025).

38. Lasso-Palomino, R. E., Medina, D., Franco, A., Soto-Aparicio, M. J., Tarapues, E. M., Muñoz, D. M., Salazar, E., *et al.* (2024). Outcomes within 100 days of hematopoietic cell transplantation in pediatric patients: Insights from an intensive care unit in Colombia. *Frontiers in Pediatrics, 12.* https://www.semanticscholar.org/paper/e09b014a08089a541c490b6b7477570824860e15 (accessed on 30th June 2025).

39. Mehta, C. K., Malaisrie, S. C., Budd, A. N., Okita, Y., Matsuda, H., Fleischman, F., Ueda, Y., *et al.* (2020). Triage and management of aortic emergencies during the coronavirus disease 2019 (COVID-19) pandemic: A consensus document supported by the American Association for Thoracic Surgery (AATS) and Asian Society for Cardiovascular and Thoracic Surgery (ASCVTS). *Journal of Thoracic and Cardiovascular Surgery, 161*, 48–53. https://doi.org/10.1016/j.jtcvs.2020.06.004 (accessed on 30th June 2025).

40. Merchant, R. M., Topjian, A. A., Panchal, A. R., Cheng, A., Aziz, K., Berg, K. M., Lavonas, E. J., *et al.* (2020). Part 1: Executive summary: 2020 American Heart Association guidelines for cardiopulmonary resuscitation and emergency cardiovascular care. *Circulation, 142.* https://doi.org/10.1161/cir.0000000000000918 (accessed on 30th June 2025).

41. Moizés, A. S., Shiotsu, C. H., & Takashi, M. H. (2016). Profile of patients admitted in a cardiovascular hospital. *Journal of Nursing UFPE Online, 10*, 2595–2603. https://www.semanticscholar.org/paper/7d8a8b3801c8fba644a273817fd5fa05c3229dd5 (accessed on 30th June 2025).

42. Nabih, I., Idbaha, Y., & Aissaoui, O. (2025). *Ralstonia pickettii*: Two cases of bacteremia in a Moroccan pediatric intensive care unit. *Cureus, 17.* https://www.semanticscholar.org/paper/202383ad0466488f6bd864038feedbe1eaf9c378 (accessed on 30th June 2025).

43. Özdemir, Ü., Kaymakçı, E., Abbasoğlu, B., İrdem Köse, Ü. N., Çataroğlu, C. K., Çevik, H., Şenlikçi, A., *et al.* (2025). The observations and experience of the surgical disaster response team from Ankara Etlik City Hospital in the earthquakes of February 6, 2023 in Türkiye. *Turkish Journal of Trauma & Emergency Surgery, 31*, 375–380. https://www.semanticscholar.org/paper/fbfeeb5ecd15293a0d1b577be5dcc573ed947346 (accessed on 30th June 2025).

44. Prekker, M. E., Brunsvold, M. E., Bohman, J. K., Fischer, G., Gram, K. L., Litell, J. M., Saavedra-Romero, R., *et al.* (2020). Regional planning for extracorporeal membrane oxygenation allocation during coronavirus disease 2019. *CHEST Journal, 158*, 603–607. https://doi.org/10.1016/j.chest.2020.04.026 (accessed on 30th June 2025).

45. Schlapbach, L., & Kissoon, N. (2018). Defining pediatric sepsis. *JAMA Pediatrics, 172*(4), 312–314. https://www.semanticscholar.org/paper/1ff18d07c27e46fa8913227a0167553d0064e820 (accessed on 30th June 2025).

46. Schneider, B. J., Naidoo, J., Santomasso, B., Lacchetti, C., Adkins, S., Anadkat, M. J., Atkins, M. B., *et al.* (2021). Management of immune-related adverse events in patients treated with immune checkpoint inhibitor therapy: ASCO guideline update. *Journal of Clinical Oncology, 39*, 4073–4126. https://doi.org/10.1200/jco.21.01440 (accessed on 30th June 2025).

47. Sehgal, A., Buckingham, M. R., Hyland, R. M., & McNamara, P. J. (2025). Diagnostic and therapeutic precision in cardiovascular diseases in the neonatal intensive care. *Journal of Perinatology: Official Journal of the California Perinatal Association.* https://www.semanticscholar.org/paper/074544e20c703c6269570be5382178a558501237 (accessed on 30th June 2025).

48. Selmanoğlu, A., Çelik, H. I., Genis, C., Koçkuzu, E., Emeksiz, Z., & Mısırlıoğlu, E. (2025). Evaluation of asthma course in patients hospitalized in pediatric intensive care unit due to severe asthma exacerbation. *Medicina, 61.* https://www.semanticscholar.org/paper/990e7253760ad5b87817923952a5d061e51a9db9 (accessed on 30th June 2025).

49. Sen, K., Harrar, D., Pariseau, N., Tucker, K., Keenan, J. S., Zhang, A., & Gropman, A. (2024). Seizure characteristics and EEG features in intoxication type and energy deficiency neurometabolic disorders in the pediatric intensive care unit: Single-center experience over 10 years. *Neurocritical Care.* https://www.semanticscholar.org/paper/02dc66faa2943c47b025dbdf79579f0304ba43b6 (accessed on 30th June 2025).

50. Singer, M., Deutschman, C. S., Seymour, C. W., Shankar-Hari, M., Annane, D., Bauer, M., Bellomo, R., *et al.* (2016). The third international consensus definitions for sepsis and septic shock

(Sepsis-3). *JAMA, 315*, 801–801. https://doi.org/10.1001/jama.2016.0287 (accessed on 30th June 2025).

51. Şık, N., Arslan, G., Akça Çağlar, A., Ülgen Tekerek, N., Fidancı, İ., Tolu Kendir, Ö., Bal, A., *et al.* (2024). The use of point-of-care ultrasound in pediatric emergency departments and intensive care units. *Pediatric Emergency Care, 40*, 796–800. https://www.semanticscholar.org/paper/b06360b480d3b94d25f0f210024f35a6cec2e78b (accessed on 30th June 2025).

52. Talwar, S., Bhende, V. V., Krishnakumar, M., Tandon, K., & Patel, P. R. (2025). Is surgery for congenital heart defects in neonates, infants, and children more challenging and demanding than surgery for acquired heart defects in adults? *Cureus, 17.* https://www.semanticscholar.org/paper/9bb3735cac3b263a8f5717c33b31c009c4b62ca2 (accessed on 30th June 2025).

53. Truong, D. T., Dionne, A., Muniz, J. C., McHugh, K. E., Portman, M. A., Lambert, L. M., Thacker, D., *et al.* (2021). Clinically suspected myocarditis temporally related to COVID-19 vaccination in adolescents and young adults: Suspected myocarditis after COVID-19 vaccination. *Circulation, 145*, 345–356. https://doi.org/10.1161/circulationaha.121.056583 (accessed on 30th June 2025).

54. Whelton, P. K., Carey, R. M., Aronow, W. S., Casey, D. E., Collins, K. J., Dennison Himmelfarb, C., DePalma, S. M., *et al.* (2017). 2017 ACC/AHA/AAPA/ABC/ACPM/AGS/APhA/ASH/ASPC/NMA/PCNA guideline for the prevention, detection, evaluation, and management of high blood pressure in adults: A report of the American College of Cardiology/American Heart Association Task Force on Clinical Practice Guidelines. *Hypertension, 71.* https://doi.org/10.1161/hyp.0000000000000065 (accessed on 30th June 2025).

55. Haar Zeida, L., Prakash, R., Foster, S., Li, X., Bhaskar, P., Lasa, J., Raman, L., *et al.* (2024). Abstract Sa808: Validation of a modified pediatric sequential organ failure assessment score following cardiac arrest in children with cardiac disease. *Circulation.* https://www.semanticscholar.org/paper/3f691ff86c29beff8b43b3ba20cd4fd3b6ca1d69 (accessed on 30th June 2025).

NEUROLOGICAL EMERGENCIES

5

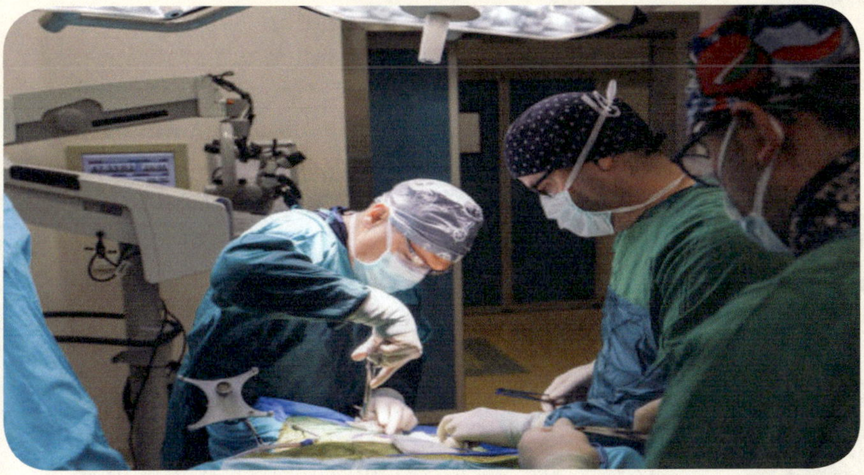

LEARNING OBJECTIVES

After studying this chapter, you will be able to:

1. Understand Types of Neurological Emergencies.
2. Explain Diagnosis and Assessment.
3. Describe Management and Treatment.

Introduction

Neurological emergencies in pediatric intensive care create a unique problem that is of an urgent nature and requires specialized knowledge. Seizures, stroke, and traumatic brain injury are hazardous to the developing brain, considering their emergent onset, which underscores the importance of quick and effective intervention. Since healthcare practitioners aim to achieve the best outcomes for the affected children, the processes responsible for these neurological conditions must be clarified. Current research emphasizes collaborative strategies used by medical teams to maximize the capacity for acting in time during emergencies (Alyea *et al.*, 2010). Furthermore, advances in resuscitation science give practitioners the necessary guides, especially on the diagnosis and management of pediatric patients with acute neurological distress (Aickin *et al.*, 2019). This chapter examines the complexity of diagnosing and managing emergencies and discusses best practices and new research that serve to advance pediatric care (Figure 5.1).

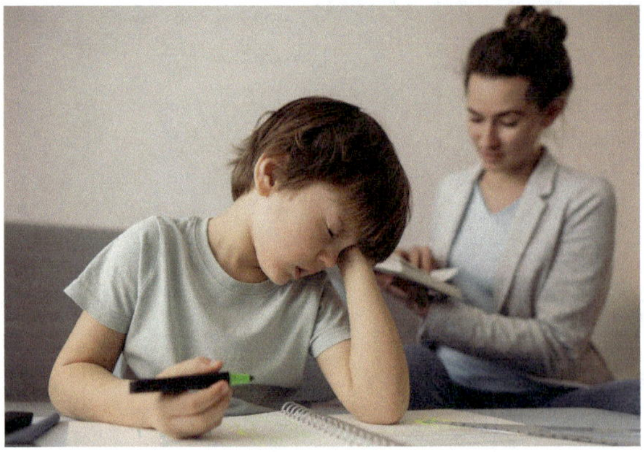

Figure 5.1. The rapid onset of conditions such as seizures, stroke, and traumatic brain injury poses significant risks to the developing brain, underscoring the importance of prompt and effective intervention.

Source: https://aayush-hospitals.com/wp-content/uploads/2024/05/child-being-tired-while-tutored-home-scaled.jpg.

5.1. Types of Neurological Emergencies

Learning Outcome

1. Focus on seizures in pediatric patients.
2. Describe acute stroke in children.
3. Discuss traumatic brain injury.
4. Explain meningitis and encephalitis.
5. Understand hydrocephalus.
6. Know brain tumors.
7. Identify neuromuscular disorders.
8. Explain status epilepticus.
9. Discuss neurogenic shock.

Neurological pediatric emergencies include a range of disorders that can require immediate treatment for their potentially deadly nature. The most frequent among them are febrile convulsions, unprovoked seizures, and an altered state of consciousness, which altogether represent a high percentage of pediatric emergency referrals. A study of 7670 children who presented at a pediatric emergency department found that 4.5% of them complained of neurological conditions, with 49% complaining of headache and nearly 15% having unprovoked seizures (Attard *et al.*, 2016). This finding points to the importance of early assessment, as children complaining of unprovoked seizures had higher admission rates—75.5%—compared to those who complained of headache (Attard *et al.*, 2016). Also, altered consciousness and other neurological presentations, though less common, also necessitate immediate evaluation due to their possible implications on the global health and welfare of the child. Familiarity with the neurologic emergencies is essential for the best management in pediatric critical care settings.

5.1.1. Seizures in Pediatric Patients

Seizure presentation in children needs careful assessment due to the variety of etiologies as well as the risk of significant morbidity. Seizures are very common among complaints brought by children presenting to pediatric emergency departments, and a good proportion of them comprise seizures. Seizures have been recognized as an emergent problem in pediatric acute care, where unprovoked seizures account for 15.3% of neurological presentations and febrile convulsions account for 14.4% of cases, a study shows (Attard *et al.*, 2016). Moreover, admission to hospital has a considerably different likelihood based on the seizure, with 75.5% of children admitted for further management with presentation of unprovoked seizures (Attard *et al.*, 2016). In the context of emergency medical services, mistriage poses a serious concern, especially in neurological cases, where 24% of target patients for intensive care presented themselves with neurological presentations, underlining the critical role played by accurate assessment in pediatric settings (Figure 5.2).

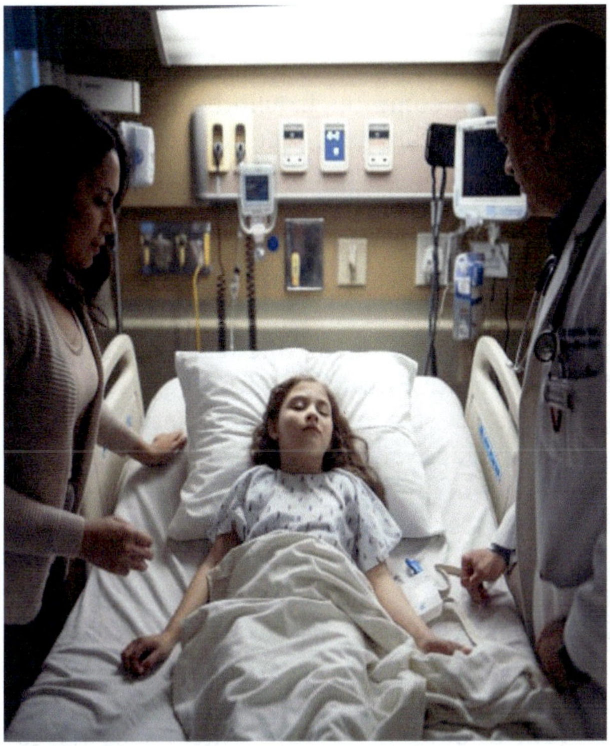

Figure 5.2. The presentation of seizures in pediatric patients necessitates careful evaluation due to the variety of underlying causes and the potential for significant morbidity.

Source: https://i0.wp.com/iem-student.org/wp-content/uploads/2025/01/a-photo-of-a-7-year-old-girl.jpg?fit=500%2C500&ssl=1.

5.1.2. Acute Stroke in Children

The acute stroke syndrome in children, while comparatively rare as a fraction of the adult population, is uniquely challenging within the pediatric intensive care setting. Pediatric stroke may be due to myriad etiologic conditions, including congenital heart disease, infection, and hematologic abnormalities, such that a nuanced approach to pathophysiology is needed to direct successful management strategies. Although prognosis in children who experience strokes is better, long-term effects on neurodevelopment, including impairment of cognition and potential disability, remain of concern. Many of these strokes are treated with a multi-disciplinary approach, including thrombolytic therapy or anticoagulation in certain cases, again illustrative of the emergent need for prompt diagnosis and intervention. Moreover, improving evidence emphasizes tight control of blood glucose as important in maximizing outcomes in critically ill children, similar to findings in adults (Ceriello *et al.*, 2010). It is thus important to grasp the varied presentations and optimal treatment of acute stroke in children to maximize the overall prognosis and developmental outcomes (Attarbaschi *et al.*, 2016).

5.1.3. Traumatic Brain Injury

Traumatic brain injury (TBI) management in the pediatric intensive care unit is particularly problematic given the developmental and physiological differences among children and adults. Identification and intervention early are extremely critical since untreated TBI can lead to grave complications like elevated intracranial pressure (ICP) and imminent herniation of the brain.

Decompressive craniectomy (DC) is now an available surgery in cases where medical management cannot sustain severe ICP, an indicator of its effectiveness in handling TBI in various resource environments (Adeleye *et al.*, 2019). Also, ongoing education and training of health professionals are essential in improving their proficiency in managing emergencies, as indicated by studies that show considerable benefits in practice and know-how through planned educational interventions (Aini *et al.*, 2021).

With emphasis on both the educational and surgical details, pediatric intensive care is better equipped to safeguard against the devastating impact of TBI, leading to better outcomes for the affected children (Figure 5.3).

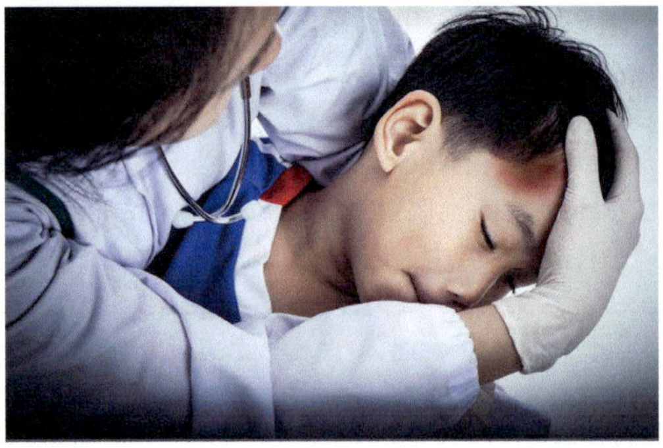

Figure 5.3. The management of traumatic brain injury (TBI) in pediatric intensive care presents unique challenges due to the physiological and developmental differences in children compared to adults.

Source: https://medicine.washu.edu/app/uploads/2017/02/KidHeadInjury.jpg.

5.1.4. Meningitis and Encephalitis

Encephalitis and meningitis are frequent neurological emergencies that need to be treated and diagnosed early to prevent the dangerous consequences. Meningitis is an inflammation of the central nervous system's protective membranes. It comes with high morbidity when left untreated in a timely manner. Pediatric patients may have special symptoms that include fever, irritability, and lethargy, among others.

Encephalitis, on the other hand, involves direct inflammation of brain tissue, typically as a result of viral infection and requiring immediate treatment with supportive therapy and therapeutics. Management protocol varies according to local epidemiology and available resources; hence, Caruso *et al.* (2013) emphasize that one needs to look at the applicability of formulated guidelines in areas of high HIV prevalence. Further, enhancement of treatment protocol for both conditions is of prime importance, as noted in Beeching *et al.* (2016), highlighting a better method of investigation and treatment in treating acute cases.

5.1.5. Hydrocephalus

Hydrocephalus is a neurological emergency that is very common in children admitted to the intensive care unit, and it is characterized by an abnormal accumulation of cerebrospinal fluid (CSF) within the ventricles of the brain. Hydrocephalus leads to increased intracranial pressure (ICP), which, in turn, leads to serious complications if not adequately diagnosed and treated. For instance, one case highlighted hydrocephalus-induced pathology following the removal of a brain tumor, with a patient aged 6 years showing profuse pulmonary edema from neurogenic causes, an example of the systemic presentation of the disease (Nakata *et al.*, 2024). Additionally, in the event of hydrocephalus occurring with other neurological conditions, such as aneurysms, it is very important to treat early. A two-year-old patient with acute hydrocephalus due to a brain aneurysm revealed the necessity for immediate external ventricular drainage to treat pressure and prevent neurological deterioration (Lagos-Servellon *et al.*, 2021). The treatment should be done promptly, as there can be chronic morbidity in children left behind if not treated early (Figure 5.4).

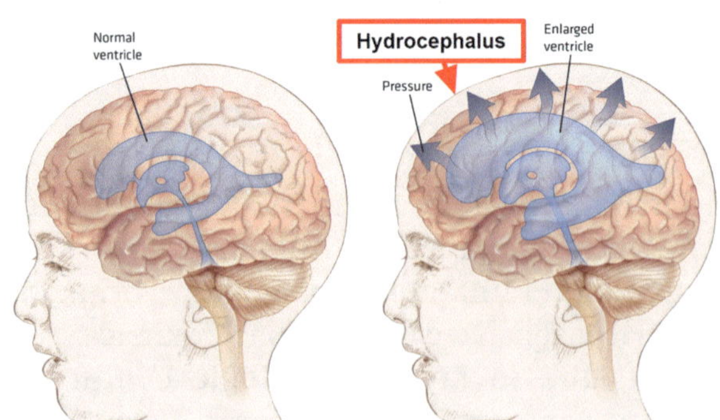

Figure 5.4. Hydrocephalus represents a critical neurological emergency often encountered in pediatric intensive care settings, characterized by an abnormal accumulation of cerebrospinal fluid (CSF) within the ventricles of the brain.

Source: https://healthjade.com/wp-content/uploads/2018/03/hydrocephalus.jpg.

5.1.6. Brain Tumors

Diagnosis and treatment of brain tumors are central aspects of intensive care unit pediatric care since tumors have a propensity to lead to neurological emergencies that require urgent treatment. Brain tumors, for example, gliomas and medulloblastomas, may result in elevated intracranial pressure and abrupt development of neurological deficits, thus presenting specific challenges to the health professionals. Imaging modalities' early detection is crucial, as delay can complicate patients' conditions and render treatment difficult. While resection surgery remains a cornerstone for the majority of tumors, combination with therapies such as chemotherapy and radiation is also pertinent, particularly when complete resection cannot be achieved. Expert consensus indicates that personalized plans of management must be followed, particularly in the setting of the increasing recognition of immune-related treatment adverse events (Bryan *et al.*, 2021). Also, knowledge of the burden of tumors at the epidemiological level emphasizes the need for systematic management and monitoring in this vulnerable population (Donna *et al.*, 2019).

5.1.7. Neuromuscular Disorders

Neuromuscular illnesses are a leading category of neurological emergencies in pediatric intensive care, since they have a tendency to induce acute respiratory failure on the basis of their effect on muscle function and on the respiratory device. From congenital myopathies to autoimmune conditions like myasthenia gravis, these illnesses often present with abrupt impairment of respiratory capacity, requiring immediate medical intervention. The respiratory distress from bulbar compromise and weakness of the muscles can result in hypercapnia, retained secretions, and associated consequences of pneumonia, eventually aggravating the child's morbidity and mortality risk. Acute presentation of chronic respiratory failure necessitates timely identification, particularly in the slowly progressive neuromuscular disorders, as well as immediate treatment of sudden-onset respiratory failure in more acute progressive illnesses. Proper management interventions like noninvasive ventilation and manual facilitation of cough are crucial in mitigating such complications and ensuring the best outcome among infected children's patients (Mongini *et al.*, 2019; Caliskan *et al.*, 2017) (Figure 5.5).

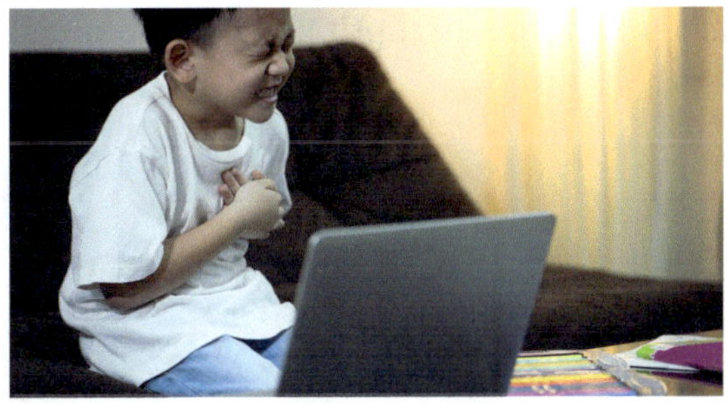

Figure 5.5. Neuromuscular disorders represent a significant category of neurological emergencies within pediatric intensive care settings, as they often lead to acute respiratory failure due to their impact on muscle function and respiratory system.

Source: https://cdn3.rainbowhospitals.in/blog/banner_desktop_images/7BWfukUS2g4OHYQnQqTs7SgPOsDxRE29QKQ6Ngz8.jpg.

5.1.8. Status Epilepticus

Among neurological emergencies, status epilepticus (SE) is a condition that demands urgent intervention, especially in pediatric intensive care units. Defined as seizures lasting or recurring with no return of consciousness in between, SE carries serious risks such as permanent neurological damage. Among the recent studies, one highlighted that approximately 15.3% of children presenting to emergency rooms with neurological complaints were experiencing unprovoked seizures, which indicates the prevalence of such presentations in pediatric patients (Attard *et al.*, 2016). In addition, the impact of prolonged seizure activity among children is not only associated with the acute presentation but also leads to cognitive impairment, affects development as a whole, and, in some extreme instances, leads to fatalities. The strong need for effective treatment protocols is otherwise illustrated by the relationship of neurological sequelae from seizure disorders, as seen in acute cases of preeclampsia impacting the brain's function (Emonts *et al.*, 2016). Immediate recognition and therapy of status epilepticus in pediatric care, therefore, is a matter of utmost significance.

5.1.9. Neurogenic Shock

Neurogenic shock is a dangerous and complex issue in pediatric intensive care, resulting primarily from an extreme disruption of autonomic pathways due to spinal cord trauma or other neurologic insult.

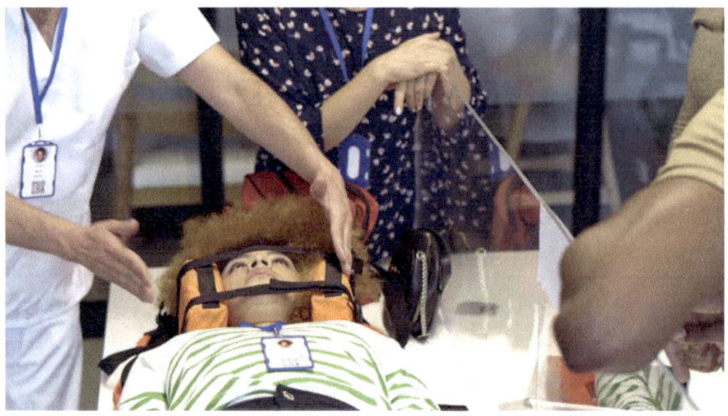

Figure 5.6. Neurogenic shock represents a significant and complex challenge within the realm of pediatric intensive care, primarily resulting from a severe disruption of autonomic pathways following spinal cord injury or other neurological insults.

Source: https://media.gettyimages.com/id/1665875282/video/professional-doctor-immobilizes-the-head-of-one-of-the-employees-of-an-office-to-whom-he-is.jpg?s=640x640&k=20&c=Lno6dKi4LRtjizo2iyf9JO3xJtpRFee8V2xk1mVV3kc=.

It is a process that involves loss of sympathetic tone and leads to severe hypotension and bradycardia, potentially risking perfusion to vital organs. Optimal management of neurogenic shock requires a sharp understanding of the pathophysiological rationale and the initiation of targeted therapeutic interventions. For instance, precise administration of inotropes may be used to ensure hemodynamic stability, as demonstrated by Bhambre *et al.* (2025), whereas fluid resuscitation is required to restore circulation and avoid secondary organ damage. Additionally, clinicians must exercise caution in observing and making adjustments to the treatment regimens based on the response of different patients, highlighting the importance of evidence-based practice while adequately managing this critical condition (Alers *et al.*, 2020) (Figure 5.6).

Test Your Knowledge

1. How is acute bacterial meningitis recognized as a neurological emergency in children?
2. What types of traumatic brain injury (TBI) are most common in pediatric patients?

5.2. Diagnosis and Assessment

Learning Outcome

1. Understand clinical presentation of neurological emergencies.
2. Know the importance of history taking.
3. Learn neurological examination techniques.
4. Focus on imaging studies.
5. Discuss laboratory tests and their relevance.
6. Describe electroencephalogram (EEG) usage.
7. Know differential diagnosis considerations.
8. Understand the role of telemedicine in assessment.
9. Discuss the importance of rapid assessment protocols.

Accurate diagnosis and estimation are precious components in the treatment of pediatric intensive care neurological emergencies since they determine patient outcomes to some extent. The initial evaluation includes meticulous history-taking and detailed physical examination to identify the emergent presentation of neurological signs, such as altered consciousness or seizures. Furthermore, sophisticated diagnostic tools, like neuroimaging modalities and continuous monitoring, play a critical role in identifying the underlying causes of these emergencies. With the complexities that are associated with pediatric neurological conditions, medical practitioners are aided by using clinical judgment and established guidelines in navigating these evaluations. For instance, untimely triage and misdiagnosis within emergency settings can lead to incorrect treatment, as evidenced by findings that neurological illnesses were the most commonly misdiagnosed conditions in intensive care, constituting 24% of the patients (Bucher *et al.*, 2020). Early identification of risk factors, including hypertension among children, can also permit interventions at the appropriate time, which are essential for good outcomes (Agabiti-Rosei *et al.*, 2016).

5.2.1. Clinical Presentation of Neurological Emergencies

Presentation of neurological emergencies in children is typically a mixture of acute symptoms and signs necessitating emergent medical assessment. Common presentations may be changes in level of consciousness, seizure, and focal neurological deficit, and are expressions of underlying pathologies such as encephalitis, traumatic brain injury, or vascular injury. For instance, preeclampsia, severe in its nature, is complicated by neurological presentation such as posterior reversible encephalopathy syndrome (PRES) that can present with sudden visual disturbances and potentially permanent injury if not managed (Emonts *et al.*, 2016). Furthermore, hypertension (HTN) is now a prominent problem in this group, and it results in the development of cerebrovascular events and underlines the need for early detection and intervention strategies (Agabiti-Rosei *et al.*, 2016). Given the diversity of clinical presentation, it is critical that clinicians who work in pediatric intensive care understand these emergencies deeply (Figure 5.7).

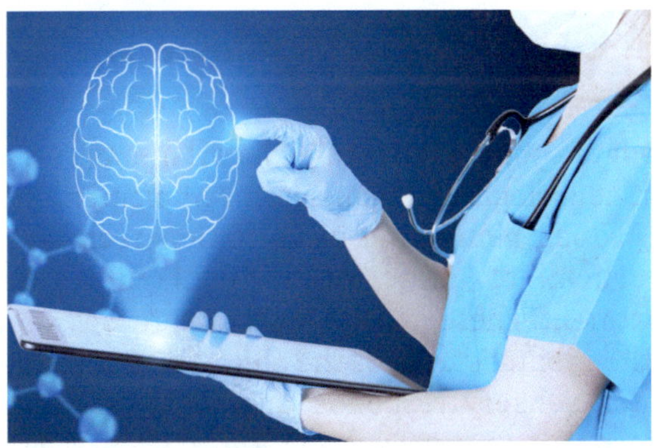

Figure 5.7. The clinical presentation of neurological emergencies in pediatric patients often encompasses a range of acute symptoms that necessitate immediate medical attention.

Source: https://idreamcareer.com/wp-content/uploads/2023/04/how-to-become-a-neurologist.webp.

5.2.2. Importance of History Taking

In relation to neurological emergencies in pediatric intensive care, the importance of getting a proper history cannot be overstated. Proper patient history is key to establishing an acute presentation's underlying conditions that may be adding to it, such as hypertension or renal problems. Hypertension, for instance, is becoming increasingly considered a primary health concern for children and is most commonly linked to grave consequences if left untreated (Agabiti-Rosei *et al.*, 2016). In cases where secondary hypertension is suspected, such as in renal vascular diseases, taking history is important in the diagnosis of conditions such as renovascular disease, which can present with signs and symptoms such as failure to thrive or muscle weakness (Dionísio *et al.*, 2015). By gaining accurate histories of the child's past medical history, genetic predispositions, and novel changes in behavior or physical status, clinicians are able to accelerate pertinent interventions and target organ damage risks, highlighting the role of history-taking in the management of children.

5.2.3. Neurological Examination Techniques

From the point of view of pediatric intensive care unit neurologic emergencies, the implementation of proper neurologic examination techniques is crucial to allow for early diagnosis and treatment. These include systematic assessment of the mental status of the child, cranial nerves, motor, sensory response, and reflexes. Adding a focused airway examination, particularly in those with recognized anatomical derangements, is necessary to avoid sedation-associated complications, as highlighted in Charles *et al.* (2019). Additionally, one cannot overstate the importance of size- and age-related equipment to facilitate adequate neurological assessment, as this allows clinicians to adequately screen for possible neurological deficits in children. Improving the precision of such an evaluation may also depend on concerted action of multidisciplinary teams according to guidelines issued by specialist agencies to strengthen clinical practice (Paul *et al.*, 2017). Such an integrated approach ultimately allows for proper and timely management of severe neurological disease in children (Figure 5.8).

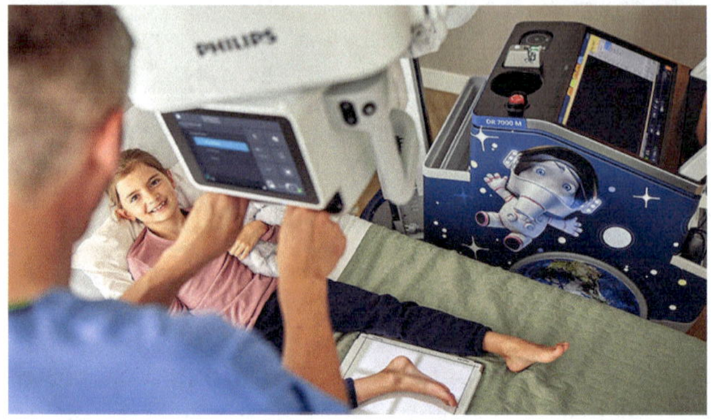

Figure 5.8. The importance of age- and size-appropriate equipment for effective neurological assessment cannot be overstated, ensuring that clinicians can accurately evaluate potential neurological deficits in pediatric patients.

Source: https://www.philips.com/c-dam/corporate/newscenter/global/standard/resources/healthcare/2024/q-and-a-with-atul-gupta-md/dr-7000-m-application-tech-pediatric-eth.jpg.

5.2.4. Imaging Studies (CT, MRI)

In pediatric intensive care, imaging tests such as CT and MRI are solely responsible for diagnosing and managing neurological emergencies. The fine capability of these imaging techniques enables healthcare personnel to see and classify various types of intracranial pathologies, thereby determining treatment. For instance, subpial hemorrhages, which are a common occurrence in neonates, are best assessed by MRI to assess their size and location, which are strongly predictive of motor outcome (Martinez-Correa *et al.*, 2025). Additionally, follow-up assessment of midline shift on CT provides useful information on intracranial pressure, which is required for the guidance of urgent therapeutic management (Kartik *et al.*, 2024). The ability of imaging studies to reveal accurate anatomical and pathological information not only helps achieve accurate identification of emergent disorders but also greatly impacts the overall management and progression of pediatric patients with neurological catastrophes. This emphasizes the utility of imaging in pediatric neurocritical care as unavoidable.

5.2.5. Laboratory Tests and Their Relevance

Laboratory tests form a critical part of the treatment of pediatric intensive care neurological emergencies because they provide critical information needed for diagnosis and management. Laboratory tests enable clinicians to diagnose underlying metabolic derangements, which are frequent in emergencies such as inborn errors of metabolism and acute lymphoblastic leukemia (ALL).

For instance, the findings of a study uncovered that a significant percentage of children with metabolic disorders exhibited background abnormalities and seizures apparent on electroencephalograms (EEGs), hence guiding therapy interventions (Sen *et al.*, 2024). Additionally, laboratory markers such as levels of leukocytes and inflammatory cytokines like CRP and procalcitonin have been shown to be correlated with worsening in ALL patients, hence serving as predictors for clinical deterioration (Kurakbayev *et al.*, 2024). Such findings highlight the necessity of monitoring through laboratory assessments on a regular basis to initiate timely interventions that could potentially improve the outcomes of the patient within the PICU setting (Figure 5.9).

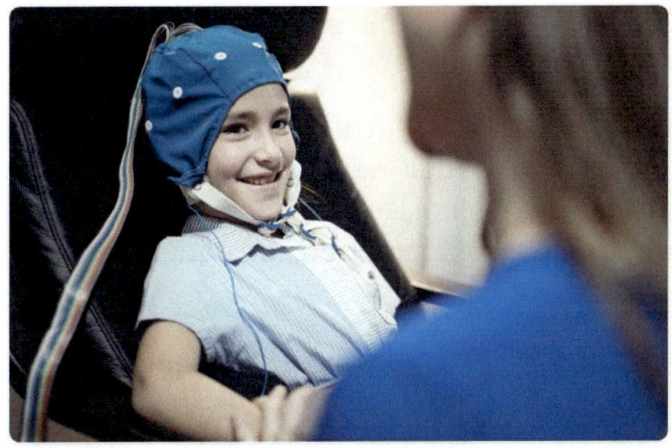

Figure 5.9. Laboratory tests play a crucial role in the management of neurological emergencies in pediatric intensive care, as they provide essential data for diagnosis and treatment.

Source: https://www.news-medical.net/image-handler/picture/2021/4/shutterstock_1260284200.jpg.

5.2.6. Electroencephalogram (EEG) Usage

In pediatric intensive care, the use of Electroencephalogram (EEG) technology has been an indispensable diagnostic and management tool in the treatment of neurological emergencies. EEG is also crucial to the detection of seizure activity and other abnormal brain activities that are most often predictors of severe neurological conditions. For example, for patients suffering from severe preeclampsia resulting in Posterior Reversible Encephalopathy Syndrome (PRES), EEG can be used to offer critical information about the patient's brain activity, allowing for prompt interventions to prevent long-term injury (Emonts *et al.*, 2016). Furthermore, the application of EEG in an interdisciplinary context, e.g., Neurointensive Care Nurseries (NICN), allows for comprehensive monitoring of high-risk infants to maximize treatment regimens and improve outcomes (Ferriero *et al.*, 2019). Application of EEG thus not only aids in early diagnosis but also allows for overall management of pediatric patients with catastrophic neurological emergencies.

5.2.7. Differential Diagnosis Considerations

Under pediatric intensive care settings, which come under neurological emergencies, differential diagnosis must be done taking great care of clinical presentation and pathophysiology.

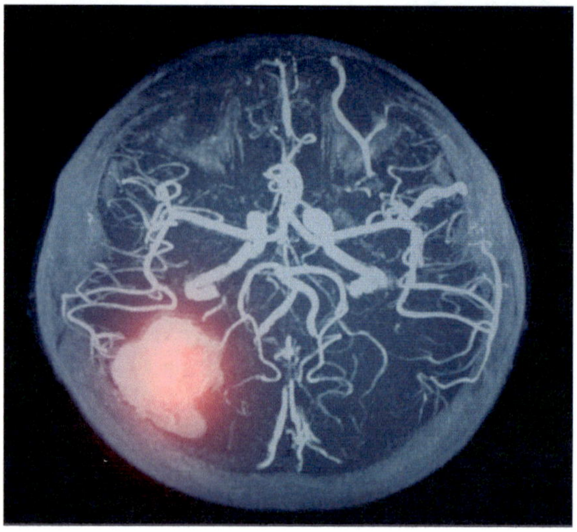

Figure 5.10. Effective evaluation employs tools such as the Glasgow Coma Scale and immediate imaging, such as head CT and MRI, to rule out structural or ischemic causes.

Source: https://chblob.icloudhospital.com/images/3-b540e3d4-59c6-476b-82d2-06448f52a936.jpg.

Signs such as metabolic illnesses, exemplified by propionic acidemia, can have multiple presentations, including hypotonia and neurological dysfunction, more likely to complicate the clinical presentation and to mimic that of other life-threatening diseases such as botulism or acute inflammatory demyelinating polyneuropathy (Allison *et al.*, 2024). Therefore, timely diagnosis is crucial in an effort to identify reversible causes and minimize long-term neurological sequelae (Sanchez-Albisua, 2023). Adequate assessment employs tools such as the Glasgow Coma Scale and urgent imaging, including head CT and MRI, to rule out structural or ischemic causes. By identifying the wide variety of possible conditions that can produce a child's altered neurologic status, pediatric intensivists can create tailored interventions aimed at minimizing morbidity and maximizing outcomes (Figure 5.10).

5.2.8. Role of Telemedicine in Assessment

Telemedicine incorporation in pediatric intensive care neurological emergencies assessment is a shift from traditional healthcare provision with emphasis on urgency and effectiveness of patient assessment. Telemedicine provides quick access to specialty care, which is critical in emergency situations where interventions with immediate needs can become the difference in outcome.

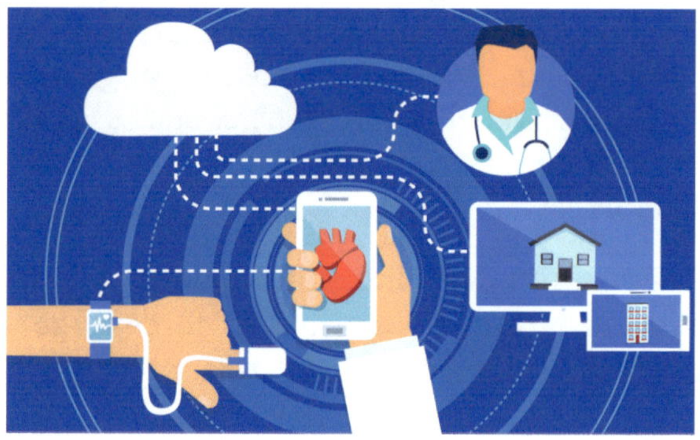

Figure 5.11. Telemedicine facilitates immediate access to specialized care, which is particularly crucial in emergencies where time-sensitive interventions can significantly influence outcomes.

Source: https://blog.pepid.com/wp-content/uploads/2024/05/shutterstock_1467777668-Converted-1-1080x675.png.

As Antodaro *et al.* (2023) explains, this technology enables a care model that is focused on accessibility, wherein families are in a position to access healthcare professionals from other locations. Moreover, eradicating geographic limitations is imperative when handling pediatric neurological emergencies, such that there is prompt consultation and evaluation. This points to the need for research into telemedicine's' efficacy and safety beyond the controlled research environments as described by Burner *et al.* (2021), where there is a clear agenda for research into telehealth solutions in emergency medicine. In the end, Pediatric intensive care can enhance its capabilities of assessment through telemedicine that assist patients in the most severe cases (Figure 5.11).

5.2.9. Importance of Rapid Assessment Protocols

In pediatric intensive care situations of neurological emergencies, utilization of rapid assessment protocols plays a crucial role in helping deliver interventions promptly and effectively. The protocols enable one to rapidly identify life-threatening situations that can be used in informed decision-making at high-stress levels. For instance, rapid assessments can facilitate the immediate evaluation of the neurological status of a child, which can influence prognosis and treatment outcomes. The ability to triage patients quickly not only aids in resource utilization but also allows for multidisciplinary treatment among healthcare teams, aligning with the complexities of pediatric critical care. Additionally, as it has been discovered in trauma care practice, teachings about events that require immediate intervention, such as those referenced in contemporary studies, highlight the significance of organized approaches in handling acute illnesses (Murray *et al.*, 2020). By and large, rapid assessment protocols are a central aspect in improving the delivery of care to children with neurological emergencies (Agabiti-Rosei *et al.*, 2016).

Test Your Knowledge

1. What role does neuroimaging (CT, MRI) play in diagnosing neurological emergencies in children?
2. What bedside monitoring tools (e.g., EEG, ICP monitoring) are commonly used in PICU for neurological assessment?

5.3. Management and Treatment

Learning Outcome

1. Explain initial stabilization of the patient.
2. Understand pharmacological interventions.
3. Know surgical options for emergencies.
4. Discuss supportive care measures.
5. Focus on a multidisciplinary approach to treatment.
6. Describe the role of rehabilitation in recovery.
7. Focus on family involvement in care.
8. Explain ethical considerations in treatment.
9. Understand long-term management strategies.

Effective management and treatment of pediatric intensive care neurological emergencies are crucial because these conditions can call for prompt and proper intervention. Prehospital treatment by emergency medical services (EMS) can influence outcomes to a large extent, especially when advanced life support (ALS) is utilized in stabilizing the patients before their hospitalization in critical care centers (Bucher *et al.*, 2020). When admitted to pediatric intensive care units, physicians must properly triage and assess neurological symptoms that range from febrile seizures to spontaneous seizures and altered mental status. Interestingly, it has been seen that among children who visit emergency departments, approximately 4.5% of them have neurological disorders, thereby confirming the need for correct workups to guide treatment (Attard *et al.*, 2016). Ultimately, early intervention can increase the recovery rate and decrease complications, thus emphasizing the significance of well-structured management protocols in the pediatric critical care environment.

5.3.1. Initial Stabilization of the Patient

Initial stabilization of an injured child in a case of a neurological emergency is crucial to optimal outcomes and mitigating any potential long-term consequences. It begins with a swift assessment of airway, breathing, and circulation—most commonly known as the ABCs of trauma care. In severe injury, that is, motor vehicle collisions, the severity scores of injury and lab values must be closely monitored since they can forecast the evolution of acute kidney injury (AKI), which takes place in approximately one-third of such children (Kuok *et al.*, 2022). Further, early interventions such as intubation and management of critical lab values are vital. It is of paramount importance to manage immediate interventions alongside continuous observation in order to modify treatment approaches effectively, with the assurance that vital signs are stabilized prior to transferring the patient to a more advanced care environment (Song *et al.*, 2021). Finally, careful and anticipatory stabilization lays the groundwork for additional intensive care management (Figure 5.12).

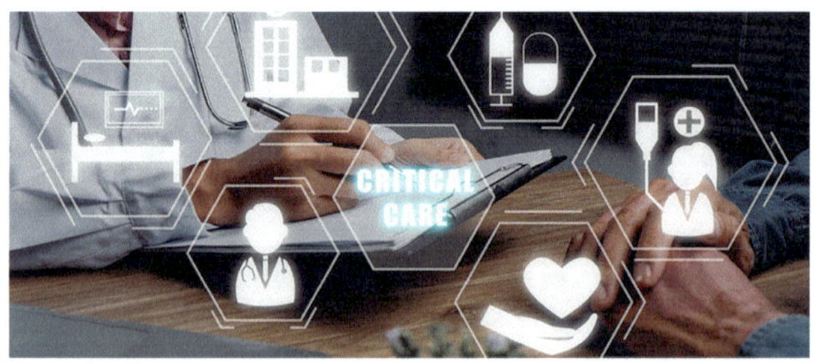

Figure 5.12. Timely interventions, including intubation and managing critical laboratory values, are essential.

Source: https://www.diginerve.com/blogs/wp-content/uploads/2023/09/22.jpg.

5.3.2. Pharmacological Interventions

Pharmacotherapy plays a pivotal role in treating neurological emergencies within pediatric intensive care units, particularly with the handling of such conditions as severe hypertension. The increased prevalence of hypertension among children's populations necessitates special treatment measures aimed at eliminating the threat of target organ damage; uncontrolled hypertension can lead to serious complications involving neurological dysfunctions and cardiovascular emergencies (Agabiti-Rosei *et al.*, 2016). In cases of secondary hypertension due to underlying disease, such as renovascular disease, the demand for efficacious pharmacologic intervention becomes even more critical. For instance, one notable example involved a 13-month-old with a refractory hypertensive emergency that was unresponsive to multiple antihypertensive regimens, highlighting the importance of timely and proper adjustment of medications (Dionísio *et al.*, 2015). A tailored pharmacological treatment, thus, not only facilitates timely relief from symptoms but also contributes to improved long-term management in children with neurological emergencies, underlining the importance of such treatments in critical care.

5.3.3. Surgical Options for Emergencies

Within the context of neurological emergencies in pediatric intensive care, surgery generally becomes unavoidable to correct acute conditions such as traumatic brain injury or cerebrovascular accident. Emergency surgical options are guided by recommendations that prioritize clinical necessity and the safeguarding of patients and medical staff. For instance, in an intracranial hemorrhage that is life-threatening, immediate decompressive craniectomy may be indicated to decompress and prevent further neurological damage. Treatment of infections, such as brain abscesses, can also be achieved through surgical drainage in order to prevent severe complications. It is essential to adhere to protocols in place in order to limit respiratory risk, especially in the context of infectious disease, as described in more recent literature emphasizing strict infection control in the operating room (Liang *et al.*, 2020). Essentially, effective surgical care not only aims to stabilize the patient but also preserves neurological function, so an individualized treatment plan is essential in critical care cases (Paul *et al.*, 2017) (Figure 5.13).

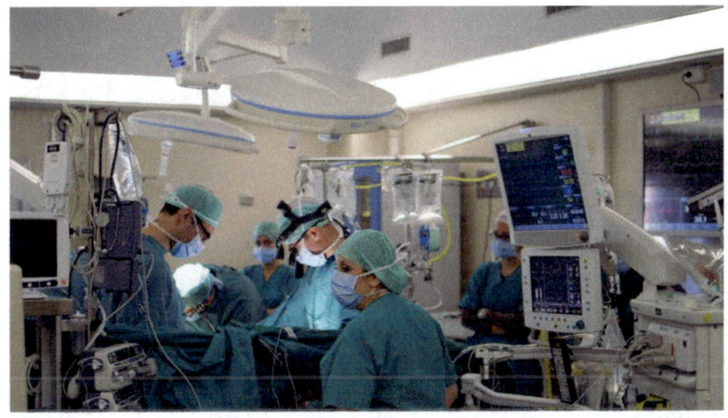

Figure 5.13. Emergency surgical options are guided by principles that prioritize clinical urgency and the protection of both patients and healthcare workers.

Source: https://upload.wikimedia.org/wikipedia/commons/thumb/2/2e/Cardiac_surgery_operating_room.jpg/1200px-Cardiac_surgery_operating_room.jpg.

5.3.4. Supportive Care Measures

In pediatric intensive care, supportive care measures are crucial to stabilize the patient and aid recovery in the event of neurological emergencies. The supportive care consists of respiratory and hemodynamic stability management, which is vital in managing the conditions that can lead to acute or chronic neurological impairment. For instance, in a 2-month-old infant case that highlighted the importance of ongoing supportive care, the patient exhibited worsening breathing difficulties despite initial provision of supportive care, which ultimately required hospitalization and admission to an intensive care unit (Patel *et al.*, 2013). Similarly, yet another significant case illustrated how supportive care would avert life-threatening complications of heatstroke in children, where aggressive management ameliorated multiple organ failures and neurologic insults (Ozcetin *et al.*, 2012). These cases illustrate the central role of supportive care not only in early stabilization but also in theprevention of long-term neurological sequelae in children with critical illness.

5.3.5. Multidisciplinary Approach to Treatment

The diversified character of neurological emergencies in pediatric intensive care calls for a treatment approach that considers the intricacy of the patient's needs via multidisciplinary care. In situations such as those caused by *Neisseria meningitidis*, the rapid manifestation of neurological symptoms necessitates immediate treatment by experts like pediatric intensivists, neurologists, and infectious disease experts.

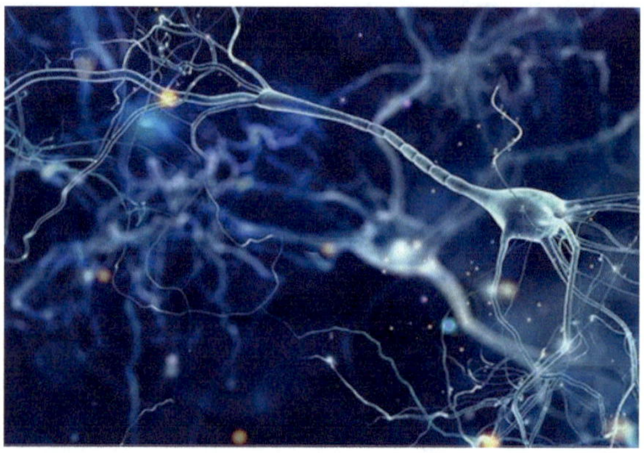

Figure 5.14. In cases such as those involving *Neisseria meningitidis*, the rapid onset of neurological symptoms requires immediate intervention from various specialists, including pediatric intensivists, neurologists, and infectious disease experts.

Source: https://images.medicinenet.com/images/article/main_image/multiple-sclerosis.jpg?output-quality=75.

Early communication of these specialists is to blame for the institution of appropriate antibiotic treatment and managing patients' complications, thereby reducing mortality and long-term neurological morbidity. Secondly, because the prevalence of chronic disease rises in pediatric populations, the demands for coordinated care continue to increase, which underscores the benefits of concerted, multidisciplinary teams in the intensive care setting. Literature indicates that these collaborative models benefit patient outcomes and also inform palliative care decision-making, allowing families to navigate challenging end-of-life conditions (G-A *et al.*, 2025; Sanderson *et al.*, 2020) (Figure 5.14).

5.3.6. Role of Rehabilitation in Recovery

The role of rehabilitation in the recovery of pediatric patients from neurological emergencies is crucial in achieving optimal outcomes. Rehabilitation not only contributes to physical recovery but also contributes to mental and emotional enhancement, which is highly significant for holistic recovery following critical illness. Services tailored to the particular requirements of children, such as speech and occupational therapy, are also highly significant in overcoming developmental problems that may arise following an injury or illness. Besides, progress in supportive care treatments like extracorporeal membrane oxygenation (ECMO) has transformed survival rates among critically ill children to a great extent, as statistics have revealed 80% survival among patients treated with ECMO therapy for severe lung injuries, which facilitates successful rehabilitation efforts (Elahi *et al.*, 2017). As shown through recent interventions, the addition of broad-based rehabilitation services can lead to substantial gains in quality of life, highlighting its central role within the recovery process.

5.3.7. Family Involvement in Care

In the context of pediatric intensive care neurological emergencies, family involvement in care is a very important factor that determines patient outcomes decisively. Families tend to be an important support system, providing emotional stability and consistency for the child during crucial medical interventions. For instance, in the treatment of such diseases as Guillain-Barré syndrome, which is treatable by multifaceted therapeutic strategies like plasmapheresis, as discussed in Indrawan *et al.* (2025), inclusion of the family in decision-making and care processes can enhance compliance with treatment and satisfaction in general. Moreover, conditions like pediatric multi-system inflammatory syndrome (MIS-C) demonstrate that family involvement is key to effective treatment of complex symptoms, including neurological symptoms, in a manner that ensures families are informed and prepared for the long-term care required during hospital stay, as highlighted in Botan *et al.* (2023). A family-centered approach thus guarantees holistic person-centered attention, advancing enhanced health and resilience in both the parent and the child (Figure 5.15).

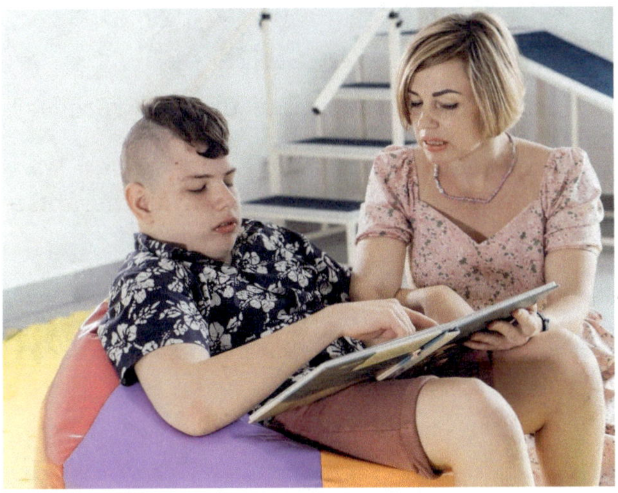

Figure 5.15. Families often serve as a vital support system, providing emotional stability and continuity for the child during critical medical interventions.

Source: https://ldnetwork.org/fixefybo/2024/11/family-involvement-in-transition.webp.

5.3.8. Ethical Considerations in Treatment

Where pediatric intensive care neurological emergencies are involved, ethical concerns come to the fore, particularly with regard to prognostication and management decisions. The mortal-peril nature of brain injuries in the majority of cases presents challenges to approximating possible recovery outcomes, where the stigma of inaccurate projections is critical. Misevaluation will lead to either unjustified withdrawal of life-support therapy or seeking futile interventions, both encompassing consequential ethical dilemmas on the quality of life and the family's wishes. American Heart Association's findings highlight the need for improvements in neurological prognostication practices, pointing out the poor quality of existing evidence and the resulting uncertainty in results (Romergryko *et al.*, 2019). In addition, with treatment practices evolving further, for example, the more recent advent of ketamine infusions as a treatment for acute pain, there is a necessity to create consensus guidelines to encourage ethical practice, minimize risks, and optimize care for vulnerable child patients (Eric *et al.*, 2018).

5.3.9. Long-Term Management Strategies

Successful long-term management strategies are crucial within the treatment of children who present with neurological emergencies since they will have significant implications for recovery and quality of life. Following acute neurological injury, long-term follow-up care must include regular review by multidisciplinary teams to monitor neurological function, intellectual growth, and emotional stability. Incorporation of formalized programs of rehabilitation will aid in optimal recovery, with physical and neurological rehabilitation addressed as appropriate to individual needs. Interventions must also go towards addressing the psychosocial needs of care because involvement of the patient and parent in treatment facilitates triggering of resilience as well as adaptation to changes in health conditions. As is evident from studies aimed at burnout in clinicians, proper adherence to long-term management protocols can alleviate stress from healthcare professionals, hence enhancing the quality of care being delivered (Downing *et al.*, 2018). Developing harmonious working relationships among care teams is essential, harmonizing strategies in accordance with ordered guidelines that ensure consistency and effectiveness in management of complex cases (Paul *et al.*, 2017) (Figure 5.16).

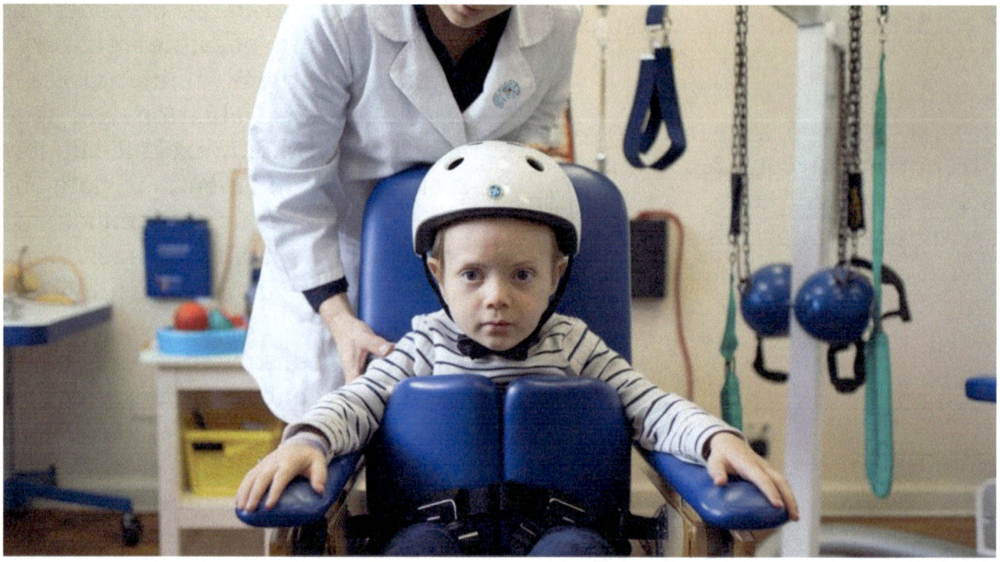

Figure 5.16. Incorporating structured rehabilitation programs can facilitate optimal recovery, promoting physical and neurological rehabilitation tailored to needs.

Source: https://ptkids.co.uk/wp-content/uploads/2024/11/a-photo-of-a-pediatric-physiotherapist-working-wit-w80QUBFEQpClot1AAwNFag-0cx4dlrNSOiZGW0Clj7LNQ-1024x574.jpeg.

Test Your Knowledge

1. How are infections such as bacterial meningitis and encephalitis managed in the PICU?
2. What are the indications for sedation and neuromuscular blockade in children with severe brain injury?

SUMMARY

Pediatric intensive care setting analysis of neurologic emergencies highlights the utmost significance of proper triage and appropriate handling of patients presenting with neurological manifestations. It is substantiated by statistics that a significant number of children, approximately 4.5%, present to emergency departments with neurological complaints, the most common being headache and seizure (Attard *et al.*, 2016). Also, the triage practice study reveals a concerning trend whereby 2% of patients misclassified as Basic Life Support (BLS) were admitted to the critical care units, demonstrating the serious consequences of misclassification (Bucher *et al.*, 2020). This underlines the value of improved protocols and training for healthcare professionals to enhance decision-making in the event of emergencies. Ultimately, strategically managing such challenges can lead to better results for pediatric patients and guarantee that the emergent nature of neurological emergencies is met with the corresponding level of care.

In the context of pediatric intensive care neurologic emergencies, several key aspects arise that reflect the intricacies involved in managing such acute conditions. First and foremost, the increasing prevalence of hypertension in children emphasizes the need for heightened vigilance and prompt action, given its long-term impact on cardiovascular health in children (Agabiti-Rosei *et al.*, 2016). Furthermore, the recent advances in resuscitation science identify the importance of evidence-based recommendations, including the use of dispatcher-assisted cardiopulmonary resuscitation and the establishment of cardiac arrest centers. The methods are important in improving outcomes following cardiac events in adults and children (Aickin *et al.*, 2019). In addition, it is important to understand cardiovascular risk factor clustering in order not to delay management and prevention initiatives. Generally, these results highlight the necessity for ongoing research and policy-making to enhance children's care in the occurrence of neurological emergencies, thereby enhancing health outcomes in vulnerable populations.

KEY TERMS FROM THIS CHAPTER

- Seizures
- Traumatic brain injury
- Headache
- Infection
- Pathophysiology
- Cognition
- Anticoagulation
- Decompressive craniectomy (DC)
- Stroke
- Febrile convulsions
- Consciousness
- Hematologic abnormalities
- Neurodevelopment
- Thrombolytic therapy
- Intracranial pressure (ICP)
- Meningitis

CRITICAL THINKING QUESTIONS

1. **What is the most common cause of altered mental status in pediatric patients?**
   a. Stroke
   b. Seizures
   c. Hypoglycemia
   d. Trauma
2. **A child presents with status epilepticus. What is the first-line treatment?**
   a. Phenobarbital
   b. Phenytoin
   c. Midazolam or Lorazepam
   d. Mannitol
3. **Which clinical sign indicates increased intracranial pressure (ICP)?**
   a. Hypothermia
   b. Bradycardia and hypertension
   c. Tachycardia and hypotension
   d. Fixed miosis
4. **What is the most appropriate initial imaging for a child with a sudden onset of focal neurological deficits?**
   a. MRI with contrast
   b. X-ray of the skull
   c. Non-contrast CT head
   d. EEG
5. **In a suspected case of bacterial meningitis, what is the priority before lumbar puncture?**
   a. Administer corticosteroids
   b. Perform EEG
   c. Administer empiric antibiotics
   d. Wait for MRI

Short Answer Questions

1. What are the common types of neurological emergencies encountered in the pediatric intensive care setting?
2. How do seizures and status epilepticus present differently in children compared to adults?
3. What are the key elements of neurological examination in critically ill children?
4. How is the Glasgow Coma Scale (GCS) adapted for pediatric patients?
5. What is the initial management approach to status epilepticus in pediatric patients?
6. How are elevated intracranial pressure and cerebral edema treated in the PICU?

Answers to Critical Thinking Questions

1. (c) 2. (c) 3. (b) 4. (c) 5. (c)

REFERENCES

1. Adeleye, A. O., Clavijo, A., Johnson, E. D., *et al.* (2019). The role of decompressive craniectomy in limited resource environments. https://core.ac.uk/download/487079900.pdf (accessed on 30th June 2025).
2. Agabiti-Rosei, E., Cruickshank, J. K., Dominiczak, A., *et al.* (2016). 2016 European Society of Hypertension guidelines for the management of high blood pressure in children and adolescents. https://core.ac.uk/download/46165193.pdf (accessed on 30th June 2025).
3. Ahmad, A., Imran, M., & Ahsan, H. (2023). Biomarkers as biomedical bioindicators: Approaches and techniques for the detection, analysis, and validation of novel biomarkers of diseases. *Pharmaceutics, 15*, 1630. https://doi.org/10.3390/pharmaceutics15061630 (accessed on 30th June 2025).
4. Aickin, R., Andersen, L. W., Atkins, D. L., *et al.* (2019). 2019 international consensus on cardiopulmonary resuscitation and emergency cardiovascular care science with treatment recommendations: Summary from the Basic Life Support; Advanced Life Support; Pediatric Life Support; Neonatal Life Support; Education, Implementation, and Teams; and First Aid Task Forces.
5. Aini, D. N., Alfaray, R. I., Batsaikhan, S., *et al.* (2021). The effectiveness of classic lecture and workshop as interventions to improve primary health care providers' knowledge and skill on the management of pediatric emergencies: A case study. https://core.ac.uk/download/386288335.pdf (accessed on 30th June 2025).
6. Alers, A., Bendas, C., Dammann, K., *et al.* (2020). Resuscitation endpoints in traumatic shock: A focused review with emphasis on point-of-care approaches. https://core.ac.uk/download/322580765.pdf (accessed on 30th June 2025).
7. Alyea, J. M., Kochhar, K., & Zollinger, T. W. (2010). Report of responses to the 2004, 2006, and 2008 Physician Assistant Re-Licensure Surveys. https://core.ac.uk/download/46959932.pdf (accessed on 30th June 2025).
8. Anderson, B. R., Ivascu, N. S., Brodie, D., Weingarten, J. A., Manoach, S., Smith, A., Millerman, K., *et al.* (2020). Breaking silos: The team-based approach to coronavirus disease 2019 pandemic staffing. *Critical Care Explorations, 2*, e0265–e0265. https://doi.org/10.1097/cce.0000000000000265 (accessed on 30th June 2025).
9. Antodaro, F., Argentiero, A., Bassi, M., *et al.* (2023). Use of telemedicine healthcare systems in pediatric assistance at territorial level: Consensus document of the Italian Society of Telemedicine (SIT), of the Italian Society of Preventive and Social Pediatrics (SIPPS), of the Italian Society of Pediatric Primary Care (SICuPP), of the Italian Federation of Pediatric Doctors (FIMP), and of the Syndicate of Family Pediatrician Doctors (SIMPeF). https://core.ac.uk/download/554207100.pdf (accessed on 30th June 2025).
10. Attarbaschi, A., Barzilai, S., Escherich, G., *et al.* (2016). Consensus definitions of 14 severe acute toxic effects for childhood lymphoblastic leukemia treatment: A Delphi consensus. https://core.ac.uk/download/42370388.pdf (accessed on 30th June 2025).
11. Attard, S., Cappello, A., Duca, B., *et al.* (2016). A review of attendances at Pediatric Accident and Emergency Department at Mater Dei Hospital for neurological complaints patient. https://core.ac.uk/download/46603887.pdf (accessed on 30th June 2025).

12. Bakry, M., Hoffmann, P., Prematunga, R., Keightley, P., & Subramaniam, K. (2024). The transitioning from pediatric to adult inflammatory bowel disease services: A qualitative study of adolescents and their parents. *Gastroenterology Research, 17,* 146–149. https://www.semanticscholar.org/paper/ca87862c90f552c5b208a67b4e37f886c027e5f2 (accessed on 30th June 2025).

13. Balistreri, K. A., Hagan, M. B., Canavera, K., Marik, P., Smith, J., Balistreri, S. E., Barakat, L., *et al.* (2025). Evaluation of psychology practice models in the pediatric intensive care unit. *Clinical Practice in Pediatric Psychology.* https://www.semanticscholar.org/paper/ae726a705455aa284133138bddc0a6ae383796c4 (accessed on 30th June 2025).

14. Batra, R., Edgeworth, J., Eziefula, A. C., *et al.* (2008). Throat and rectal swabs may have an important role in MRSA screening of critically ill patients.

15. Beeching, N. J., Borrow, R., Cohen, J., *et al.* (2016). The UK joint specialist societies guideline on the diagnosis and management of acute meningitis and meningococcal sepsis in immunocompetent adults. https://core.ac.uk/download/pdf/81942013.pdf (accessed on 30th June 2025).

16. Bhambre, A. S., Bhise, P. P., Gawali, P. F., Sugriv, S., *et al.* (2025). A comparative study of inotropes and vasopressin in critical care unit. https://core.ac.uk/download/655504141.pdf (accessed on 30th June 2025).

17. Boland, A. C., Wind, A., & Alkhoujah, M. (2024). Unusual presentation of propionic acidemia mimicking botulism in an infant: A case report and literature review. *Cureus, 16.* https://www.semanticscholar.org/paper/a1d4f8cd4a18ba46f71ac4e9c15769202209a99c (accessed on 30th June 2025).

18. Botan, E., Ay, M., Boyraz, M., Bako, D., & Yüce, S. (2023). Neurological complications in MIS-C: Case report. *Pediatric Academic Case Reports.* https://www.semanticscholar.org/paper/e1d6550448743524963af69b50f834c304c3c852 (accessed on 30th June 2025).

19. Bucher, J., Feldman, D., & Joseph, J. (2020). Mistriaged advanced life support patients in a two-tiered, suburban emergency medical services system. https://core.ac.uk/download/287621993.pdf (accessed on 30th June 2025).

20. Burner, E., Chandra, S., Chang, B., Clark, E., *et al.* (2021). Telehealth in emergency medicine: A consensus conference to map the intersection of telehealth and emergency medicine. https://core.ac.uk/download/612397236.pdf (accessed on 30th June 2025).

21. Caliskan, E. (2017). Neonatal care for anesthesiologists. https://core.ac.uk/download/322433592.pdf (accessed on 30th June 2025).

22. Caruso, N., Chandra, A., Goldfarb, D., Haas, M., *et al.* (2013). CT before lumbar puncture in suspected meningitis in Botswana: How established guidelines may not apply / Tomodensitométrie avant ponction lombaire en cas de suspicion de méningite au Botswana: Comment les directives classiques peuvent ne pas s'appliquer. https://core.ac.uk/download/76392048.pdf (accessed on 30th June 2025).

23. Ceriello, A., Ceriello, A., Ceriello, A., Chiaretti, A., Rovlias, A., Russo, A., Russo, A., *et al.* (2010). Control of hyperglycemia in pediatric intensive care (CHiP): Study protocol. https://core.ac.uk/download/20330333.pdf (accessed on 30th June 2025).

24. Coté, C. J., & Wilson, S. (2019). Guidelines for monitoring and management of pediatric patients before, during, and after sedation for diagnostic and therapeutic procedures. *Pediatrics, 143.* https://doi.org/10.1542/peds.2019-1000 (accessed on 30th June 2025).

25. Di Sarno, L., Caroselli, A., Tonin, G., Graglia, B., Pansini, V., Causio, F. A., Gatto, A., *et al.* (2024). Artificial intelligence in pediatric emergency medicine: Applications, challenges, and future perspectives. *Biomedicines, 12*, 1220. https://doi.org/10.3390/biomedicines12061220 (accessed on 30th June 2025).

26. Dionísio, T., Gomes, C., Jerónimo, M., Neves, M., *et al.* (2015). Renovascular hypertension: A case with atypical neurological signs. https://core.ac.uk/download/61498613.pdf (accessed on 30th June 2025).

27. Downing, N. L., Bates, D. W., & Longhurst, C. (2018). Physician burnout in the electronic health record era: Are we ignoring the real cause? *Annals of Internal Medicine, 169*, 50–50. https://doi.org/10.7326/m18-0139 (accessed on 30th June 2025).

28. Elahi, M. M., & Matata, B. (2017). Meeting report on the International Conference of ECMO-Life Support for Pakistan in 21st Century held May 11–12, 2017, Lahore. https://core.ac.uk/download/131166373.pdf (accessed on 30th June 2025).

29. Emonts, P., Kridelka, F., Lambert, G., Maquet, J., *et al.* (2016). A reversible posterior leucoencephalopathy syndrome including blindness caused by preeclampsia. http://orbi.ulg.ac.be/bitstream/2268/207252/1/Vandenbossche%20G%20FVVinObGyn-8-173.pdf (accessed on 30th June 2025).

30. Ferriero, D. M., Fullerton, H. J., Bernard, T. J., Billinghurst, L., Daniels, S. R., DeBaun, M. R., deVeber, G., *et al.* (2019). Management of stroke in neonates and children: A scientific statement from the American Heart Association/American Stroke Association. *Stroke, 50.* https://doi.org/10.1161/str.0000000000000183 (accessed on 30th June 2025).

31. Ferriero, D. M., Glass, H. C., Rowitch, D. H., Shimotake, T., *et al.* (2019). The neurointensive nursery: Concept, development, and insights gained. https://core.ac.uk/download/200999838.pdf (accessed on 30th June 2025).

32. Geocadin, R. G., Callaway, C. W., Fink, E. L., Golan, E., Greer, D. M., Ko, N., Lang, E., *et al.* (2019). Standards for studies of neurological prognostication in comatose survivors of cardiac arrest: A scientific statement from the American Heart Association. *Circulation, 140.* https://doi.org/10.1161/cir.0000000000000702 (accessed on 30th June 2025).

33. Indrawan, K., & Manggala, S. (2025). Plasmapheresis and multidisciplinary intensive care management for Guillain-Barré syndrome with prolonged mechanical ventilation: A case report. *Proceedings Book of International Conference and Exhibition on The Indonesian Medical Education Research Institute.* https://www.semanticscholar.org/paper/5d52fb4f41c387954e8721bc31674976c7585852 (accessed on 30th June 2025).

34. Jalbă (Sîrbu), G. A., Coreţchi, D., Moraru, P. I., Peptine, L., Răileanu, C. R., & Nechita, A. (2025). Severe pediatric sepsis caused by *Neisseria meningitidis*: A case report. *The Annals of Dunarea de Jos University of Galati Fascicle XV Physical Education and Sport Management.* https://www.semanticscholar.org/paper/5de4335c36bad06df9b81062c7754e3065f5459d (accessed on 30th June 2025).

35. Kahveci, F., Ocak, B. O., Gün, E., Gurbanov, A., Uçmak, H., Durak Aslan, A., Ceran, A., *et al.* (2023). Impact of the COVID-19 pandemic on diabetic ketoacidosis management in the pediatric

intensive care unit. *Acute and Critical Care, 38*, 371–379. https://www.semanticscholar.org/paper/fea5ac13e7ec5bc24c3c16fd226fdf31766c27e3 (accessed on 30th June 2025).

36. Kartik, M., Sunil Kumar, N., Jupally, R., & Suryaprakash, Y. (2024). Transcranial ultrasound guided assessment of brain midline shifts *in neuro* intensive care unit. *National Board of Examinations Journal of Medical Sciences.* https://www.semanticscholar.org/paper/11cf05ca0cd3b9ed6aceb3093be05053a2c061c5 (accessed on 30th June 2025).

37. Kleinpell, R., Grabenkort, W. R., Boyle, W. A., Vines, D., & Olsen, K. M. (2021). The Society of Critical Care Medicine at 50 years: Interprofessional practice in critical care: Looking back and forging ahead. *Critical Care Medicine, 49*, 2017–2032. https://doi.org/10.1097/ccm.0000000000005276 (accessed on 30th June 2025).

38. Koser, L. (2015). Ultra-early blood pressure control in aneurysmal subarachnoid hemorrhage. https://core.ac.uk/download/159576761.pdf (accessed on 30th June 2025).

39. Kuok, C., & Chan, W. (2022). Motor vehicle collision and acute kidney injury in children. *Pediatric Emergency Care, 38*, 545–549. https://www.semanticscholar.org/paper/7dec0d0dc465b4291182683b2c12b1dbfdb32280 (accessed on 30th June 2025).

40. Kurakbayev, Y., Turdaliyeva, B., Manzhuova, L., Schukin, V., Aimakhanova, A., & Aitbayev, K. (2024). Acute lymphoblastic leukemia in children hospitalized in the intensive care unit: A retrospective analysis. *Oncologic I Radiologic Kazakhstani.* https://www.semanticscholar.org/paper/4b669717083c2cc1eda8b6c1dd06f05a4846b05f (accessed on 30th June 2025).

41. Lagos-Servellon, J., Zelaya, V., Escalante-Lanza, G., Zelaya, M., Murillo, T. P., & Servellon, D. (2021). Abstract 1122-000017: Giant brain aneurysm: A case report in a pediatric patient. *Stroke: Vascular and Interventional Neurology.* https://www.semanticscholar.org/paper/c2a6890c224e2a7943079fc32bc5663b4289b63d (accessed on 30th June 2025).

42. Liang, Z., Chong, M., Sim, M. A., Lim, J. L., Castañeda, P., Green, D. W., Fisher, D., *et al.* (2020). Surgical considerations in patients with COVID-19. *Journal of Bone and Joint Surgery, 102*, e50. https://doi.org/10.2106/jbjs.20.00513 (accessed on 30th June 2025).

43. Martinez-Correa, S., Rafful, P. P., Ramirez-Suarez, K. I., Viaene, A., Beslow, L. A., Agarwal, S., Whitehead, M. T., *et al.* (2025). Imaging patterns of neonatal subpial hemorrhage–Provisional statements on neurological outcomes. *AJNR. American Journal of Neuroradiology.* https://www.semanticscholar.org/paper/f7db8ece81e13cdc916c7df615c69a431382505e (accessed on 30th June 2025).

44. Mongini, T., Racca, F., Ruggeri, P., *et al.* (2019). Practical approach to respiratory emergencies in neurological diseases. https://core.ac.uk/download/268911808.pdf (accessed on 30th June 2025).

45. Murray, K., Roth, R. N., Tobias, A. Z., Weiss, S., *et al.* (2020). Tree of Life Synagogue shooting in Pittsburgh: Preparedness, prehospital care, and lessons learned. https://core.ac.uk/download/287621999.pdf (accessed on 30th June 2025).

46. Nakata, Y., Takasaki, Y., Nandate, H., Hida, A., Sekiya, K., Abe, N., Nishihara, T., *et al.* (2024). Pediatric neurogenic pulmonary edema after brain tumor removal complicated with severe myocardial injury: A case report. *The American Journal of Case Reports, 25*, e943645-1–e943645-5. https://www.semanticscholar.org/paper/ba509358145bce9831eb2367c0bd6eb64c2244f5 (accessed on 30th June 2025).

47. Ozcetin, M., Arslan, M., Yilmaz, R., & Yildirim, A. (2012). Rare cause of cerebral damage: Child with heatstroke found inside an enclosed vehicle. *Hong Kong Journal of Emergency Medicine, 19*, 126–129. https://www.semanticscholar.org/paper/ed4e447528ec846570ec9e1786f83255d7242cf2 (accessed on 30th June 2025).

48. Patel, P., Swamy, N., Klimovich, G., Marcus, M., & Holleman, R. (2013). A 2-month-old female infant with failure to thrive. *Pediatric Annals, 42*(5), 191–193. https://www.semanticscholar.org/paper/deaa5ba4cca50cf8ca6301312d1dc76e5930998e (accessed on 30th June 2025).

49. Raches, D., Gajjar, A., Robinson, G. W., Ashford, J., Bryndziar, M., Huggins, A., Lockett, S., *et al.* (2024). Intensive interdisciplinary rehabilitation in the pediatric hematology/oncology setting: Feasibility and perceived benefit of the Acute Neurological Injury Service. *Cancers, 16.* https://www.semanticscholar.org/paper/b9debe09515f49c53b1c5edee751c906aedb9ad8 (accessed on 30th June 2025).

50. Sanchez-Albisua, I. (2023). Impaired consciousness in the pediatric intensive care unit: Etiology and diagnostics—English version. *Clinical Epileptology, 36*, 120–124. https://www.semanticscholar.org/paper/fffd781c3a7dd5d3f6f0927580a1a20d557ab5ac (accessed on 30th June 2025).

51. Sanderson, A., & Burns, J. (2020). Is it time to move beyond observational studies of the epidemiology and mode of PICU deaths? *Pediatric Critical Care Medicine.* https://www.semanticscholar.org/paper/46bd832b448396102341096c52f268cecc71cbb7 (accessed on 30th June 2025).

52. Schneider, B. J., Naidoo, J., Santomasso, B., Lacchetti, C., Adkins, S., Anadkat, M. J., Atkins, M. B., *et al.* (2021). Management of immune-related adverse events in patients treated with immune checkpoint inhibitor therapy: ASCO guideline update. *Journal of Clinical Oncology, 39*, 4073–4126. https://doi.org/10.1200/jco.21.01440 (accessed on 30th June 2025).

53. Schwenk, E. S., Viscusi, E. R., Buvanendran, A., Hurley, R. W., Wasan, A. D., Narouze, S., Bhatia, A., *et al.* (2018). Consensus guidelines on the use of intravenous ketamine infusions for acute pain management from the American Society of Regional Anesthesia and Pain Medicine, the American Academy of Pain Medicine, and the American Society of Anesthesiologists. *Regional Anesthesia & Pain Medicine.* https://doi.org/10.1097/aap.0000000000000806 (accessed on 30th June 2025).

54. Scott, K., Beckham, S. W., Gross, M., Pariyo, G., Rao, K. D., Cometto, G., & Perry, H. B. (2018). What do we know about community-based health worker programs? A systematic review of existing reviews on community health workers. *Human Resources for Health, 16.* https://doi.org/10.1186/s12960-018-0304-x (accessed on 30th June 2025).

55. Sen, K., Harrar, D., Pariseau, N., Tucker, K., Keenan, J. S., Zhang, A., & Gropman, A. (2024). Seizure characteristics and EEG features in intoxication type and energy deficiency neurometabolic disorders in the pediatric intensive care unit: Single-center experience over 10 years. *Neurocritical Care.* https://www.semanticscholar.org/paper/02dc66faa2943c47b025dbdf79579f0304ba43b6 (accessed on 30th June 2025).

56. Song, J., Kim, Y., & Kim, I. C. (2021). Successful treatment of post-myocardial infarction ventricular septal rupture. *International Journal of Heart Failure, 3*, 200–204. https://www.semanticscholar.org/paper/36f40c82d7058d59662f42389d6eb1ad1ede73b4 (accessed on 30th June 2025).

57. Whelton, P. K., Carey, R. M., Aronow, W. S., Casey, D. E., Collins, K. J., Dennison Himmelfarb, C., DePalma, S. M., *et al.* (2017). 2017 ACC/AHA/AAPA/ABC/ACPM/AGS/APhA/ASH/ASPC/NMA/PCNA guideline for the prevention, detection, evaluation, and management of high blood pressure in adults: A report of the American College of Cardiology/American Heart Association Task Force on Clinical Practice Guidelines. *Hypertension, 71.* https://doi.org/10.1161/hyp.0000000000000065 (accessed on 30th June 2025).

RENAL AND ELECTROLYTE MANAGEMENT

6

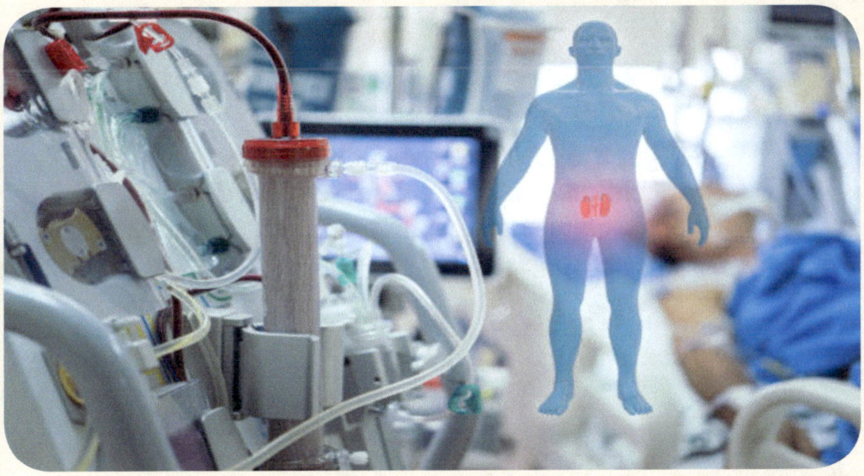

LEARNING OBJECTIVES

After studying this chapter, you will be able to:

1. Understand Physiology of Renal Function in Children.
2. Explain Common Electrolyte Imbalances in Pediatric Patients.
3. Describe Renal Replacement Therapy in Pediatric Intensive Care.
4. Focus on Multidisciplinary Approach to Renal and Electrolyte Management.

Introduction

In the world of pediatric intensive care, renal and electrolyte management is a progressively crucial element directly affecting patient outcomes. With the susceptibility of children being treated for numerous acute illnesses, the risk for acute kidney injury (AKI) is prevalent, making their overall clinical management more problematic. The international standards developed by the Kidney Disease: Improving Global Outcomes have sought to create a uniform approach to understanding AKI, such as definitions, risk evaluation, prevention, and treatment (Kellum *et al.*, 2013). In addition, the nephrotoxicity of certain pediatric chemotherapy, such as that used in treating acute lymphoblastic leukemia, points to the delicate balance between maintaining renal function and avoiding harmful side effects (Attarbaschi *et al.*, 2016). This interrelationship between renal function and more broad-based therapy interventions points to the need for pediatric therapy teams to be well-versed in renal physiology as well as the relevance of electrolyte derangements, thereby enhancing safe and effective patient care in such vulnerable populations.

6.1. Physiology of Renal Function in Children

Learning Outcome

1. Understand developmental differences in renal anatomy.
2. Focus on glomerular filtration rate (GFR) in pediatric patients.
3. Explain tubular function and electrolyte reabsorption.
4. Know the impact of age on renal function.
5. Describe renal response to stress and illness.
6. Learn differences in fluid balance in children.
7. Focus on hormonal regulation of renal function.
8. Identify renal function assessment methods.
9. Focus on implications of renal physiology on treatment.

Knowledge of the physiology of renal function in children is vital to efficiently manipulate the kidneys and electrolytes in pediatric intensive care units. The physiology of the kidney in children differs from that of adults, with clearly demarcated anatomical and functional patterns because of the immaturity of the kidneys, which mature throughout life. This progressive maturation affects glomerular filtration rate and tubular function, leading to alterations in managing electrolytes, particularly sodium (Na^+) and potassium (K^+) levels. Alterations in these electrolytes have significant implications since they are needed for a variety of body functions, including the transmission of nerves and muscle contraction (Lombardi *et al.*, 2022). Moreover, recent evidence indicates that slight variations from normal ranges of electrolytes may be a significant contributor to influencing patient outcomes and that a sense of maintaining vigilant observation of these alterations is crucial in children's survival in intensive care units (Balarama *et al.*, 2020). Therefore, a complex appreciation of pediatric renal physiology provides the basis for maximizing clinical interventions in this vulnerable group (Figure 6.1).

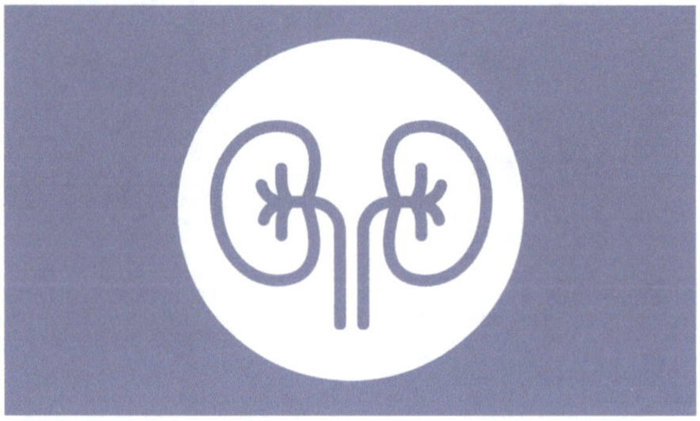

Figure 6.1. The physiology of renal function in children is crucial for effective renal and electrolyte management in pediatric intensive care settings.

Source: https://www.emjreviews.com/wp-content/uploads/2021/11/NEPH.png.

6.1.1. Developmental Differences in Renal Anatomy

Recognition of developmental variation in renal anatomy is crucial for effective renal and electrolyte management in pediatric intensive care. The kidneys of the neonate and young child exhibit significant anatomical and physiological variation compared to adults, including differences in size, shape, and vascular supply. In the infant, the renal cortex is relatively thicker and nephrons are less mature, affecting filtration rates and electrolyte management. There are additional developmental variations in renal anatomy that are present during childhood. In addition, the renal tubules in children that have not reached maturity have a poor ability to concentrate urine and therefore create challenges when balancing fluid and electrolyte homeostasis in illness. All these anatomical features present specific challenges that require individualized approaches in anesthetic care and acute management of children, given that their unique renal patterns influence the pharmacokinetics of drugs used in critical care (Carter *et al.*, 2017). Furthermore, understanding of the interaction of renal function with co-morbidities, such as acute lung injury, underscores the necessity of individualized interventions to obtain the best results in children (Chimbira *et al.*, 2001).

6.1.2. Pediatric Patients' Glomerular Filtration Rate (GFR)

In children, glomerular filtration rate (GFR) is a measure that plays a crucial role in renal and electrolyte disease management, particularly in the intensive care unit. GFR reflects kidney function and may indicate potential abnormalities, such as acute kidney injury (AKI), which is often compounded by multiple factors, including antecedent illness and medication therapies.

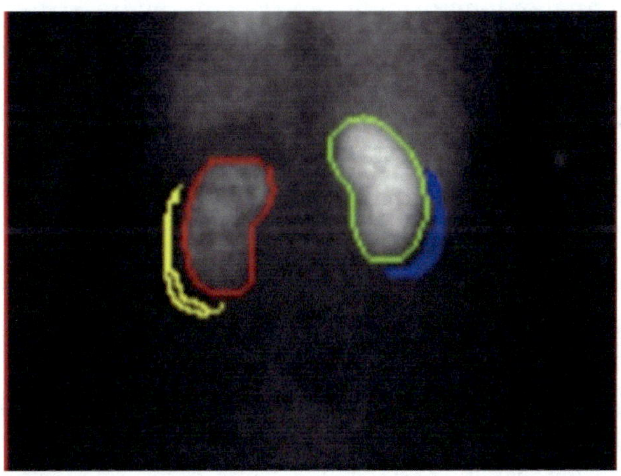

Figure 6.2. In pediatric patients, the assessment of glomerular filtration rate (GFR) is crucial for managing renal and electrolyte abnormalities, particularly in critical care settings.

Source: https://www.mdpi.com/applsci/applsci-12-00698/article_deploy/html/images/applsci-12-00698-g001.png.

Quantitative assessment of GFR in this group is challenging, considering the growth and development with changing renal function. Equations to estimate GFR, such as the Schwartz equation, have to be calibrated carefully in children to avoid discrepancies. Furthermore, newer evidence has identified that aggressive management strategies can make a strong contribution to outcomes in children presenting with impaired GFR, reflecting evidence obtained from studies on chronic kidney disease in adults (Hsu *et al.*, 2019). Moreover, some of the challenges posed by comorbid disease, such as cancers, necessitate an individualized approach to electrolyte management in pediatric intensive care (Benoit *et al.*, 2016) (Figure 6.2).

6.1.3. Tubular Function and Electrolyte Reabsorption

In pediatric critical care, an understanding of the tubular function and electrolyte reabsorption is vital to effective renal management. The renal tubules are responsible for fluid and electrolyte balance, particularly sodium and chloride, which play a crucial role in overall homeostasis. Imbalance within this system can lead to disorders such as dyschloremia, which has been linked with elevated morbidity and mortality in critical care patients. Specifically, hyperchloremia exacerbates hemodynamic instability and is responsible for acute renal injury, necessitating renal replacement therapy in some cases (Ali *et al.*, 2022). Furthermore, local mechanisms such as intrarenal dopamine also play a significant role in tubular function through the augmentation of sodium excretion and avoidance of renal vasculature from inflammatory damage (Choi *et al.*, 2015). Therefore, an in-depth understanding of these mechanisms is absolutely critical for pediatric clinicians to optimize renal outcomes and guide therapeutic interventions in critically ill patients.

6.1.4. Impact of Age on Renal Function

Renal function demonstrates impressive changes throughout various periods of life, particularly in children, wherein age can be an important factor in renal physiology as well as in treating renal disease. In infancy and early childhood, the kidneys are in development, thus causing heterogeneity in glomerular filtration rate (GFR) and tubular function compared to children above that age and adults.

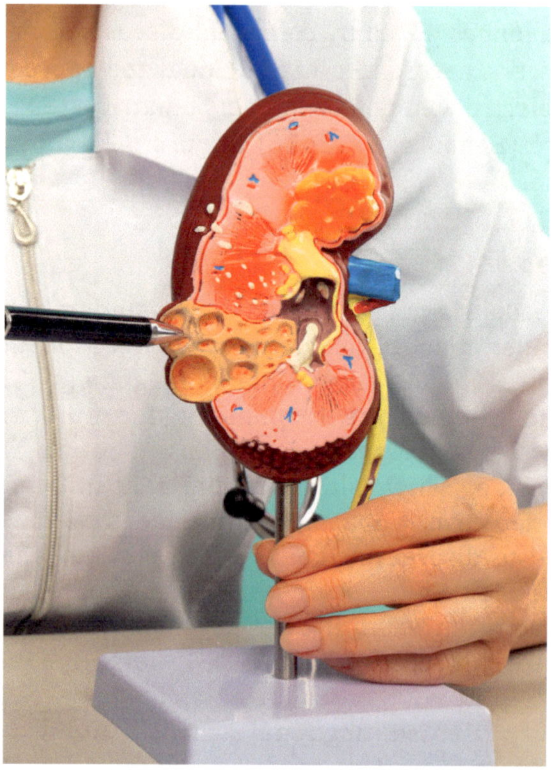

Figure 6.3. Renal function exhibits significant changes throughout various stages of life, particularly in pediatric populations.

Source: https://www.worldkidneyday.org/wp-content/uploads/2023/11/Your-Amazing-Kidneys-World-Kidney-Day-732x1024.jpg.

The immature kidney also poses the risk of exposing the neonate to acute kidney injury (AKI) and complicating pediatric intensive care unit management. For instance, the risk of nephrotoxicity due to drugs also augments with developmental age, and dosing and monitoring renal function in younger patients, especially those undergoing treatment for acute lymphoblastic leukemia, need to be approached carefully. Moreover, Kidney Disease: Improving Global Outcomes recommendations bring attention to individual risk stratification and the use of preventive interventions that are tailored to the age-related frailty of renal function (Kellum *et al.*, 2013). Understanding these dynamics is crucial to maximizing renal and electrolyte management in critically ill children (Figure 6.3).

6.1.5. Renal Response to Stress and Illness

Renal response to stress and disease is a significant consideration in the intensive care management of children. During acute stress, for example, acute illness or trauma, the kidney reorganizes its function to maintain homeostasis through mechanisms like increased activity of the renin-angiotensin-aldosterone system (RAAS), which eventually leads to renal vasoconstriction and altered filtration dynamics.

This bodily response, even though it is protective initially, can have the possibility of causing events like acute kidney injury (AKI), especially in high-risk individuals such as children. AKI is characterized by a sudden deterioration of renal function, often occurring in combination with other systemic stressors and diseases, and is critically discussed in terms of its definitions and staging (Dewitte *et al.*, 2017). Furthermore, the regulation of renal responses, for example, blocking adrenal crises due to stress, is essential for improving patient outcomes (Falhammar *et al.*, 2019). Such interdependent processes are important to understand to achieve the best clinical interventions.

6.1.6. Fluid Balance Differences in Children

Awareness of variation in fluid status in children is central to pediatric intensive care, where renal and electrolyte status management hinges on such variations. Pediatric patients are special due to their stage of development; premature infants and neonates, for instance, have very much higher fluid and nutritional requirements per kilogram body weight than children who are older and adults.

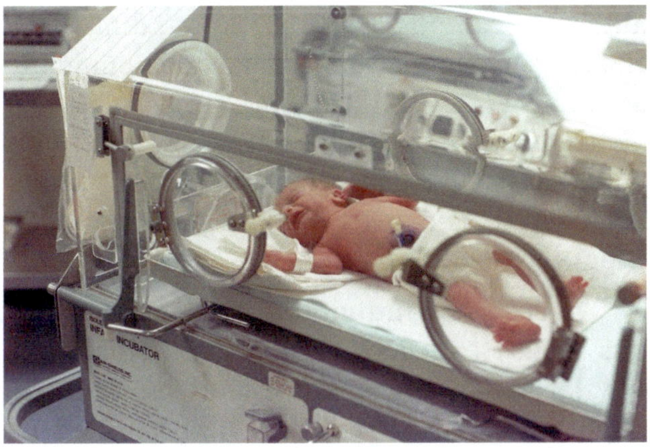

Figure 6.4. Pediatric patients present unique challenges due to their developmental stage; for instance, premature infants and newborns have distinctly higher fluid and nutrient requirements per kilogram compared to older children and adults.

Source: https://upload.wikimedia.org/wikipedia/commons/thumb/e/ee/Infant-Incubator-wBaby-1978-USA.jpg/1200px-Infant-Incubator-wBaby-1978-USA.jpg.

This physiological characteristic demands precise calculations rather than assumptions during parenteral nutrition administration, as inefficient fluid balance will lead to long-term metabolic derangements. In addition, age and conditions such as multiorgan failure significantly influence fluid management strategies. It is documented that children undergoing continuous renal replacement therapy (CRRT) after cardiac surgery exhibit different fluid balance needs, which affect mortality and clinical outcomes (Bellón *et al.*, 2013). This diversity underlines the necessity for customized fluid management strategies to cater to the broad spectrum of pediatric patient needs (Figure 6.4).

6.1.7. Hormonal Regulation of Renal Function

Hormonal regulation is at the forefront of renal function preservation, particularly in the pediatric intensive care setting. The kidney's function to clear blood and maintain electrolyte balance is delicately adapted to several hormones such as aldosterone, antidiuretic hormone (ADH), and natriuretic peptides. The role of these hormones in sodium reabsorption, water retention, and fluid balance in general is crucial in managing pediatric patients at risk for acute renal failure. Literature indicates that dysregulation of hormones is capable of exacerbating renal impairment, particularly when organ impairment is a complex interaction, like acute respiratory distress syndrome (Arriagada *et al.*, 2015). Furthermore, conditions like diabetes insipidus, which are prevalent among critically ill children, demonstrate the importance of proper hormonal regulation in preventing secondary complications and preserving renal integrity. Hence, awareness of these hormonal mechanisms is essential for the best renal and electrolyte management in this vulnerable population.

6.1.8. Methods of Renal Function Assessment

In pediatric intensive care, appropriate assessment of renal function is important for optimal management of both acute and chronic kidney disease. Several methods are employed, including serum creatinine measurements, the estimated glomerular filtration rate (eGFR), and monitoring urine output. Serum creatinine, although commonly used, may be insensitive in children due to variation in muscle mass, and therefore, eGFR estimates that can provide a more precise measure of renal function in terms of age, sex, and body surface area must be employed. Urine output is also a critical parameter, particularly in critical illness, which can manifest early in the disease course, indicating renal compromise. Kidney Disease: Improving Global Outcomes guidelines place emphasis on these assessment methods for enhancing patient outcomes in acute kidney injury (AKI) and treatment success (Kellum *et al.*, 2013). Hence, a holistic approach based on these assessment methods is the requirement in pediatric intensive care units to ensure improved renal management and electrolyte balance (Dahl *et al.*, 2014) (Figure 6.5).

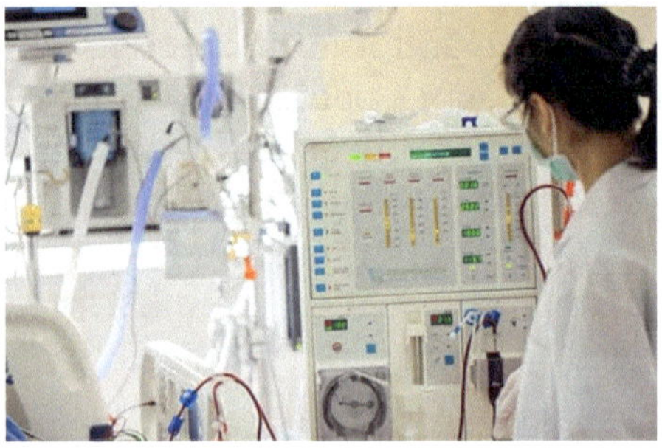

Figure 6.5. In pediatric intensive care, accurate assessment of renal function is crucial for effective management of both acute and chronic kidney conditions.

Source: https://stemcellthailand.org/wp-content/uploads/2019/06/dialysis-thailand.jpg.webp.

6.1.9. Implications of Renal Physiology on Treatment

In pediatric intensive care, an understanding of renal physiology is crucial in optimizing treatment modalities, particularly in fluid and electrolyte imbalances.

Age groups demand varying metabolic needs; e.g., premature infants have a much greater fluid and nutrient demand per kilogram when compared to older children and adolescents, and require precise calculation to avoid parenteral nutrition complications. Compounding such challenges, hyponatremia is far too commonly a secondary disorder following intravenous fluid management in post-operative children, with potentially life-threatening effects on sodium homeostasis and general electrolyte regulation (Aperia *et al.*, 2011).

Therefore, individualizing therapy to this distinctive renal function and electrolyte regulation in this population is of vital importance. Such treatment programs on an individual basis not only lower the risk of long-term metabolic programming but also enhance clinical outcomes, underscoring the value of close monitoring and titration of renal-associated therapies in children's critical care units.

Test Your Knowledge

1. How does glomerular filtration rate (GFR) change with age in pediatric patients?
2. What role do the kidneys play in acid-base balance in children?

6.2. Common Electrolyte Imbalances in Pediatric Patients

Learning Outcome

1. Explain an overview of key electrolytes such as sodium, potassium, and calcium.
2. Identify causes of hyponatremia in children.
3. Explain causes of hyperkalemia in pediatric patients.
4. Focus on hypocalcemia and its clinical significance.
5. Describe management of electrolyte imbalances.
6. Monitor protocols for electrolyte levels.
7. Discuss the role of nutrition in electrolyte balance.
8. Know the impact of medications on electrolyte levels.

Electrolyte disturbances are particularly prevalent in children, often from several associated conditions and treatments. Hyponatremia, hyperkalemia, and hypocalcemia are common disturbances that all present significant risks to this patient group. Hyponatremia, for instance, can lead to cerebral edema, while hyperkalemia may lead to deadly cardiac arrhythmias. Pediatric patients, especially intensive care patients, tend to develop such imbalances due to reasons such as acute kidney injury and intravenous fluid or medication administration. Effective management depends on the rapid detection and correction of such disturbances to prevent permanent complications such as renal impairment. Further, the ensuing, almost suffocating stress of critical illness has the potential to exacerbate such electrolyte imbalances, and timely monitoring in the pediatric intensive care unit setting is therefore especially critical. Resolving these issues is critical towards optimizing survival rates and overall outcome in such patients (Chawla *et al.*, 2012; BOSCATO *et al.*, 2023).

6.2.1. Overview of Key Electrolytes: Sodium, Potassium, Calcium

In pediatric intensive care, awareness of the role of significant electrolytes—sodium, potassium, and calcium—is crucial for efficient renal and electrolyte management. Sodium plays a role in the control of osmotic equilibrium and fluid homeostasis, while derangement leads to extreme neurological implications. Potassium, required for myocardial and skeletal muscle activity, plays a critical role in the control of cardiac rhythm, while derangements can lead to extreme arrhythmias, particularly in the event of renal impairment in children. Calcium is similarly important, affecting neuromuscular excitability and mineral metabolism of bone; levels are tightly regulated, reflecting underlying renal function. Balance between these electrolytes has to be carefully regulated, particularly in post-transplant care, where electrolyte imbalance can worsen the patient's condition. Effective management strategies, like frequent monitoring and early intervention, are critical to support favorable outcomes among this vulnerable population (Huffer *et al.*, 2017; David-Neto *et al.*, 2014) (Figure 6.6).

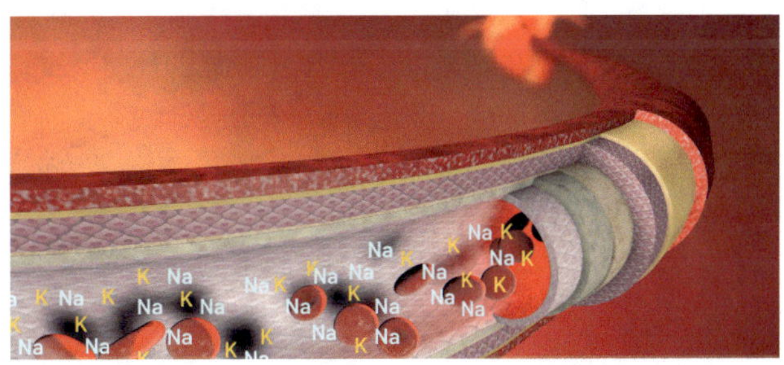

Figure 6.6. Potassium, essential for myocardial and skeletal muscle function, plays a vital role in cardiac rhythm, and disturbances can result in severe arrhythmias, particularly in children with renal dysfunction.

Source: https://rnareset.com/cdn/shop/articles/potassium-sodium-balance-for-heart-health_54acc7d1-23f2-4da6-a65e-dfee9f32c770.png?v=1739395505.

6.2.2. Causes of Hyponatremia in Children

The pathogenesis of hyponatremia in children is multifactorial and generally a complex interaction of baseline medical and environmental conditions. Some of the most common etiologies of hyponatremia in pediatric intensive care are overhydration, inappropriate antidiuretic hormone secretion (SIADH), gastrointestinal losses, and renal pathologies. As an example, heart failure can lead to hypervolemic hyponatremia through excess fluid that allows for sodium dilution (지종현, 2022). In addition, gastrointestinal upset, especially in acute conditions, is capable of inducing tremendous electrolyte imbalance via vomiting or diarrhea, thereby contributing to a fall in serum sodium (Huffer *et al.*, 2017). In ensuring timely and proper interventions are implemented for such critically ill children, it is critical that the reason why hyponatremia occurs be known (Huffer *et al.*, 2017). Ultimately, early diagnosis and targeted treatment of the etiologies can improve outcomes in this vulnerable group.

6.2.3. Pediatric Etiologies of Hyperkalemia

Hyperkalemia in children is caused by various underlying pathologies and, therefore, is a significant renal and electrolyte illness within intensive care units. Acute kidney injury (AKI) is one of the primary causes and leads to abnormal excretion of potassium due to renal compromise. This can be due to a variety of etiologies, including acute tubular necrosis that can be secondary to rhabdomyolysis, muscle damage that also increases potassium.

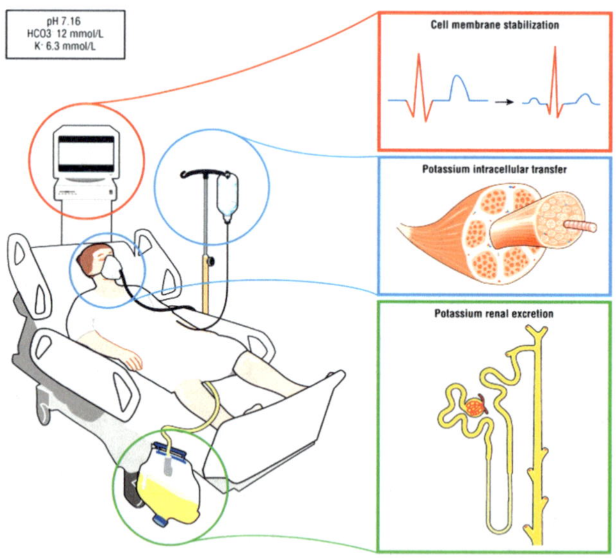

Figure 6.7. The incidence of hyperkalemia in pediatric patients can be attributed to various underlying conditions, making it a critical aspect of renal and electrolyte management in intensive care settings.

Source: https://media.springernature.com/lw685/springer-static/image/art%3A10.1186%2Fs13613-019-0509-8/MediaObjects/13613_2019_509_Fig5_HTML.png.

Metabolic disorders and drugs can also contribute to worsening hyperkalemia by facilitating the release of potassium from cells or altering renal handling of electrolytes. Proper management of hyperkalemia in critically ill children is vital since inadequate management of hyperkalemia can lead to life-threatening cardiac conditions, which emphasizes the need for accurate diagnosis and urgent intervention (Kellum *et al.*, 2013). Knowing these causes is thus vital for improving patient outcomes among this vulnerable population (Figure 6.7).

6.2.4. Hypocalcemia and Its Clinical Significance

Hypocalcemia, which is low serum calcium levels, is a significant clinical issue in the pediatric intensive care unit as it has the potential to worsen a number of underlying diseases and reduce overall metabolic activities. Hypocalcemia in critically ill children can be caused by a variety of etiologies, including nutritional deficiencies, acute illnesses, or endocrine disturbances. Interestingly, its occurrence is generally associated with other disturbances in electrolytes, such as hypomagnesemia, which is also a frequent finding among critically ill patients, highlighting the use of combined electrolyte management practices (Abdollahi *et al.*, 2025). The effect of hypocalcemia is also important since it can have symptoms ranging from muscle cramps to cardiac dysrhythmias and influence patient outcomes. Apart from this, perinatal asphyxia disorders have also been associated with endocrine disturbances, including disturbances in calcium homeostasis, which also predispose to hypocalcemia and hence the need for close monitoring and immediate intervention (Aversa *et al.*, 2023).

6.2.5. Management of Electrolyte Imbalances

Electrolyte imbalance management is crucial in pediatric intensive care, particularly among patients with acute renal failure or multi-organ dysfunction syndrome. The reason that electrolyte homeostasis in children is so tightly regulated requires attentive assessment and strict monitoring because imbalance results in severe complications like cardiac arrhythmias and neurological disturbances.

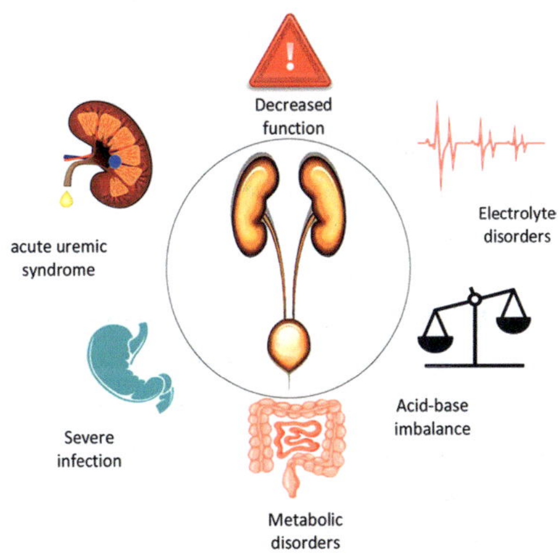

Figure 6.8. Strategies such as continuous renal replacement therapy (CRRT) have been demonstrated to successfully correct these imbalances by facilitating the gradual removal or replacement of electrolytes as needed.

Source: https://images-provider.frontiersin.org/api/ipx/w=1200&f=png/https://www.frontiersin.org/files/Articles/1122778/fphar-14-1122778-HTML/image_m/fphar-14-1122778-g001.jpg.

Methods such as CRRT have proven to be effective in addressing these imbalances through a process of sequential removal or substitution of electrolytes where appropriate (Baker *et al.*, 2005). Additionally, the evolution of EBPTs has provided further avenues for treatment of these issues, but the variability of clinical practice towards these interventions reflects the need for protocol standardization (Bayrakci *et al.*, 2025). Overall, there is a comprehensive approach with early intervention and identification of emerging therapies that can ensure substantial success for pediatric patients against electrolyte imbalance in intensive care units (Figure 6.8).

6.2.6. Monitoring Protocols for Electrolyte Levels

Monitoring of serum electrolytes is required for pediatric intensive care unit patients to maintain homeostasis and prevent renal impairment complications. Monitoring of serum electrolytes is generally performed every four to six hours post-surgery, such as kidney transplantation, to intervene rapidly in case of imbalance (Abu-Sultaneh *et al.*, 2017).

This proactive approach allows clinicians to continue to evolve fluid therapies and electrolyte replacement based on real-time data, which is of utmost importance in the context of high within-patient variability of response to treatment. Besides, application of standardized protocols also allows pediatric intensivists to prevent clinical inhomogeneities and promote global patient outcomes (Bernasconi *et al.*, 2019). This sustained watchfulness in the regulation of electrolytes is not only best practice in pediatric care but also reflects the interdisciplinary enthusiasm to optimize outcomes in high-risk groups, affirming the rationale for stringent observation as an integral part of renal and electrolyte management strategies.

6.2.7. The Role of Nutrition in Maintaining Electrolyte Balance

Nutrition is an integral part of electrolyte balance in pediatric critical care, and it, in turn, is responsible for optimal renal function and overall health outcomes in critically ill children. Essential electrolytes such as sodium, potassium, calcium, and magnesium are responsible for various physiological processes, like nerve transmission and muscle contraction.

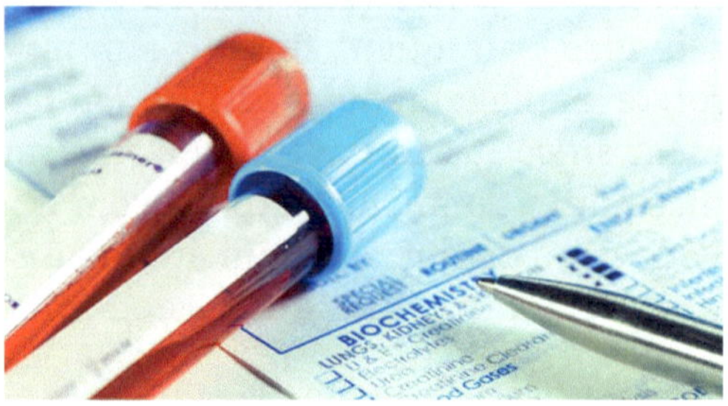

Figure 6.9. Inadequate nutrition can lead to electrolyte imbalances, heightening the risk of complications such as arrhythmias and impaired renal function.

Source: https://www.lifeextension.com/-/media/lef/images/protocols/images/hero/2015_prot_kidneydisease_hero.jpg.

Malnutrition can lead to electrolyte imbalance, predisposing the patient to complications such as arrhythmias and impaired renal function. For instance, it has been established through studies that trace element deficiencies, such as selenium and manganese overload, are prevalent among parenteral nutrition patients, a type of intravenous feeding that is prevalent in intensive care units (Dodington *et al.*, 2025). Moreover, an understanding of malnutrition's impact on electrolyte homeostasis is essential, as cancer patients in old age have proven that malnutrition would exacerbate metabolic derangements, thus highlighting the need for tailored nutritional assessment (Bullock *et al.*, 2022). Hence, nutrition management is essential for maintaining and creating electrolyte balance in pediatric patients (Figure 6.9).

6.2.8. Impact of Medications on Electrolyte Levels

In pediatric intensive care, some medications have significant impacts on electrolyte status, complicating renal and electrolyte management. For instance, chemotherapy for acute lymphoblastic leukemia (ALL) can produce metabolic abnormalities, including serum electrolyte changes, with effects on the outcome of treatment. Specifically, studies have shown that children who are administered forceful induction chemotherapy tend to experience alterations in significant electrolyte levels, including serum bicarbonate and blood urea nitrogen (BUN), which are specifically related to the hospitalization period as well as general recovery (Althouse *et al.*, 2018). Furthermore, the poisonous effects of drugs, such as methotrexate, may exacerbate these disturbances by inducing nephrotoxicity and interfering with renal function, hence augmenting electrolyte imbalances (Attarbaschi *et al.*, 2016). Such a complicating interaction highlights the necessity for proper monitoring and tailored therapeutic interventions to reverse the undesirable effects of drugs on electrolyte homeostasis in children undergoing intensive care.

Test Your Knowledge

1. How is hyperkalemia typically managed in the PICU setting?
2. What causes hypocalcemia in pediatric intensive care patients?

6.3. Renal Replacement Therapy in Pediatric Intensive Care

Learning Outcome

1. Know indications for renal replacement therapy (RRT).
2. Identify types of RRT.
3. Explain pediatric considerations in RRT.
4. Know complications associated with RRT.
5. Understand timing and initiation of RRT.
6. Explain monitoring and management during RRT.
7. Learn long-term outcomes of RRT in children.
8. Discuss innovations in RRT technology.
9. Describe ethical considerations in pediatric RRT.

For pediatric intensive care, renal replacement therapy (RRT) is a severe treatment for acute kidney injury (AKI), an illness that has grave consequences in severely ill children. RRT is applied to balance electrolytes and filter out waste products that the kidneys cannot properly filter, thereby restoring homeostasis. The frequency of AKI in pediatric patients warrants rigorous adherence to guidelines that encompass the evaluation and treatment of this condition, as well as RRT guidelines. Surprisingly, a multi-disciplinary approach has been recommended in practice, emphasizing the need to introduce evidence-based methods to the care of AKI in children. These methods must appreciate physiological problems in children that are not similar to adults, since their response to nephrotoxins differs significantly from that of adults. Thus, it is important to understand the nuances of RRT in children to minimize complications and improve outcomes in this vulnerable group (Kellum *et al.*, 2013; Benoit *et al.*, 2016).

6.3.1. Indications for Renal Replacement Therapy (RRT)

Indications in pediatric intensive care for renal replacement therapy (RRT) are multifactorial and critical in the management of acute kidney injury (AKI). Initiation of RRT is often indicated by several clinical signs, including the presence of persistent anuria, frank fluid overload, and life-threatening electrolyte derangements such as hyperkalemia. In addition, acute tumor lysis syndrome, a common situation in children with cancer, requires emergent treatment to prevent additional renal injury (Benoit *et al.*, 2016). Choice of the RRT modality—intermittent hemodialysis, peritoneal dialysis, or continuous renal replacement therapy—is based on the individual patient profile, the patient's clinical presentation, and the capability of the institution (Airede *et al.*, 2008). Early and adequate RRT not only enhances the immediate result of renal failure but also significantly lowers the prognosis, particularly in critically ill children, and emphasizes the significance of accurate assessment and urgent decision-making within the pediatric intensive care unit (Figure 6.10).

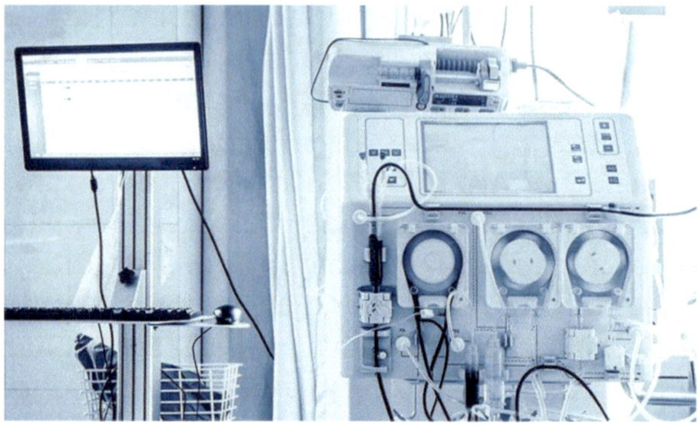

Figure 6.10. The indications for renal replacement therapy (RRT) are multifaceted and critical for managing acute kidney injury (AKI).

Source: https://mobildialysis.net/wp-content/uploads/2024/10/Continuous-Renal-Replacement-Therapy-CRRT-1200x720-1.jpg.

6.3.2. Types of RRT: Hemodialysis Versus Peritoneal Dialysis

For children, in the scenario of renal replacement therapy (RRT), peritoneal dialysis versus hemodialysis has significant implications for patient care and management. Hemodialysis, being the most widespread modality, necessitates the removal of waste products through an external machine, in most instances necessitating more frequent intervention and access management with opportunities of difficult vascular access in pediatric patients (Tupper *et al.*, 2016). Conversely, peritoneal dialysis utilizes the peritoneal membrane for filtration and has advantages in the form of greater autonomy and lesser dietary restriction, and thus is preferable for young patients (Tupper *et al.*, 2016). However, even with its advantages, peritoneal dialysis cannot be easily implemented as a result of limitations like catheter-related infections as well as caregiver training. As the RRT horizon continues to evolve, knowledge of the distinct features and implications of every modality remains critical to providing optimal outcomes in pediatric critical care settings.

6.3.3. Pediatric Issues in RRT

In the pediatric population, initiation of renal replacement therapy (RRT) necessitates a delicate understanding of pharmacological and physiological considerations unique to the pediatric age group.

Incomplete renal function in neonates and young children can markedly affect drug pharmacokinetics, necessitating thoughtful dose adjustment to avoid either toxicity or subtherapeutic effect. For example, it is important to monitor carefully patients on antibiotic drugs like cefepime for acute kidney injury (AKI), as in one case where neurotoxicity arose secondary to unaltered dosing during the context of AKI (Andreoli *et al.*, 2011). Furthermore, perioperative integration recognizes the requirement for stability and homeostasis in procedures that may compromise renal function and hence underscores the absolute necessity of tailored approaches in the management of such vulnerable patients (Banerji *et al.*, 2017). Thus, an integrated approach ensures effective and safe RRT tailored to the needs of the pediatric patient (Figure 6.11).

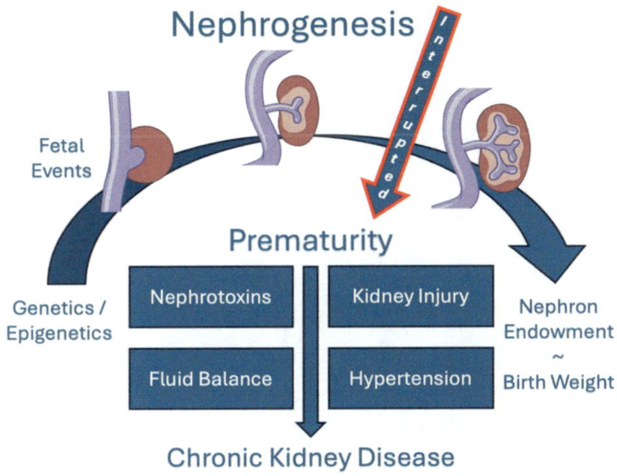

Figure 6.11. In pediatric patients, the initiation of renal replacement therapy (RRT) necessitates a nuanced understanding of both physiological and pharmacological factors unique to the youth population.

Source: https://www.mdpi.com/children/children-12-00339/article_deploy/html/images/children-12-00339-g001.png.

6.3.4. Complications Associated with RRT

The use of renal replacement therapy (RRT) in pediatric intensive care units is fraught with a wide range of possible complications that can profoundly affect patient outcomes.

The complications could either result from the very technical complexity of managing critically ill children or from the physiological alterations required during RRT. For instance, drug pharmacokinetic changes caused by the impact of extracorporeal therapeutic processes can lead to less-than-optimal drug effect or harmful side effects, which contribute to the clinician's challenges (Aebi *et al.*, 2017). Furthermore, children with predisposing states such as cancer are particularly at risk of acute kidney injury (AKI), typically enhanced by nephrotoxic treatment or acute tumor lysis syndrome (Benoit *et al.*, 2016).

Thus, acknowledgment of the different intricacies of these complications will be necessary to optimize renal and electrolyte management methods, ultimately for improved safety and effectiveness in RRT in this vulnerable group.

6.3.5. Timing and Initiation of RRT

Initiation and timing of renal replacement therapy (RRT) in the pediatric intensive care units are of paramount relevance in patient outcomes for acute kidney injury (AKI). Early RRT has been associated with higher survival rates and better overall recovery, and hence, identification of the best time of intervention is of utmost relevance.

Clinical practice guidelines, such as those of Kidney Disease: Improving Global Outcomes, emphasize the value of tailored treatment that considers the individual patients clinical circumstance, such as the severity of AKI and AKI-associated complications (Kellum *et al.*, 2013). Furthermore, the past protocols were created to offer timely and effective RRT initiation to correct fluid and electrolyte disorders and the accumulation of toxins (ADQI 26 workgroup *et al.*, 2024). Consequently, timely intervention and a structured management approach are required in maximizing renal results and overall paths to recovery among critically ill children (Figure 6.12).

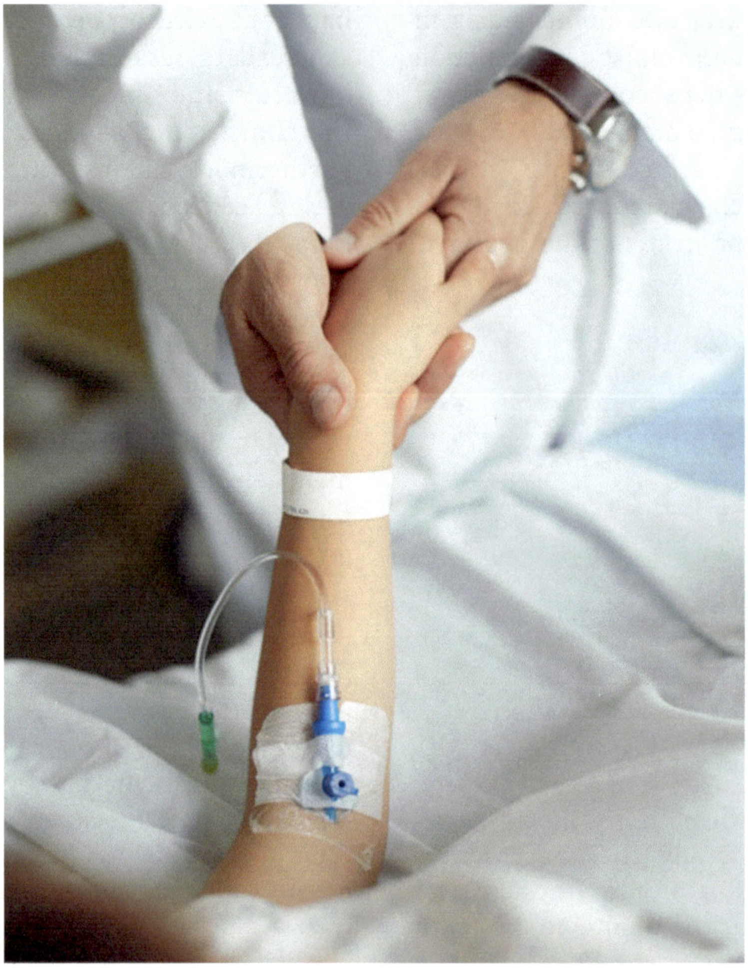

Figure 6.12. The timing and initiation of renal replacement therapy (RRT) in pediatric intensive care settings is a critical factor influencing patient outcomes in acute kidney injury (AKI).

Source: https://usbcci.baxter.com/sites/g/files/ebysai2396/files/2019-04/Acute_Kidney_Injury_HPlargetile.jpg.

6.3.6. Monitoring and Management During RRT

Effective monitoring and management during renal replacement therapy (RRT) are key components in maximizing pediatric patients with acute kidney injury. Ongoing monitoring of vital parameters, fluid balance, and biochemical markers is crucial in ensuring RRT is tailored to each child's unique needs, thereby preventing therapy-related complications. For instance, keeping a proper electrolyte balance and managing potential toxic effects of therapy can improve patient safety as well as chances for recovery significantly. Some protocols highlight the importance of countering acute toxic effects such as nephrotoxicity and its related complications, particularly in this high-risk population (Kellum *et al.*, 2013). Furthermore, the characterization of the frequency and severity of these toxic effects supports the need for multidisciplinary collaboration in formulating effective management plans. By committing to the adoption of established standards and enhancing treatment protocols, healthcare providers can significantly enhance the quality of renal and electrolyte management in pediatric critical care settings (Attarbaschi *et al.*, 2016).

6.3.7. Long-Term Outcomes of RRT in Children

Long-term consequences of renal replacement therapy (RRT) in infants and children are of special concern in renal and electrolyte management in the intensive care unit. Experience shows that children who receive RRT have long-term morbidity of unknown severity, such as growth failure and cardiovascular disease, which can manifest as significant issues to quality of life.

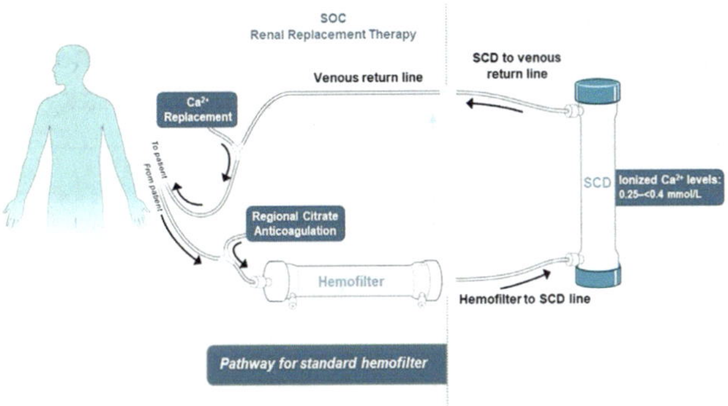

Figure 6.13. Children who undergo RRT are at risk for varying degrees of long-term morbidity, including growth impairment and cardiovascular complications.

Source: https://www.kidneymedicinejournal.org/cms/10.1016/j.xkme.2024.100792/asset/cdc19c18-0361-487e-ab2f-3cd920124aa8/main.assets/gr1_lrg.jpg.

The clinical guidelines developed by Kidney Disease: Improving Global Outcomes emphasize the significance of a proper assessment and management plan to decrease such outcomes, particularly in the case of acute kidney injury (AKI) (Kellum *et al.*, 2013).

On top of that, the need for individualized care pathways is emphasized, as the development level of the patients not only could influence their reaction to the treatment to start with but also their recovery in the long run (Kellum *et al.*, 2013). Such long-term implications need to be taken into account by healthcare professionals when planning holistic care for the vulnerable population (Figure 6.13).

6.3.8. Innovations in RRT Technology

As RRT technology evolves, pediatric critical care units are increasingly equipped to provide individualized and efficient treatment for children with acute kidney injury. Developments such as miniaturized, portable dialysis machines and continuous renal replacement therapies enable the provision of RRT in a more patient-focused manner in line with the trend toward individualized treatment in pediatric nephrology.

These technologies expand the flexibility of treatment approaches, allowing clinicians to better match them to varied patient needs and stabilize hemodynamic conditions during courses of critical care.

Furthermore, as highlighted in discourse regarding dialysis initiation and modality choice, integration of innovative patient-centered approaches has the potential to have a significant impact on the outcome for the pediatric patient with end-stage kidney disease (ESKD) (Davenport *et al.*, 2019). Better monitoring and automation in RRT procedures also promise to increase the quality and level of safety required in pediatric intensive care environments, ultimately to offer improved support to high-risk patient populations (Boscato *et al.*, 2023).

6.3.9. Ethical Issues in Pediatric RRT

The ethical aspects of renal replacement therapy (RRT) in pediatric patients are increasingly becoming significant in critical care. Physicians are faced with complex challenges in determining whether to initiate RRT in children, mostly weighing the chances against the risks, such as hemodynamic instability and long-term effects.

This decision-making is also compounded by an absence of randomized controlled trials pertaining to pediatric RRT, and thus, clinicians are left without tangible guidelines that can direct their decisions (Basu *et al.*, 2011). Further, the well-being of children and the potential for irreversible neurological damage caused by electrolyte imbalances, such as hyponatremia, also must be accorded priority (Aperia *et al.*, 2011). Thus, the pediatric RRT ethical landscape is marked by the necessity of informed guardianship consent and the application of multidisciplinary teams to ensure that treatment is in the patient's best interests. Lastly, such ethical subtleties necessitate the fine balance between intervention and careful monitoring within the risky context of the pediatric intensive care unit (Figure 6.14).

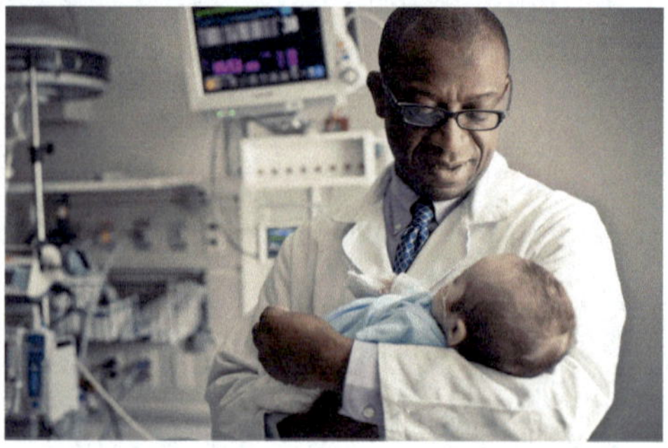

Figure 6.14. Physicians face complex dilemmas when deciding to initiate RRT for children, often weighing potential benefits against risks, such as hemodynamic instability and long-term outcomes.

Source: https://www.akronchildrens.org/images-general/84570/image/large/forbes-1481.png.

Test Your Knowledge

1. What challenges are specific to vascular access in pediatric patients requiring RRT?
2. How is fluid balance managed during RRT in infants and young children?

6.4. Multidisciplinary Approach to Renal and Electrolyte Management

Learning Outcome

1. Discuss the role of nephrologists in pediatric care.
2. Know the importance of nursing in electrolyte management.
3. Focus on collaboration with dietitians for nutritional support.
4. Discuss involvement of pharmacists in medication management.
5. Explain psychological support for pediatric patients and families.
6. Describe education and training for healthcare providers.
7. Understand family-centered care in the PICU.
8. Learn case management and follow-up care.
9. Explain research and advancements in pediatric nephrology.

Pediatric intensive care renal and electrolyte management complexities call for an interdisciplinary model of care involving multiple healthcare professionals, such as pediatric nephrologists, intensivists, nurses, and dietitians. Such a multimodal model provides for comprehensive and customized patient care adaptive to the unique needs of critically ill children.

As reported by recent studies, involvement of pediatric nephrologists in postoperative care in the immediate period following kidney transplant in the recipient is nearly universal at 97% of institutions (Abu-Sultaneh *et al.*, 2017). Furthermore, guidelines on acute kidney injury underscore the value of coordinated multidisciplinary care to optimize outcomes by evidence-based interventions (Kellum *et al.*, 2013). By facilitating effective communication and shared decision-making, the healthcare providers are able to bridge the complicated problems of renal and electrolyte imbalances and thereby enhance patient safety and recovery pathways in pediatric intensive care units.

6.4.1. Nephrologist's Role in Pediatric Care

Nephrologists play a crucial role in pediatric care with regard to the management and treatment of renal and electrolyte conditions, particularly in critical care.

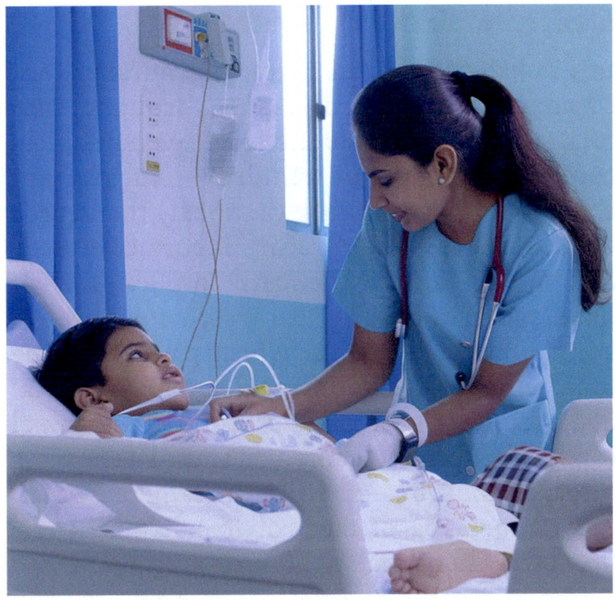

Figure 6.15. Role of nephrologists in pediatric care.

Source: https://www.dheehospitals.com/wp-content/uploads/2024/10/Paditrics.jpg.

Their expertise is crucial when it comes to diagnosing and managing conditions such as acute kidney injury (AKI), which are prevalent among critically ill children and need to be addressed immediately. The preferred modality of dialysis—intermittent hemodialysis, peritoneal dialysis, or continuous renal replacement therapy (CRRT)—depends on several patient and provider variables; thus, the involvement of nephrologists becomes essential (Airede *et al.*,

2008). The establishment of specialized renal teams, such as nephrologists and pediatric intensivists, has been shown to enhance the efficacy and efficiency of CRRT among children since there are greater rates of utilization after the deployment of such teams. Nephrologists have a significant role to play in creating care protocols that mirror evolving guidelines and thus ensure optimal kidney care in the intensive care unit (Figure 6.15).

6.4.2. Importance of Nursing in Electrolyte Management

In intensive care pediatrics, the nursing task of managing electrolytes is brought into focus because of the delicate physiological requirements of ill children. Nurses are charged with monitoring cautiously the degree of electrolytes, interpreting laboratory tests, and understanding delicate implications of imbalances caused by the treatment of acute lymphoblastic leukemia, which presents some toxic effects like nephrotoxicity and arterial hypertension (Attarbaschi *et al.*, 2016). As initial caregivers, nurses not only deliver the appropriate interventions but also inform families about the importance of electrolyte balance. Their proactive involvement in assessing hydration status and delivering timely interventions can prove to be a crucial step towards minimizing the risk of electrolyte disturbances, which are commonly observed in this high-risk population. Also, teamwork in their practice ensures that they appropriately convey vital information to the interdisciplinary care team, improving patient outcomes and the quality of care in the pediatric intensive care setting.

6.4.3. Teamwork with Dietitians for Nutritional Care

Effective coordination with dietitians is quite crucial in providing maximum nutritional care to pediatric intensive care, particularly for children suffering from renal problems. The intricate dynamic between nutrition and kidney function necessitates frequent alteration of dietary plans that have to be malleable enough to accommodate the variable nature of acute kidney injury (AKI) and other renal diseases. Through the efforts of interprofessional teams, for example, healthcare professionals and dietitians, individualized medical nutrition therapies can help in avoiding undesirable metabolic effects while helping cater to the needs of individual pediatric patients. Existing recommendations by the Pediatric Renal Nutrition Taskforce emphasize the importance of interprofessional partnership to ensure that nutritional care is synchronized with the individual medical treatments that are being provided (Anderson *et al.*, 2023). Furthermore, application of new interactive technologies in dietetic training enables active learning by the students, thereby improving the quality of care delivered by dietetic interns as they learn key skills in nutritional care (Litchfield *et al.*, 2000). Such an integrative approach thus enables improved patient outcomes in the pediatric intensive care setting (Figure 6.16).

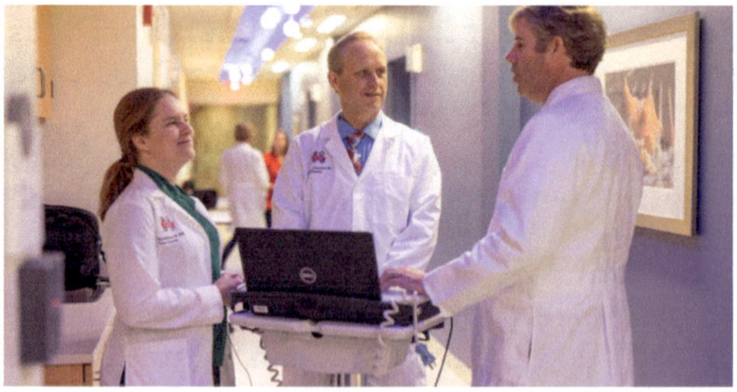

Figure 6.16. Effective collaboration with dietitians is crucial for providing optimal nutritional support in pediatric intensive care, particularly for children facing renal challenges.

Source: https://cdn.rileychildrens.org/content/_850x450_crop_center-center_none/pediatric_nephrology_team.jpg.

6.4.4. Involvement of Pharmacists in Medication Management

The role of pharmacists in drug management is of the highest priority, especially as it relates to renal and electrolyte management in pediatric intensive care units. Their professional judgment ensures effective and safe medication use, which is critical given the heightened risk of adverse effects among this vulnerable group. Pharmacists conduct medication reviews extensively, actively identifying potential drug interactions and managing drug pharmacokinetics in patients with impaired renal function. Active practice by pharmacists not only enhances patient safety but also optimizes the therapeutic effect. Moreover, in the delivery of sophisticated therapies such as parenteral nutrition, pharmacists have a key role in minimizing procedure-related risks through the rigorous practice of prescribed consensus guidelines encompassing prescribing and compounding processes (Adams *et al.*, 2014). They are essential in the personalized drug counseling and education, thus improving the multidisciplinary team's capability to provide quality care appropriate to the special needs of pediatric patients (Brophy *et al.*, 2005).

6.4.5. Psychological Support of Pediatric Patients and Their Families

Psychological management of the pediatric patients and their families is the most significant priority in pediatric intensive care from the perspective of renal and electrolyte management. Chronic illnesses, such as end-stage kidney disease, place huge psychological and emotional burdens, not only on the children, but on the caregivers as well. As highlighted within the recent arguments over the treatment of end-stage kidney disease, an interdisciplinary approach including psychological management can improve results overall by addressing the psychosocial expressions of the patient (Brennan *et al.*, 2020). Furthermore, adequate support mechanisms and interaction are also crucial to minimizing anxiety and fear over hospital admission and surgical procedures. Provision of comprehensive psychological care enables families to better cope with the emotional stressors that are linked to their child's condition, and with higher resilience and quality of life. Besides facilitating emotional well-being for the patient, this combination of care also maximizes the overall adherence of the patient to the treatment, which is central in pediatric settings (Kazuyoshi *et al.*, 2018) (Figure 6.17).

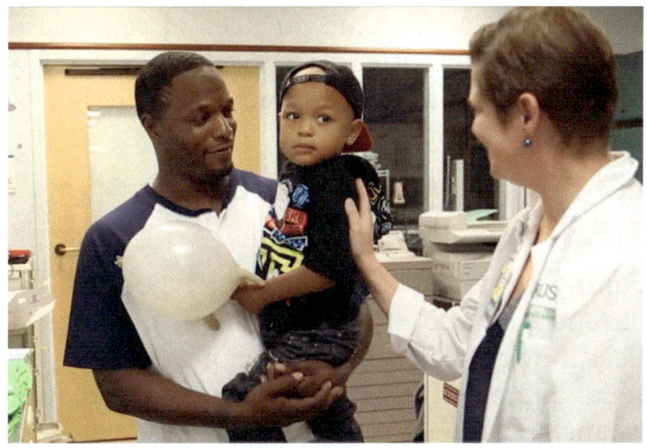

Figure 6.17. Chronic illnesses, such as end-stage kidney disease, impose significant emotional and psychological challenges, not only for the children but also for their caregivers.

Source: https://www.rush.edu/sites/default/files/inline-images/pediatric-nephrology-program-min.jpg.

6.4.6. Education and Training for Healthcare Providers

Whole-person education and professional training of healthcare workers are important in ensuring optimal renal and electrolyte management in the pediatric intensive care unit. The complexity of pediatric nephrology requires continuous professional development that enables healthcare workers to keep abreast with evolving practice and patient-centered care. Secondly, the increasing global burden of end-stage kidney disease (ESKD) also brings into focus the importance of customization in the treatment, as the KDIGO conference deliberations of the variation in dialysis initiation practices across the world (Davenport *et al.*, 2019). In addition, interventions on training that involve resources such as the Provider Bull's-Eye Tool (PBT) have been discovered to enhance more clinical reasoning and communication among nurse practitioners, thereby having a positive effect on patient experience and outcomes along key transitions of care (Zaworski *et al.*, 2019). By these competencies, healthcare providers are able to manage the nuances of renal care in pediatric intensive care, ultimately leading to increased quality and safety in care delivery.

6.4.7. Family-Centered Care in the PICU

Family-centered care has emerged as an essential model for enhancing the overall health of critically ill children, particularly for renal and electrolyte management in pediatric intensive care units (PICUs). Family-centered care is a recognition of the family's role in taking care of their children and making them understand and be involved in the medical decisions made. Through active involvement with families, the healthcare professionals can gather vital information regarding a child's medical background and tastes and make interventions more individualized. Notably, studies have highlighted advancements in critical care practices that significantly facilitate family involvement, as recorded in recent pediatric care progress reviews (Bernasconi *et al.*, 2019). In doing this, inclusion of family-centered principles not only promotes emotional health but also enhances clinical success, which is a testament to the need for ongoing practice to strengthen collaboration among healthcare workers and families in the PICU setting (Bernasconi *et al.*, 2019) (Figure 6.18).

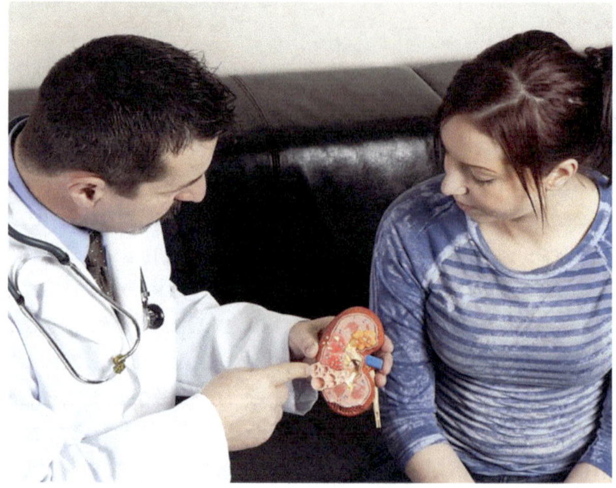

Figure 6.18. By actively engaging families, healthcare providers can gather valuable insights about a child's medical history and preferences, thus tailoring interventions more effectively.

Source: https://cdn.prod.website-files.com/6265a955fd624c60a9c38baa/6297e1eddab9bd11464464d4_gipokaliemiya-diagnostika.webp.

6.4.8. Case Management and Follow-Up Care

Effective follow-up care and case management are an essential part of the overall strategy for renal and electrolyte management in pediatric intensive care. With the heterogeneity of pathologies within renal disease in children, a firm case management plan is required to provide for the different requirements of this vulnerable group. It involves personalized treatment plans, systematic monitoring, and interprofessional team communication, such that the child's all conditions are considered. Follow-up treatment not only offers proper monitoring of renal function and homeostasis of electrolytes but also promotes early intervention against potential treatment toxicity complications, as research on acute toxic effects in children with acute lymphoblastic leukemia highlights (Attarbaschi *et al.*, 2016). Besides, recent pediatrics advancements provide valuable information on the improvement of patient outcomes through the augmentation of increased follow-up mechanisms, thereby enabling the inclusion of effective preventive practices (Bernasconi *et al.*, 2019).

6.4.9. Research and Advances in Pediatric Nephrology

Extensive research and advancements in the field of pediatric nephrology have fallen into prominence, particularly in managing acute kidney injury (AKI) in pediatric intensive care unit settings. Further refinements in continuous renal replacement therapy (CRRT) have been shown to be pivotal in the management of multi-organ dysfunction syndrome in children, showing that early initiation of CRRT combined with effective fluid management can enhance survival in critically ill children (Baker *et al.*, 2005). Along with this, the development in specialized extracorporeal dialysis technologies that are suited for neonate and infant-specific physiology is reflective of the advancements in this field. The newer models minimize the volume of blood used for therapies such as hemodialysis and continuous KRT so that solute clearance is improved without any compromise in hemodynamic stability (Ceschia *et al.*, 2023). Combined, these advances herald a scientific revolution in pediatric nephrology to improve clinical outcomes through evidence-based, targeted therapeutic interventions and technology-based solutions.

Test Your Knowledge

1. How is communication coordinated among the multidisciplinary team in complex renal cases?
2. What family education and support considerations are important in pediatric renal emergencies?

SUMMARY

Renal and electrolyte management in pediatric intensive care highlights the utmost importance of uniform guidelines to enhance outcomes in children with the condition. As evident from recent data, the prevalence of acute kidney injury (AKI) underscores pivotal challenges with which clinical professionals have to deal, necessitating firm compliance with evidence-based methods as prescribed by the international clinical practice guidelines for AKI (Kellum *et al.*, 2013). Furthermore, heterogeneity in early post-transplant management in pediatric kidney transplant patients is an indicator of the absence of pediatric-specific guidelines, and this demonstrates the imperative for centers to take a similar route towards streamlining management strategies (Abu-Sultaneh *et al.*, 2017). The inclusion of such guidelines enables better monitoring and therapeutic interventions and, notably, enhances recovery pathways. Therefore, continuous communication and research on best practices are necessary in order to minimize disparities and strengthen the quality of care delivered in pediatric intensive care environments so that all patients can be provided with optimum renal and electrolyte management.

Renal function and electrolyte management are an important part of pediatric intensive care due to the high susceptibility of children to acute kidney injury (AKI) complications and electrolyte balance abnormalities. Renal management directly influences a child's overall clinical outcome because compromised renal function exacerbates fluid overload and blunts acid-base balance and has serious repercussions on health. Dialytic treatments, whether intermittent hemodialysis, peritoneal dialysis, or continuous renal replacement therapy, must be tailored to the patient's unique profile and clinical needs, a service informed by well-refined criteria such as the profile framework (Airede *et al.*, 2008). Furthermore, guidelines like the Japanese Clinical Practice Guidelines for Management of Sepsis and Septic Shock also recognize the need to include renal and electrolyte management within overall treatment protocols (Kazuyoshi *et al.*, 2018). By having such a general approach, health care providers are better equipped to address the complex issues of severely ill children.

KEY TERMS FROM THIS CHAPTER

- Electrolyte management
- Risk evaluation
- Chemotherapy
- Sodium
- Electrolytes
- Muscle contraction
- Dyschloremia
- Acute lymphoblastic leukemia
- Acute kidney injury (AKI)
- Nephrotoxicity
- Kidneys
- Potassium
- Nerves
- Glomerular filtration rate (GFR)
- Hyperchloremia
- Renin-angiotensin-aldosterone system (RAAS)

CRITICAL THINKING QUESTIONS

1. **What is the most common cause of acute kidney injury (AKI) in critically ill children?**
   a. Congenital anomalies
   b. Hypovolemia and sepsis
   c. Nephrotoxic medications
   d. Urinary tract obstruction
2. **Which electrolyte disturbance is most commonly associated with cardiac arrhythmias in PICU patients?**
   a. Hypernatremia
   b. Hypokalemia
   c. Hypercalcemia
   d. Hypomagnesemia
3. **What is the primary goal of fluid management in pediatric patients with acute kidney injury?**
   a. Achieve negative fluid balance immediately
   b. Maintain adequate perfusion without causing overload
   c. Restrict all fluids until dialysis
   d. Give large volume boluses regardless of status
4. **Which of the following is a common sign of hyponatremia in critically ill children?**
   a. Polyuria
   b. Seizures
   c. Hypertension
   d. Bradycardia
5. **In a child with hyperkalemia, which treatment is used to stabilize cardiac membranes rapidly?**
   a. Sodium bicarbonate
   b. Calcium gluconate
   c. Insulin and glucose
   d. Furosemide

Short Answer Questions

1. How does renal function in neonates differ from that in older children and adults?
2. What are the key stages of kidney maturation in infancy and early childhood?
3. What are the most common electrolyte disturbances seen in critically ill pediatric patients?
4. What are the clinical manifestations of hyponatremia in children?
5. What are the main indications for initiating renal replacement therapy (RRT) in children?
6. What roles do nephrologists, intensivists, and nurses play in managing pediatric renal failure?
7. How does the dietitian contribute to electrolyte and fluid management in the PICU?

Answers to Critical Thinking Questions

1. (b) 2. (b) 3. (b) 4. (b) 5. (b)

REFERENCES

1. Abdollahi, M., Ahmadi, A., Ghaini, M. R., Mojtahedzadeh, M., *et al.* (2025). The role of magnesium sulfate in the intensive care unit. https://core.ac.uk/download/pdf/141827972.pdf (accessed on 30th June 2025).
2. Abu-Sultaneh, S., Goggins, W. C., Hobson, M. J., Lutfi, R., *et al.* (2017). Practice variation in the immediate postoperative care of pediatric kidney transplantation: A national survey. https://core.ac.uk/download/158967822.pdf (accessed on 30th June 2025).
3. Adams, S., American Society for Parenteral and Enteral Nutrition, Ayers, P., Boullata, J., *et al.* (2014). A.S.P.E.N. parenteral nutrition safety consensus recommendations. https://core.ac.uk/download/62428919.pdf (accessed on 30th June 2025).
4. ADQI 26 Workgroup, Arikan, A. A., Askenazi, D. J., Basu, R., *et al.* (2024). Programs and processes for advancing pediatric acute kidney support therapy in hospitalized and critically ill children: A report from the 26th Acute Disease Quality Initiative (ADQI) consensus conference. https://core.ac.uk/download/604217787.pdf (accessed on 30th June 2025).
5. Aebi, A., Shah, G., Anderson, M., Arlt, W., Barr, J., Barthelemy, R., Beiderlinden, M., *et al.* (2017). Medication complications in extracorporeal membrane oxygenation. https://core.ac.uk/download/129191716.pdf (accessed on 30th June 2025).
6. Airede, A., Akcan-Arikan, A., Auron, A., Sehic, A., Sehic, A., Alarabi, A. A., Arieff, A. I., *et al.* (2008). Dialysis and pediatric acute kidney injury: Choice of renal support modality. https://core.ac.uk/download/pdf/8335291.pdf (accessed on 30th June 2025).
7. Ali, A. A. A., Badawy, F. A., Esmail, N. S., HelmyAbdelhady, M., *et al.* (2022). Hyperchloremia in critically ill patients in ICU: Review article. https://core.ac.uk/download/524771712.pdf (accessed on 30th June 2025).
8. Althouse, S. K., Batra, S., Rahrig, A., Rupenthal, L., *et al.* (2018). Factors associated with a prolonged hospital stay during induction chemotherapy in newly diagnosed high risk pediatric acute lymphoblastic leukemia. https://core.ac.uk/download/160755266.pdf (accessed on 30th June 2025).
9. Anderson, C. E., Cerminara, D., Desloovere, A., Greenbaum, L. A., *et al.* (2023). Nutritional management of children with acute kidney injury—Clinical practice recommendations from the Pediatric Renal Nutrition Taskforce. https://core.ac.uk/download/613946687.pdf (accessed on 30th June 2025).
10. Andreoli, S. P., Brown, D. M., Knoderer, C. A., Nichols, K. R., *et al.* (2011). Cefepime neurotoxicity in an adolescent cystic fibrosis patient with aminoglycoside-induced acute kidney injury. https://core.ac.uk/download/62428828.pdf (accessed on 30th June 2025).
11. Aoyama, K., Azuhata, T., Doi, K., Matsuyuki, D., Egi, M., Fujimura, N., Fujishima, S., *et al.* (2018). The Japanese clinical practice guidelines for management of sepsis and septic shock 2016 (J-SSCG 2016). https://core.ac.uk/download/154950014.pdf (accessed on 30th June 2025).
12. Aperia, A., Au, A., Durward, A., Leaf, A., Steele, A., Arieff, A. I., Arieff, A. I., *et al.* (2011). The efficacy of hypotonic and near-isotonic saline for parenteral fluid therapy given at low maintenance rate in preventing significant change in plasma sodium in post-operative pediatric patients: Protocol for a prospective randomized non-blinded study. https://core.ac.uk/download/pdf/8601016.pdf (accessed on 30th June 2025).

13. Arriagada, D. S., Cruces, P. R., & Donoso, A. F. (2015). Pulmonary-renal crosstalk in the critically ill patient. https://core.ac.uk/download/288915683.pdf (accessed on 30th June 2025).

14. Attarbaschi, A., Barzilai, S., Escherich, G., Frandsen, B., *et al.* (2016). Consensus definitions of 14 severe acute toxic effects for childhood lymphoblastic leukemia treatment: A Delphi consensus. https://core.ac.uk/download/42370388.pdf (accessed on 30th June 2025).

15. Aversa, T., Capalbo, D., Cozzolino, M., de Sanctis, L., del Pistoia, M., Dituri, F., Garbetta, G., *et al.* (2023). Perinatal asphyxia and hypothermic treatment from the endocrine perspective. https://core.ac.uk/download/638799899.pdf (accessed on 30th June 2025).

16. Baker, C., Barnett, J., Baum, M. A., Blowey, D., *et al.* (2005). Pediatric patients with multi-organ dysfunction syndrome receiving continuous renal replacement therapy. https://core.ac.uk/download/pdf/82334978.pdf (accessed on 30th June 2025).

17. Balaraman, V., Osmani, V., & Sheikhalishahi, S. (2020). Benchmarking machine learning models on multi-centre eICU critical care dataset. https://core.ac.uk/download/543474288.pdf (accessed on 30th June 2025).

18. Banerji, A., Farooqi, S., Haug, S., Hopper, S., *et al.* (2017). Perioperative care of the neonate. https://core.ac.uk/download/322429716.pdf (accessed on 30th June 2025).

19. Basu, R. K., Doughty, L., Goldstein, S., Wheeler, D., *et al.* (2011). Acute renal replacement therapy in pediatrics. https://core.ac.uk/download/pdf/8582363.pdf (accessed on 30th June 2025).

20. Bayrakci, B., Bianzina, S., Bottari, G., Briassoulis, G., *et al.* (2025). Extracorporeal blood purification in European pediatric intensive care units. https://core.ac.uk/download/646220868.pdf (accessed on 30th June 2025).

21. Bellón, J. M., del Castillo, J., López-Herce, J., Santiago, M. J., *et al.* (2013). Continuous renal replacement therapy in children after cardiac surgery. https://core.ac.uk/download/pdf/82530454.pdf (accessed on 30th June 2025).

22. Benoit, D., Lameire, N., Van Biesen, W., Vanholder, R., *et al.* (2016). Acute kidney injury in critically ill cancer patients: An update. https://core.ac.uk/download/55807820.pdf (accessed on 30th June 2025).

23. Bernasconi, S., Borrelli, M., Caffarelli, C., Corsello, G., *et al.* (2019). Report on advances for pediatricians in 2018: Allergy, cardiology, critical care, endocrinology, hereditary metabolic diseases, gastroenterology, infectious diseases, neonatology, nutrition, respiratory tract disorders and surgery. https://core.ac.uk/download/pdf/237170258.pdf (accessed on 30th June 2025).

24. Boscato, S. (2023). Risk factors and outcomes of oncohematologic patients admitted to pediatric intensive care unit: ONCOTIPNET, an Italian multicenter study. https://core.ac.uk/download/588606296.pdf (accessed on 30th June 2025).

25. Brennan, F., Davidson, B., Krause, R., Wearne, N., *et al.* (2020). Renal palliative and supportive care in South Africa–A consensus statement. https://core.ac.uk/download/386359520.pdf (accessed on 30th June 2025).

26. Brophy, G. M., Erstad, B. L., Haas, C. E., Jacobi, J., *et al.* (2005). Key articles and guidelines relative to intensive care unit pharmacology—2004. https://deepblue.lib.umich.edu/bitstream/2027.42/90189/1/phco.25.4.585.61024.pdf (accessed on 30th June 2025).

27. Bullock, A. F. (2022). The detection and assessment of malnutrition, sarcopenia and cachexia, in older adults with cancer. https://core.ac.uk/download/595480920.pdf (accessed on 30th June 2025).
28. Carter, H., Leiter, P., Nour, C., Vadi, V., *et al.* (2017). Anesthetic management of the newborn surgical patient. https://core.ac.uk/download/322429460.pdf (accessed on 30th June 2025).
29. Ceschia, G., Parolin, M., & Vidal, E. (2023). New perspectives in pediatric dialysis technologies: The case for neonates and infants with acute kidney injury. https://core.ac.uk/download/576928440.pdf (accessed on 30th June 2025).
30. Chawla, L. S., Kellum, J. A., & Ronco, C. (2012). Permissive hypofiltration. https://core.ac.uk/download/78482785.pdf (accessed on 30th June 2025).
31. Chimbira, W., Crawford, H., Gupta, S., Legg, J., *et al.* (2001). Acute lung injury in pediatric intensive care: Course and outcome. https://core.ac.uk/download/pdf/8715345.pdf (accessed on 30th June 2025).
32. Choi, M. R., Fernandez, B. E., Kouyoumdzian, N. M., Kravetz, D., *et al.* (2015). Renal dopaminergic system: Pathophysiological implications and clinical perspectives. https://core.ac.uk/download/52483298.pdf (accessed on 30th June 2025).
33. Dahl, E. M., Hutchinson, D., & Prescott, W. A. (2014). Education in pediatrics in US colleges and schools of pharmacy. https://core.ac.uk/download/287923247.pdf (accessed on 30th June 2025).
34. Davenport, A., Liew, A., Nadeau-Fredette, A., Tong, A., Bleyer, A. J., Abu-Alfa, A. K., Wang, A. Y., *et al.* (2019). Dialysis initiation, modality choice, access, and prescription: Conclusions from a kidney disease: Improving Global Outcomes (KDIGO) Controversies Conference. https://core.ac.uk/download/201752561.pdf (accessed on 30th June 2025).
35. David-Neto, E., Nahas, W. C., Torricelli, F. C. M., Watanabe, M., *et al.* (2014). Current management issues of immediate postoperative care in pediatric kidney transplantation. https://core.ac.uk/download/268269329.pdf (accessed on 30th June 2025).
36. Dewitte, A., Ishani, A., Ishani, A., Morden, A., Pai, A. B., Schneider, A. G., Lewington, A. J., *et al.* (2017). Acute kidney disease and renal recovery: Consensus report of the Acute Disease Quality Initiative (ADQI) 16 Workgroup. https://core.ac.uk/download/84041861.pdf (accessed on 30th June 2025).
37. Dodington, S. (2025). Nutritional abnormalities in patients receiving long-term home parenteral nutrition. https://core.ac.uk/download/444041684.pdf (accessed on 30th June 2025).
38. Falhammar, H., Rushworth, R. L., & Torpy, D. J. (2019). Adrenal crisis. https://core.ac.uk/download/228075100.pdf (accessed on 30th June 2025).
39. Hsu, C. Y., Ku, E., Lin, F., McCulloch, C. E., *et al.* (2019). Effect of blood pressure control on long-term risk of end-stage renal disease and death among subgroups of patients with chronic kidney disease. https://core.ac.uk/download/323072766.pdf (accessed on 30th June 2025).
40. Huffer, K. (2017). Improving new graduate critical care nurse practitioner knowledge and retention using a dedicated orientation and mentoring program. https://core.ac.uk/download/217321337.pdf (accessed on 30th June 2025).

41. Kellum, J. A., & Lameire, N. (2013). Contrast-induced acute kidney injury and renal support for acute kidney injury: A KDIGO summary (part 2). https://core.ac.uk/download/55800526.pdf (accessed on 30th June 2025).
42. Litchfield, R. E. (2000). Implementation and evaluation of interactive online instruction in the dietetic internship. https://core.ac.uk/download/38904923.pdf (accessed on 30th June 2025).
43. Lombardi, G. (2022). Electrolyte's variability and clinical outcomes, in-hospital mortality and acute kidney injury. https://core.ac.uk/download/543577182.pdf (accessed on 30th June 2025).
44. Tupper, H. (2016). Confronting the growing burden of kidney disease: The sub-Saharan landscape. https://open.bu.edu/bitstream/2144/19210/1/Tupper_bu_0017N_11986.pdf (accessed on 30th June 2025).
45. Zaworski, T. (2019). Implementation of the Provider Bull's-eye: A tool to guide clinical reasoning and communication for nurse practitioners. https://core.ac.uk/download/215176916.pdf (accessed on 30th June 2025).

ENDOCRINE AND METABOLIC EMERGENCIES

7

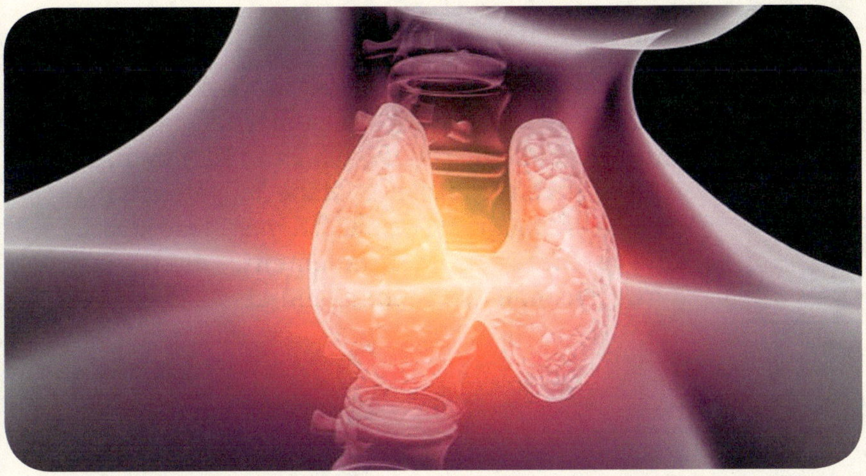

LEARNING OBJECTIVES

After studying this chapter, you will be able to:

1. Understand Common Endocrine Emergencies in Pediatrics.
2. Explain Metabolic Emergencies in Pediatric Patients.
3. Describe Diagnosis and Management Strategies.

Introduction

The heightened perceptions of endocrine and metabolic emergencies in pediatric patients require a distinct appreciation of their complications in the intensive care unit. With an increase in conditions such as diabetes mellitus and hypertension, healthcare providers are faced with daunting challenges in early management and diagnosis. The prevalence of hypertension among children and adolescents has emerged as a serious public health problem, with attention directed at its long-term cardiovascular consequences, as highlighted in Agabiti-Rosei *et al.* (2016). Concurrently, diabetes mellitus, particularly its acute manifestations, diabetic ketoacidosis and hyperosmolar hyperglycemic state, is fraught with extreme peril in children and demands urgent therapies including fluid replacement and insulin infusion (Gort *et al.*, 2020). This chapter aims to explain the salient characteristics of these metabolic and endocrine disasters and emphasize the need for advanced protocols and enhanced vigilance in pediatric intensive care units for improved patient outcomes (Figure 7.1).

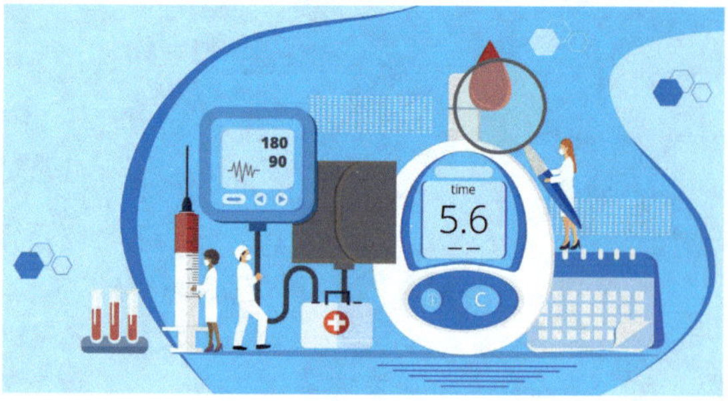

Figure 7.1. Diabetes mellitus and hypertension escalate, healthcare professionals face significant challenges in timely diagnosis and management.

Source: https://www.mdanderson.org/images/publications/cancerwise/D/CW-diabetes-iStock-1168613048.jpg.

7.1. Common Endocrine Emergencies in Pediatrics

Learning Outcome

1. Understand diabetic ketoacidosis.
2. Explain hyperglycemic hyperosmolar state.
3. Focus on adrenal crisis.
4. Discuss thyroid storm and hypoglycemia.
5. Describe pheochromocytoma crisis.
6. Know growth hormone deficiency emergencies.
7. Explain congenital adrenal hyperplasia.
8. Focus on Cushing's syndrome in children.

In pediatric critical care, frequent endocrine emergencies tend to present abruptly and may threaten the lives of vulnerable children. Of such conditions, adrenal crises are most urgent, which are severe glucocorticoid deficiency that requires immediate treatment to avert fatal consequences. As noted in recent literature, the incidence of adrenal crisis has been shown to increase, despite the presence of effective preventive measures, calling for greater awareness among clinicians (Falhammar *et al.*, 2019). In addition, elevated blood pressure in children and adolescents has become a serious public health concern, posing cardiovascular complications if left untreated. The increasing recognition of pediatric hypertension highlights the need for correct diagnosis and initiation of overall management regimens considering emerging risk factors and vascular phenotypes (Agabiti-Rosei *et al.*, 2016). Overall, these endocrine emergencies highlight the need for better awareness and active management in pediatric intensive care units.

7.1.1. Diabetic Ketoacidosis (DKA)

Diabetic ketoacidosis (DKA) is a potentially fatal emergency among the pediatric endocrine and metabolic disorders, which predominantly affects juvenile Type 1 diabetic patients. It results from insulin insufficiency, leading to severe metabolic derangements, including hyperglycemia, ketonemia, and acidosis.

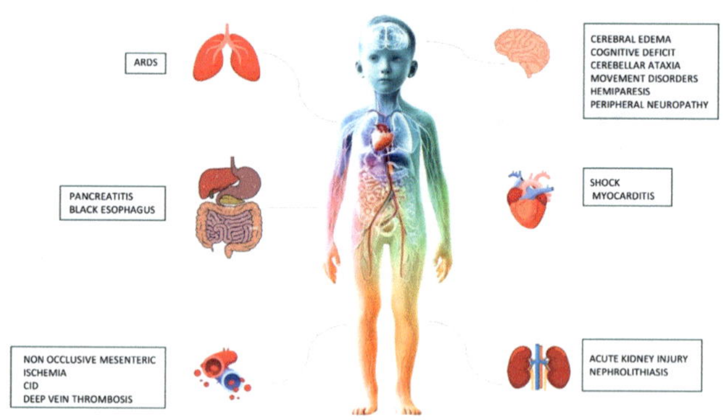

Figure 7.2. Diabetic ketoacidosis (DKA) represents a critical emergency within the spectrum of pediatric endocrine and metabolic disorders, predominantly affecting young individuals with Type 1 diabetes mellitus.

Source: https://pub.mdpi-res.com/children/children-12-00110/article_deploy/html/images/children-12-00110-g002.png?1737273085.

Treatment is urgent, with mortality up to 1–2% in developed environments but much increased in the developing world, implying the necessity for early clinical presentation

(Abdulrazzaq *et al.*, 2016). DKA occurs in approximately a quarter of new-onset diabetes in the child and usually in the context of infections or inadequate insulin control on intercurrent illness (Gort *et al.*, 2020). In addition, children, and particularly adolescent females, are at increased risk of recurrence in the event of previous episodes.

Therefore, accurate identification of the symptoms of DKA and understanding of its pathogenesis is required to appropriate management in the pediatric intensive care unit (Figure 7.2).

7.1.2. Hyperglycemic Hyperosmolar State (HHS)

The hyperglycemic hyperosmolar condition (HHS) is a formidable challenge in pediatric intensive care, mostly in those with type 2 diabetes mellitus, but also being increasingly seen in children with type 1 diabetes. Marked by profound hyperglycemia, increased serum osmolality, and relative lack of ketoacidosis, HHS can result in catastrophic neurological complications if not timely managed. Diagnosis relies on clinical presentation of polyuria, polydipsia, and alteration in mental status supplemented by laboratory data of hyperglycemia >600 mg/dL and serum osmolality >320 mOsm/kg (Gort *et al.*, 2020). The case of a male patient presenting with extreme hyperglycemia and hyperosmolarity underscores the need for caution and swift response in managing HHS due to the fact that misdiagnosis has potentially disastrous results (Chun *et al.*, 2022).

Early detection and aggressive treatment measures, that is, intravenous fluid therapy and insulin therapy, are also crucial in maximizing the outcome in such precarious circumstances.

7.1.3. Adrenal Crisis

Adrenal crisis is a critical condition in pediatric intensive care characterized by an acute deficiency in glucocorticoids that can lead to severe hypotension, shock, and ultimately death if not promptly diagnosed and treated. Adrenal crisis commonly occurs in children with adrenal insufficiency, particularly during physiological stress, for instance, disease or surgery.

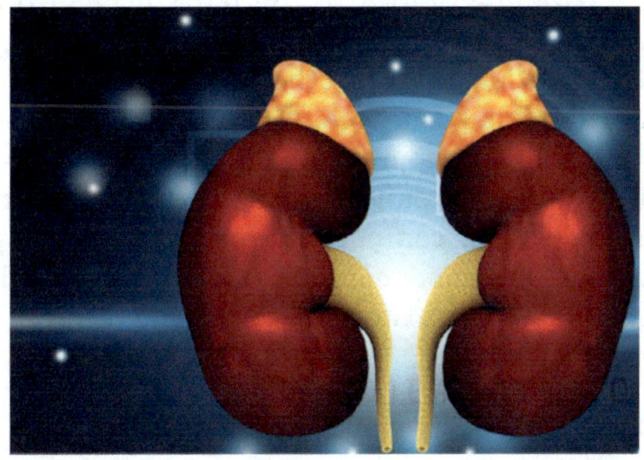

Figure 7.3. Adrenal crisis represents a critical challenge in pediatric intensive care, characterized by a severe deficiency of glucocorticoids that can lead to profound hypotension, shock, and even death if not promptly recognized and treated.

Source: https://www.emra.org/siteassets/emresident/images/articles/2022/02-february/49-1-pediatric-adrenal-insufficiency.png?w=600.

Despite improvement in glucocorticoid replacement therapy that has boosted survival rates since the 1950s for patients suffering from adrenal insufficiency, the frequency of adrenal crisis is alarming, which reflects inadequate preventive measures and monitoring (Falhammar *et al.*, 2019). The need to assess carefully and intervene early is exemplified by the complexity in the regulation of adrenal hormones in children, such that every patient may have very divergent responses. Last but not least, familiarity with adrenal crisis pathophysiology and treatment guidelines is important for medical professionals in guaranteeing the health of vulnerable pediatric patients (Agabiti-Rosei *et al.*, 2016) (Figure 7.3).

7.1.4. Thyroid Storm

Thyroid storm represents a critical endocrine emergency that primarily arises from uncontrolled hyperthyroidism, characterized by an exacerbation of hypermetabolic processes, including severe tachycardia, fever, and altered mental status. In pediatric intensive care, timely recognition and intervention are paramount, as the condition can lead to multiorgan dysfunction if left untreated. The pathophysiology of thyroid storm involves profound disturbances in hormonal regulation, particularly in the hypothalamic-pituitary-thyroid (HPT) axis, which can also overlap with the dysregulation seen in other endocrine emergencies, such as severe sepsis, where alterations in the HPA axis occur (Mehdi *et al.*, 2025). The complexities of managing thyroid storm necessitate a multifaceted approach, combining antithyroid medications, beta-blockers, and supportive care to stabilize the patient's metabolic state. Furthermore, the catecholamine surge associated with thyroid storm can provoke paroxysmal sympathetic hyperactivity, further complicating clinical outcomes (Nasa *et al.*, 2024). Thus, a thorough understanding and prompt intervention are crucial in managing this life-threatening condition.

7.1.5. Hypoglycemia

Treatment of hypoglycemia in pediatric intensive care is essential because the condition will cause severe neurological damage if not timely and appropriately intervened.

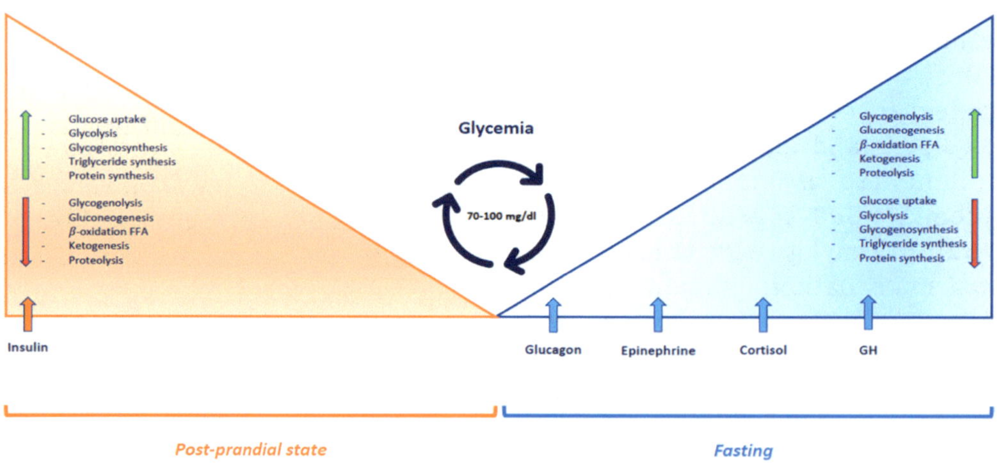

Figure 7.4. The management of hypoglycemia in pediatric intensive care is critical, as this condition can lead to severe neurological impairment if not promptly addressed.

Source: https://www.mdpi.com/nutrients/nutrients-15-03544/article_deploy/html/images/nutrients-15-03544-g001.png.

Hypoglycemia in children, particularly with associated endocrine disease such as diabetes mellitus, most commonly happens because of inappropriately administered insulin therapy or even inadequate carbohydrate replenishment. Keen monitoring is required because early detection of hypoglycemia will prevent the onset of more severe complications, such as seizures and brain injury, causing unconsciousness. Research identifies that hypoglycemia may be accompanied by adrenal crises in children with adrenal insufficiency, in whom low glucocorticoid levels once again complicate metabolic instability (Falhammar *et al.*, 2019). In addition, diabetic children of all types, particularly those with Type 1 diabetes, need to be cautious about the ratio between insulin injections and food consumption to prevent hypoglycemic episodes, further emphasizing the necessity of multidimensional management strategies in pediatric intensive care units (Gort *et al.*, 2020) (Figure 7.4).

7.1.6. Pheochromocytoma Crisis

Pheochromocytoma crisis is a catastrophic endocrine emergency that can seriously compromise pediatric patients and necessitate prompt identification and management. Being bypassed by catecholamine release-induced paroxysms of severe hypertension, the crisis can lead to catastrophic consequences in the form of hypertensive emergencies that are capable of inducing end-organ injury. The awareness of hypertension in pediatric populations has increased, and heightened detection of primary arterial hypertension (PAH) is now a common finding among adolescents, highlighting the need for vigilance when assessing the differential reasons for hypertensive events (Akingbola *et al.*, 2012). Although pheochromocytoma is rare in children, its presentation can mimic primary forms of hypertension, complicating clinical decision-making (Agabiti-Rosei *et al.*, 2016). Early diagnosis through biochemical investigations and imaging, followed by management that may consist of antihypertensive therapy and surgery, is imperative to prevent complications of this lethal condition. The severity of pheochromocytoma crisis dictates the provision of expertise within the pediatric intensive care unit.

7.1.7. Growth Hormone Deficiency Emergencies

In pediatric intensive care, emergencies due to growth hormone deficiency can present challenging situations, necessitating rapid and successful intervention.

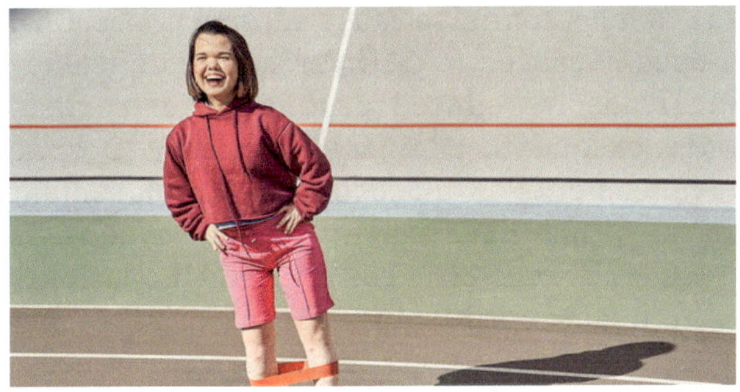

Figure 7.5. Growth hormone deficiency (GHD) manifests not only as stunted growth but also as a predisposition to other metabolic derangements, including altered glucose metabolism.

Source: https://ai-care.id/photos/dr%20 arifin/63c52302889cf.jpeg.

Growth hormone deficiency (GHD) is not merely manifested as growth retardation but also in susceptibility to other derangements in metabolism, e.g., deranged glucose metabolism. This dual effect induces identical concerns as those faced in diabetic ketoacidosis, in which disturbances in endocrines lead to potentially fatal physiological disequilibria that spiral out of control when they are not treated with priority (Abdulrazzaq *et al.*, 2016). Furthermore, the prevalence of child hypertension may be worsened by long-term GHD and therefore correlates with total cardiovascular risk in the children's population (Agabiti-Rosei *et al.*, 2016). Consequently, clinicians must possess an increased index of suspicion for GHD among the high-risk patients and implement prompt diagnosis and treatment regimens to counteract the threat of potentially life-threatening complications in the exposed population (Figure 7.5).

7.1.8. Congenital Adrenal Hyperplasia (CAH)

Among endocrine and metabolic emergencies in pediatric intensive care, Congenital Adrenal Hyperplasia (CAH) is of special clinical interest due to its potential to cause adrenal crises. CAH is usually caused by 21-hydroxylase deficiency and leads to reduced production of cortisol and subsequently adrenal insufficiency. Despite advancements in glucocorticoid replacement therapy that have maximized survival rates since the mid-20th century, CAH patients remain susceptible to adrenal crises—life-threatening conditions characterized by acute adrenal insufficiency (Falhammar *et al.*, 2019). Further, with cases of child hypertension with CAH emerging, the complexity in the management of this disorder includes cardiovascular complications, and thus attention and intervention need to be exercised carefully (Agabiti-Rosei *et al.*, 2016). Hence, knowledge of CAH's pathophysiology and its application in the critical care setting is required to achieve optimal outcomes for children so impacted.

7.1.9. Cushing's Syndrome in Children

Cushing's syndrome, with its hypercortisolism, is a very challenging condition in pediatric intensive care, particularly since it has varied etiologies and may possess serious complications. The syndrome in children is most commonly caused by endogenous factors such as an adrenal tumor, or more commonly, a pituitary adenoma leading to Cushing's disease. The physical presentation among young patients could be represented by rapid weight gain, hypertension, and growth retardation, which, if not appreciated, result in extreme long-term morbidities and increased mortality risks (Broersen *et al.*, 2019). The complex dilemma of Cushing's syndrome involves the obligation of clinicians to possess an acute awareness of physical as well as psychological aftermaths resulting from prolonged hypercortisolism. Treatment requires a thorough and multidisciplinary approach that is appropriate to each child's needs, with particular emphasis on the necessity for increased awareness and knowledge of this endocrine crisis in children's clinics and hospitals (Association, 1962) (Figure 7.6).

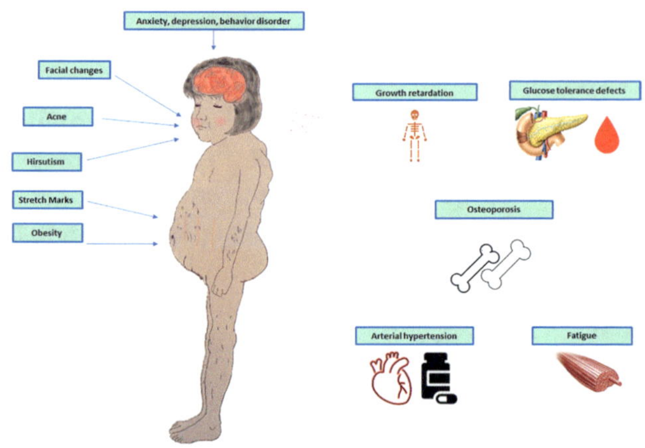

Figure 7.6. Cushing's syndrome, characterized by excess cortisol levels, presents a notably challenging scenario within pediatric intensive care.

Source: https://www.frontiersin.org/files/Articles/1329082/fendo-14-1329082-HTML/image_m/fendo-14-1329082-g001.jpg.

Test Your Knowledge

1. How is congenital hypothyroidism identified and managed in critically ill neonates?
2. What is thyroid storm, and how does it differ from hyperthyroidism in presentation and severity?

7.2. Metabolic Emergencies in Pediatric Patients

Learning Outcome

1. Understand inborn errors of metabolism.
2. Explain acute liver failure.
3. Describe urea cycle disorders.
4. Focus on fatty acid oxidation disorders.
5. Discuss organic acidemias.
6. Explain electrolyte imbalances.
7. Explain metabolic acidosis.
8. Focus on metabolic alkalosis.
9. Understand hyperammonemia.

The control of metabolic emergencies in children is of utmost importance when viewed from the perspective of pediatric intensive care because these conditions readily develop into extreme complications if not monitored. Two of the most significant metabolic emergencies are diabetic ketoacidosis (DKA) and hypertension, both of which pose significant threats to the well-being of children. DKA is most prominently exhibited in children with Type 1 diabetes mellitus in the form of high serum glucose levels and metabolic acidosis, which has to be treated immediately to correct metabolic balance (Gort *et al.*, 2020). On the other hand, the rising rate of hypertension in pediatric patients calls for greater awareness and active countermeasures, particularly as hypertension left untreated could result in chronic cardiovascular disease (Agabiti-Rosei *et al.*, 2016). Standardized treatment protocols and order sets for such metabolic emergencies can enhance patient outcomes, eventually reducing hospital length of stay and optimizing recovery trajectories in the intensive care environment, and make meticulous care coordination critical.

7.2.1. Inborn Errors of Metabolism

Inborn errors of metabolism (IEM) are a significant category of endocrine and metabolic emergencies that one would encounter in pediatric intensive care and need to be identified and treated promptly. These genetic disorders, typically secondary to enzymatic deficiencies, are capable of causing severe metabolic dysregulation and acute clinical presentations, including neurological deteriorations and secondary systemic complications. These studies have found organic acidemias such as propionic acidemia and methylmalonic acidemia to be prevalent forms of IEM with daunting mortality rates that illustrate their severity (Famori *et al.*, 2016). Early diagnosis through newborn screening programs is critical, as early treatment has the potential to dramatically alter the course, illustrating the importance of proper metabolic workup in high-risk populations. Furthermore, the synergy of environmental factors and genetic predispositions, particularly in populations of high consanguinity, highlights the need for increased screening measures and targeted public awareness in an effort to improve prognostic outcomes for affected individuals (Figure 7.7).

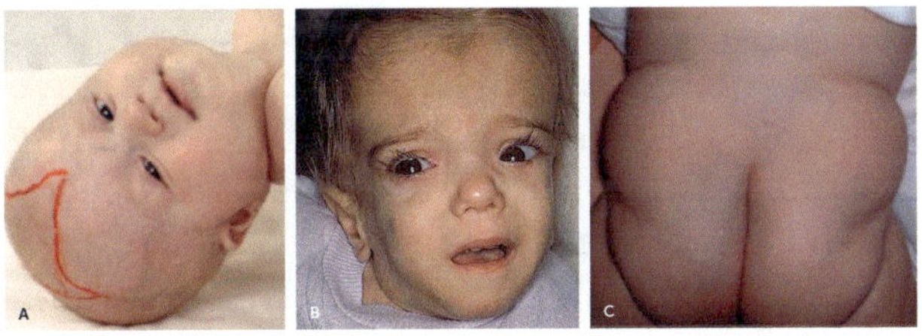

Figure 7.7. Inborn errors of metabolism (IEM) represent a significant subset of endocrine and metabolic emergencies encountered in pediatric intensive care, necessitating prompt recognition and intervention.

Source: https://www.aafp.org/content/dam/brand/aafp/pubs/afp/issues/2019/0101/p25-f1.jpg.

7.2.2. Acute Liver Failure

Acute liver failure represents an acute medical emergency in children with the rapid development of decreasing hepatic function typically caused by viral infections, metabolic disease, or drug overdose. It presents clinically with jaundice, coagulopathy, and encephalopathy, and consists of urgent care to prevent severe morbidity and mortality. Management of acute liver failure in the pediatric intensive care unit includes multi-modal treatment consisting of supportive management, monitoring of vital parameters, and early identification of underlying etiology. Of special importance are concomitant metabolic derangements, which tend to aggravate hepatic function and lead to fatal complications. It is essential to have some knowledge regarding the pathophysiological correlation between acute liver failure and metabolic disturbances for effective treatment. In general, identification and proper management of this condition can greatly enhance outcomes for kids presenting with this potentially life-threatening condition (Akingbola *et al.*, 2012; Gort *et al.*, 2020).

7.2.3. Urea Cycle Disorders

Urea cycle disorders (UCDs) refer to a group of congenital, rare genetic diseases that compromise the body's ability to remove ammonia, thus resulting in life-threatening metabolic crises in children. They are usually characterized by hyperammonemia, which, if left untreated promptly in an intensive care unit, may result in extensive neurological damage and death. The clinical presentation may be accompanied by vomiting, somnolence, and changes in consciousness, which are mimicked by other acute critical illnesses. These conditions make it difficult to diagnose and treat. Rapid diagnosis and treatment are crucial in pediatric intensive care, as treatments like ammonia scavenger therapy and protein restriction in diet are commonly required to mitigate the toxic effects of ammonia accumulation. Furthermore, UCDs could coincide with other metabolic crises, and this requires multidisciplinary treatment that recognizes both immediate and long-term impacts of these conditions on the development and health of a child. Apparently, it is imperative to offer integrated management strategies that could include supportive therapy and follow-up assessments to monitor long-term courses and prevent recurrent crises (Gort *et al.*, 2020; Baldassare *et al.*, 2020) (Figure 7.8).

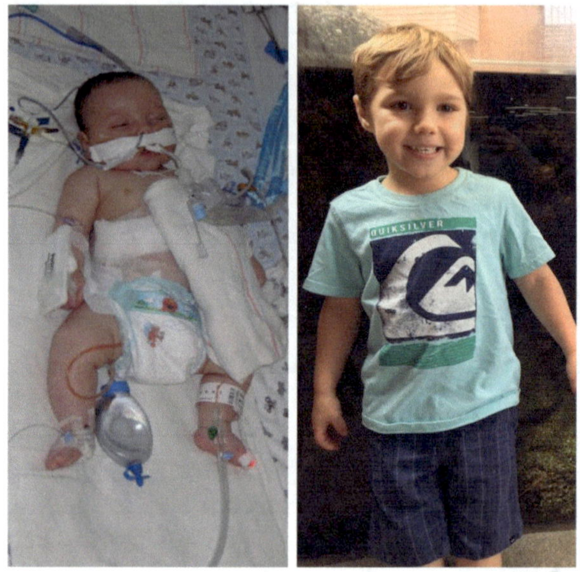

Figure 7.8. Urea cycle disorders (UCDs) represent a group of rare genetic conditions that disrupt the body's ability to remove ammonia, which can lead to significant metabolic crises in pediatric patients.

Source: https://cdn.greatnonprofits.org/images/uploads/organizations/051916.JPG.

7.2.4. Fatty Acid Oxidation Disorders

In pediatric intensive care, fatty acid oxidation disorders (FAODs) represent serious metabolic problems that can lead to acute and potentially life-threatening crises. The disorders are genetically caused and disrupt the body's ability to oxidize fatty acids, resulting in fasting state, exercise, or infection-induced energy shortages. Clinically, the patient can have, for instance, hypoglycemia, liver dysfunction, and myocardial disease, which require immediate management. Treatment is usually in the form of rapid diagnosis and intravenous dextrose administration to reverse hypoglycemia, with urinary metabolite close monitoring to decide on proper continued management. In light of the complexity of FAODs, it is important that whole follow-up programs, such as the Iowa Newborn Screening Program, are integrated to ensure early diagnosis and control. In children, early intervention is crucial because untreated metabolic crises are dangerous to life if not treated early. These include irreversible neurological damage (Gort *et al.*, 2020).

7.2.5. Organic Acidemias

In pediatric intensive care, the evolution of organic acidemias presents both a diagnostic and a management challenge. Organic acidemias, metabolic illnesses due to the accumulation of organic acids as a result of enzymatic deficiencies, can result in severe neurological and developmental effects unless addressed early in the course of the condition.

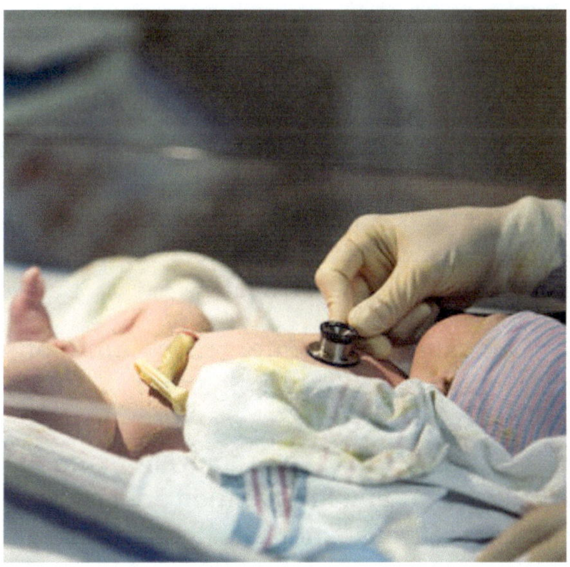

Figure 7.9. Organic acidemias.

Source: https://wp.drgreene.com/wp-content/uploads/Propionic-Acidemia-dreamstime_s_69752321-340x338.jpeg.

Recent studies highlight that methylmalonic acidemia and propionic acidemia are among the most prevalent forms, with a high mortality rate of 18.8% for infected patients, depicting the severity of early diagnosis and treatment protocols (Famori *et al.*, 2016). Further, the prevailing presence of consanguinity within populations complicates diagnosis, underlining the need for proper screening programs capable of improving outcomes through early interventions. In pediatric intensive care settings, it is essential to be familiar with symptoms of organic acidemias for improving prognostic outcomes and reducing morbidity associated with such metabolic emergencies (Figure 7.9).

7.2.6. Electrolyte Imbalances

Electrolyte imbalance is a life-threatening complication of general occurrence in pediatric intensive care units, particularly in endocrine and metabolic crises such as diabetic ketoacidosis (DKA). The balance of electrolytes such as sodium, potassium, and chloride is crucial to maintaining cellular function and fluid status. In pediatric DKA, the type and volume of intravenous fluids administered can have a direct effect on the electrolyte levels. Most significantly, research indicates that the fluctuation of sodium content of rehydration fluids is not indicated by a disparity in sodium plasma concentrations or other metabolic markers between children with DKA, demonstrating that close monitoring remains of utmost concern (Gönül Öçal *et al.*, 2013). In addition, the risks of premature fluid therapy, such as cerebral edema, demonstrate the necessity for a nuanced treatment approach (Marella, 2022). Lastly, identification and management of electrolyte imbalances are essential to maximize outcomes in critically ill children.

7.2.7. Metabolic Acidosis

Metabolic acidosis is a severe metabolic emergency that is often encountered in pediatric intensive care, typically secondary to underlying endocrine illness such as diabetes mellitus. Diabetic ketoacidosis (DKA) in children can lead to severe metabolic acidosis, characterized by low arterial blood pH and bicarbonate, primarily due to insulin deficiency and the generation of ketone bodies (Abdulrazzaq *et al.*, 2016). The necessity of treating such acid-base disturbances cannot be overemphasized, since uncomplicated metabolic acidosis can have unfavorable effects on organ function and overall physiological stability. The presence of disturbances in electrolytes complicates clinical treatment and demands a multidimensional treatment approach that includes intravenous fluid correction, insulin therapy, and careful monitoring of electrolytes (Gort *et al.*, 2020). Early intervention is critical because the prognosis enormously improves with early detection and treatment of the key causes of metabolic acidosis in children, reinforcing the necessity for vigilant surveillance in intensive care (Figure 7.10).

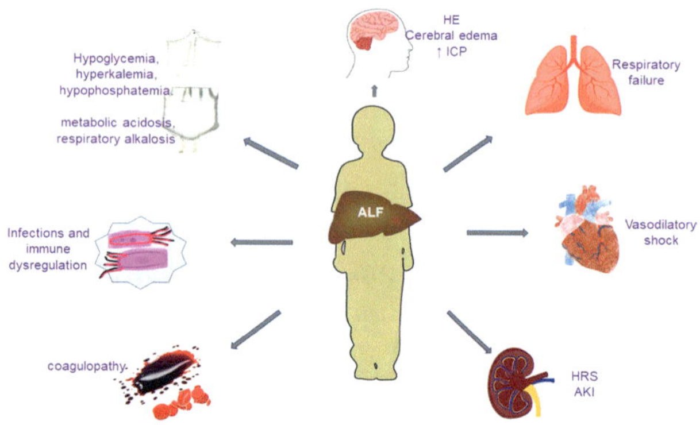

Figure 7.10. Metabolic acidosis represents a significant metabolic emergency frequently encountered in pediatric intensive care, often arising from underlying endocrine disorders such as diabetes mellitus.

Source: https://www.pediatric.theclinics.com/cms/10.1016/j.pcl.2022.02.003/asset/6ce5554c-9e7b-4664-9578-e3cb0c5c4b7e/main.assets/gr1_lrg.jpg.

7.2.8. Metabolic Alkalosis

Metabolic alkalosis is the emergent disorder of the pediatric intensive care world that needs urgent correction. It is most commonly brought about by the excessive loss of hydrogen ions or the addition of bicarbonate and ultimately results in an elevated blood pH, with the resultant marked effect on a child's physiological status. Underlying causes like vomiting, diuretic treatment, and mineralocorticoid excess can also be superimposed upon the intrinsic nature of other endocrine illnesses. Considering the rising incidence of hypertension and diabetes in kids, early identification of metabolic alkalosis is crucial for effective treatment regimens in intensive care units (Agabiti-Rosei *et al.*, 2016). The condition is generally treated by addressing the underlying cause, and fluid and electrolyte resuscitation is cautiously administered in an attempt to restore balance. There can be a delay in the diagnosis and management of metabolic alkalosis, ultimately impacting the health status of vulnerable pediatric patients (Abdulrazzaq *et al.*, 2016).

7.2.9. Hyperammonemia

Hyperammonemia is an acute, severe illness that is most often encountered in pediatric intensive care and is characterized by an elevated blood concentration of ammonia that can cause extreme neurological injury and, if left untreated, coma or death.

This metabolic emergency most often occurs secondary to congenital metabolic disease, such as disorders of the urea cycle, that negatively affect the removal of ammonia. Early diagnosis and intervention are important; elevated levels of ammonia lead to an imbalance of neurotransmitters, which can result in seizures and mental impairment. In a report highlighting early diagnosis, hyperammonemia was reported to occur in conditions of organic acidemia frequently, highlighting the significance of good screening among affected groups (Famori *et al.*, 2016). In addition, advancements in point-of-care technology for measuring ammonia will enable greater instantaneous clinical decision-making (Authors, 2018). Accordingly, hyperammonemia will require a multi-faceted approach that incorporates rapid diagnosis, appropriate management, and prevention of long-term neurologic consequences (Figure 7.11).

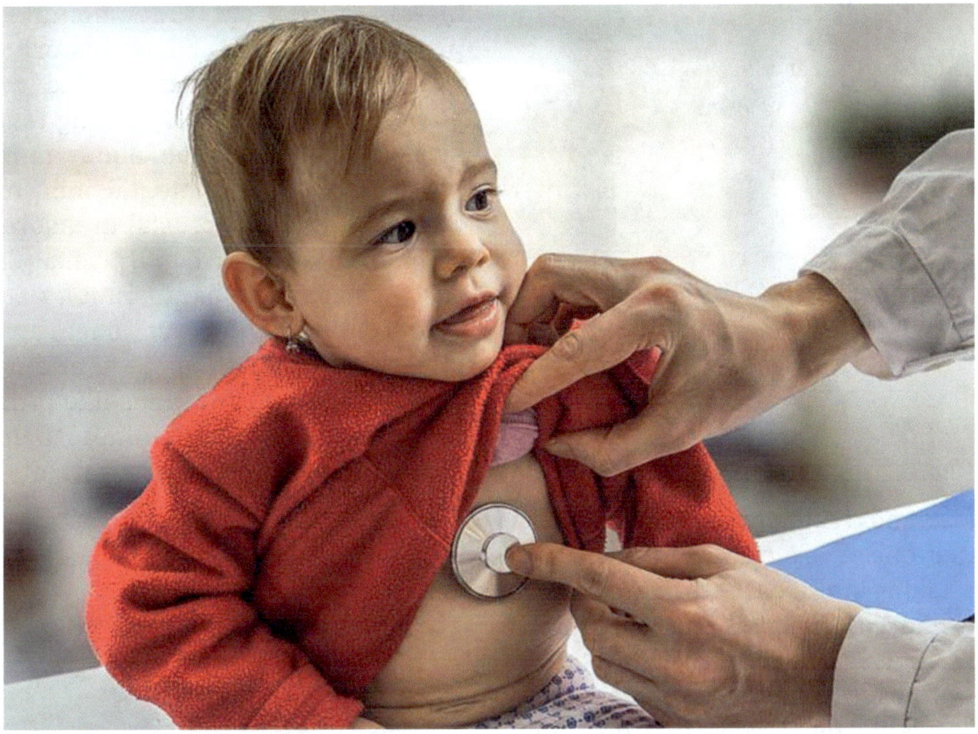

Figure 7.11. Hyperammonemia.

Source: https://media.post.rvohealth.io/wp-content/uploads/2020/09/toddler_doctor-732x549-thumbnail-732x549.jpg.

Test Your Knowledge

1. How is hypoglycemia managed in neonates and infants presenting with seizures?
2. What is the typical metabolic presentation of diabetic ketoacidosis in children?

7.3. Diagnosis and Management Strategies

Learning Outcome

1. Understand clinical assessment and history taking.
2. Explain laboratory tests and imaging studies.
3. Focus on the role of continuous glucose monitoring.
4. Discuss fluid and electrolyte management.
5. Know pharmacological interventions.
6. Discuss nutritional support and dietary management.
7. Learn a multidisciplinary approach in treatment.
8. Focus on monitoring and follow-up care.
9. Understand family education and support.

Careful diagnosis and treatment of endocrine and metabolic emergencies are critical in pediatric intensive care, taking into account the differential physiology of children. Clinicians must recognize signs of adrenal crises, which in spite of better therapeutic options, remain a life-threatening condition, as evident from recent literature. The application of timely glucocorticoid replacement therapy is vital, but only if it isas effective as the right diagnosis and monitoring modalities to prevent crisis generation (Falhammar *et al.*, 2019). Additionally, hypertension in children requires a comprehensive intervention including identification of emerging risk factors and application of new measurement techniques for accurate blood pressure assessment (Agabiti-Rosei *et al.*, 2016). By incorporating clinical recommendations and research findings, health professionals can develop individualized management plans that not only alleviate short-term symptoms but also consider the long-term implications of endocrine and metabolic disorders, thereby improving the health outcomes in this high-risk group.

7.3.1. Clinical Assessment and History Taking

In pediatric intensive care, particularly in endocrine and metabolic emergencies, intense clinical assessment and meticulous history taking are fundamental. Such steps provide a robust medical history that guides subsequent interventions and management plans. Successful history taking tends to reveal important information about family medical history and developmental milestones, issues that are especially crucial in disorders such as congenital adrenal hyperplasia (CAH), where early detection is paramount to achieving the best results. Health practitioners are required to integrate care in an effort to attain the holistic management of conditions like CAH, which has been stressed in guidelines to improve the broken care that defines patients with long-term illnesses (Aisenberg *et al.*, 2010).

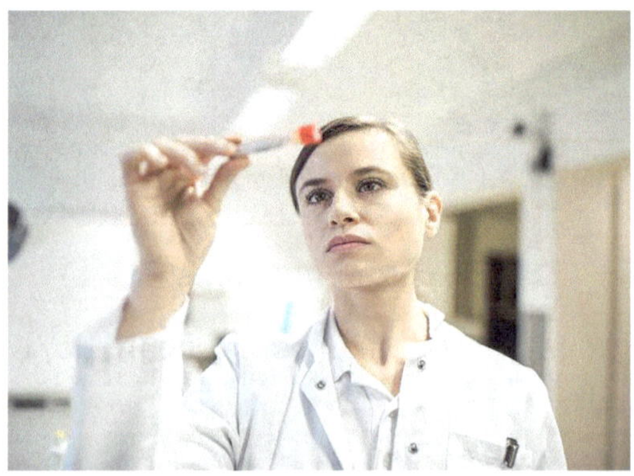

Figure 7.12. Effective history taking often unveils critical information regarding family medical history and developmental milestones, which are particularly significant in conditions like congenital adrenal hyperplasia (CAH) where early diagnosis is crucial for optimal outcomes.

Source: https://media.post.rvohealth.io/wp-content/uploads/2020/09/1215-Blood_Poisoning-732x549-thumbnail-1-732x549.jpg.

It is also important to understand the increasing hypertension in children, which requires important assessment techniques and tailored treatments based on clinical guidelines (Agabiti-Rosei *et al.*, 2016). Hence, the clinical history taking and evaluation can significantly influence patient outcomes for critically ill patients (Figure 7.12).

7.3.2. Laboratory Tests and Imaging Studies

Of all diagnostic modalities in the realm of pediatric intensive care, and in particular endocrine and metabolic emergencies, laboratory tests and imaging studies play a critical role in diagnosis and management. These diagnostic modalities permit the detection of many hormonal disturbances and metabolic derangements such that immediate and proper intervention can be undertaken. For instance, some laboratory tests can measure hormone levels such as cortisol and thyroid-stimulating hormone, which can uncover intrinsic endocrine disturbances brought about by central nervous system infections or other metabolic stressors (Buonsenso *et al.*, 2025). Imaging tests such as CT and MRI scans can be useful to identify underlying anatomical irregularities or lesions that are causing hormonal derangement. On top of that, given the increasing burden of hypertension among youth populations, as highlighted by contemporary recommendations, a comprehensive evaluation through these means is significant in averting long-term cardiovascular morbidity (Agabiti-Rosei *et al.*, 2016). Lastly, coordination among laboratory and imaging testing plays a crucial role in optimizing pediatric patient outcomes in intensive care.

7.3.3. Role of Continuous Glucose Monitoring

While in pediatric intensive care, the use of continuous glucose monitoring (CGM) takes the forefront role in the management of endocrine and metabolic emergencies, particularly in children at risk for diabetic ketoacidosis (DKA). CGM systems provide real-time glucose readings, which allow for prompt adjustments in treatment plans, something that is crucial because early detection of DKA reduces morbidity and mortality associated with the condition (Zyl *et al.*, 2008). Furthermore, the use of CGM in medical facilities enhances the capacity of medical professionals to recognize fluctuating levels of glucose, thereby allowing for prompt interventions. This is even more relevant in a pediatric setting where hypertension and other metabolic problems may be widespread, emphasizing the need for an all-encompassing approach to glucose management (Agabiti-Rosei *et al.*, 2016). By creating an environment of anticipatory monitoring, CGM not only enhances real-time clinical decision-making but also contributes to overall stabilization of vulnerable pediatric patients, ultimately optimizing outcomes in intensive care units (Figure 7.13).

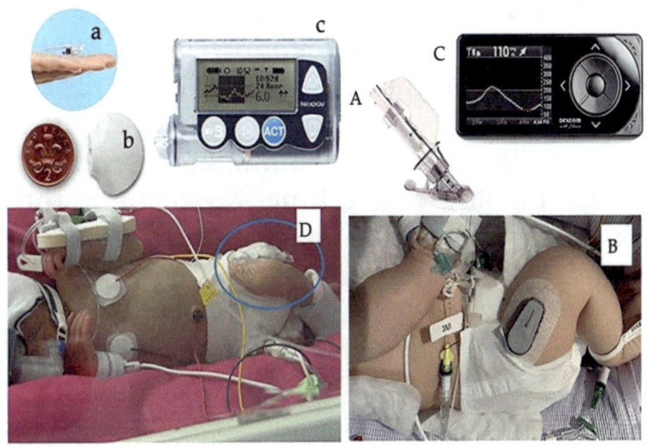

Figure 7.13. The role of continuous glucose monitoring (CGM) emerges as a pivotal element in managing endocrine and metabolic emergencies, particularly for children at risk for diabetic ketoacidosis (DKA).

Source: https://images-provider.frontiersin.org/api/ipx/w=1200&f=png/https://www.frontiersin.org/files/Articles/1115228/fped-11-1115228-HTML-r1/image_m/fped-11-1115228-g001.jpg.

7.3.4. Fluid and Electrolyte Management

Appropriate fluid and electrolyte management is important in pediatric critical care, especially in endocrine and metabolic emergencies such as diabetic ketoacidosis (DKA) and hyperosmolar hyperglycemic state (HHS). The conditions most often need urgent intravenous fluid resuscitation and proper electrolyte replacement to normalize and prevent further complications. DKA patients tend to be hyperglycemic and have metabolic acidosis, with the need for vigorous fluid resuscitation to reconstitute fluid status and correct chemistry. HHS, despite the severe hyperglycemia with little or no appreciable ketoacidosis, needs to have electrolytes carefully managed to avoid complications such as cerebral edema. Implementation of standardized treatment protocols or order sets has been associated with improved patient outcomes, including reduced hospital and intensive care unit length of stay and improved compliance with treatment guidelines (Gort *et al.*, 2020). Also, correct and timely intervention in cardiogenic shock will minimize detrimental effects on end-organ function further, thus underlining the value of aggressive fluid and electrolyte management (Candini *et al.*, 2020).

7.3.5. Pharmacological Interventions

Pharmacotherapies have an important role to play in the management of pediatric intensive care endocrine and metabolic emergencies. They are particularly important in disorders such as diabetic ketoacidosis (DKA) and hyperosmolar hyperglycemic state (HHS), where early insulin therapy has a dramatic effect on patient prognosis. For DKA, which is most commonly observed in children with Type 1 diabetes, insulin therapy in combination with severe fluid replacement and correction of electrolytes is essential for the normalization of glucose levels in the blood and the correction of metabolic acidosis (Gort *et al.*, 2020). Similarly, HHS also often needs careful pharmacologic attention to treat the severely increased amounts of glucose found in patients, prompting clinicians to find a balance between insulin treatment and observation to prevent hypoglycemic events. Moreover, identification of rising hypertension in children emphasizes the importance of tailored pharmacologic therapies to manage blood pressure and mitigate the long-term cardiovascular risk (Agabiti-Rosei *et al.*, 2016). Such combined pharmacologic treatments are non-negotiable to promote recovery in children with endocrine and metabolic emergencies (Figure 7.14).

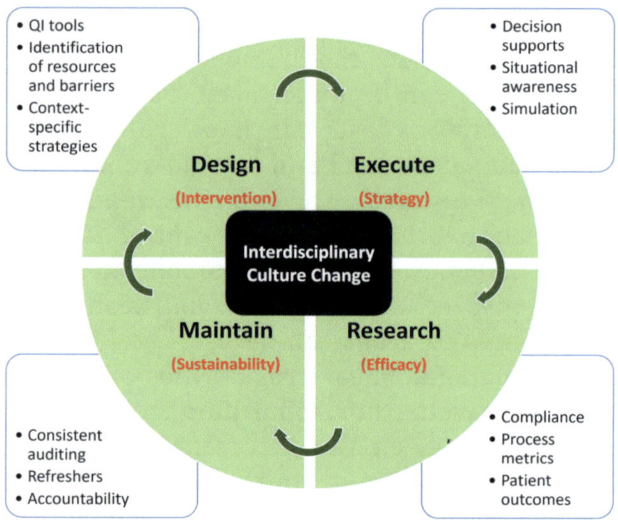

Figure 7.14. Pharmacological interventions play a critical role in managing endocrine and metabolic emergencies within pediatric intensive care settings.

Source: https://www.frontiersin.org/files/Articles/864029/fped-10-864029-HTML/image_m/fped-10-864029-g001.jpg.

7.3.6. Nutritional Support and Dietary Management

Effective management and nutritional therapy are crucial to the treatment and cure of pediatric intensive care unit patients with endocrine and metabolic emergencies. Proper nutritional therapy not only addresses the acute metabolic need secondary to the acute process but also affects long-term outcome. As has been documented by several studies, e.g., increasing rates of hypertension in young individuals, dietary changes can significantly diminish cardiovascular disease and risk factors for metabolic disorders (Agabiti-Rosei *et al.*, 2016). Moreover, children with cancer are at higher risk of developing malnutrition due to the severe side effects of therapy. Malnutrition has harmful effects on tolerance to therapy as well as survival (Esposito *et al.*, 2023). Recognition of the role of nutritional status on outcome spells the need for a planned management of diet in pediatric intensive care to make nutritional interventions an integral part of comprehensive patient care.

7.3.7. Multidisciplinary Approach in Treatment

Endocrine and metabolic emergencies in pediatric intensive care demand a multidisciplinary process that effectively integrates the various healthcare providers' inputs. Such collaborative systems are indispensable, particularly for complex conditions like congenital adrenal hyperplasia (CAH), where fractured care is linked with poor outcomes.

By encouraging collaboration among pediatric endocrinologists, urologists, surgeons, and mental health professionals, the treatment plans could be tailored to suit the specific requirements of involved children and families.

This process is also supported by the inclusion of patients and families in care discussions, as was achieved at an important meeting dedicated to planning ambitious care centers. Recommendations of this team identify the need to formulate comprehensive health care plans targeting the diverse needs of CAH patients as an anchor for future pediatric care service development (Aisenberg *et al.*, 2010). Ultimately, these integrated strategies provide an avenue for enhanced patient and family outcomes within the environment of pediatric intensive care.

7.3.8. Monitoring and Follow-up Care

Appropriate monitoring and follow-up care are the essential components in treating endocrine and metabolic emergencies in pediatric critical care, where the result could dramatically affect a child's recovery course. Constant monitoring of vital signs and metabolic status must be done, particularly in disorders like diabetic ketoacidosis (DKA) and hypertension that need to be treated promptly before severe complications arise.

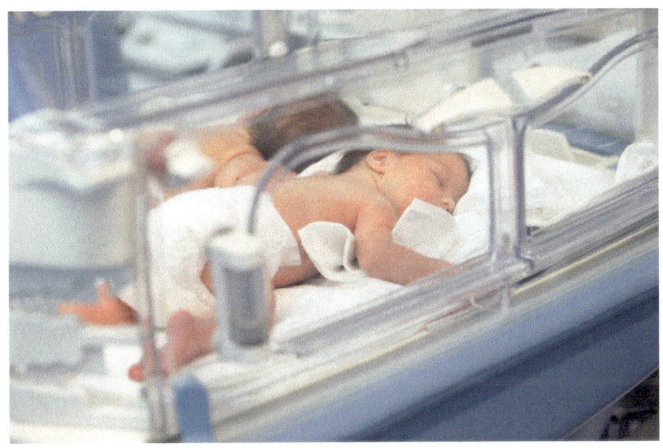

Figure 7.15. Effective monitoring and follow-up care are critical components in managing endocrine and metabolic emergencies in pediatric intensive care, where the stakes can significantly impact a child's recovery trajectory.

Source: https://neonest.in/wp-content/uploads/2024/01/newborn-children-are-boxes-hospital-1024x683-1.jpg.

A detailed follow-up plan, including evidence-based suggestions, enables healthcare providers to treat potential recurrences and deal with the chronic implications of such disorders. For instance, DKA management protocols need to be carefully monitored for serum glucose and electrolyte concentrations in a way that enables responsive modifications in therapy, with attempts to standardize protocols as highlighted in recent treatment guidelines. Additionally, putting the spotlight on childhood hypertension, as done in recent recommendations, places importance on regular follow-up to minimize long-term cardiovascular risk (Agabiti-Rosei *et al.*, 2016; Gort *et al.*, 2020). Hence, established monitoring systems are essential for optimizing gains in this high-risk group (Figure 7.15).

7.3.9. Family Education and Support

In the field of endocrine and metabolic emergencies within pediatric intensive care, patient outcomes are guaranteed through family support and education. Family caregivers and members often encounter a high-stakes setting of medical information and treatment protocols, necessitating intensive educational processes provided by medical practitioners. Research emphasizes that well-informed families can more effectively recognize symptoms and react to treatment plans, particularly in conditions like hypertension and Type 1 Diabetes (T1D), where interventions undertaken in a timely way can have a profound impact on prognoses (Agabiti-Rosei *et al.*, 2016; McFarling *et al.*, 2020). Moreover, integrating family dynamics within the management of these diseases provides a supportive environment, which enhances the child's emotional and psychological resilience. In this way, multidisciplinary care focused on involving family members not only improves clinical results but also empowers families such that they can successfully advocate for their child's health at times of crisis and thereafter.

Test Your Knowledge

1. What role does insulin infusion play in DKA, and how is the rate titrated?
2. How is hypernatremia managed in diabetes insipidus, and what complications must be avoided?

SUMMARY

Pediatric intensive care endocrine and metabolic emergencies are a critical component of maximizing patient outcomes and fulfilling the unique requirements of this vulnerable population. Through their understanding of the complexities of conditions such as diabetic ketoacidosis (DKA) and hyperosmolar hyperglycemic state (HHS), as evidenced in clinical practice, healthcare providers can implement effective treatments to maximize recovery rates and minimize complications (Gort *et al.*, 2020). Moreover, with the rising incidence of primary arterial hypertension (PAH) in children, especially adolescents, the risk of hypertensive emergencies calls for heightened awareness and targeted interventions in order to curb morbidity and mortality of such crises (Akingbola *et al.*, 2012). Standardized order sets and guidelines can also ensure timely interventions and, hence, equip health teams with the appropriate skills to manage such critical emergencies effectively. In summary, ongoing education and evidence-based care are still of paramount importance to progress pediatric intensive care.

In pediatric critical care, the understanding of endocrine and metabolic emergencies is central to intervention and management. Key points in recent literature reveal the increasing prevalence and clinical effects of hypertension and diabetes mellitus among children. Hypertension, often underdiagnosed, is a key stimulus for the cardiovascular epidemic that occurs in this age bracket and deserves more awareness and treatment as described in Agabiti-Rosei *et al.* (2016). Moreover, diabetes mellitus, particularly type 2 and type 1, may lead to severe complications like diabetic ketoacidosis and hyperosmolar hyperglycemic state that require instant medical attention due to their life-threatening potential. As elaborated in Gort *et al.* (2020), effective management of these diseases mostly relies on well-documented practices such as order sets that enhance patient outcomes through standardized care pathways. Therefore, ongoing education and policy formation are of primary importance in managing such vital health conditions in the pediatric patient.

KEY TERMS FROM THIS CHAPTER

- Hypertension
- Diabetes mellitus
- Hyperosmolar hyperglycemic state
- Insulin infusion
- Awareness
- Vascular phenotypes
- Polyuria
- Adolescents
- Diabetic ketoacidosis
- Fluid replacement
- Endocrine disasters
- Clinicians
- Ketonemia
- Polydipsia

CRITICAL THINKING QUESTIONS

1. **What is the most common endocrine emergency in pediatric patients?**
   a. Thyroid storm
   b. Hypoglycemia
   c. Diabetic ketoacidosis (DKA)
   d. Adrenal crisis
2. **Which of the following is a hallmark finding in diabetic ketoacidosis (DKA)?**
   a. Respiratory alkalosis
   b. Hypernatremia
   c. Metabolic acidosis with high anion gap
   d. Hypercalcemia
3. **What is the first priority in managing a child presenting with DKA?**
   a. Administer insulin immediately
   b. Correct potassium before anything else
   c. Initiate IV fluid resuscitation
   d. Give sodium bicarbonate
4. **What life-threatening complication must be monitored during treatment of DKA in children?**
   a. Myocardial infarction
   b. Cerebral edema
   c. Pulmonary embolism
   d. Liver failure
5. **A child with Addison's disease is brought to the PICU in shock. What is the most likely cause?**
   a. Adrenal crisis due to cortisol deficiency
   b. Hypoglycemia from insulin overdose
   c. Congenital heart block
   d. Hyperthyroidism

Short Answer Questions

1. What are the most frequent endocrine emergencies encountered in the PICU?
2. How does diabetic ketoacidosis (DKA) typically present in children?
3. What are the common metabolic emergencies seen in pediatric intensive care?
4. How do inborn errors of metabolism typically present in acutely ill infants?
5. What are the critical laboratory investigations for a child presenting with a suspected endocrine or metabolic emergency?
6. How should fluid therapy be initiated and adjusted in a child with DKA?

Answers to Critical Thinking Questions

1. (c) 2. (c) 3. (c) 4. (b) 5. (a)

REFERENCES

1. Abdulrazzaq, N. F., Abdulwahid, M. K., & Hadi, A. A. (2016). Clinical profile of pediatric diabetic ketoacidosis in Karbala City, Iraq. https://core.ac.uk/download/234656369.pdf (accessed on 30th June 2025).
2. Agabiti-Rosei, E., Cruickshank, J. K., Dominiczak, A., Erdine, S., *et al.* (2016). 2016 European Society of Hypertension guidelines for the management of high blood pressure in children and adolescents. https://core.ac.uk/download/46165193.pdf (accessed on 30th June 2025).
3. Aisenberg, J., Alger Lin, G., Auchus, R. J., Azziz, R., *et al.* (2010). Guidelines for the development of comprehensive care centers for congenital adrenal hyperplasia: Guidance from the CARES Foundation initiative. https://core.ac.uk/download/pdf/8517177.pdf (accessed on 30th June 2025).
4. Akingbola, O., El-Dahr, S., Singh, D., Yosypiv, I., *et al.* (2012). Emergency management of hypertension in children. https://core.ac.uk/download/pdf/8723168.pdf (accessed on 30th June 2025).
5. Aznar-Lain, G., Bibic, I., Bibic, V., Cross, J. H., *et al.* (2024). Unraveling unmet needs in ketogenic dietary services: An ERN EpiCARE survey. https://core.ac.uk/download/624202972.pdf (accessed on 30th June 2025).
6. Baldassarre, M. E., Borrelli, O., Cordelli, D. M., Di Nardo, M., *et al.* (2020). Cyclic vomiting syndrome in children. https://core.ac.uk/download/541251781.pdf (accessed on 30th June 2025).
7. Bassett, B. (2023). Modifiable and non-modifiable factors associated with DKA among children and adolescents with type 1 diabetes: A machine learning exploration using the T1D Exchange Data Set. https://core.ac.uk/download/548683853.pdf (accessed on 30th June 2025).
8. Broersen, L. H. A. (2019). Clinical consequences of endogenous and exogenous glucocorticoid excess. https://core.ac.uk/download/388637294.pdf (accessed on 30th June 2025).
9. Buonsenso, D., Camporesi, A., Cannioto, Z., Cipolla, C., *et al.* (2025). Endocrinologic dysfunctions and neuropsychiatric sequelae in pediatric patients with a history of central nervous system infection (ENDLESS): A prospective monocentric study. https://core.ac.uk/download/656528398.pdf (accessed on 30th June 2025).
10. Candini, N. A., Indrianto, Y. L., Koentartiwi, D., Suwarnianty, E., *et al.* (2020). Management of cardiogenic shock in pediatric patients. https://core.ac.uk/download/352916346.pdf (accessed on 30th June 2025).
11. Chun, S. H., Hwang, J. S., & Lee, H. S. (2022). Hyperosmolar hyperglycemic state as the first manifestation of type 1 diabetes mellitus in an adolescent male: A case report. https://core.ac.uk/download/628902548.pdf (accessed on 30th June 2025).
12. Esposito, S., Leardini, D., Masetti, R., Massa, G., *et al.* (2023). Role of nutrition in pediatric patients with cancer. https://core.ac.uk/download/573436042.pdf (accessed on 30th June 2025).
13. Falhammar, H., Rushworth, R. L., & Torpy, D. J. (2019). Adrenal crisis. https://core.ac.uk/download/228075100.pdf (accessed on 30th June 2025).

14. Famori, F., Ghazavi, M., Hashemipour, M., Moafi, A., *et al.* (2016). Demographic and clinical findings in pediatric patients affected by organic acidemia. https://core.ac.uk/download/483633477.pdf (accessed on 30th June 2025).
15. Gönül Öçal, G., & Bilir, P. (2013). Diabetic ketoacidosis. *Journal of Clinical Research in Pediatric Endocrinology.* https://core.ac.uk/download/322420998.pdf (accessed on 30th June 2025).
16. Gort, S. (2020). Effectiveness of order sets in the management of diabetic ketoacidosis and hyperosmolar hyperglycemia. https://core.ac.uk/download/328112832.pdf (accessed on 30th June 2025).
17. Hood, D. G. (2012). The nature and meaning of insulin pump use in emerging adults with type 1 diabetes. https://core.ac.uk/download/235237529.pdf (accessed on 30th June 2025).
18. Marella, S. (2022). When treating canine diabetic ketoacidosis, do balanced crystalloids provide superior outcomes compared to 0.9% saline? https://core.ac.uk/download/560759360.pdf (accessed on 30th June 2025).
19. McFarling, K. (2020). Factors that impact glycemic control in adolescents with type 1 diabetes. https://core.ac.uk/download/347421721.pdf (accessed on 30th June 2025).
20. Mehdi, S. F., Qureshi, M., Shahid, S., Kumari, K., Saji, E., Shah, M., Abdullah, A., *et al.* (2025). Endocrine and metabolic alterations in response to systemic inflammation and sepsis: A review article. *Molecular Medicine, 31.* https://doi.org/10.1186/s10020-025-01074-z (accessed on 30th June 2025).
21. Nasa, P., Abdul Majeed, N., & Juneja, D. (2024). Paroxysmal sympathetic hyperactivity after traumatic brain injury: Current understanding and therapeutic options. *Indian Journal of Critical Care Medicine, 28,* 97–99. https://doi.org/10.5005/jp-journals-10071-24647 (accessed on 30th June 2025).
22. Zyl Van, D. G. (2008). Diagnosis and treatment of diabetic ketoacidosis. https://core.ac.uk/download/478306597.pdf (accessed on 30th June 2025).

GASTROINTESTINAL AND HEPATIC DISORDERS

8

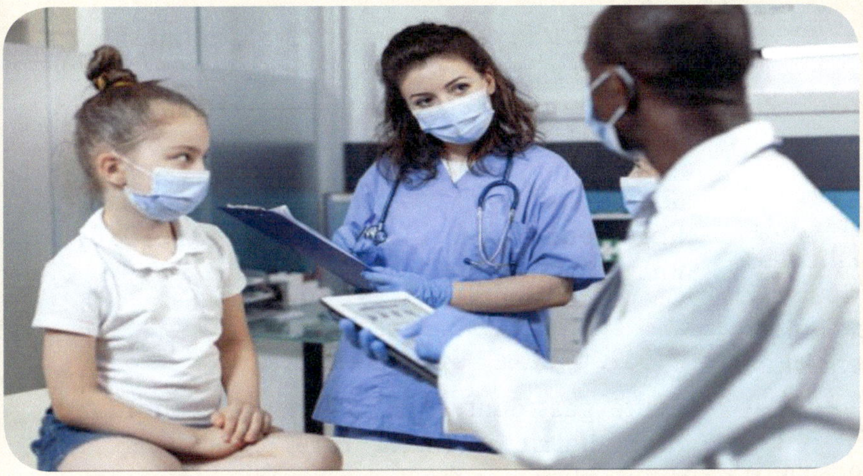

LEARNING OBJECTIVES

After studying this chapter, you will be able to:

1. Understand Common Gastrointestinal Disorders in Pediatric Patients.
2. Explain Hepatic Disorders in Pediatric Patients.
3. Describe Diagnostic Approaches in Pediatric Intensive Care.
4. Focus on Management Strategies for Gastrointestinal and Hepatic Disorders.

Introduction

The pediatric patient presents unique challenges in the context of gastrointestinal and hepatic illnesses, particularly in the intensive care setting. These illnesses vary from simple gastrointestinal infection to complex liver disease, such as ascites and hepatic encephalopathy, and demand a delicate understanding of pediatric physiology and the specific clinical presentation that is seen in children as compared to adults. One of the key concerns is the low survival associated with such conditions; e.g., the development of ascites in children can greatly reduce survival and make treatment challenging (Scott et al., 2021). Additionally, geographical variations in disease incidence, such as in hepatocellular carcinoma, emphasize the need for locally derived treatment plans that take into account varying medical settings and epidemiological environments (Omata et al., 2017). Hence, understanding the subtleties of gastrointestinal and liver illness within pediatric intensive care is the key to optimizing the potential of patients and guiding successful management practices.

8.1. Common Gastrointestinal Disorders in Pediatric Patients

Learning Outcome

1. Understand acute gastroenteritis.
2. Explain inflammatory bowel disease.
3. Describe gastroesophageal reflux disease.
4. Focus on constipation and fecal impaction.
5. Discuss intestinal obstruction.
6. Know celiac disease.
7. Understand necrotizing enterocolitis.
8. Describe short bowel syndrome.
9. Focus on functional gastrointestinal disorders.

In children, gastrointestinal disorders have unique requirements due to special challenges that need special treatment, particularly in the intensive care unit. Among the most prevalent disorders are acute gastroenteritis, which refers to inflammation of the stomach and intestines, most often caused by viral or bacterial infections, and can lead to severe dehydration and electrolyte disturbances. Further, disorders like gastroesophageal reflux disease (GERD) and functional abdominal pain are frequent occurrences, impacting growth as well as quality of life. Disorders can also be present concomitantly with more serious syndromes, e.g., multisystem inflammatory syndrome in children (MIS-C), which can be associated with gastrointestinal manifestations of diarrhea and abdominal pain as discussed by Shaigany *et al.* (2020). Furthermore, liver diseases like hepatocellular carcinoma (HCC) are increasingly being diagnosed in children and mirror regional variations in prevalence, in this case, areas seen to be presenting high rates of HCC, as seen in Omata *et al.* (2017). Understanding such diseases is essential for effective management in the pediatric intensive care unit (Figure 8.1).

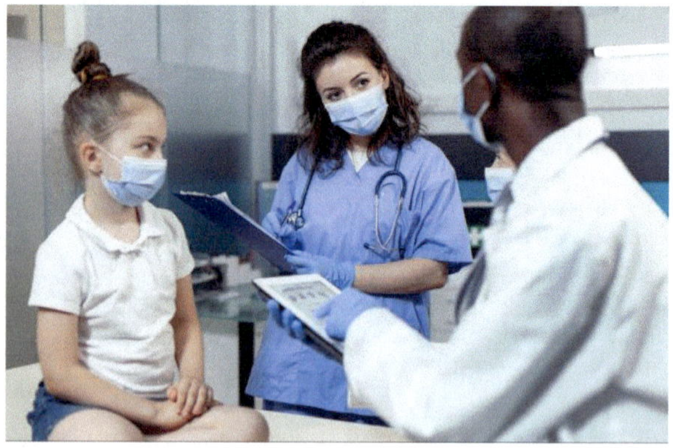

Figure 8.1. In pediatric patients, gastrointestinal disorders present unique challenges that necessitate specialized care, particularly in intensive care settings.

Source: https://www.geetanjalihospital.co.in/img/media/cache/blogs/02/825x408/1010/image2%20(5).jpg.

8.1.1. Acute Gastroenteritis

Acute gastroenteritis is a critical condition in pediatric intensive care, presenting as inflammation of the gastrointestinal tract with resultant violent diarrhea and vomiting. Acute gastroenteritis can be caused by viral, bacterial, or parasitic infections and lead to dehydration, electrolyte imbalance, and admission to the hospital. Acute gastroenteritis needs to be treated urgently in children because it occurs rapidly, and young children are prone to fluid loss. Furthermore, acute gastroenteritis presentation with extrapulmonary symptoms has previously been reported with conditions such as COVID-19, highlighting the need for whole-picture diagnostic approaches (Elrobaa *et al.*, 2021). Secondly, one must also take into consideration the pathophysiology behind such a presentation, as proper management and hydration therapy will significantly affect patient outcomes (Hedi *et al.*, 2021). Thus, effective treatment measures should be framed to lower the complications of acute gastroenteritis in critically ill children, making it a priority in pediatric healthcare units.

8.1.2. Inflammatory Bowel Disease

Inflammatory bowel disease (IBD) is a group of chronic inflammatory disorders, most notably Crohn's disease and ulcerative colitis, and is being increasingly recognized as a critical issue in the pediatric intensive care setting. IBD in children is often likely to lead to multifaceted clinical presentations and complications that are not only varied but may also substantially impact growth and development.

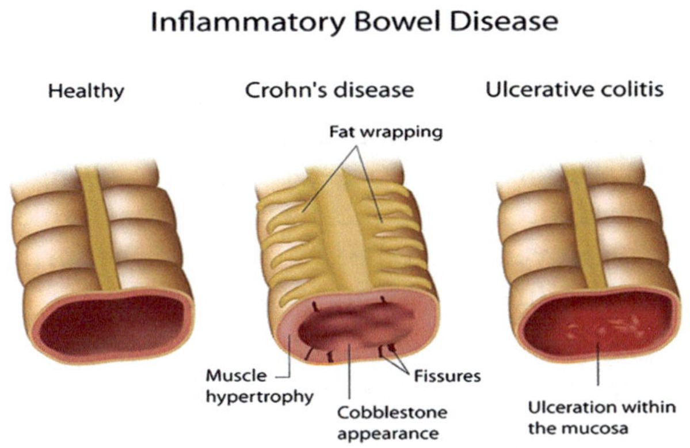

Figure 8.2. Inflammatory bowel disease (IBD) encompasses a spectrum of chronic inflammatory conditions, primarily Crohn's disease and ulcerative colitis, and is increasingly recognized as a significant concern within pediatric intensive care settings.

Source: https://www.ibdrelief.com/uploads/files/ibd1_gallery_image_924_131.jpg.

Accordingly, new therapeutic approaches, including stem cell therapy, are promising to reverse the inflammatory features of IBD. As emphasized in recent achievements, human pluripotent stem cells (hPSCs) and multipotent mesenchymal stem cells (MSCs) have promise for application in regenerative medicine for inflammatory conditions, offering new hope for treatment regimens (Duc *et al.*, 2022). Furthermore, the use of probiotics to manage gastrointestinal symptoms has been another area of focus, where evidence suggests that they can aid in mucosal barrier function and immune system modulation, thereby contributing to the overall management of IBD in children (Stavropoulou *et al.*, 2020). This approach implies that there is a necessity to undertake further research to achieve improved clinical outcomes in children with IBD (Figure 8.2).

8.1.3. Gastroesophageal Reflux Disease (GERD)

Gastroesophageal reflux disease (GERD) is a frequent condition in children that is very difficult to control in intensive care settings. Retrograde movement of gastric contents into the esophagus characterizes GERD and may result in annoying symptoms such as vomiting, irritability, and intolerance to feeds in children. The condition not only impairs the process of taking nutrients but also can cause more serious effects in the form of esophagitis and respiratory problems. Management of GERD in critically ill children often requires multimodal management, such as the use of pharmacologic therapy with the addition of dietary modifications and positional maneuvers. Notably, recent evidence further delineated correlations between GERD and other gastrointestinal disorders, and yet again, further. comprehensive assessments are advised for maximum. treatment. Moreover, since there is a multifaceted interplay of determinants influencing GERD, physicians must be watchful for comorbidities that may exacerbate the condition, particularly in vulnerable groups such as infants and children with pre-existing conditions (Kimura *et al.*, 2024; Júlia Balthazar *et al.*, 2022).

8.1.4. Constipation and Fecal Impaction

Of the gastrointestinal disorders, constipation and fecal impaction are of primary concern in pediatric intensive care. Both are potential causes of significant distress, potential bowel obstruction, and complications such as abdominal distension and pain. The etiology of constipation in children is multifactorial and could be related to dietary deficiencies, inadequate fluid intake, and changes in activity levels. In addition, conditions like obesity, which are prevalent in children, make it even more severe because it is caused by inactivity and unhealthy eating habits, as referenced in Dennis *et al.* (2017). Hardened stools can accumulate due to untreated constipation, resulting in painful bowel movements as well as hospitalization. Avoidance of such problems can result in long-term gastrointestinal problems, highlighting the importance of timely intervention and appropriate treatment measures in an effort to provide the best care for patients involved in intensive care units (Andrade *et al.*, 2021) (Figure 8.3).

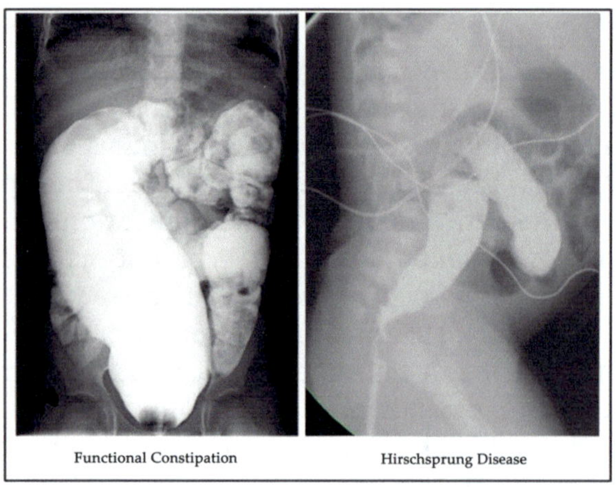

Figure 8.3. Within the realm of gastrointestinal disorders, constipation and fecal impaction represent significant concerns in pediatric intensive care settings.

Source: https://www.mdpi.com/children/children-10-01078/article_deploy/html/images/children-10-01078-g001.png.

8.1.5. Intestinal Obstruction

Intestinal obstruction is a significant problem in the context of gastrointestinal illness among pediatrics, particularly in the intensive care unit. It can be secondary to many etiologies, such as mechanical etiologies like adhesions, tumors, or congenital anomalies, and functional etiologies like motility disorders. Early diagnosis and management of intestinal obstruction in the pediatric intensive care unit (PICU) is critical since delays may cause severe complications like bowel ischemia and perforation. The presentation may be variable, but most often includes abdominal distension, vomiting, and alteration in bowel habits, and needs careful evaluation and management. Moreover, PICU patients are especially sensitive to acid-base and electrolyte disturbances that can further complicate the clinical condition of intestinal obstruction (Khairunnisa *et al.*, 2025). In this regard, efforts to negate such imbalances must be incorporated into the overall treatment plan for improved outcomes in children suffering from the disease (Chung *et al.*, 2025).

8.1.6. Celiac Disease

Celiac disease, an autoimmune chronic illness resulting from the consumption of gluten, presents certain challenges in pediatric intensive care. A disorder that is the outcome of an abnormal immune response to gluten, it inflicts widespread damage to the intestine, malabsorption of nutrients, and long-term complications such as growth retardation and osteoporosis. In sick children who are admitted to intensive care units, the treatment for celiac disease calls for a multidisciplinary intervention, especially considering the nutritional deficiency that also complicates their illness. The convergence of gastrointestinal health with immune processes in the system underscores the importance of intestinal integrity; hence, probiotics have emerged as a possible adjunctive therapy. They are able to enhance mucosal barrier function and regulate the immune system, potentially treating gastrointestinal symptoms of celiac disease (Stavropoulou *et al.*, 2020). As the link between microbiota and immune health is revealed, it bears witness to the importance of holistic care protocols in celiac disease treatment within the context of gastrointestinal and hepatic disease (Jane *et al.*, 2018) (Figure 8.4).

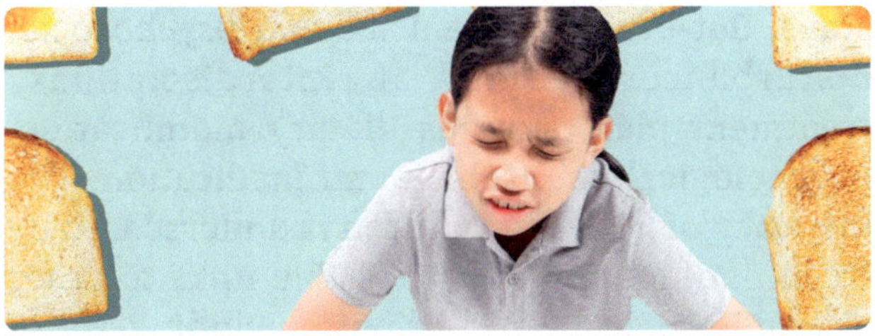

Figure 8.4. Celiac disease, a chronic autoimmune disorder triggered by gluten consumption, presents unique challenges in pediatric intensive care settings.

Source: https://womenandchildren.avisena.com.my/wp-content/uploads/2025/03/article-celiac-disease-intro.jpg.

8.1.7. Necrotizing Enterocolitis

Necrotizing enterocolitis (NEC) is a critical gastrointestinal disease that predominantly affects preterm infants in pediatric intensive care units. NEC is characterized by inflammation and necrosis of intestinal tissue, whereby NEC is linked to severe threats such as systemic infections and long-term morbidity. Pathogenesis of NEC is multifactorial and involves a number of causes, including gut microbiota dysbiosis and feeding practices. Recent studies have explored the application of probiotics to lower the risk of NEC, with live and heat-killed preparations both being considered for their immunomodulatory effects and intestinal barrier function improvement (Núria Piqué *et al.*, 2019). Furthermore, the dysbiosed gut microbiota-diet interaction has been identified as an etiology of various diseases, pointing to a greater impact of gastrointestinal health on general infant development, primarily in autism spectrum disorders, in which the inflammation in the gut may be an environmental cause of the disease (Derrick, 2015). The effective prevention and cure of NEC remain critical for the improvement of outcomes in high-risk infant and pediatric patients.

8.1.8. Short Bowel Syndrome

Short bowel syndrome (SBS) is an important problem in the setting of gastrointestinal pathologies presenting to pediatric intensive care. Malabsorption following massive resection of the small intestine, SBS can lead to severe nutritional deficiencies and fluid imbalance. The syndrome most often presents in neonates with congenital defects or those being operated on for disease of the intestine.

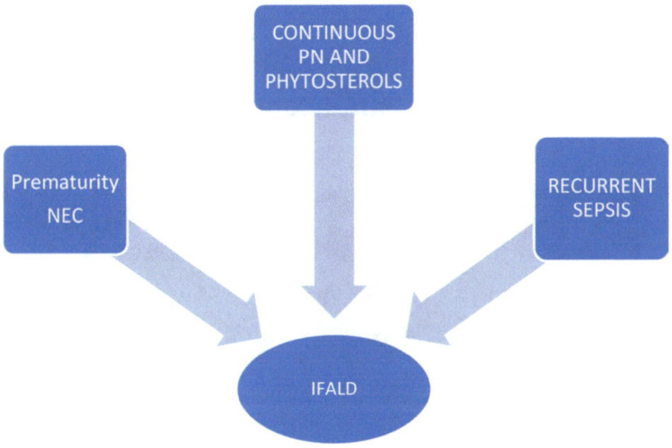

Figure 8.5. Short bowel syndrome (SBS) represents a significant concern within the realm of gastrointestinal disorders encountered in pediatric intensive care.

Source: https://pub.mdpi-res.com/nutrients/nutrients-15-02341/article_deploy/html/images/nutrients-15-02341-g003.png?1684302040.

Treatment of SBS in critically ill children involves a comprehensive approach with nutritional support, e.g., parenteral nutrition, to compensate for malabsorption and allow growth and development. Novel therapeutic intervention with probiotics, e.g., heat-killed bacteria, is being researched for positive influence on gut health and complication prevention, as discussed under the overall context of gastrointestinal disease (Núria Piqué *et al.*, 2019). Successful management of SBS not only addresses the immediate nutritional requirements but also plays a key role in long-term health outcomes among this high-risk population (Melamed *et al.*, 2023) (Figure 8.5).

8.1.9. Functional Gastrointestinal Disorders

Functional gastrointestinal disorders (FGIDs) are a serious issue within pediatric intensive care since they significantly impact children's overall well-being and recovery. They are characterized by the absence of structural abnormality but with debilitating symptoms such as abdominal pain, constipation, and irritable bowel syndrome. They will tend to complicate the treatment of an acute gastrointestinal illness. Children with FGIDs can have increased stress and anxiety, creating a vicious cycle that may result in deteriorating symptoms and increased hospital stays. Gut-brain mechanisms and psychosocial disturbances require an interdisciplinary treatment plan, such as dietary modification, psychological counseling, and medication. The intricacy of FGIDs in children is underscored by fresh findings revealing possible links to other systemic medical conditions, including those with post-COVID status, affecting other organ systems, including gastrointestinal and liver involvement (Scott *et al.*, 2021; Andrade *et al.*, 2021). Holistic treatment of FGIDs is crucial to achieve the best results in the pediatric intensive care unit.

Test Your Knowledge

1. What signs and symptoms suggest a diagnosis of intussusception in a young child?
2. How is functional constipation distinguished from obstructive GI pathologies in the PICU?

8.2. Hepatic Disorders in Pediatric Patients

Learning Outcome

1. Understand hepatitis (viral and autoimmune).
2. Explain biliary atresia.
3. Focus on fatty liver disease, Wilson's disease, hemochromatosis, and liver tumors.
4. Identify metabolic liver diseases.
5. Explain acute liver failure.
6. Discuss chronic liver disease.

Child liver disorders are a major pediatric critical care problem, which demands an interdepartmental approach to achieve optimum outcomes. Liver dysfunction can be due to numerous etiologies, like metabolic, infectious, and autoimmune conditions, often superimposed on pre-existing gastrointestinal conditions. For instance, obesity in childhood has been recognized as a significant risk factor for liver diseases, and an estimated 17% of children and adolescents in the United States suffer from obesity, which could lead to hepatic steatosis and other complex liver diseases (David *et al.*, 2017). In addition, in regions where hepatocellular carcinoma (HCC) is prevalent, particularly in the Asia-Pacific region, it is critical to understand the patient-specific features and management protocols for pediatric patients suffering from hepatic malignancies (Omata *et al.*, 2017). As the pediatric age category has different physiology in terms of fluctuating liver function, treatment modalities must be tailored to individual needs to effectively treat these complex conditions in intensive care units (Figure 8.6).

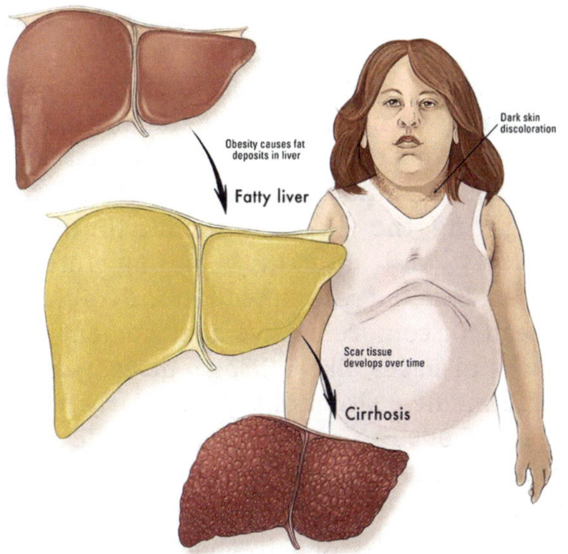

Figure 8.6. Hepatic dysfunction can arise from various etiologies, including metabolic, infectious, and autoimmune disorders, often complicating existing gastrointestinal issues.

Source: https://www.nash24x7.com/wp-content/uploads/2018/06/Why-you-should-not-delay-diagnosis-of-NAFLD-in-kids.jpg.

8.2.1. Hepatitis (Viral and Autoimmune)

Both viral and autoimmune hepatitis present serious challenges in the practice of pediatric intensive care and require careful understanding of their pathophysiology and management. Viral hepatitis, primarily caused by Hepatitis A, B, C, D, and E viruses, is well recognized to precipitate acute and chronic liver disease with varied clinical presentations, such as hepatocellular carcinoma or liver failure, particularly in endemic regions like Asia-Pacific, where hepatocellular carcinoma prevalence is notably high, as discussed by Omata *et al.* (2017). Autoimmune hepatitis, where there is an immune-mediated attack on liver cells, is likely to complicate the typical presentations of viral infections, and thus early diagnosis and management are crucial. Emerging advances in regenerative medicine, e.g., stem cell therapy, have been promising in the management of hepatic conditions, opening new windows of therapy for diseases that were otherwise deemed difficult to manage, as viewed in relevant clinical trials and stem cell use considerations discussed in Duc *et al.* (2022).

8.2.2. Biliary Atresia

Biliary atresia is a pediatric liver disease characterized by gradual obliteration of bile ducts, cholestasis, and severe hepatic damage if left untreated early. Biliary atresia usually happens in infants and should be addressed immediately to prevent irreversible liver failure. Unless surgery, such as the Kasai procedure, is performed, babies must be subjected to liver transplantation due to ensuing complications, which may be growth failure, nutritional deprivation, and biliary cirrhosis.

The complex interaction between biliary atresia and intestinal health only contributes to the complexity of patient outcomes, with children with the disease having an increased chance of developing intestinal failure, a severe condition that undermines the process of nutrient absorption and can culminate in systemic complications (Goulet *et al.*, 2019). Recent advances in regenerative medicine, particularly with stem cell treatment, offer promising paths to new therapies that seek to restore liver function and the quality of life for afflicted infants (Duc *et al.*, 2022) (Figure 8.7).

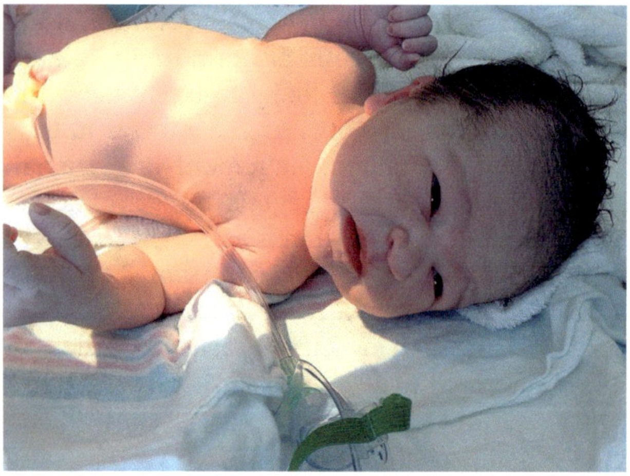

Figure 8.7. Biliary atresia.

Source: https://midsouthliveralliance.org/wp-content/uploads/2021/07/Biliary-Atresia.jpg.

8.2.3. Fatty Liver Disease

In pediatric intensive care, fatty liver disease is also a significant issue, particularly as obesity rates in children increase. As approximately 17% of youths in the United States are found to be affected by obesity, the risk of developing nonalcoholic fatty liver disease (NAFLD) increases greatly. This syndrome is characterized by abnormal fat accumulation in the liver in the absence of alcohol consumption and is typically associated with metabolic diseases such as insulin resistance and dyslipidemia. The manifestation of FLD in children has extrahepatic effects on the liver, which can have undesirable outcomes such as cardiovascular disease and type 2 diabetes in adulthood (Duc *et al.*, 2022). While scientists explore the therapeutic value of novel treatments, such as stem cell therapy, obesity needs to be understood in the context of fatty liver in an attempt to develop an intervention that targets the etiology of this disorder (Duc *et al.*, 2022).

8.2.4. Wilson's Disease

Wilson's disease, which is a genetic condition with abnormal copper metabolism, represents a major challenge in the field of pediatric hepatic and gastrointestinal disorders. Wilson's disease causes the deposition of copper in organs, especially the liver and brain, causing hepatic failure and neurological manifestations. In the pediatric intensive care unit, early intervention and diagnosis are essential in preventing the following life-threatening complications of hepatic failure, which have been reported following cirrhosis and hepatocellular carcinoma (HCC), thus highlighting the disorder's contribution to morbidity and mortality among infected children. Existing recommendations emphasize the need for comprehensive management plans for liver diseases, like Wilson's disease, across diverse medical situations, particularly in high HCC prevalence areas of the Asia–Pacific region (Omata *et al.*, 2017). Detection of metabolic disorders like Wilson's disease is also important for effective intervention because, left untreated, these individuals will experience irreversible harm (Dennis *et al.*, 2017). This is a pointer to the need for heightened alertness and aggressive screening in pediatrics (Figure 8.8).

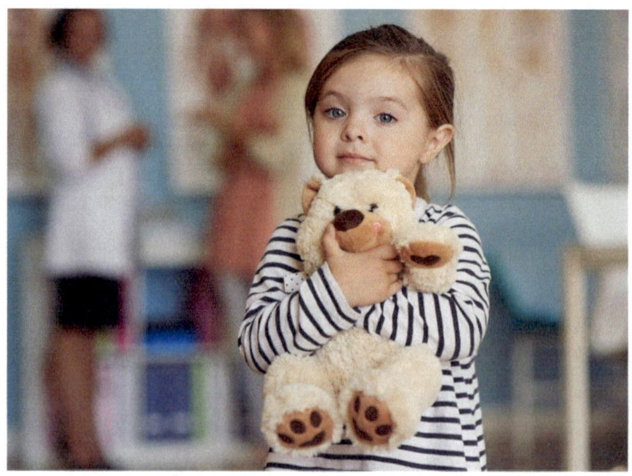

Figure 8.8. Wilson's disease.

Source: https://careoptionsforkids.com/wp-content/uploads/2025/04/Wilsons-Disease-1.jpg.

8.2.5. Hemochromatosis

Hemochromatosis, an iron overload, poses serious challenges for pediatric intensive care, particularly due to the fact that it also has the potential to damage gastrointestinal and hepatic function. Hemochromatosis in children may be caused by genetic mutations affecting iron absorption, leading to systemic toxicity, damaging multiple organ systems. Early detection is essential as it avoids the possibility of severe complications such as liver cirrhosis and diabetes, both of which place long-term burdens on health. Therapy for hemochromatosis typically involves therapeutic phlebotomy to reduce the iron stores and regular monitoring of micronutrient deficiency, which can be augmented both by the disease process and treatment (Mette *et al.*, 2024). The severity of such an illness necessitates an interdisciplinary approach, with regular monitoring of the liver's functioning and adequate nutritional supplementation based on the individual's needs, to allow for optimal recovery in a pediatric intensive care unit (Hasenmajer *et al.*, 2023).

8.2.6. Liver Tumors

Liver masses in children present severe challenges in the intensive care unit because of their potential for aggressive development and life-compromising complications. These masses, ranging from hepatoblastoma, the most common primary liver cancer in children, to metastatic masses, can induce disastrous hepatic failure and multi-organ failure if not timely intervened upon. The complex interplay of pediatric health with liver tumors necessitates multidisciplinary opinion from oncologists, hepatologists, and intensivists. New trends in treatment, including stem cell therapies, have been explored as emerging therapeutic strategies that can augment regenerative potential and enhance patient outlook (Duc *et al.*, 2022). In addition, the effect of severe systemic diseases like COVID-19 can become a more aggressive liver tumor clinical presentation, making careful observation and treatment of pediatric patients with intrinsic gastrointestinal and hepatic pathologies necessary (Andrade *et al.*, 2021). Understanding these dynamics is vital to achieving maximum care in the pediatric intensive care unit (Figure 8.9).

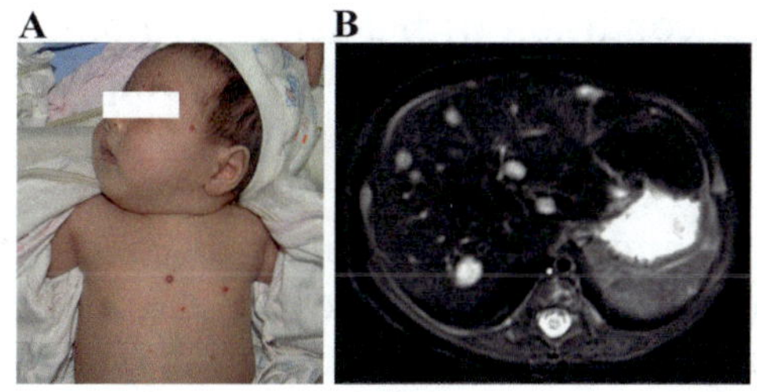

Figure 8.9. Liver tumors in pediatric patients.

Source: https://media.springernature.com/full/springer-static/image/art%3A10.1038%2Fsrep31744/MediaObjects/41598_2016_Article_BFsrep31744_Fig1_HTML.jpg.

8.2.7. Metabolic Liver Diseases

Metabolic liver diseases, including a range of genetic diseases affecting the liver's function in metabolizing compounds, are complex conditions found in pediatric intensive care units. These diseases, like urea cycle disorders, maple syrup urine disease, and fatty acid oxidation disorders, can cause severe acute metabolic crises that require immediate and sophisticated treatment. Notably, technological innovations such as liver elastography have enhanced diagnostic capabilities in neonatal intensive care units (NICUs), providing non-invasive approaches to quantify liver stiffness and diagnose illnesses like cholestatic diseases and metabolic disorders (Angel Zapata *et al.*, 2025). Moreover, the occurrence of seizures and deranged mental status among patients with metabolic liver diseases emphasizes the necessity for keen observation, as indicated by evidence that depicts a high frequency of neurological presentation with metabolic crisis

(Sen *et al.*, 2024). In general, awareness and management of metabolic liver diseases are necessary to enhance outcomes among critically ill children.

8.2.8. Acute Liver Failure

Acute liver failure (ALF) in children is a serious medical condition with a generally non-sudden onset and potential for serious complications. The etiology of ALF may be multifactorial, with a range of etiologies from viral hepatitis to drug toxicity and metabolic liver diseases. Early diagnosis is required because the condition can progress quickly to hepatic encephalopathy and multi-organ failure, necessitating intensive care treatment and management. Later research emphasizes careful monitoring and early intervention in PICUs to support better patient outcomes.

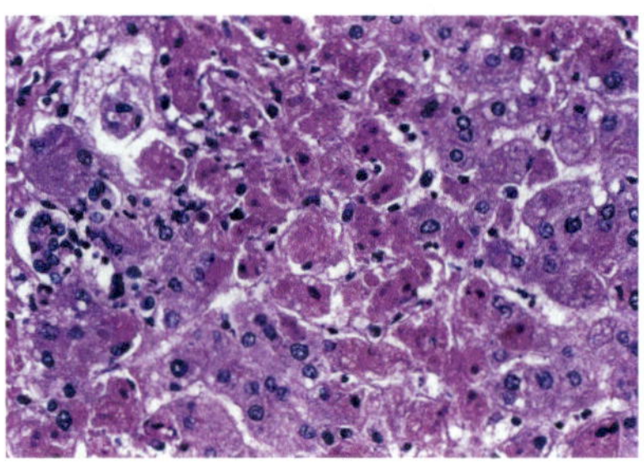

Figure 8.10. Acute liver failure (ALF) in pediatric patients.

Source: https://upload.wikimedia.org/wikipedia/commons/4/42/Marburg_virus_liver_injury.jpg.

This is complemented by evolving trends in liver transplantation discussed in recent conferences, where new advances in treatment approaches to ALF were central, showcasing innovations that meet urgent care demands in this group (Mathew *et al.*, 2024). Additionally, the relevance of symptoms such as multisystem inflammatory syndrome (MIS-C) following COVID-19 may complicate the clinical picture, necessitating wary observation of gastrointestinal and hepatic presentations (Sica *et al.*, 2021) (Figure 8.10).

8.2.9. Chronic Liver Disease

Chronic liver disease creates a challenge of substantial magnitude in the intensive care of children since it involves a range of complex disorders that often translate into considerable morbidity and mortality. The etiology of chronic liver disease in children is multifactorial, involving metabolic disorders, viral diseases, and congenital abnormalities that need an interdisciplinary approach in management to resolve the complexities of such disorders well.

Chronic liver disease in children may lead to growth failure, nutritional deprivation, and developmental delay, which will further deteriorate the health status and complicate the treatment course. Moreover, as the literature has shown, diseases leading to liver transplantation account for a considerable percentage of chronic diseases managed in pediatric palliative care settings, emphasizing the necessity of early intervention and ongoing treatment (Spolador *et al.*, 2024). In extreme instances, these complications, such as hepatic encephalopathy and coagulopathy, may necessitate urgent intervention in the pediatric intensive care unit, illustrating the need for specialist care in such a vulnerable subgroup (Dorleta López-Suso *et al.*, 2022).

Test Your Knowledge

1. What is the most common cause of chronic liver disease in infants?
2. What laboratory tests indicate impaired liver synthetic function in children?

8.3. Diagnostic Approaches in Pediatric Intensive Care

Learning Outcome

1. Understand clinical assessment and history taking.
2. Explain laboratory tests and biomarkers.
3. Learn imaging studies.
4. Describe endoscopy and biopsy techniques.
5. Discuss the role of multidisciplinary teams.
6. Identify challenges in diagnosis.
7. Know the importance of timely intervention.
8. Learn the use of scoring systems for severity assessment.
9. Focus on follow-up and monitoring strategies.

In pediatric intensive care, accurate and timely diagnosis is very important, particularly when managing gastrointestinal and hepatic diseases. Diagnostic methods, such as abdominal ultrasound and paracentesis, can provide important information about diseases like ascites and portal hypertension, which are inevitabilities in children with liver disease. As emphasized in recent guidelines, ascites serum albumin gradient measurement is an important consideration for the differentiation of ascites secondary to portal hypertension from others, aiding in planning appropriate management (Scott *et al.*, 2021). Moreover, multidisciplinary care by pediatric gastroenterologists, intensivists, and nutritionists optimizes diagnosis through detailed assessment and management of primary conditions. As rates of obesity among young individuals continue to rise, screening for comorbidity has become of specific importance, and hence it is imperative that healthcare providers stay current regarding the latest guidelines and interventions tailored for pediatric patients with such complex diseases (Dennis *et al.*, 2017) (Figure 8.11).

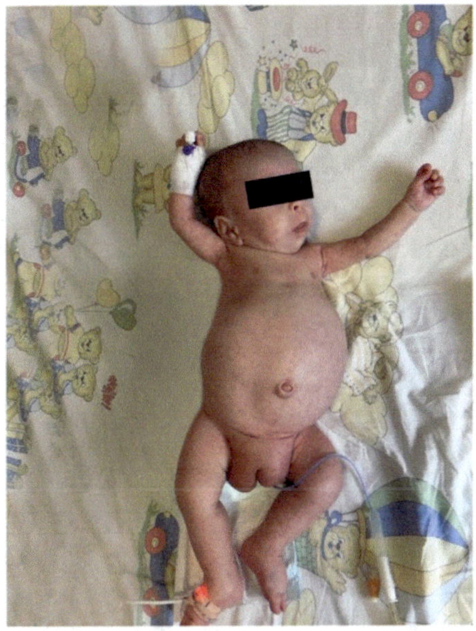

Figure 8.11. Assessing the serum albumin ascites gradient plays a pivotal role in differentiating portal hypertension-related ascites from other causes, contributing to effective management strategies.

Source: https://media.springernature.com/lw685/springer-static/image/art%3A10.1007%2Fs00467-021-05010-1/MediaObjects/467_2021_5010_Fig1_HTML.jpg.

8.3.1. Clinical Assessment and History Taking

Effective clinical assessment and history taking are essential in the treatment of gastrointestinal and liver diseases in pediatric intensive care units. An effective understanding of a child's medical, nutritional, and family history is essential in the diagnosis of predisposing conditions that can cause acute or chronic gastroenterological conditions. Specifically, assessment needs to consider patterns of growth and obesity comorbidities, which have been seen to affect a significant proportion of US children (David *et al.*, 2017). Moreover, this evidence base allows for individualized assessment and intervention to occur based on the unique situations for each child's case (Jane *et al.*, 2018). Through taking a comprehensive interview and physical examination, medical professionals are able to acquire a clear clinical picture, thereby maximizing the effectiveness of treatment interventions and patient outcomes. In the end, robust history taking and clinical assessment are fundamental cornerstones in the delivery of excellent care in pediatric intensive care units.

8.3.2. Laboratory Tests and Biomarkers

In pediatric intensive care, laboratory investigations and biomarkers are critical to the diagnosis and management of gastrointestinal and liver illness. They help in the identification of underlying pathology as well as the monitoring of disease progression, something that in a pediatric context is particularly valuable because presentations can be nonspecific and subtle.

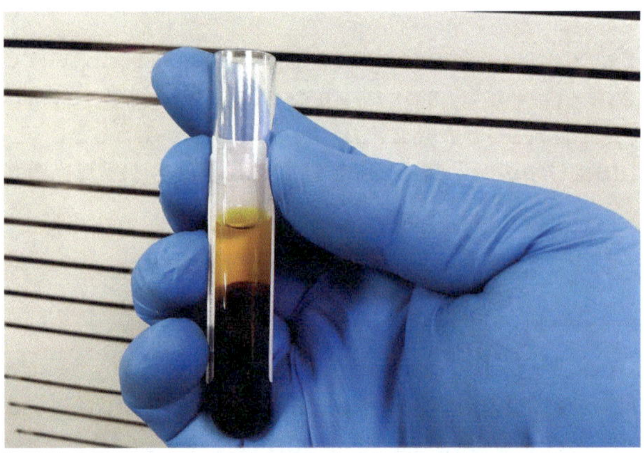

Figure 8.12. Biomarkers can aid in evaluating liver function, as alterations in enzyme levels may indicate hepatic injury or biliary obstruction.

Source: https://cdn.royalcanin-weshare-online.io/qehQlpMBaPOZra8qoUAq/v9/vf-342-article-6-figure-2.

As an illustration, biomarkers may be employed to evaluate liver function because alterations in the concentration of enzymes may indicate hepatic damage or bile duct obstruction. Some new findings have also enhanced our understanding of congenital adrenal hyperplasia (CAH), which may frequently present in children with abnormal genitals or adrenal crises, raising diagnostic precision with improved genotyping and steroid profiling techniques (Hedi *et al.*, 2021). Furthermore, the research on stem cell therapies raises the potential for regenerative treatment in cases where conventional methods are not effective, as observed with active clinical trials (Duc *et al.*, 2022). Together, these laboratory tests and biomarkers enhance the quality of treatment for critically ill pediatric patients (Figure 8.12).

8.3.3. Imaging Studies (Ultrasound, CT, MRI)

In pediatric intensive care, within the context of gastrointestinal and hepatic illness, imaging studies such as ultrasound, computed tomography (CT), and magnetic resonance imaging (MRI) have significant roles as diagnostic and monitoring tools. Ultrasound is usually the first imaging method because it is a non-invasive modality that offers real-time imaging and is therefore well-suited for assessing fluid collections, organ size, and vascular structures in children. CT scanning can generate cross-sectional views with high resolution, facilitating more accurate intra-abdominal pathology assessment, especially in the context of acute pancreatitis or appendicitis. Conversely, MRI is capable of providing improved soft tissue contrast, which is beneficial in the understanding of complex liver disease as well as inflammatory changes of adjacent structures. For instance, imaging investigations' findings have been directing attention towards associations of SARS-CoV-2 infection with gastrointestinal manifestations, and precise imaging is needed to guide management and treatment strategies in critically ill children (Salamanna *et al.*, 2020; Dolhnikoff *et al.*, 2020).

8.3.4. Endoscopy and Biopsy Techniques

Endoscopy and biopsy play an essential role in the diagnosis and care of gastrointestinal and liver disease in pediatric intensive care. Direct visualization of the gut with endoscopy and biopsy tissue facilitates simple diagnosis of conditions such as inflammatory bowel disease, neoplasia, and infection. Advances in endoscopic technology have made it possible for children to have minimally invasive treatments that are less painful and that shorten recovery times.

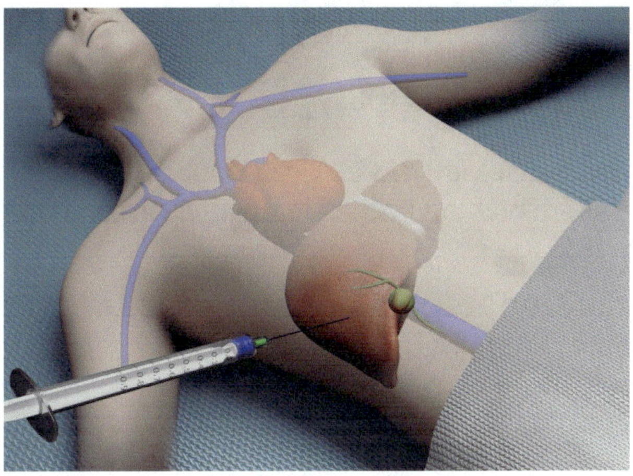

Figure 8.13. Endoscopy and biopsy techniques play a pivotal role in diagnosing and managing gastrointestinal and hepatic disorders in pediatric intensive care.

Source: https://www.mdpi.com/diagnostics/diagnostics-13-00784/article_deploy/html/images/diagnostics-13-00784-g001.png.

The integration of endoscopic information with molecular profiling, as seen in the recent study, contributes to further insight into various gastrointestinal pathologies, including familial adenomatous polyposis (FAP) and extraintestinal manifestations of it (Dinarvand *et al.*, 2019). Endoscopic methods also play a crucial part in therapeutic interventions such as polypectomy or dilation of a stricture, highlighting their usefulness in treating children (Duc *et al.*, 2022). Thus, endoscopy and biopsy remain key to optimizing care in this vulnerable population (Figure 8.13).

8.3.5. Role of Multidisciplinary Teams

The complexity in managing gastrointestinal and liver illnesses in pediatric intensive care units projects the role of multidisciplinary teams in a central position. The pediatricians, gastroenterologists, hepatologists, nurses, nutritionists, and social workers form a team to work together and give comprehensive and efficient patient care. This process of coordination facilitates early detection and intervention, leading to improved outcomes. For instance, in cases of severe pneumonia with recurrent gastrointestinal reactions, a multidisciplinary intervention not only helps to manage the respiratory failure but also provides nutritional support and drugs specifically tailored to prevent multidrug-resistant bacteria-related complications (Yuan *et al.*, 2025). Apart from that, some disorders like Rett syndrome show that there is a need for multidisciplinary care, where the interventions of various specialties are required to enhance the patient's quality of life despite gradual deterioration (Lozano *et al.*, 2025). Therefore, effective collaboration in these healthcare facilities is essential to enhance treatment strategies and patient safety.

8.3.6. Challenges in Diagnosis

In pediatric intensive care, diagnosing gastrointestinal and hepatic illnesses presents a significant challenge in that they share common symptoms and complex diseases in nature. The multidimensional presentation of the diseases has a tendency to make clinical assessment challenging, yielding to risks of misdiagnosis or delayed treatment. For instance, conditions such as nonalcoholic fatty liver disease (NAFLD) can mimic other metabolic conditions, hence need strict screening methods to precisely differentiate them (Miriam *et al.*, 2016). Additionally, when diagnosing primary adrenal insufficiency in critically ill children, the clinicians' detection threshold is low, highlighting the need for careful assessments in order not to miss this potentially life-threatening disorder (Stefan *et al.*, 2016). The variables in clinical presentation, the equipment for diagnosis, and the need for specialized information make the diagnosis all the more complex, and therefore, it is imperative that strict guidelines are laid down to ensure early detection and effective management (Figure 8.14).

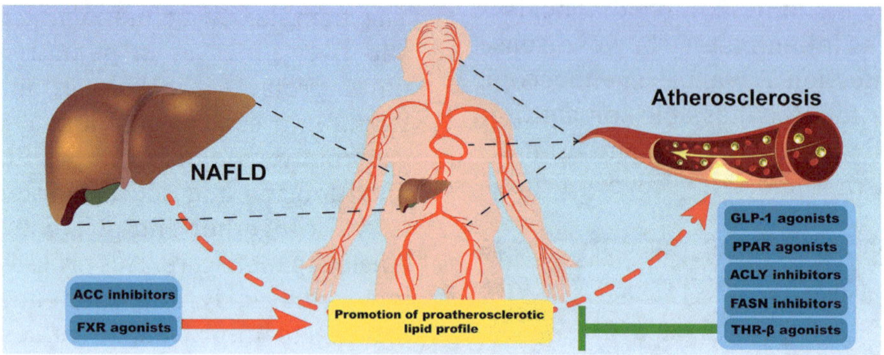

Figure 8.14. Conditions such as nonalcoholic fatty liver disease (NAFLD) can appear similar to other metabolic disorders, thereby necessitating rigorous screening protocols to differentiate them accurately.

Source: https://www.atherosclerosis-journal.com/cms/10.1016/j.atherosclerosis.2022.07.010/asset/623f3371-ea84-4a0a-b247-318343674022/main.assets/ga1_lrg.jpg.

8.3.7. Importance of Timely Intervention

Prompt handling of gastrointestinal and liver diseases in the pediatric intensive care unit (PICU) is critical to improve patient outcomes in addition to preventing long-term complications. Early detection and management of the diseases may reduce mortality and morbidity rates among children, particularly those who are critically ill. Studies depict that early treatment of gastrointestinal symptoms is likely to prevent the onset of more dangerous complications, such as hemorrhage or septic shock, which are common risks among this vulnerable group. In addition, with the rising burden from post-acute sequelae following viral infections such as COVID-19, acknowledging the importance of timely clinical assessment and intervention becomes more imperative, as patients are likely to exert lasting impacts on numerous organ systems. The interprofessional workflow outlined in clinical guidelines emphasizes the integration of timely evaluation and interaction among various professionals, which is required to ensure that pediatric patients receive appropriate and effective treatment as per their unique needs (Melamed *et al.*, 2023; Timothy *et al.*, 2018).

8.3.8. Use of Scoring Systems for Severity Assessment

The application of scoring systems for the evaluation of severity is a significant component of the management of gastrointestinal and liver diseases in pediatric intensive care settings. Such standardized evaluations enable stratification of patients based on the severity of illness, thereby guiding therapeutic interventions and resource allocation. For instance, the Child-Pugh score and the Model for End-Stage Liver Disease (MELD) score are key in determining liver function and the urgency of liver transplant in hepatic decompensation. Accurate estimation by these scoring systems not just enhances decision-making clinically but also with patient outcomes, including mortality and risk for complications like hepatic encephalopathy and spontaneous bacterial peritonitis (Scott *et al.*, 2021). Consequently, effective application of these scoring systems can potentially provide more individualized and focused treatment plans, ultimately better care for critically ill children with hepatic and gastrointestinal illnesses (George *et al.*, 2018) (Figure 8.15).

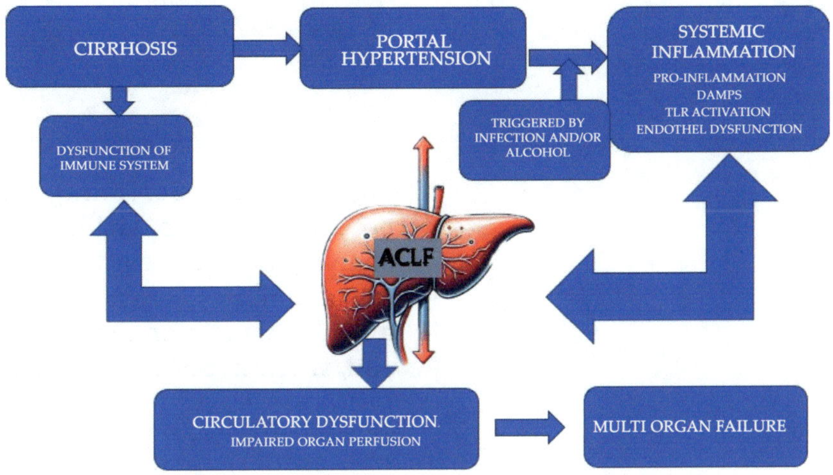

Figure 8.15. The incorporation of scoring systems for severity assessment plays a crucial role in managing gastrointestinal and hepatic disorders within pediatric intensive care settings.

Source: https://www.mdpi.com/jcm/jcm-13-00506/article_deploy/html/images/jcm-13-00506-g001.png.

8.3.9. Follow-Up and Monitoring Strategies

In pediatric intensive care, close monitoring and follow-up are most crucial in managing gastrointestinal and hepatic illness to maximize patient outcomes. It enables clinicians to identify complications early and subsequently adjust therapy accordingly. For instance, the utilization of interdisciplinary teams can be used to monitor multisystem inflammatory response patients, such as those with PIMS-TS, where gastrointestinal and cardiac involvement is prevalent (Fernández-Sarmiento *et al.*, 2021). Moreover, constant monitoring of biochemical markers and clinical features can be used to inform therapeutic interventions, allowing for early intervention in response to altering conditions (Rocha-e-Silva, 2009). Establishing a solid follow-up schedule ensures that healthcare providers can monitor disorder progress more effectively and implement required care plan adjustments, thus significantly improving overall care of affected pediatric patients in intensive care settings.

Test Your Knowledge

1. What is the role of point-of-care ultrasound (POCUS) in diagnosing GI emergencies?
2. How are stool studies used in the evaluation of acute diarrhea in hospitalized children?

8.4. Management Strategies for Gastrointestinal and Hepatic Disorders

Learning Outcome

1. Understand nutritional support and dietary management.
2. Explain pharmacological treatments.
3. Discuss surgical interventions.
4. Know the role of liver transplantation.
5. Describe palliative care considerations.
6. Describe family-centered care approaches.
7. Focus on psychological support for patients and families.
8. Discuss education and training for healthcare providers.
9. Know future directions in management.

Pediatric intensive care treatment of gastrointestinal and liver diseases requires evidence-based, multimodal management of the diverse range of problems presented by these conditions. Effective interventions involve early diagnosis and intervention to prevent complications like nonalcoholic fatty liver disease (NAFLD), which has become increasingly prevalent in children due to increased obesity rates caused by insulin resistance (Miriam *et al.*, 2016). Screening strategies need to be established to enable early diagnosis, enabling the use of management strategies that encompass dietary interventions, lifestyle modifications, and, where necessary, pharmacotherapy. Psychological effects also need to be addressed in relation to such conditions, for example, pediatric obesity, using guidelines requesting psychological screening and intervention (Dennis *et al.*, 2017). Such an integrated management system aims not only to treat the immediate clinical manifestations but also to provoke long-term health benefits and avoid recurrence of hepatic and gastrointestinal disease in high-risk children (Figure 8.16).

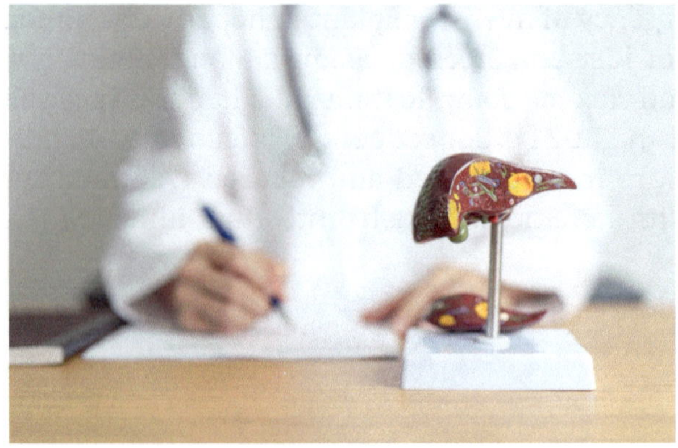

Figure 8.16. Screening protocols should be established to facilitate timely diagnosis, enabling healthcare practitioners to implement management strategies that encompass nutritional interventions, lifestyle modifications, and, when necessary, pharmacotherapy.

Source: https://www.drsandeepsatsangi.com/wp-content/uploads/2023/10/doctor-with-human-liver-anatomy-model-liver-cance-2023-06-19-23-39-27-utc-scaled.jpg.

8.4.1. Nutritional Support and Dietary Management

Nutritional management and dietary therapy are essential in the pediatric intensive care unit, particularly in children with gastrointestinal and hepatic disturbances. The complications typically complicate nutrient digestion and place them at risk for malnutrition, requiring special dietary treatment. Moderate dietary sodium restriction is vital in use since it helps to control fluid overload and ascites in patients with cirrhosis in the pediatric population, enhancing their overall therapeutic regimen. Furthermore, the inclusion of probiotics, especially heat-killed probiotics, has a promising method of immunomodulation and intestinal barrier integrity, particularly valuable in pediatric patients with gastrointestinal diseases (Núria Piqué *et al.*, 2019). Studies show that enteral nutrition through specific feeds also contributes significantly to nutritional status while minimizing hospitalization and complication rates of such diseases. Consequently, a multidimensional approach with diet restrictions and supplementary nutrition is a must to achieve optimal treatment and recovery in pediatric intensive care patients (Scott *et al.*, 2021).

8.4.2. Pharmacological Treatments

Pharmacological management is the cornerstone of the management of gastrointestinal and hepatic disease in children on intensive care, particularly in complicated clinical scenarios. Pharmacological management usually takes the form of an array of drugs that are employed to manage the symptoms, the causative pathology, and prevent complications.

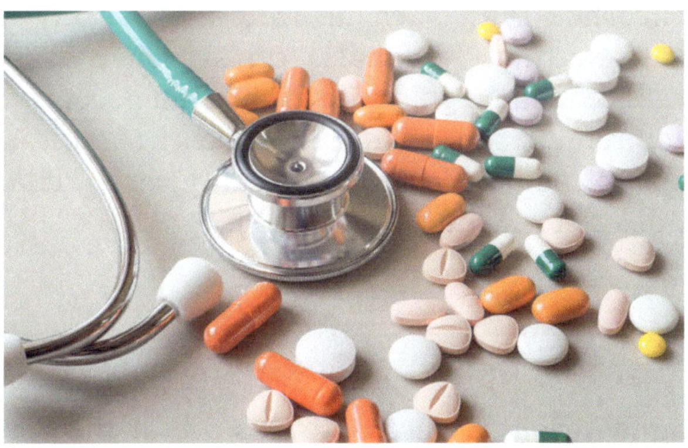

Figure 8.17. Pharmacological treatments play a pivotal role in managing gastrointestinal and hepatic disorders in pediatric intensive care, particularly in addressing complex clinical presentations.

Source: https://medlux.net.ua/wp-content/uploads/2021/07/medikamentoznoe-lechenie-narkomanii-tabletki.jpg.

For instance, proton pump inhibitors are now employed on a regular basis to manage acid-related disorders, while medications such as lactulose and rifaximin are employed to manage hepatic encephalopathy, a disease that is seen frequently in children with liver disease. Steroid therapy can also be indicated in inflammatory bowel diseases, a recognition of the need for an individualized pharmacological approach depending on each child's unique requirements. The success of these therapies is significantly dependent on the judicious application of appropriate dosages and careful monitoring for potential side effects, with caution to ensure that the therapeutic effect is more than the risk in this vulnerable population. As research becomes more advanced, application of new drug therapies will continue to enhance the patients' outcomes in such intensive care units (Dennis *et al.*, 2017; Stefan *et al.*, 2016) (Figure 8.17).

8.4.3. Surgical Interventions

Surgical procedures have a central role in pediatric intensive care in the treatment of hepatic and gastrointestinal diseases, particularly when treatment conservatively fails. They can vary from low-invasive procedures such as laparoscopic surgery to major procedures such as liver transplantation and resections for HCC. Case complexity typically necessitates a multidisciplinary team made up of surgical experts and allied imaging and supportive care to optimize outcomes. For instance, the Toward Revision of the Asian Pacific Association for the Study of the Liver (APASL) HCC Guidelines emphasizes evidence-based management that is particularly pertinent in light of the geographical prevalence of HCC in the Asia–Pacific region, where the disease has significant public health relevance (Omata *et al.*, 2017). Besides, there are still evolving newer techniques of surgery, in line with the significance of ongoing adaptation and questioning towards improved outcomes and survival levels in children with these powerful diseases (Dennis *et al.*, 2017).

8.4.4. Role of Liver Transplantation

Liver transplantation is also a life-saving measure for advanced hepatic diseases, particularly in children who might have biliary atresia and metabolic liver diseases, to be cured through surgery. Failure of the liver can lead to multi-organ failure, and hence early transplantation is an important solution to restore liver function to attain survival. Pediatric patients with hepatocellular failure caused by cirrhosis are at increased morbidity and mortality; hence, identification for transplantation is essential during their clinic assessment. Referral for liver transplant evaluation is warranted when patients experience manifestations of hepatic decompensation, e.g., ascites or encephalopathy, that are associated with worse survival (Scott *et al.*, 2021). Also, revised guidelines highlight the need for early intervention and appropriate management planning in such patients, especially as per the distinct complexities in pediatric patients according to the recent APASL guidelines (Omata *et al.*, 2017). Lastly, liver transplant is a last-resort life-saving procedure to manage advanced liver disease in children (Figure 8.18).

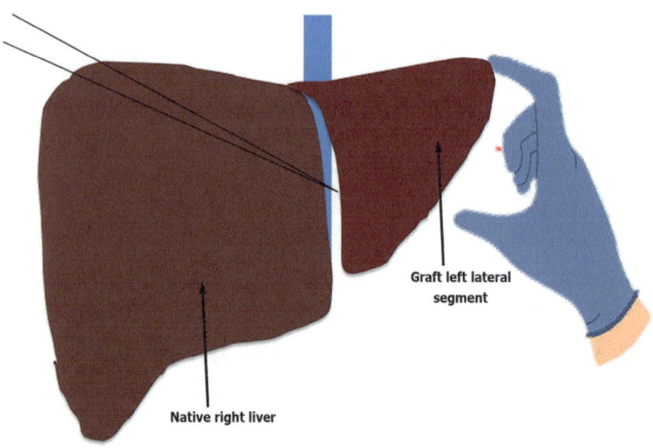

Figure 8.18. Liver transplantation plays a critical role in managing severe hepatic disorders, particularly in pediatric patients where conditions like biliary atresia and metabolic liver diseases often necessitate surgical intervention.

Source: https://f6publishing.blob.core.windows.net/3dcd2809-7d1b-49ce-9494-f79a3758f9cd/WJH-13-1351-g002.png.

8.4.5. Palliative Care Considerations

In children with gastrointestinal and hepatic disease, the palliative care concerns are secondary to enhancing the patients' quality of life and also that of their families. Effective palliative care should cover relief of not just the physical effects of these diseases, such as pain and ascites, but also the emotional and psychological problems arising from treatment. Utilization of a multidisciplinary model, with pediatric experts along with palliative care teams, is critical for the management of complex medical needs and psychosocial factors. For instance, multimodal analgesia, careful discussion about prognosis, and addressing family members are essential in the provision of informed decision-making and pain relief for the patient. With the complexities concerned with such disorders, especially in acute settings, emphasis on evidence-based practice in managing pain in children becomes a requirement because its lack makes a significant contribution to decreasing quality care (Stefan *et al.*, 2019; Scott *et al.*, 2021).

8.4.6. Family-Centered Care Approaches

Family-oriented care practices are at the core of maximizing the experience and outcomes of pediatric patients with gastrointestinal and hepatic disease within the pediatric intensive care setting. If families are integrated into decision-making, providers are more effective in creating an environment that is respectful to their informational and emotional needs, and promotes a holistic approach to care. As emphasized in recent literature, effective interprofessional interventions in the ICU concern patients' family inclusion in care planning to facilitate effective communication and collaboration among team members with the goal of enhancing patient outcomes (Kleinpell *et al.*, 2021). Moreover, addressing the specific needs of the family, especially where there are complex medical conditions involved, is significant in improving on minimizing stress and building resilience among pediatric patients. This is in accordance with evidence-based management guidelines for liver-related complications, which are prevalent among pediatric patients, particularly those from the Asia-Pacific region (Omata *et al.*, 2017). Overall, the integration of family-centered care principles significantly enhances the quality of pediatric intensive care (Figure 8.19).

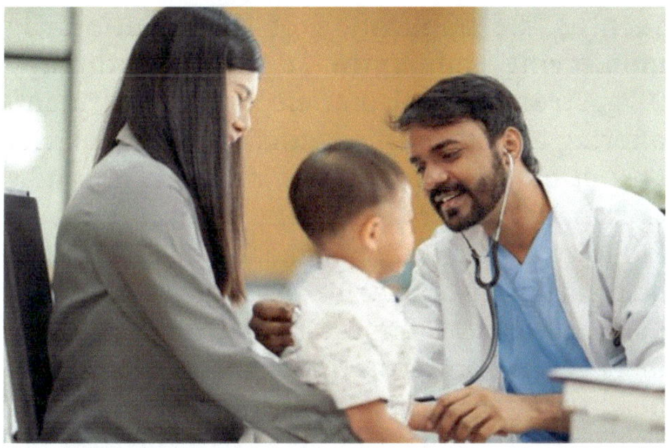

Figure 8.19. Family-centered care approaches are pivotal in enhancing the experiences and outcomes of children facing gastrointestinal and hepatic disorders in the pediatric intensive care setting.

Source: https://s3.amazonaws.com/utep-uploads/wp-content/uploads/online-regis-college/2018/03/24030126/pediatric_nurse.jpg.

8.4.7. Psychological Support for Patients and Families

In pediatric intensive care for hepatic and gastrointestinal illnesses, psychological support to families and patients is of utmost significance. The emotional and mental toll of critical illness can have a significant impact on recovery outcomes and overall family well-being. Firm psychological support encompasses good communication, empathy, and family engagement in decision-making, which can generate a sense of security and confidence. Literature has identified that family involvement in multidisciplinary rounds not only enhances decision-making but also enhances emotional resilience during the patient's hospital stay (Kleinpell *et al.*, 2021). Furthermore, incorporation of spiritual care and social work in the ICU team attests to responding to the psychological aspect of care, thereby mitigating the emotional turmoil that results from complex treatment modalities (Arslanian *et al.*, 2018). Lastly, a general plan of psychological intervention can help heal and build the coping capacity of the family during negative circumstances.

8.4.8. Education and Training for Healthcare Providers

In the provision of optimal care to pediatric patients suffering from hepatic and gastrointestinal disease, training and education of healthcare professionals are given prominence. This involves an integrated program that addresses interprofessional collaboration, since the healthcare teams must have several specialties in order to address the multilateral needs of such critically ill children. Effective education initiatives set out to create competency in the utilization of high-level technology equipment, such as mobile ultrasound machines, that have proven to be useful in pediatric settings, enabling improved diagnostics and patient monitoring (Nielsen *et al.*, 2018). Also, interprofessional models of care, explained by SCCM, respond to the requirement for effective care and communication among team members so that all providers' skills are leveraged to improve patients' outcomes (Kleinpell *et al.*, 2021). By laying emphasis on multidisciplinary education and continuous professional growth, clinicians can better prepare themselves, hence being able to deliver high-standard, evidence-based care to adolescents with severe hepatic and gastrointestinal challenges in intensive care settings (Figure 8.20).

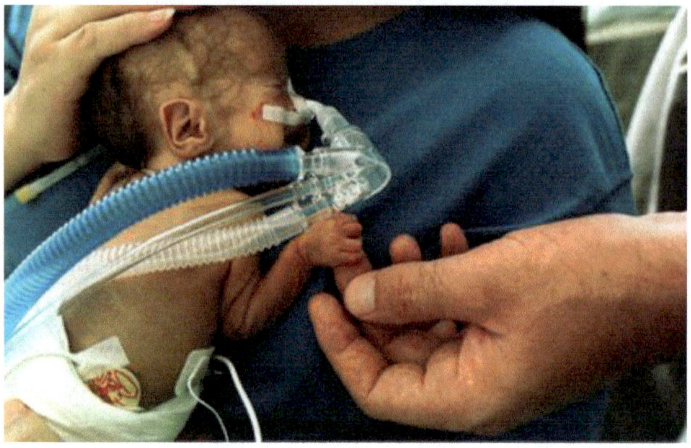

Figure 8.20. In providing optimal care for pediatric patients with gastrointestinal and hepatic disorders, the education and training of healthcare providers are paramount.

Source: https://www.physio-pedia.com/images/thumb/9/92/Infant_CPAP.jpeg/400px-Infant_CPAP.jpeg.

8.4.9. Future Directions in Management

With increasingly sophisticated pediatric intensive care in the future, initiatives to treat gastrointestinal and hepatic illness must factor in therapeutic progress and the unique complexity of this patient population. Multidisciplinary approaches are called for; a multidisciplinary team approach between intensivists, gastroenterologists, and clinical pharmacists can optimize treatment effectiveness by incorporating consideration of the intricate pharmacokinetics and pharmacodynamics of medication in critically ill children. Notably, advances in the field of personalized medicine, such as the application of therapeutic drug monitoring, can optimize pharmacotherapy in gastrointestinal and hepatic impairment, offering optimal dosing with minimized toxicity (Via *et al.*, 2025). Secondly, research into new therapeutic approaches like combined liver-kidney transplantation in metabolic disease can be a savior for otherwise refractory conditions, bringing out the importance of individualized management protocols that change as per patient needs (Ishtiaq, 2025). This advancement reflects the need for ongoing research and flexible treatment protocols in pediatric intensive care units.

Test Your Knowledge

1. What are the treatment goals for children with necrotizing enterocolitis?
2. How is hepatic encephalopathy managed in pediatric patients?

SUMMARY

The complexity of gastrointestinal and hepatic illness in pediatric intensive care necessitates the use of a range of strategies in managing patients. In addition to contributing to the complexity of the clinical picture, these illnesses exert profound impacts on outcome. As testified to by work conducted at Rajendra Institute of Medical Sciences, electrolyte disturbances are frequent in critically ill children, with diseases such as conditions covering systemic diseases, such as pneumonia and central nervous system diseases, being particularly prominent (Sahu *et al.*, 2025). Moreover, newer studies indicate that probiotics like Lactobacillus GG can also be of significant importance in avoiding complications like antibiotic-associated diarrhea, which may potentially improve overall length of stay and quality of care in the PICU (Chung *et al.*, 2025). Therefore, it is essential to adopt proactive identification as well as intervention practices to ensure an improved recovery pathway for affected children to further improve pediatric critical care practices.

In general, the care of gastrointestinal and liver illness in Pediatric Intensive Care is specifically troublesome and calls for overall, coordinated care approaches. Central to this approach is the recognition of complex conditions like beta-thalassemia that need lifetime management and require specialized care teams to address personalized clinical requirements (Farmakis *et al.*, 2022). Also, new dietary treatments like the ketogenic diet are now explored for therapeutic use in other pediatric disorders apart from epilepsy, a possible pathway to therapeutic innovation (Zhu *et al.*, 2022). Evidence-based practice and current research combined into new therapies ensure the best standard of care for the pediatric patient, an indication of an interest in optimal outcomes. As healthcare professionals navigate these multifaceted disorders, a multidisciplinary approach remains crucial for addressing both the medical and psychosocial needs of affected children and their families.

KEY TERMS FROM THIS CHAPTER

- Hepatic illnesses
- Ascites
- Hepatocellular carcinoma
- Intestines
- Gastroesophageal reflux disease (GERD)
- Acute gastroenteritis
- Crohn's disease
- Multipotent mesenchymal stem cells (MSCs)
- Gastrointestinal infection
- Hepatic encephalopathy
- Stomach
- Dehydration
- Positional maneuvers
- Inflammatory bowel disease (IBD)
- Ulcerative colitis
- Probiotics

CRITICAL THINKING QUESTIONS

1. **Which of the following is a common cause of upper gastrointestinal bleeding in critically ill children?**
   a. Appendicitis
   b. Stress-related mucosal disease
   c. Intussusception
   d. Hirschsprung's disease
2. **A child with liver failure presents with confusion and altered mental status. What is the most likely diagnosis?**
   a. Sepsis
   b. Hepatic encephalopathy
   c. Diabetic ketoacidosis
   d. Brain abscess
3. **What is the most specific lab test for evaluating liver synthetic function?**
   a. ALT
   b. AST
   c. Prothrombin time (PT)/INR
   d. Alkaline phosphatase
4. **Which of the following conditions is a surgical emergency and a common cause of bilious vomiting in neonates?**
   a. Pyloric stenosis
   b. Gastroesophageal reflux
   c. Malrotation with volvulus
   d. Hirschsprung's disease
5. **What is the preferred method of nutritional support in a critically ill child with a functional GI tract?**
   a. Parenteral nutrition
   b. Enteral nutrition via NG or NJ tube
   c. Nothing by mouth (NPO)
   d. Intravenous glucose only

Short Answer Questions

1. What are the most common causes of gastrointestinal bleeding in pediatric ICU patients?
2. How does necrotizing enterocolitis (NEC) typically present in neonates?
3. What are the early clinical signs of acute liver failure in children?
4. How does hepatic encephalopathy present in pediatric patients?
5. What imaging modalities are most useful for evaluating suspected abdominal pathology in PICU patients?
6. How is abdominal distension assessed and monitored in critically ill children?
7. What are the key steps in stabilizing a child with upper GI bleeding?
8. How is fluid and electrolyte balance managed in children with vomiting and diarrhea in the PICU?

Answers to Critical Thinking Questions

1. (b) 2. (b) 3. (c) 4. (c) 5. (b)

REFERENCES

1. Abdullah, I. (2025). Joint liver-kidney transplantation for primary hyperoxaluria and other metabolic conditions. *Health Sciences AUS.* https://www.semanticscholar.org/paper/ae0e63ce23734eade7f364748ae0e70dde1953e1 (accessed on 30th June 2025).

2. Allison, C., Sehgal, M., Gavrilita, C., Falkos, S., & Vidal, R. (2025). Lactobacillus GG in the prevention of antibiotic-associated diarrhea in the pediatric intensive care unit: A prospective randomized, double-blind placebo-controlled intervention. *The Journal of Pediatric Pharmacology and Therapeutics: JPPT: The Official Journal of PPAG, 30*(1), 47–51. https://www.semanticscholar.org/paper/f92eef872894bafe4a8531e4be22fa55f016f3e8 (accessed on 30th June 2025).

3. Andrade, B., Siqueira, S., Rodrigues de Assis Soares, W., de Souza Rangel, F., Oliveira Santos, N., dos Santos Freitas, A., Silveira, P. R., *et al.* (2021). Long-COVID and post-COVID health complications: An up-to-date review on clinical conditions and their possible molecular mechanisms. *Viruses, 13*, 700–700. https://doi.org/10.3390/v13040700 (accessed on 30th June 2025).

4. Arslanian, S., Bacha, F., Grey, M., Marcus, M. D., White, N. H., & Zeitler, P. (2018). Evaluation and management of youth-onset type 2 diabetes: A position statement by the American Diabetes Association. *Diabetes Care, 41*, 2648–2668. https://doi.org/10.2337/dci18-0052 (accessed on 30th June 2025).

5. Balthazar, J. A., & Chehter, E. Z. (2022). Acute pancreatitis and COVID-19: A new target for infection? *Einstein (São Paulo), 20*. https://doi.org/10.31744/einstein_journal/2022rw6667 (accessed on 30th June 2025).

6. Berger, M. M., Shenkin, A., Dizdar, O. S., Amrein, K., Augsburger, M., Biesalski, H. K., Bischoff, S. C., *et al.* (2024). ESPEN practical short micronutrient guideline. *Clinical Nutrition, 43*, 825–857. https://doi.org/10.1016/j.clnu.2024.01.030 (accessed on 30th June 2025).

7. Biggins, S. W., Angeli, P., García-Tsao, G., Ginès, P., Ling, S. C., Nadim, M. K., Wong, F., *et al.* (2021). Diagnosis, evaluation, and management of ascites, spontaneous bacterial peritonitis and hepatorenal syndrome: 2021 practice guidance by the American Association for the Study of Liver Diseases. *Hepatology, 74*, 1014–1048. https://doi.org/10.1002/hep.31884 (accessed on 30th June 2025).

8. Bornstein, S. R., Allolio, B., Arlt, W., Barthel, A., Don-Wauchope, A., Hammer, G. D., Husebye, E. S., *et al.* (2016). Diagnosis and treatment of primary adrenal insufficiency: An Endocrine Society clinical practice guideline. *The Journal of Clinical Endocrinology & Metabolism, 101*, 364–389. https://doi.org/10.1210/jc.2015-1710 (accessed on 30th June 2025).

9. Chiang, J. L., Maahs, D. M., Garvey, K. C., Hood, K. K., Laffel, L. M., Weinzimer, S. A., Wolfsdorf, J. I., *et al.* (2018). Type 1 diabetes in children and adolescents: A position statement by the American Diabetes Association. *Diabetes Care, 41*, 2026–2044. https://doi.org/10.2337/dci18-0023 (accessed on 30th June 2025).

10. Claahsen-van der Grinten, H. L., Speiser, P., Ahmed, S. F., Arlt, W., Auchus, R. J., Falhammar, H., Flück, C. E., *et al.* (2021). Congenital adrenal hyperplasia—Current insights in pathophysiology, diagnostics, and management. *Endocrine Reviews, 43*, 91–159. https://doi.org/10.1210/endrev/bnab016 (accessed on 30th June 2025).

11. Dinarvand, P., Davaro, E., Doan, J. V., Ising, M., Evans, N. R., Phillips, N. J., Lai, J., *et al.* (2019). Familial adenomatous polyposis syndrome: An update and review of extraintestinal manifestations. *Archives of Pathology & Laboratory Medicine, 143*, 1382–1398. https://doi.org/10.5858/arpa.2018-0570-ra (accessed on 30th June 2025).

12. Dolhnikoff, M., Ferranti, J. F., Monteiro, R. A. de A., Duarte-Neto, A. N., Gomes-Gouvêa, M. S., Degaspare, N. V., Delgado, A. F., *et al.* (2020). SARS-CoV-2 in cardiac tissue of a child with COVID-19-related multisystem inflammatory syndrome. *The Lancet Child & Adolescent Health, 4*, 790–794. https://doi.org/10.1016/s2352-4642(20)30257-1 (accessed on 30th June 2025).

13. Elrobaa, I., & New, K. J. (2021). COVID-19: Pulmonary and extra pulmonary manifestations. *Frontiers in Public Health, 9*. https://doi.org/10.3389/fpubh.2021.711616 (accessed on 30th June 2025).

14. Farmakis, D., Porter, J. B., Taher, A., Cappellini, M. D., Angastiniotis, M., & Eleftheriou, A. (2022). 2021 Thalassemia International Federation guidelines for the management of transfusion-dependent thalassemia. *Hemisphere, 6*, e732–e732. https://doi.org/10.1097/hs9.0000000000000732 (accessed on 30th June 2025).

15. Fernández-Sarmiento, J., de Souza, D. D., Jabornisky, R., González, G., Arias López, M. A., & Palacio, G. (2021). Pediatric inflammatory multisystem syndrome temporally associated with COVID-19 (PIMS-TS): A narrative review and the viewpoint of the Latin American Society of Pediatric Intensive Care (SLACIP) Sepsis Committee. *BMJ Pediatrics Open, 5*. https://www.semanticscholar.org/paper/c12008aea72fc66d51db59ad5628f446aa68a624 (accessed on 30th June 2025).

16. Friedrichsdorf, S. J., & Goubert, L. (2019). Pediatric pain treatment and prevention for hospitalized children. *PAIN Reports, 5*, e804–e804. https://doi.org/10.1097/pr9.0000000000000804 (accessed on 30th June 2025).

17. Goulet, O., Abi Nader, E., Pigneur, B., & Lambe, C. (2019). Short bowel syndrome as the leading cause of intestinal failure in early life: Some insights into the management. *Pediatric Gastroenterology Hepatology & Nutrition, 22*, 303–303. https://doi.org/10.5223/pghn.2019.22.4.303 (accessed on 30th June 2025).

18. Grossman, D. C., Bibbins-Domingo, K., Curry, S. J., Barry, M. J., Davidson, K. W., Doubeni, C. A., Epling, J. W., *et al.* (2017). Screening for obesity in children and adolescents. *JAMA, 317*, 2417–2417. https://doi.org/10.1001/jama.2017.6803 (accessed on 30th June 2025).

19. Hasenmajer, V., Ferrigno, R., Minnetti, M., Pellegrini, B., Isidori, A. M., Lenzi, A., Salerno, M., *et al.* (2023). Rare forms of genetic pediatric adrenal insufficiency: Excluding congenital adrenal hyperplasia. *Reviews in Endocrine and Metabolic Disorders, 24*, 345–363. https://doi.org/10.1007/s11154-023-09784-7 (accessed on 30th June 2025).

20. Hoang, D. M., Pham, P. T., Bach, T. Q., Ngo, A. T., Nguyen, Q. T., Phan, T. K. T., Nguyễn Hoàng Giang, *et al.* (2022). Stem cell-based therapy for human diseases. *Signal Transduction and Targeted Therapy, 7*. https://doi.org/10.1038/s41392-022-01134-4 (accessed on 30th June 2025).

21. Kahaly, G. J., Bartalena, L., Hegedüs, L., Leenhardt, L., Poppe, K., & Pearce, S. H. S. (2018). 2018 European Thyroid Association guideline for the management of Graves' hyperthyroidism. *European Thyroid Journal, 7*, 167–186. https://doi.org/10.1159/000490384 (accessed on 30th June 2025).

22. Khairunnisa, A. R., Peryoga, S., & Widiasta, A. (2025). Acid-base and electrolytes profile in critically ill pediatric patients admitted to pediatric intensive care unit (PICU). *Majalah Kedokteran Bandung*. https://www.semanticscholar.org/paper/519cacc0de025c0b6fb52adf707b07e139d9d531 (accessed on 30th June 2025).

23. Kimura, Y., Suzukawa, M., Jo, T., Hashimoto, Y., Kumazawa, R., Ishimaru, M., Matsui, H., *et al.* (2024). Epidemiology of patients with severe asthma in Japan: A nationwide descriptive study. *ERJ Open Research, 10*, 00122–2024. https://doi.org/10.1183/23120541.00122-2024 (accessed on 30th June 2025).

24. Kleinpell, R., Grabenkort, W. R., Boyle, W. A., Vines, D., & Olsen, K. M. (2021). The Society of Critical Care Medicine at 50 years: Interprofessional practice in critical care: Looking back and forging ahead. *Critical Care Medicine, 49*, 2017–2032. https://doi.org/10.1097/ccm.0000000000005276 (accessed on 30th June 2025).

25. Via La , L., Marino, A., Cuttone, G., Nunnari, G., Deana, C., Tesauro, M., Voza, A., *et al.* (2025). Critical care pharmacology of antiretroviral therapy in adults. *European Journal of Drug Metabolism and Pharmacokinetics, 50*, 105–118. https://www.semanticscholar.org/paper/d828e064fc5332d94060006b5c5112641503aa79 (accessed on 30th June 2025).

26. Zapata Lancharro , Á., Aguado del Hoyo, A., Sánchez Gómez de Orgaz, M. del C., Ortega, M., & León Luís, J. A. (2025). Technical notes on liver elastography: A guide for use in neonates in intensive care units. *Journal of Clinical Medicine, 14*. https://www.semanticscholar.org/paper/da2f4b17a9e6ca65bdfe27145b994c85a8e25659 (accessed on 30th June 2025).

27. López-De Suso, D., García-Salido, A., Andión-Catalán, M., Leoz-Gordillo, I., Lassaleta-Atienza, Á., & Sirvent-Cerdá, S. (2022). Methotrexate-induced stroke-like neurotoxicity: Case report, 8 years of experience, and literature review. *Pediatric Blood & Cancer, 69*. https://www.semanticscholar.org/paper/71374fadf66b4b9f8cdbdda3e57982479f5e9864 (accessed on 30th June 2025).

28. MacFabe, D. F. (2015). Enteric short-chain fatty acids: Microbial messengers of metabolism, mitochondria, and mind: Implications in autism spectrum disorders. *Microbial Ecology in Health and Disease, 26*. https://doi.org/10.3402/mehd.v26.28177 (accessed on 30th June 2025).

29. Mathew, J. S., Shingina, A., Khan, M. Q., Wilson, E. A., Syn, N., Rammohan, A., Alconchel, F., *et al.* (2024). Proceedings of the 28th Annual Congress of the International Liver Transplantation Society. *Liver Transplantation, 30*, 544–554. https://www.semanticscholar.org/paper/b06fd667586c33d0abd52101e2a19e86a0be439b (accessed on 30th June 2025).

30. Melamed, E., Rydberg, L., Ambrose, A. F., Bhavaraju-Sanka, R., Fine, J. S., Fleming, T. K., Herman, E., *et al.* (2023). Multidisciplinary collaborative consensus guidance statement on the assessment and treatment of neurologic sequelae in patients with post-acute sequelae of SARS-CoV-2 infection (PASC). *PM&R, 15*, 640–662. https://doi.org/10.1002/pmrj.12976 (accessed on 30th June 2025).

31. Nielsen, M. B., Cantisani, V., Sidhu, P. S., Badea, R., Batko, T., Carlsen, J. F., Claudon, M., *et al.* (2018). The use of handheld ultrasound devices–An EFSUMB position paper. *Ultra Schall in der Medizing–European Journal of Ultrasound, 40*, 30–39. https://doi.org/10.1055/a-0783-2303 (accessed on 30th June 2025).

32. Omata, M., Cheng, A.-L., Kokudo, N., Kudo, M., Lee, J. M., Jia, J., Tateishi, R., *et al.* (2017). Asia–Pacific clinical practice guidelines on the management of hepatocellular carcinoma: A 2017 update. *Hepatology International, 11*, 317–370. https://doi.org/10.1007/s12072-017-9799-9 (accessed on 30th June 2025).

33. Piqué, N., Berlanga, M., & Miñana-Galbis, D. (2019). Health benefits of heat-killed (tantalized) probiotics: An overview. *International Journal of Molecular Sciences, 20*, 2534–2534. https://doi.org/10.3390/ijms20102534 (accessed on 30th June 2025).

34. Rocha-e-Silva, M. (2009). In the December 2009 issue of Clinics. *Clinics, 64*, 1137–1138. https://www.semanticscholar.org/paper/234ef1360fb9b919e5b809557485e693b14202da (accessed on 30th June 2025).

35. Sahu, U. P., Farooquee, M. R., Hasan, O., Ehtesham, S., & Hasan, R. (2025). A cross-sectional study on the observation of clinical profiles and associated electrolyte disturbances in patients admitted to the pediatric intensive care unit (PICU) at a tertiary care center. *Cureus, 17*. https://www.semanticscholar.org/paper/22003d439baa58d6056185eef7e10ffada024130 (accessed on 30th June 2025).

36. Salamanna, F., Maglio, M., Landini, M. P., & Fini, M. (2020). Body localization of ACE-2: On the trail of the keyhole of SARS-CoV-2. *Frontiers in Medicine, 7*. https://doi.org/10.3389/fmed.2020.594495 (accessed on 30th June 2025).

37. Lozano Salazar, H. E., Pérez León, A. K., Pérez León, M. D., Pérez León, A. C., & Atapuma Madrid, D. F. (2025). Rett syndrome in a pediatric patient: Progressive clinical presentation and genetic confirmation via MECP2 mutation. *Arandu UTIC*. https://www.semanticscholar.org/paper/5df18c75c838c1ee802de430856e11a1feed7a2f (accessed on 30th June 2025).

38. Sen, K., Harrar, D., Pariseau, N., Tucker, K., Keenan, J. S., Zhang, A., & Gropman, A. (2024). Seizure characteristics and EEG features in intoxication type and energy deficiency neurometabolic disorders in the pediatric intensive care unit: Single-center experience over 10 years. *Neurocritical Care*. https://www.semanticscholar.org/paper/02dc66faa2943c47b025dbdf79579f0304ba43b6 (accessed on 30th June 2025).

39. Shaigany, S., Gnirke, M., Guttmann, A., Chong, H. L., Meehan, S., Raabe, V., Louie, E., *et al.* (2020). An adult with Kawasaki-like multisystem inflammatory syndrome associated with COVID-19. *The Lancet, 396*, e8–e10. https://doi.org/10.1016/s0140-6736(20)31526-9 (accessed on 30th June 2025).

40. Sica, R., Pennoni, S., Penta, L., Riccioni, S., Di Cara, G., & Verrotti, A. (2021). Gastrointestinal and hepatic involvement during COVID-19 pandemic: A focus on pediatric population and possible future implications. *World Journal of Gastroenterology, 27*, 7000–7004. https://www.semanticscholar.org/paper/415b14f3e4c972ddae053b5a8eeac8772460bdee (accessed on 30th June 2025).

41. Spolador, G. M., Bastos, F., Polastrini, R. T. V., Zoboli, I., Henrique, A. C., Vieira Filho, J. P., Marcondes da Silveira, M. R., *et al.* (2024). Epidemiological assessment of a pediatric palliative care clinic at a Brazilian quaternary hospital: 20 years of experience. *Journal of Palliative Medicine*. https://www.semanticscholar.org/paper/28b0c09ed6da59b610508333d084a9238793dfa5 (accessed on 30th June 2025).

42. Stavropoulou, E., & Bezirtzoglou, E. (2020). Probiotics in medicine: A long debate. *Frontiers in Immunology, 11*. https://doi.org/10.3389/fimmu.2020.02192 (accessed on 30th June 2025).

43. Styne, D. M., Arslanian, S., Connor, E. L., Farooqi, I. S., Murad, M. H., Silverstein, J., & Yanovski, J. A. (2017). Pediatric obesity—Assessment, treatment, and prevention: An Endocrine Society clinical practice guideline. *The Journal of Clinical Endocrinology & Metabolism, 102*, 709–757. https://doi.org/10.1210/jc.2016-2573 (accessed on 30th June 2025).

44. Uyeki, T. M., Bernstein, H. H., Bradley, J. S., Englund, J. A., File, T. M., Fry, A. M., Gravenstein, S., *et al.* (2018). Clinical practice guidelines by the Infectious Diseases Society of America: 2018 update on diagnosis, treatment, chemoprophylaxis, and institutional outbreak management of seasonal influenza. *Clinical Infectious Diseases, 68*, e1–e47. https://doi.org/10.1093/cid/ciy866 (accessed on 30th June 2025).

45. Vos, M. B., Abrams, S. H., Barlow, S. E., Caprio, S., Daniels, S. R., Kohli, R., Mouzaki, M., *et al.* (2016). NASPGHAN clinical practice guideline for the diagnosis and treatment of nonalcoholic fatty liver disease in children. *Journal of Pediatric Gastroenterology and Nutrition, 64*, 319–334. https://doi.org/10.1097/mpg.0000000000001482 (accessed on 30th June 2025).

46. Yuan, Z., Yang, Y., Liu, Q., Zhang, B., Wang, X., Huang, S., & Ma, W. (2025). Nursing care of a patient with severe pneumonia complicated with multiple disorders under a multidisciplinary team: A long-term case report. *Medicine, 104*. https://www.semanticscholar.org/paper/29ac0dd9653fee4c167fd66a70fcbb0ea3828996 (accessed on 30th June 2025).

47. Zhu, H., Bi, D., Zhang, Y., Kong, C., Du, J., Wu, X., Wei, Q., *et al.* (2022). Ketogenic diet for human diseases: The underlying mechanisms and potential for clinical implementations. *Signal Transduction and Targeted Therapy, 7*. https://doi.org/10.1038/s41392-021-00831-w (accessed on 30th June 2025).

HEMATOLOGICAL AND ONCOLOGIC ISSUES

9

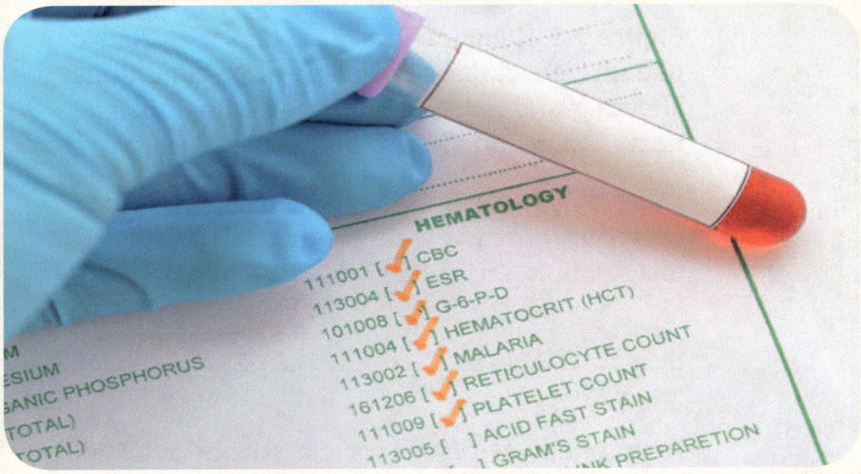

LEARNING OBJECTIVES

After studying this chapter, you will be able to:

1. Understand Hematological Disorders in Pediatric Patients.
2. Explain Oncologic Disorders in Pediatric Patients.
3. Describe Management of Hematological and Oncologic Emergencies.
4. Focus on an Interdisciplinary Approach to Care in PICU.

Introduction

Pediatric patients with hematologic and oncologic issues are often in critically unstable states and must be admitted to pediatric intensive care units (PICUs). Advances in oncology have significantly improved the survival of childhood cancer patients, but such individuals are at risk for catastrophic complications of both their disorders and underlying treatments. The complexity of their care is indicated by an increased need for intensive interventions, particularly in cases of respiratory failure and multiorgan dysfunction. Based on recent data, children undergoing treatments such as hematopoietic stem cell transplantation are a high-risk group in need of close surveillance and care management (Boscato *et al.*, 2023). In addition, the intersection of hematologic malignancies with other contemporary threats like COVID-19 has raised issues of mortality and healthcare burdens, particularly among children (Booth *et al.*, 2020). As a result, understanding the multidisciplinary challenges in PICU environments is crucial in the optimization of outcomes in these vulnerable patients.

9.1. Hematological Disorders in Pediatric Patients

Learning Outcome

1. Give an overview of hematological disorders.
2. Focus on types and causes of anemia in children.
3. Discuss implications and management of thrombocytopenia.
4. Identify diagnosis and treatment options for hemophilia.
5. Explain complications and care in sickle cell disease.
6. Describe causes and treatment strategies for aplastic anemia.
7. Focus on prevention and management of iron deficiency anemia.
8. Identify coagulation disorders.
9. Understand the role of blood transfusions in pediatric care.

Pediatric hematological diseases consist of a broad spectrum of disorders that impact the blood components, including anemia, hemophilia, and leukemias. Besides being an immediate health risk, these diseases also impact the long-term prognosis of pediatric patients, particularly when they are in intensive care. For instance, the control of hematologic complications is of paramount significance in childhood cancer chemotherapy with individualized interventions to avoid risks of low counts of blood and coagulation disorders. It is confirmed through evidence that prompt detection and intervention are of greatest significance in optimizing outcomes because tardiness will lead to life-threatening complications like infection or uncontrollable bleeding (Bryan *et al.*, 2021). Moreover, advances in molecular diagnostics to detect specific hematological diseases are relevant for the decision-making process of treatment and optimization of care in a pediatric intensive care setting (Kimberly *et al.*, 2021). Thus, control and understanding of hematological diseases are relevant to enhance the quality of life and prognosis of pediatric patients overall (Figure 9.1).

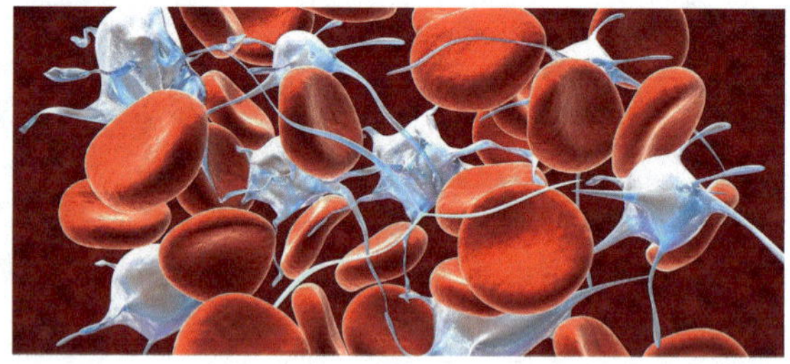

Figure 9.1. Hematological disorders in pediatric patients encompass a spectrum of conditions affecting blood components, including anemia, hemophilia, and various leukemias.

Source: https://s3-us-west-2.amazonaws.com/utsw-patientcare-web-production/original_images/GettyImages-188057859-1600x732.jpg.

9.1.1. Overview of Hematological Disorders

Hematological disorders constitute a broad category of blood and bone marrow diseases of interest in pediatric intensive care due to their complexity and challenging management. They comprise leukemias, anemias, and coagulopathies, each with clinical manifestations and a treatment pathway. Hematological cancers in children have become more common, necessitating individualized therapeutic modalities involving chemotherapy and bone marrow transplantation. Of specific mention is that patients with hematologic malignancies are likely to experience complications of acute kidney injury (AKI), which can be caused by the cancer itself as well as its therapy, and highlight the value of close observation in intensive care units (Benoit *et al.*, 2016). Furthermore, dysbiosis, or disturbance in the microbiome, can exacerbate hematologic diseases, influencing disease progression and therapeutic response through inflammatory and immune-driven mechanisms (Fattizzo *et al.*, 2020). Identification of such associations is important for the maximization of treatment strategies in affected child populations.

9.1.2. Anemia in Children: Types and Causes

Pediatric intensive care is confronted by a multifaceted challenge presented by anemia in children with numerous etiologic causes. The common types include iron-deficiency anemia, aplastic anemia, and anemia of chronic disease. Iron-deficiency anemia, which usually occurs as a consequence of inadequate dietary intake or chronic blood loss, is most prevalent among growing children, especially those with limited access to sources of dietary iron. Aplastic anemia, though less common, could develop as a result of failure of the bone marrow due to genetic disorders or toxin exposure, resulting in a reduction in blood cell production.

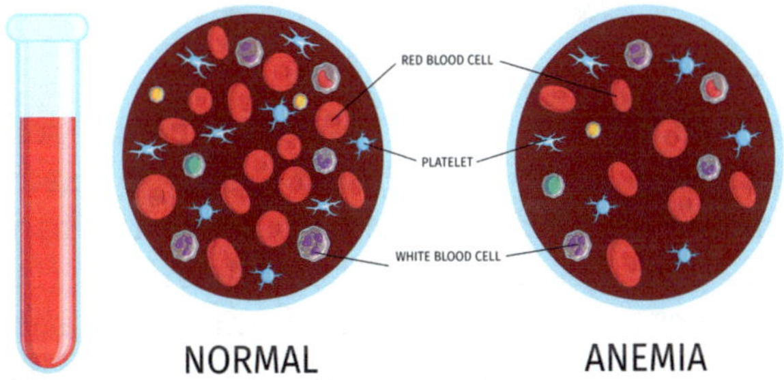

Figure 9.2. Anemia in children presents a multifaceted challenge in pediatric intensive care, stemming from various etiological factors.

Source: https://drvikasdua.com/wp-content/uploads/2022/08/Best-Pediatric-Hematologist-in-Delhi-Dr-Vikas-Dua-will-help-you-to-know-how-much-iron-is-needed-for-children-scaled.jpg.

Chronic disease anemia is also frequently seen in children with underlying disorders such as infections or malignancies, which complicates their management. As observed through research, the implications of low hemoglobin levels are urgent, particularly where treatment decisions in pediatric patients undergoing therapy like chemotherapy emphasize the necessity of blood levels in determining the permissible levels of activity (Peters *et al.*, 2011; Cugno *et al.*, 2015). Understanding these mechanisms is required for effective intervention and treatment (Figure 9.2).

9.1.3. Thrombocytopenia: Implications and Management

Thrombocytopenia, a decrease in the number of platelets, carries significant implications in pediatric intensive care patients, particularly in those with hematologic and oncologic illnesses. Therapy of thrombocytopenia necessitates a complete appreciation for its etiology, which can range from bone marrow failure to increased destruction of platelets. In children, particularly those with malignancies or undergoing treatments such as chemotherapy, the risk of hemorrhagic complications is very high, requiring strict monitoring and prompt intervention. Clinicians must balance the need for the transfusions against immune reactions and other adverse effects that come with treatments such as recombinant AAV, which, although promising, have issues such as genotoxicity and hepatotoxicity (Wang *et al.*, 2024). Furthermore, the disparity of care experienced by pediatric patients, particularly those with Down syndrome, makes the management measures even more daunting (Dimopoulos *et al.*, 2023). Therefore, an individualized, multispecialty therapeutic regimen is required to optimize the result in thrombocytopenic children.

9.1.4. Hemophilia: Diagnosis and Treatment Options

Hemophilia diagnosis and treatment are significant challenges in pediatric intensive care units due to the condition's high risk for spontaneous hemorrhage and coagulation-related complications during therapy. Diagnosis begins typically with a comprehensive history of the family, along with confirmatory coagulation tests to quantify deficiencies of clotting factors VIII or IX. Once diagnosed, the treatments have changed significantly, centered mainly around factor replacement therapy, with which the individual can receive prophylactic therapy in order to avoid bleeding episodes or on-demand intra-missive treatment during acute crises. Gene therapy is also gaining ground as a new direction, demonstrating the potential for long-term factor deficiency correction, as evidenced by recent developments. Nevertheless, immune response issues and potential side effects must be watched carefully, particularly since treatment modalities such as rAAV are the focus of current research and clinical application (Wang *et al.*, 2024). New biomarkers and diagnostic tests derived from systemic inflammatory disease studies may also enhance the diagnosis and treatment of hemophilic patients under intensive care settings (Kürti *et al.*, 2023) (Figure 9.3).

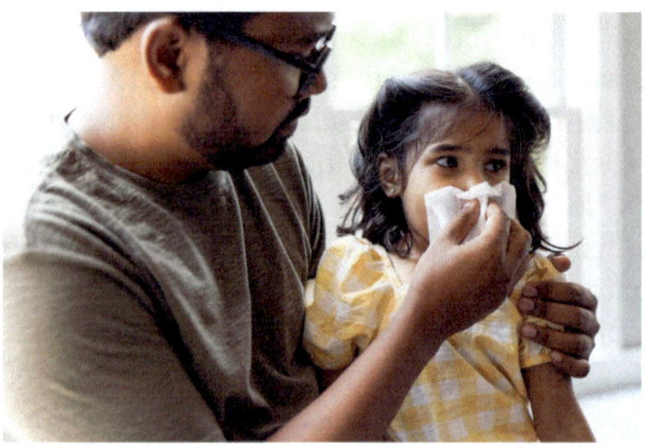

Figure 9.3. Hemophilia.

Source: https://media.post.rvohealth.io/wp-content/uploads/2023/09/3080962-What-Are-the-Symptoms-of-Hemophilia-in-Children-1296x728-header-1-1296x729.jpg.

9.1.5. Sickle Cell Disease: Complications and Care

Sickle cell disease (SCD) is characterized by its many acute and chronic complications that have an impact on pediatric patients and must be managed in intensive care with special needs. One should emphasize particularly that SCD children are at risk for severe vaso-occlusive crises, which can lead to severe morbidity if not effectively and promptly treated. Preventive strategies, including newborn screening and full care services, play a crucial role in avoiding the risk of complications such as stroke and acute chest syndrome, prevalent in this population (Colombatti *et al.*, 2016). Furthermore, the case for the availability and utilization of hematopoietic stem cell transplantation (HSCT) highlights its potential as a curative treatment, especially in middle-income countries, where resources may not be as available but outcomes can match or even exceed those of wealthier states (Faulkner *et al.*, 2021). Therefore, a multi-disciplinary approach involving early intervention and high-end treatment approaches is crucial to optimize the care of children with SCD in pediatric intensive care units.

9.1.6. Aplastic Anemia: Causes and Treatment Strategies

Aplastic anemia, with its inability of the bone marrow to produce blood cells, presents tremendous challenges in pediatric intensive care. The cause of this condition may be multifactorial, such as autoimmune disease, drug exposure, and viral illness, which interfere with hematopoiesis and result in profound cytopenias. Treatment interventions primarily focus on immunosuppressive therapy and hematopoietic stem cell transplant, both of which aim to restore normal hematopoietic function and minimize complications such as infection and organ dysfunction (Boscato *et al.*, 2023). Despite progress in the knowledge of the biological mechanisms driving aplastic anemia, which has improved outcomes for patients, the condition's nature demands an individualized approach to treatment, especially among severely ill children who can experience acute complications secondary to their underlying hematology illness (Jay *et al.*, 2022). Monitoring and intensive care are critical in modifying survival and long-term outcome (Figure 9.4).

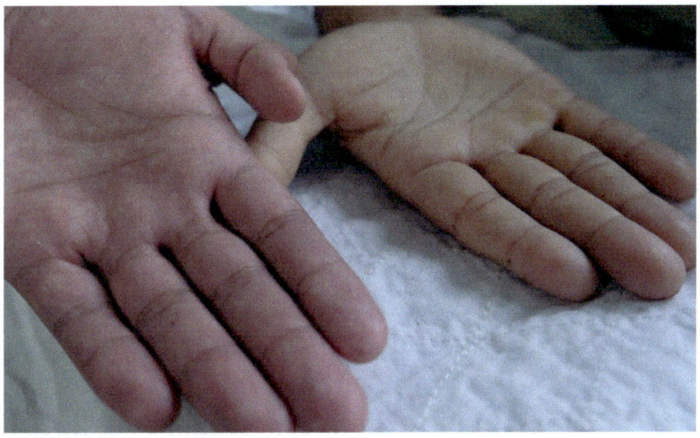

Figure 9.4. Aplastic anemia.

Source: https://drvikasdua.com/wp-content/uploads/2022/02/Aplastic-Anemia.jpg.

9.1.7. Iron Deficiency Anemia: Prevention and Management

Iron deficiency anemia (IDA) is a persistent problem of child health, particularly for intensive care units, whose treatment may complicate the prognosis of a patient. Early IDA identification is crucial, allowing for intervention in a timely manner and avert progression to complications. The study demonstrates that iron deficiency anemia was prevalent among children's patients and was a major cause of hematologic disorders in critical health situations, as discussed in the findings of the research in the context of vascular anomalies (Lucas *et al.*, 2024).

Effective prevention strategies include promoting good nutritional supplementation of iron-rich foods and, as necessary, the thoughtful supplementation with iron preparations. This is supported by recent evidence highlighting that adequate hematological and biochemical tests can facilitate early anemia diagnosis (Upadhyay *et al.*, 2022). The use of general screening programs in children, especially among those who have other health conditions, is essential in improving general management and patient outcomes among critically ill children.

9.1.8. Coagulation Disorders: Assessment and Intervention

Coagulation disorders create a significant challenge in pediatric intensive care, particularly among patients with hematological malignancies. The disorders can lead to severe complications such as bleeding or thrombosis, and hence, detailed assessment and timely intervention are necessary. Accurate assessment of coagulopathy can be achieved through the combination of clinical assessments, laboratory assessments, and the application of scoring systems for estimating the severity of the condition of the patients. Since pediatric oncology patients get exposed to invasive therapies like chemotherapy or hematopoietic stem cell transplant, they are at risk of coagulopathy as well as thrombocytopenia (Boscato *et al.*, 2023). Additionally, respiratory complications encountered in the patients can further intensify coagulation issues, making it more complex to treat them clinically (Chimbira *et al.*, 2001). As such, the implementation of targeted interventions like the careful use of clotting factors or platelet transfusions becomes paramount to optimize outcomes and minimize mortality in this risk group (Figure 9.5).

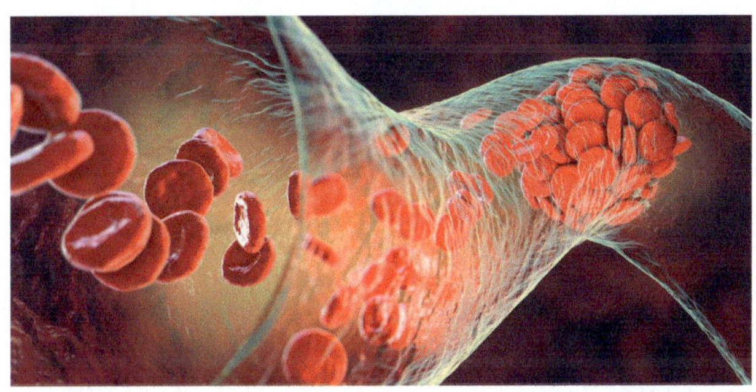

Figure 9.5. Coagulation disorders represent a significant challenge in the context of pediatric intensive care, particularly among patients with hematological malignancies.

Source: https://travelhealthpro.org.uk/media_lib/mlib-uploads/full/blood-clot-made-of-red-blood-cells-platelets-and-fibrin-protein-strands.jpg.

9.1.9. Role of Blood Transfusions in Pediatric Care

In pediatrics, blood transfusions are a significant therapeutic intervention, particularly in the treatment of hematologic and oncologic diseases, which are prevalent in intensive care units. Transfusions are of prime significance in managing superabundant blood loss resulting from trauma or surgery, and in the management of anemia of cancer patients undergoing chemotherapy. Also, having effective and safe blood products is essential in preventing procedure-related complications during procedures like central venous catheter placements that are routinely utilized in pediatric oncology (Boris Böll *et al.*, 2020). The transfusion should be determined with caution, considering the potential immune reactions and constant monitoring intra- and post-procedure (Bryan *et al.*, 2021). Lastly, appropriate and timely blood transfusions can improve rates of recovery and overall survival for this high-risk group, which makes them essential to pediatric intensive care.

Test Your Knowledge

1. What are the typical laboratory findings in hemolytic uremic syndrome (HUS)?
2. How does immune thrombocytopenia (ITP) present, and what are its treatment thresholds?

9.2. Oncologic Disorders in Pediatric Patients

Learning Outcome

1. Understand the overview of pediatric cancers.
2. Identify common types of childhood cancers.
3. Know symptoms and early detection of pediatric cancers.
4. Discuss treatment modalities: chemotherapy, radiation, and surgery.
5. Describe supportive care in pediatric oncology.
6. Focus on long-term effects of cancer treatment in children.
7. Focus on palliative care considerations in pediatric oncology.
8. Discuss the role of clinical trials in pediatric cancer treatment.
9. Understand the psychological impact of cancer on children and families.

Pediatric oncologic disorder patients are fraught with a multitude of challenges in the pediatric intensive care unit, as these children often have unique complications associated with both disease and therapy. With cancer-related intensive care unit admissions as high as 20%, these patients are at very high risk for infectious and noninfectious complications, including acute kidney injury (AKI) due to their malignancies and treatments (Benoit *et al.*, 2016). In addition, studies have shown that multi-system involvement is prevalent in critically ill children, where serious conditions such as sepsis are the leading cause of morbidity and mortality (Abbag *et al.*, 2006). The problem of oncologic disease management in this patient population calls for multidisciplinary management that addresses not just the short-term clinical needs, but also the psychosocial needs of care, with emphasis on the necessity of individualized intervention to maximize outcomes in such compromised patients (Figure 9.6).

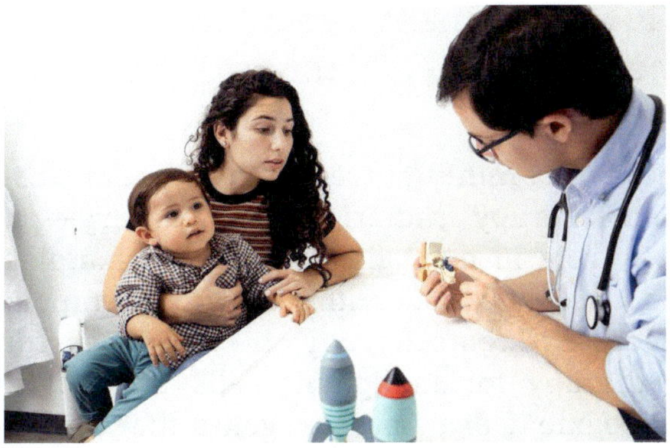

Figure 9.6. Oncologic disorders in pediatric patients present a myriad of challenges within the pediatric intensive care setting, where these children often face unique complications arising from both their disease and its treatment.

Source: https://max-website20-images.s3.ap-south-1.amazonaws.com/Pediatric_Diseases_412272b958.jpg.

9.2.1. Overview of Pediatric Cancers

Pediatric cancers present a unique set of challenges due to their varied types and biological behaviors. The most prevalent forms include hematological malignancies such as acute lymphoblastic leukemia and acute myeloid leukemia, alongside solid tumors like neuroblastoma and embryonal tumors. Collectively, these cancers affect children differently than adults, with distinct pathophysiological processes and treatment responses. Recent advancements in the understanding of cancer biology have significantly improved survival rates; however, the complexity of treatment protocols remains a salient concern, as children are more vulnerable to complications stemming from both the disease and its therapies. Research indicates that patients often require intensive care due to complications such as respiratory failure and multiorgan dysfunction, with studies highlighting the importance of risk assessment and predictive tools in these settings (Boscato *et al.*, 2023). Furthermore, long-term outcomes for children treated for cancers, especially those exposed to prenatal maternal malignancies, necessitate ongoing evaluations, emphasizing the need for comprehensive long-term follow-up care to address neurocognitive and psychosocial development (van Gerwen *et al.*, 2021).

9.2.2. Common Types of Childhood Cancers

Childhood cancers are a significant challenge in pediatric intensive care, encompassing most of the hematological and solid tumors. The most prevalent types are acute lymphoblastic leukemia (ALL), acute myeloid leukemia (AML), and other solid tumors such as neuroblastoma and Wilms tumor. ALL, representing 23% of the cases, is particularly characterized by a response to treatment but imposes high risks for therapeutic complications that often necessitate intensive care unit admission (Boscato *et al.*, 2023).

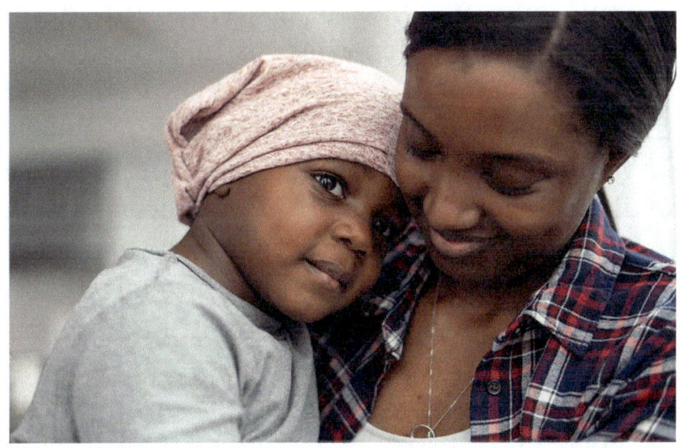

Figure 9.7. Childhood cancers are a significant concern within pediatric intensive care, encompassing various hematological and solid tumors.

Source: https://www.cancer.gov/sites/g/files/xnrzdm211/files/styles/cgov_article/public/cgov_image/media_image/2020-09/mother-of-african-descent-cuddles-her-child-who-has-cancer.jpg?h=5537fd6a&itok=ahYgaZxU.

In addition, the development of complications from therapeutic procedures, such as infection and impairment of organs, may also complicate the clinical picture of these children in intensive care units. The impact of in utero maternal cancer has possible neurodevelopmental consequences for such children, which requires long-term follow-up and psychosocial care as they grow up (van Gerwen *et al.*, 2021). These are the most common types of cancer in children, and knowing them is essential to offering focused and effective care in pediatric intensive care (Figure 9.7).

9.2.3. Symptoms and Early Detection of Pediatric Cancers

Early detection of pediatric malignancies is necessary for the optimization of patient outcomes, particularly in light of the specialized symptomatology that may occur in children. Unexplained weight loss, persistent pain, tiredness, and sudden changes in appetite are obviously potential presenting symptoms and can readily be mistaken for some minor illness. Early identification of such symptoms can result in timely diagnostic procedures, which are crucial when dealing with hematologic and oncologic problems in pediatric intensive care. Additionally, recent research identified factors of mortality and extended hospitalization in children with cancer, putting a major emphasis on early identification and strict monitoring of vulnerable patients (Boscato *et al.*, 2023). Additionally, the pandemic also posed other challenges among pediatric cancer patients, as evidenced by reports showing the impacts of SARS-CoV-2 infections on duration of treatment and survival outcomes (Berner *et al.*, 2024). In this case, therefore, a careful aspect of symptom identification and integrated management approaches remains essential for survival improvement among the vulnerable group.

9.2.4. Treatment Modalities: Chemotherapy, Radiation, and Surgery

Three prominent treatment modalities—chemotherapy, radiation, and surgery—play a key role in managing pediatric hematologic and oncologic issues in achieving therapeutic success. Chemotherapy is a cornerstone of therapy for malignant cells through the employment of cytotoxic agents that are able to efficiently bring about a decrease in tumor mass. Toxicities are involved, however, that need to be addressed with monitoring and supportive measures, particularly in the intensive care unit.

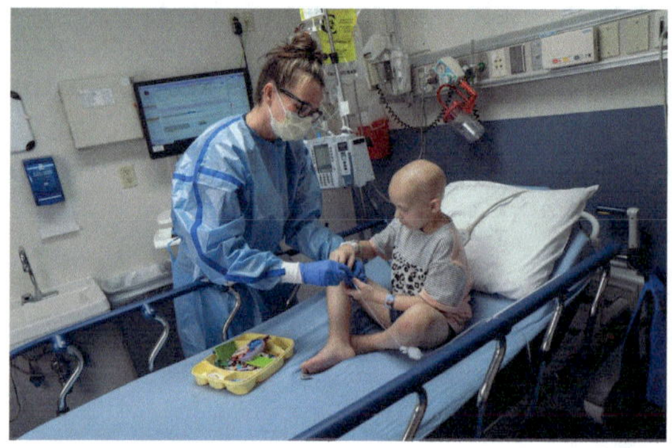

Figure 9.8. Chemotherapy serves as a cornerstone in targeting malignant cells, employing cytotoxic agents that can significantly diminish tumor burden.

Source: https://stjude.scene7.com/is/image/stjude/436606-031?fit=crop,1&wid=900.

Radiation therapy, as effective as it is in the management of localized lesions, may also cause long-term sequelae requiring complete follow-up. Surgery potentially has the benefit of providing immediate relief from obstructing masses or a complete cure of localized disease. With new treatment technologies, e.g., immune effector cell (IEC) therapies, entering the clinical arena, health practitioners must adapt how they manage new toxicities and complications arising from these new-fangled modalities (Bryan *et al.*, 2021; Marcela *et al.*, 2020). Integrating these treatment modalities must be properly orchestrated to address the multi-faceted requirements of pediatric patients and minimize adverse consequences and maximize recovery (Figure 9.8).

9.2.5. Supportive Care in Pediatric Oncology

Managing pediatric oncology's complexities requires a multifaceted approach to supportive care that aims to reverse the impacts of the disease and also its treatment. Patients with hematological malignancy in the pediatric category are particularly vulnerable to infectious complications, which is one of the biggest risks to their recovery and quality of life overall (Kjellander *et al.*, 2016). Effective supportive care measures must thus entail close observation for deterioration, where Pediatric Early Warning Systems (PEWS) can play a key role in the detection of vulnerable patients at an early stage (Kappen *et al.*, 2022). Through the provision of timely intervention, these systems can help prevent extreme consequences related to complications, underlining the value of supportive care in maximizing survivorship in pediatric oncology. In addition, strict infection surveillance and management protocols ensure effective treatment regimens, stressing the need for an integrated system to help these children in intensive care units.

9.2.6. Long-Term Effects of Cancer Treatment in Children

The long-term effect of cancer treatment among children is substantial and widespread, often far-reaching beyond the clear-cut physical challenges associated with their illness. As survival rates have improved as a consequence of advances in pediatric oncology, concern is now being directed toward the long-term effects of therapy, such as chemotherapy and radiotherapy. These treatments can lead to complications affecting several organ systems, including neurological, cardiac, and intellectual functioning. Research has demonstrated that children who have been exposed to antenatal cancer and treatment are at risk of developmental issues that need to be followed up on systematically on a long-term basis (van Gerwen *et al.*, 2021). Furthermore, research highlights complications resulting from treatment directly and how children may develop chronic physical health challenges and psychosocial problems as they mature into adulthood (Boscato *et al.*, 2023). Thus, ongoing monitoring and supportive therapies are important to maintain this high-risk subgroup's unique needs to ensure they have optimum health outcomes post-treatment (Figure 9.9).

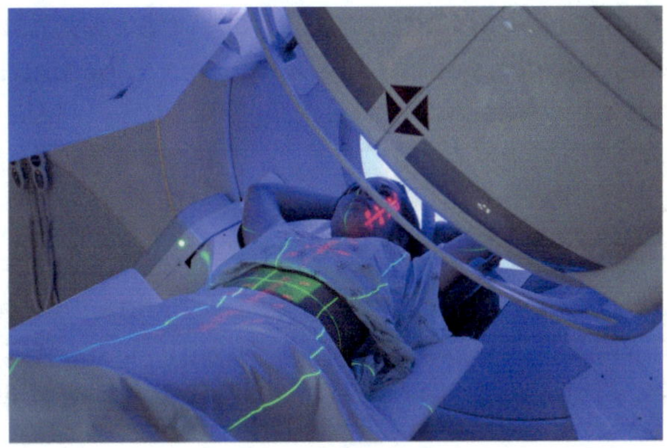

Figure 9.9. As advancements in pediatric oncology improve survival rates, the focus shifts to the enduring consequences of therapies, such as chemotherapy and radiation.

Source: https://img.ascendmedia.com/files/base/ascend/hh/image/2024/03/Picture1.65eb32147c3b7.png?auto=format%2Ccompress&fit=max&q=70&w=1200.

9.2.7. Palliative Care Considerations in Pediatric Oncology

Inclusion of palliative care into pediatric oncology is a key consideration, particularly in the context of the hematologic and oncologic issues that arise in the intensive care setting. Children with malignancies will often have complex medical issues that demand a multifaceted intervention. This encompasses not only the management of the disease but also symptom management and enhancement of quality of life. As suggested, the quality of life and prognosis following ICU admission for cancer patients are significant but not yet explored areas. These must be studied as adequate palliative care can significantly minimize suffering, provide emotional support to the family, and allow informed decision-making along difficult treatment courses (Tanhchaleun *et al.*, 2018).

Moreover, the necessity to address and combat potential prejudices against intensive care unit cancer patients, highlighted by comparable studies as well, also confirms the importance of extensive and compassionate care methods specifically applicable to pediatric oncology (van der Zee *et al.*, 2023).

9.2.8. Role of Clinical Trials in Pediatric Cancer Treatment

The role of clinical trials in the management of childhood cancers is invaluable, with not only avenues for new therapy but also critical information about the new reactions of children to cancer treatment. With the new face of pediatric oncology, there remains a need to adjust treatment based on research continuously, enhancing survival and quality of life. Notably, recent research has pointed out that early clinical trial enrollment is associated with better outcomes, particularly in the case of high-risk patients who need intensive care, highlighting the need for continuous assessments of the effectiveness of treatment (Boscato *et al.*, 2023).

Moreover, while the child mortality rate with hematologic malignancies during crises such as the COVID-19 pandemic remains concerning, studies suggest that targeted clinical measures under trial frameworks can negate risks and improve care management (Booth *et al.*, 2020). Therefore, clinical trials are not just experimental stages but also priceless components in formulating pediatric cancer care protocols (Figure 9.10).

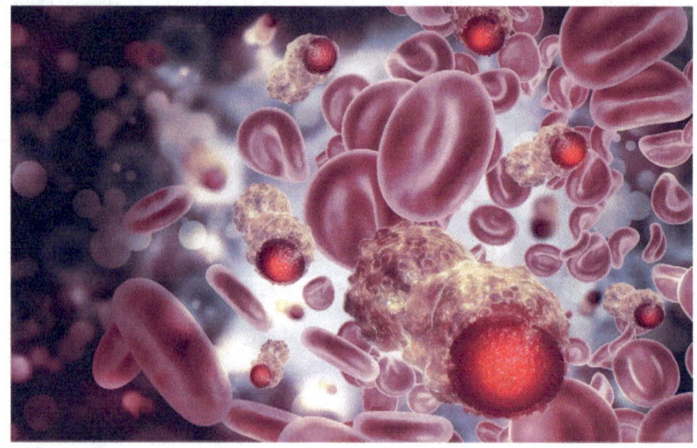

Figure 9.10. The role of clinical trials in pediatric cancer treatment is pivotal, offering not only avenues for innovative therapies but also critical insights into the unique responses of children to oncological interventions.

Source: https://blog.championsoncology.com/hubfs/Header%20Image_ASH%20MM%20Blog.webp.

9.2.9. Psychological Impact of Cancer on Children and Families

The psychological impact of cancer on children and their families is pervasive and intricate, resulting in long-term emotional problems. Children who have cancer commonly experience a spectrum of psychological problems, including depression and anxiety, that are compounded by fear of treatment and uncertainty of survival. As highlighted in research, severe acute behavioral and emotional disorders can occur as among the most significant treatment-side effects in pediatric oncology, which might necessitate the use of psychotropic drugs to manage these disorders effectively (Johanna *et al.*, 2022). Furthermore, families are not spared the psychological burdens of a diagnosis of cancer in the child; stress can complicate family functioning, leading to increased stress and potential conflict. Attention to the unique psychosocial requirements of patients and families, as outlined in adolescent and young adult oncology guidelines, is required in crafting all-inclusive care plans (Bhatia *et al.*, 2023).

Test Your Knowledge

1. What symptoms and imaging findings suggest superior mediastinal syndrome in children with lymphoma?
2. What supportive care strategies are used during intensive chemotherapy?

9.3. Management of Hematological and Oncologic Emergencies

Learning Outcome

1. Learn the definition of hematological and oncologic emergencies.
2. Focus on the identification of critical symptoms in PICU.
3. Discuss protocols for managing acute anemia.
4. Explain management of febrile neutropenia.
5. Describe the treatment of tumor lysis syndrome.
6. Address bleeding complications in hematological disorders.
7. Learn management of hyperleukocytosis.
8. Know the role of supportive care in emergencies.
9. Discuss the importance of rapid response teams in the PICU.

Effective handling of oncologic and hematologic emergencies within the pediatric intensive care environment is essential for optimizing patient outcomes. Such emergencies are commonly a complication of the underlying malignancies themselves or arising as a result of treatment and thus need to be addressed immediately and with specialty intervention. Indeed, febrile neutropenia (FN) is one of the most emergent presentations encountered as it can rapidly result in lethal sepsis if left untreated promptly (Alsharawneh *et al.*, 2019). The general evaluation of children's emergency services reflects the importance of professionals trained to cope with cancer emergencies, as indicated by a study that shows that early intervention in febrile neutropenia can generally enhance the quality of care received (André *et al.*, 2023). In addition, the frequency of symptoms such as fever also supports effective triage and rapid evaluation for facilitating proper treatments to be applied so that children receive proper and timely care in emergencies.

9.3.1. Definition of Hematological and Oncologic Emergencies

The phrase hematologic and oncologic emergencies is used to describe an array of life-threatening processes that arise in children, most commonly secondary to their own malignancy or chemotherapy. Hematologic emergencies, such as TLS, can rapidly arise and result in life-threatening metabolic derangements like hyperkalemia, which needs to be promptly corrected to prevent lethal complications. Additionally, oncologic emergencies typically present themselves in the form of infection, most often augmented by chemotherapy-related immunosuppression. These situations, as documented in studies conducted on children who are cancer patients, highlight the importance of valuing indications like fever that may indicate the urgency of the need for treatment

(André *et al.*, 2023). Moreover, such emergencies need management by an expert healthcare team capable of handling both the acute and chronic requirements of such vulnerable patients, thus optimizing results and lessening morbidity in relation to such life-altering events (Asefi *et al.*, 2018) (Figure 9.11).

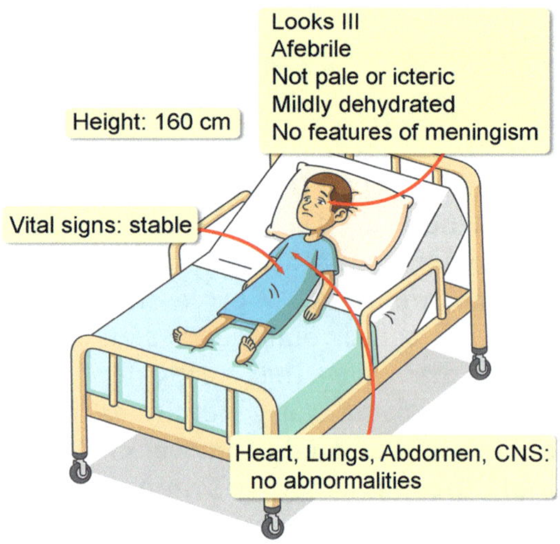

Figure 9.11. Hematological emergencies, such as tumor lysis syndrome (TLS), can manifest unexpectedly and cause severe metabolic disturbances like hyperkalemia, which may necessitate immediate intervention to prevent life-threatening complications.

Source: https://clinicalodyssey.com/storage/case-images/pd/PD-M-169_en.png.

9.3.2. Identification of Critical Symptoms in PICU

Detection of major symptoms in the Pediatric Intensive Care Unit (PICU) is extremely crucial, particularly with the multifaceted hematologic and oncologic complications of at-risk children. The early recognition of symptoms such as unexplained bleeding, repeated fevers, and profound fatigue can be indicators of conditions like coagulopathies or malignancies of the hematologic system, and immediate intervention is needed. Proper monitoring protocols, including routine checking of vital signs and lab parameters, strongly enhance the prospects of early detection. Also, coordination among multidisciplinary teams plays an important role in formulating appropriate management plans in accordance with the patient. With increasing use of advanced therapeutic interventions, care is to be taken to avoid complications arising from such treatments, according to management guidelines on immune-related adverse events in oncological settings (Wang *et al.*, 2024; Bryan *et al.*, 2021). Finally, the development of a systematic approach to symptom identification can have a direct impact on the outcome for critically ill pediatric patients in the PICU.

9.3.3. Protocols to Treat Acute Anemia

Severe anemia in children, particularly children with intensive care of neoplastic disorders, demands stringent management guidelines to avert associated hazards and complications. Treatment planning typically involves a multidisciplinary approach with careful assessment of hemoglobin level, clinical presentation, and etiology, such as chemotherapy or hematological disorders. Interestingly, the use of blood transfusion remains a pillar of therapy for acute anemia with the aim of quick restoration of oxygen-carrying capacity while having the least potential for transfusion reaction. Also, supportive therapy administration, like erythropoiesis-stimulating agents, is efficacious in stimulating red blood cell production, thereby correcting the anemia at its source (Boscato *et al.*, 2023). Close monitoring of how the patients respond to treatment is important, as it informs the need for further interventions or adjustments in the plan of management. Ultimately, an organized approach to the management of acute anemia is the foundation of the overall care provided to pediatric patients in the intensive care setting (Jay *et al.*, 2022) (Figure 9.12).

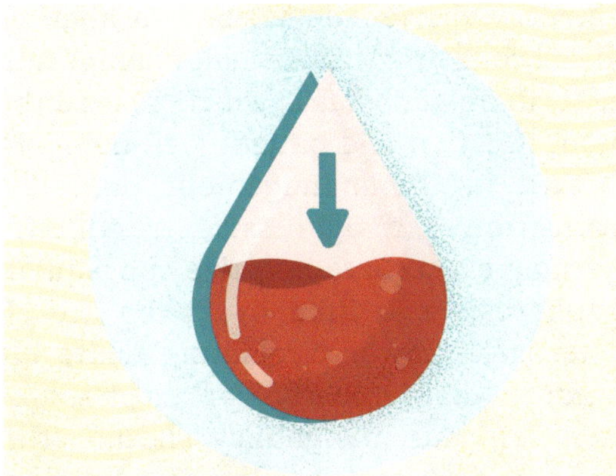

Figure 9.12. Acute anemia in pediatric patients, particularly those undergoing intensive care for oncological conditions, necessitates well-defined management protocols to mitigate associated risks and complications.

Source: https://images.everydayhealth.com/images/2025-gateway-illustrations/eh-anemia-gg-1440x810.png?sfvrsn=70a01bfc_3.

9.3.4. Management of Febrile Neutropenia

In the treatment of pediatric oncology, febrile neutropenia (FN) is an important aspect to be managed, considering its implication in high morbidity and mortality. FN often presents in those patients whose immune systems are weakened because of chemotherapy, and it requires immediate medical attention. The Canadian triage guidelines are created to offer children with FN timely and appropriate treatment; however, research has documented that mal-triage is prevalent, leading to unnecessary delay in important evaluation and antibiotic therapy, potentially aggravating patient outcomes (Alsharawneh *et al.*, 2019). In addition, the causative conditions that lead to FN, often a complication of hematologic malignancies, further complicate clinic management since such patients are at increased risk for in-hospital complications, including organ failure (Boscato *et al.*, 2023). Therefore, a comprehensive triage approach, early intervention, and constant monitoring are essential in improving health outcomes in this vulnerable population.

9.3.5. Treatment of Tumor Lysis Syndrome

Management of tumor lysis syndrome (TLS) is critical in the treatment of children with hematologic malignancies, particularly when they present with heavy tumor burdens. Extensive therapy would, therefore, ideally start with aggressive hydration to improve renal perfusion and increase urine production, thus successfully curbing hyperuricemia and attendant complications.

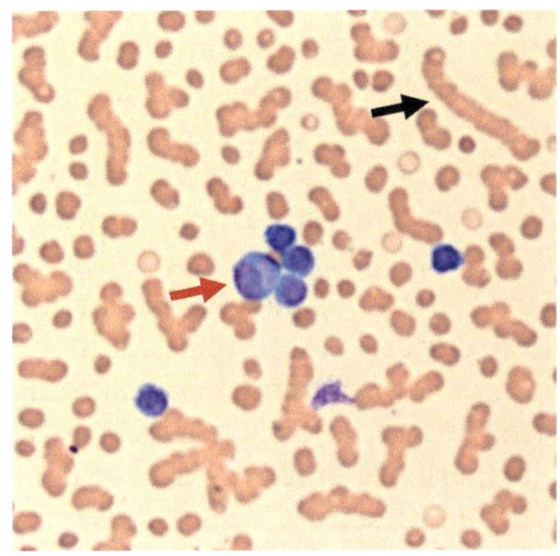

Figure 9.13. The treatment of tumor lysis syndrome (TLS) is critical in managing pediatric patients with hematologic malignancies, particularly when they present with high tumor burdens.

Source: https://casereports.bmj.com/content/bmjcr/14/2/e234122/F1.large.jpg.

Traditionally, allopurinol has been the treatment of choice in the management of elevated uric acid levels, but it is at times reduced in efficacy, and clinicians have been pushed to resort to alternatives. Rasburicase is an essential therapy since it can rapidly metabolize uric acid without leading to the accumulation of xanthine or hypoxanthine, and it is of higher utility compared to allopurinol in this context (Castellini *et al.*, 2008). This change in treatment approaches reflects a better grasp of TLS management and emphasizes the necessity for continuous improvement of care standards in pediatric intensive care patients, addressing the complications created by their underlying malignancies (Boscato *et al.*, 2023) (Figure 9.13).

9.3.6. Addressing Bleeding Complications in Hematological Disorders

Management of bleeding complications arising from hematological diseases is crucial in optimizing patient outcomes in pediatric intensive care. Hemorrhage in children with thrombocytopenia or coagulopathies is highly likely, particularly in intensive care, where multiple comorbid conditions render their management complicated. Other considerations, such as central venous line placement and acute hemostatic derangement, significantly increase the risk of bleeding events, necessitating close monitoring and active treatment (Agarwal *et al.*, 2024). Furthermore, emerging data on conditions like COVID-19 illustrate how this viral illness can be responsible for a hypercoagulable state as well as bleeding risks from coagulopathy, complicating treatment strategies (Yu *et al.*, 2023). By implementing thorough risk assessment guidelines and personalized therapy plans, medical professionals can better manage the delicate balance between preventing and treating bleeding complications to enhance the safety and effectiveness of treatment being provided to these vulnerable pediatric patients.

9.3.7. Management of Hyperleukocytosis

The treatment of hyperleukocytosis in pediatric patients requires a multi-modal plan, especially because of the increased risk during oncologic treatment. Hyperleukocytosis, or a high white blood cell count, may cause major complications in the form of leukostasis, which poses a threat to organ function and patient well-being. Most important in the management plan is the identification and aggressive treatment, as delays may exacerbate negative consequences. Leukapheresis and fluid hydration are often used to safely lower circulating white blood cells. Additionally, underlying precipitants such as infection and malignancy should still be treated to the patient's advantage. As evidenced in the literature, infection control measures need to be effective, given that the risk of sepsis in hyperleukocytosis is high (Capoferri *et al.*, 2024). Furthermore, the high-level interaction between treatment modalities and the likelihood of long-term effects emphasize the need for personalized management strategies to optimize outcomes (Óskarsson *et al.*, 2022) (Figure 9.14).

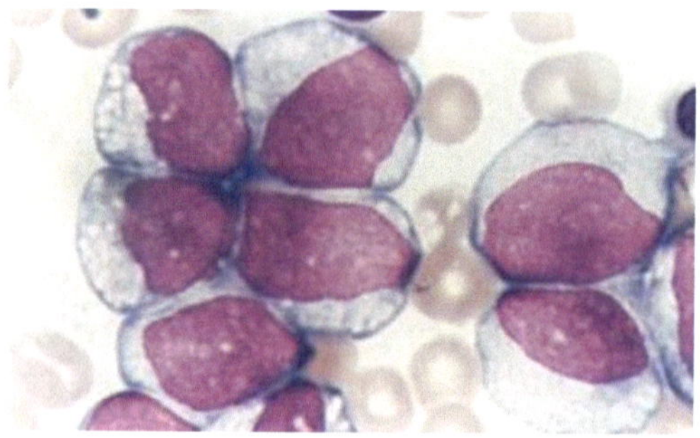

Figure 9.14. Hyperleukocytosis, characterized by elevated white blood cell counts, can lead to significant complications such as leukostasis, which poses threats to both organ function and overall patient well-being.

Source: https://www.acep.org/siteassets/sites/critical-care/media/article-images/hyperleuko-jan-2025-cover.jpg.

9.3.8. Role of Supportive Care in Emergencies

In pediatric critical care, particularly with hematologic and oncologic issues, supportive management in emergency conditions is the focus. Supportive management entails prompt management of interventions, reducing complications of cancer therapy, such as febrile neutropenia (FN), an acute syndrome predisposing to catastrophic outcomes if not managed promptly. Effective supportive care not only includes prompt medical treatments but also involves far-reaching measures for effective triage and speedy access to necessary therapies. The evidence indicates that most patients face mal-triage, which results in unwanted delays in initiating critical treatment and adverse effects on health (Alsharawneh *et al.*, 2019). Moreover, establishing pediatric emergency departments with specialist staffing greatly improves the management of cancer-related emergencies, ultimately optimizing survival and patient health (André *et al.*, 2023). Thus, integrating supportive care into emergency protocols is important for optimizing outcomes in pediatric patients with life-threatening oncological conditions.

9.3.9. Importance of Rapid Response Teams in PICU

Use of rapid response teams (RRTs) in the Pediatric Intensive Care Unit (PICU) plays a critical role in the management of emergent hematologic and oncologic complications in critically ill children. RRTs are multidisciplinary teams whose central objective is to quickly intervene in patients who have undergone acute deterioration, thus also saving them from anticipated unplanned admissions and cardiac arrests. A study conducted in King Abdulaziz University Hospital revealed the effectiveness of pediatric RRTs, which showed a significant decrease in unexpected PICU admissions post-initiation (RR = 0.552, $p < 0.0001$) and absolute elimination of non-ICU cardiac arrests (RR = 0) (Al-Harbi, 2024). Further, RRT integration not only enhances acute care of patients but also lessens family anxiety during crisis, mirroring the provision of extensive care required in pediatric oncology departments. Last but not least, RRT implementation is vital towards increased outcomes and the development of a safer care environment for vulnerable pediatric patients (Figure 9.15).

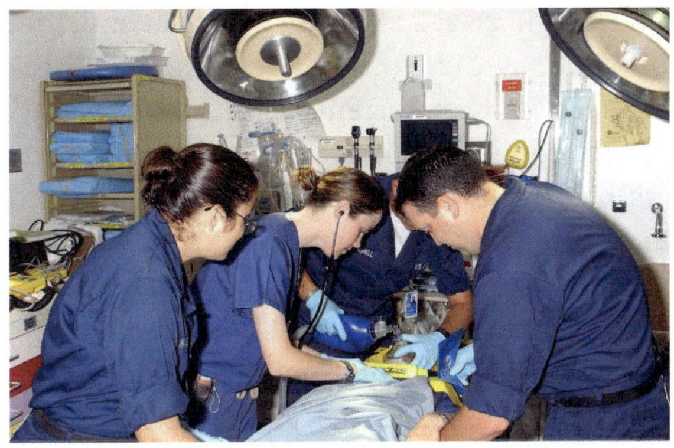

Figure 9.15. The implementation of rapid response teams (RRTs) in the Pediatric Intensive Care Unit (PICU) plays a crucial role in addressing emergent hematological and oncologic issues among critically ill children.

Source: https://www.clinicalcorrelations.org/wp-content/uploads/2018/04/RRTs.jpg.

Test Your Knowledge

1. What treatments are used to prevent renal failure in tumor lysis syndrome?
2. When is leukapheresis indicated in pediatric oncology?

SUMMARY

The complexity that goes into hematologic and oncologic issues management in pediatric intensive care necessitates a multi-dimensional approach to provide optimal outcomes in patients. The predominance of issues such as febrile neutropenia in acute myeloid leukemia among children demonstrates the absolute necessity of effective risk stratification and timely interventions, since the high morbidity associated with delays clearly suggests (Nittu *et al.*, 2024). Furthermore, the issues portrayed through foreign body aspiration cases highlight the need for timely diagnosis and intervention to prevent adverse effects in vulnerable pediatric patients (Bjerregaard *et al.*, 2025). As doctors work to advance guidelines and apply advances in genomics and clinical care, the end goal remains the same: enhancing the quality of life and reducing the healthcare burden for children with hematologic and oncologic conditions in intensive care. This commitment to improvement is essential to the future of pediatrics.

In the examination of hematologic and oncologic issues among children in intensive care, a few things become apparent that demonstrate the complexity of addressing these conditions. Hematologic crises such as hypercalcemia and hyperleukocytosis appear as emergent threats, with immediate medical action needed in order to prevent a rapid downturn and subsequent multiorgan failure, such as experienced in the necessity for urgent recognition and management intervention (Duminuco *et al.*, 2024). Also, conditions like tumor lysis syndrome and sickle cell crisis further complicate the clinical scenario, making individualized approaches necessary to optimize acute management and prevent long-term injury. Modern advances in gene therapy, particularly the application of recombinant adeno-associated virus (rAAV), have created potential for curing many diseases, but also pose questions regarding immune responses and likely side effects, calling for judicious use in clinical practice (Wang *et al.*, 2024). Hence, an in-depth understanding of these issues is needed to drive patient interests in the pediatric intensive care context.

KEY TERMS FROM THIS CHAPTER

- Hematopoietic stem cell transplantation
- Care management
- Anemia
- Leukemias
- Molecular diagnostics
- Bone marrow transplantation
- Microbiome
- Surveillance
- Hematologic malignancies
- Hemophilia
- Life-threatening
- Chemotherapy
- Dysbiosis

CRITICAL THINKING QUESTIONS

1. **What is the most common hematologic emergency in pediatric intensive care?**
    a. Hemophilia A
    b. Disseminated intravascular coagulation (DIC)
    c. Sickle cell crisis
    d. Aplastic anemia
2. **A child with leukemia presents with fever and neutropenia. What is the most urgent next step?**
    a. Blood transfusion
    b. Start broad-spectrum antibiotics immediately
    c. Wait for culture results
    d. Start chemotherapy
3. **What lab abnormality is most concerning in tumor lysis syndrome (TLS)?**
    a. Hypokalemia
    b. Hypophosphatemia
    c. Hyperuricemia
    d. Hypernatremia
4. **Which condition is associated with pancytopenia and hepatosplenomegaly in a critically ill child?**
    a. Iron-deficiency anemia
    b. Hemophagocytic lymphohistiocytosis (HLH)
    c. Immune thrombocytopenia (ITP)
    d. Hemolytic uremic syndrome (HUS)
5. **Which of the following is a common coagulopathy in children with liver failure or sepsis?**
    a. Immune thrombocytopenia
    b. DIC
    c. Von Willebrand disease
    d. Hemophilia B

Short Answer Questions

1. What are the clinical features and complications of sickle cell disease in critically ill children?
2. How is disseminated intravascular coagulation (DIC) diagnosed and managed in pediatric patients?
3. What are the most common pediatric cancers requiring ICU-level care?
4. How does tumor lysis syndrome (TLS) present and what are its early warning signs?
5. What is the initial management of acute chest syndrome in sickle cell disease?
6. How is massive transfusion protocol applied in pediatric hemorrhagic emergencies?

Answers to Critical Thinking Questions

1. (c); 2. (b); 3. (c); 4. (b); 5. (b)

REFERENCES

1. Abbag, F. I., & El Awad, M. (2006). Mortality in the pediatric intensive care units, experience from Saudi Arabia. https://core.ac.uk/download/288210307.pdf (accessed on 30th June 2025).
2. Agarwal, S., Sandiford, P. A., Stanek, J. R., O'Brien, S. H., & Kerlin, B. (2024). Development and validation of a risk assessment model for venous thromboembolism in the pediatric intensive care unit. *Blood*. https://www.semanticscholar.org/paper/bbcbe7e2f957cd5a77d32ce561e16e7f8b9914c0 (accessed on 30th June 2025).
3. Al-Harbi, S. (2024). Impact of rapid response teams on pediatric care: An interrupted time series analysis of unplanned PICU admissions and cardiac arrests. *Healthcare, 12*. https://www.semanticscholar.org/paper/ee75de7d92341394c66fa839d2641d1c85b59011 (accessed on 30th June 2025).
4. Alsharawneh, A. (2019). The effectiveness of the Canadian triage guidelines in improving the treatment outcomes of cancer patients with febrile neutropenia. https://core.ac.uk/download/237205451.pdf (accessed on 30th June 2025).
5. Araújo da Silva, A. R., da Silva Lima, F. F., da Cunha, M. O. M., Grabois, M. F., & Ferman, S. (2023). Pediatric emergency care for children and adolescents with cancer: Causes of consultation and factors associated with hospitalization. https://core.ac.uk/download/587785871.pdf (accessed on 30th June 2025).
6. Asefi, S., SadrMoharrerpour, S., Tamaddoni, A., & Tamaddoni, A. (2018). Rare presentation of renal failure related to tumor lysis syndrome. https://core.ac.uk/download/322610723.pdf (accessed on 30th June 2025).
7. Benoit, D., Lameire, N., Van Biesen, W., & Vanholder, R. (2016). Acute kidney injury in critically ill cancer patients: An update. https://core.ac.uk/download/55807820.pdf (accessed on 30th June 2025).
8. Berner, R., Lehrnbecher, T., Schlage, S., & Simon, A. (2024). SARS-CoV-2 in pediatric cancer: A systematic review. https://core.ac.uk/download/617878290.pdf (accessed on 30th June 2025).
9. Bhatia, S., Pappo, A. S., Acquazzino, M., Allen-Rhoades, W., Barnett, M., Borinstein, S. C., Casey, R., *et al.* (2023). Adolescent and young adult (AYA) oncology, Version 2.2024, NCCN clinical practice guidelines in oncology. *Journal of the National Comprehensive Cancer Network, 21*, 851–880. https://doi.org/10.6004/jnccn.2023.0040 (accessed on 30th June 2025).
10. Bjerregaard, A. T., Holm, J. K., & Clausen, N. G. (2025). Time from suspected foreign body aspiration to bronchoscopy at Odense University Hospital during a 5-year period. *Acta Anesthesiologic Scandinavica, 69*. https://www.semanticscholar.org/paper/4835799f5c70a01c083ecc945bb05d192ea49dc6 (accessed on 30th June 2025).
11. Blom, J. M. C., Barisone, E., Bertolotti, M., Caprino, D., Cellini, M., Clerici, C. A., Colliva, C., *et al.* (2022). The use of psychotropic medication in pediatric oncology for acute psychological and psychiatric problems: Balancing risks and benefits. *Children, 9*, 1878–1878. https://doi.org/10.3390/children9121878 (accessed on 30th June 2025).
12. Böll, B., Schalk, E., Buchheidt, D., Hasenkamp, J., Kiehl, M., Kiderlen, T. R., Kochanek, M., *et al.* (2020). Central venous catheter–related infections in hematology and oncology: 2020 updated guidelines on diagnosis, management, and prevention by the Infectious Diseases Working Party (AGIHO) of the German Society of Hematology and Medical Oncology (DGHO).

Annals of Hematology, 100, 239–259. https://doi.org/10.1007/s00277-020-04286-x (accessed on 30th June 2025).

13. Booth, S., Chatzikonstantinou, T., Cook, G., & Fattizzo, B. (2020). Outcomes of patients with hematologic malignancies and COVID-19: A systematic review and meta-analysis of 3377 patients. https://core.ac.uk/download/372995672.pdf (accessed on 30th June 2025).
14. Boscato, S. (2023). Risk factors and outcomes of oncohematologic patients admitted to pediatric intensive care unit: ONCOTIPNET, an Italian multicenter study. https://core.ac.uk/download/588606296.pdf (accessed on 30th June 2025).
15. Capoferri, G., Esposito, S., Leardini, D., & Masetti, G. (2024). Managing the risk of foodborne infections in pediatric patients with cancer: Is the neutropenic diet still an option? https://core.ac.uk/download/611936133.pdf (accessed on 30th June 2025).
16. Carrard, V. C., Martins, M. D., Martins, M. A. T., & Neves, F. (2021). Analysis of referrals to the stomatology service in a Southern Brazilian hospital: A retrospective study. https://core.ac.uk/download/548518305.pdf (accessed on 30th June 2025).
17. Castellini, C., Melchionda, F., & Pession, A. (2008). Pitfalls, prevention, and treatment of hyperuricemia during tumor lysis syndrome in the era of rasburicase (recombinant urate oxidase). https://core.ac.uk/download/pdf/8319012.pdf (accessed on 30th June 2025).
18. Chimbira, W., Crawford, H., Gupta, S., & Legg, S. (2001). Acute lung injury in pediatric intensive care: Course and outcome. https://core.ac.uk/download/pdf/8715345.pdf (accessed on 30th June 2025).
19. Colombatti, R., Montanaro, M., & Sainati, L. (2016). A global perspective on milestones of care for children with sickle cell disease. https://core.ac.uk/download/322427799.pdf (accessed on 30th June 2025).
20. Cugno, C., Deola, S., Filippini, P., & Rutella, S. (2015). Granulocyte transfusions in children and adults with hematological malignancies: Benefits and controversies. https://core.ac.uk/download/46562816.pdf (accessed on 30th June 2025).
21. Dimopoulos, K., Constantine, A., Clift, P., Condliffe, R., Moledina, S., Jansen, K., Inuzuka, R., *et al.* (2023). Cardiovascular complications of Down syndrome: Scoping review and expert consensus. *Circulation, 147*, 425–441. https://doi.org/10.1161/circulationaha.122.059706 (accessed on 30th June 2025).
22. Docking, R., Kinsella, J., Moss, L., Sim, R., *et al.* (2012). An investigation into the effects of commencing hemodialysis in the critically ill. https://core.ac.uk/download/1439066.pdf (accessed on 30th June 2025).
23. Duminuco, A., Del Fabro, V., Patanè, L., Leotta, D., Limoli, M. C., Longo, E., Nardo, A., *et al.* (2024). Emergencies in hematology: Why, when and how I treat? *Journal of Clinical Medicine, 13*, 7572–7572. https://doi.org/10.3390/jcm13247572 (accessed on 30th June 2025).
24. Fattizzo, B., Cavallaro, F., Folino, F., & Barcellini, W. (2020). Recent insights into the role of the microbiome in malignant and benign hematologic diseases. https://core.ac.uk/download/589941807.pdf (accessed on 30th June 2025).
25. Faulkner, L., Rovelli, A., the Pediatric Diseases Working Party of the European Blood and Marrow Transplantation Group, Verna, M., *et al.* (2021). Setting up and sustaining blood and marrow transplant services for children in middle-income economies: An experience-driven

position paper on behalf of the EBMT PDWP. https://core.ac.uk/download/491392132.pdf (accessed on 30th June 2025).

26. Forteza Sáez, M., & Llantà, M. del C. (2024). Oncopediatric palliative care. *Intech Open eBooks*. https://doi.org/10.5772/intechopen.1003878 (accessed on 30th June 2025).

27. Hanson, K. E., Caliendo, A. M., Diaz Arias, C. A., Hayden, M. K., Englund, J. A., Lee, M. J., Loeb, M., *et al.* (2021). The Infectious Diseases Society of America guidelines on the diagnosis of COVID-19: Molecular diagnostic testing. *Clinical Infectious Diseases, 78*, e170–e207. https://doi.org/10.1093/cid/ciab048 (accessed on 30th June 2025).

28. Jay, M. A., Selers, E. L., & Walker, S. M. (2022). Intravenous opioids for chemotherapy-induced severe mucositis pain in children: Systematic review and single-center case series of management with patient- or nurse-controlled analgesia (PCA/NCA). https://core.ac.uk/download/480395114.pdf (accessed on 30th June 2025).

29. Kalache, A., Adam, A. K., Shimabukuro-Vornhagen, A. A., Vahid, B., Khassawneh, B. Y., Reichner, C. A., Murdoch, D., *et al.* (2010). CCC meets ICU: Redefining the role of critical care of cancer patients. https://core.ac.uk/download/pdf/8491794.pdf (accessed on 30th June 2025).

30. Kappen, T. H., Lekkerkerker, C. W., Nieuwenhuis, E. E., & Soeteman, M. (2022). The predictive performance and impact of pediatric early warning systems in hospitalized pediatric oncology patients—A systematic review. https://core.ac.uk/download/519054839.pdf (accessed on 30th June 2025).

31. Kjellander, C. (2016). Bloodstream infections in patients with hematological malignancies. https://core.ac.uk/download/70343959.pdf (accessed on 30th June 2025).

32. Kürti-G Szabó, & Szakács Szilágyi. (2023). 61st National Congress of the Hungarian Society of Laboratory Medicine. *Clinical Chemistry and Laboratory Medicine (CCLM), 61*, eA57–eA114. https://doi.org/10.1515/cclm-2023-0485 (accessed on 30th June 2025).

33. Lucas, B., Malay, S., & Pateva, I. B. (2024). Frequency of hematologic and nonhematologic conditions in pediatric patients with vascular anomalies: A Pediatric Health Information System database study. *Journal of Vascular Anomalies*. https://www.semanticscholar.org/paper/23d8eaa123f8e4ff3c8d7455933e6bb871c8e7e6 (accessed on 30th June 2025).

34. Markov, Y. I., Markova, I. A., Goriainova, N., & Kuiavovych, B. M. (2023). Hematological disorders as a complication of COVID-19. *Emergency Medicine*. https://www.semanticscholar.org/paper/caa95fb690100034342f9558d43946e6644f0a01 (accessed on 30th June 2025).

35. Maus, M. V., Alexander, S., Bishop, M. R., Brudno, J. N., Callahan, C., Davila, M. L., Diamonte, C., *et al.* (2020). Society for Immunotherapy of Cancer (SITC) clinical practice guideline on immune effector cell-related adverse events. *Journal for Immunotherapy of Cancer, 8*, e001511–e001511. https://doi.org/10.1136/jitc-2020-001511 (accessed on 30th June 2025).

36. Nittu, S. R., Nguyen, N., Wang, J., Alonzo, T., Aplenc, R., Gamis, A., Kolb, A., *et al.* (2024). Gene expression profiling in pediatric AML patients with febrile neutropenia during induction therapy. *Blood*. https://www.semanticscholar.org/paper/4b5c92939a5039c883c6f9974a6d803469781ba6 (accessed on 30th June 2025).

37. Óskarsson, T. (2022). Register-based studies on childhood cancer: Relapsed childhood acute lymphoblastic leukemia and skeletal adverse events in childhood cancer survivors in the Nordic countries. https://core.ac.uk/download/516464036.pdf (accessed on 30th June 2025).

38. Peters, K., & Tice, J. (2011). Safety of physical therapy using symptomatic blood value guidelines in children being treated for cancer. https://core.ac.uk/download/200291431.pdf (accessed on 30th June 2025).

39. Schneider, B. J., Naidoo, J., Santomasso, B., Lacchetti, C., Adkins, S., Anadkat, M. J., Atkins, M. B., *et al.* (2021). Management of immune-related adverse events in patients treated with immune checkpoint inhibitor therapy: ASCO guideline update. *Journal of Clinical Oncology, 39*, 4073–4126. https://doi.org/10.1200/jco.21.01440 (accessed on 30th June 2025).

40. Soeteman, M. (2024). Identifying the critically ill pediatric oncology patient. https://doi.org/10.33540/2063 (accessed on 30th June 2025).

41. Tadros, S., Prévot, J., Meyts, I., Sánchez-Ramón, S., Hassan Erwa, N. H., Fischer, A., Lefèvre, G., *et al.* (2023). The PID Odyssey 2030: Outlooks, unmet needs, hurdles, and opportunities–Proceedings from the IPOPI global multi-stakeholders' summit (June 2022). *Frontiers in Immunology, 14*. https://doi.org/10.3389/fimmu.2023.1245718 (accessed on 30th June 2025).

42. Tanhchaleun, A. (2018). An evidence-based protocol for the assessment and management of glucocorticoid-induced hyperglycemia. https://core.ac.uk/download/211329112.pdf (accessed on 30th June 2025).

43. Traversa, P., & Loiselle, C. G. (2023). Abstract proceedings of the 38th Annual Canadian Association of Psychosocial Oncology (CAPO) Conference, June 2023. *Current Oncology, 30*, 6872–6963. https://doi.org/10.3390/curroncol30070503 (accessed on 30th June 2025).

44. Upadhyay, P., & Kanetkar, S. (2022). Clinic hematological profile of anemia in pediatric (newborn to eighteen years) age group. *International Journal of Health Sciences and Research*. https://www.semanticscholar.org/paper/9b0e858a3ca651edeb7501aa54d073ec97d8eec4 (accessed on 30th June 2025).

45. van der Zee, E. (2023). Care for critically ill cancer patients: From the perspective of the intensive care health care providers. https://core.ac.uk/download/566896104.pdf (accessed on 30th June 2025).

46. van Gerwen, M. M. A. (2021). Child development after maternal cancer diagnosis and treatment during pregnancy. https://core.ac.uk/download/489785082.pdf (accessed on 30th June 2025).

47. Wang, J. H., Gessler, D. J., Zhan, W., Gallagher, T. L., & Gao, G. (2024). Adeno-associated virus as a delivery vector for gene therapy of human diseases. *Signal Transduction and Targeted Therapy, 9*. https://doi.org/10.1038/s41392-024-01780-w (accessed on 30th June 2025).

48. Wong, H. M. (2014). Oral complications and management strategies for patients undergoing cancer therapy. https://core.ac.uk/download/205893001.pdf (accessed on 30th June 2025).

49. Yip, D., Soma, A., Pati, N., Spencer, W., Hua, B., & Jagilly, R. (2023). Building capability and capacity: The establishment of an oncology unit in the Solomon Islands. *JCO Global Oncology*. https://doi.org/10.1200/go.22.00325 (accessed on 30th June 2025).

INFECTIOUS DISEASES AND SEPSIS

10

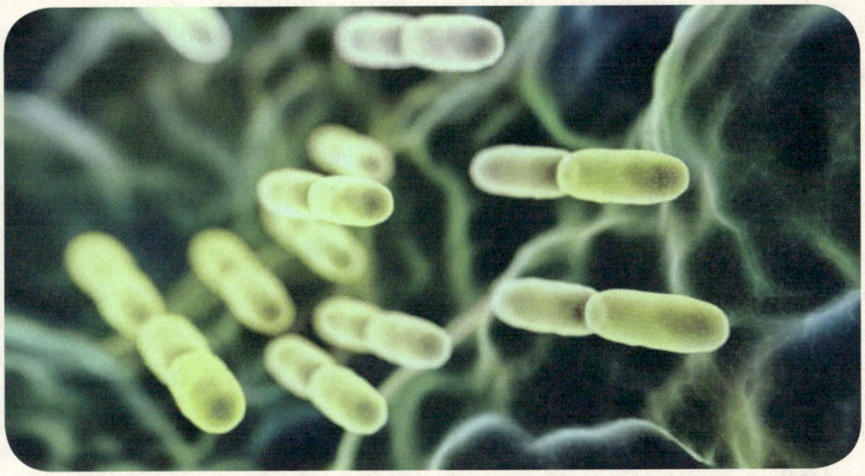

LEARNING OBJECTIVES

After studying this chapter, you will be able to:

1. Understand Infectious Diseases in Pediatrics.
2. Explain the Definition, Causes, and Risk Factors of Sepsis.
3. Describe Management of Sepsis in Pediatric Intensive Care.
4. Focus on Prevention Strategies for Infectious Diseases and Sepsis.

Introduction

Infectious disease prevalence leading to sepsis in pediatric intensive care units (PICUs) poses an emergency health situation worldwide that needs to be addressed with immediate attention to effective management. Neonatal infections alone account for nearly a million deaths annually, primarily in low-income settings, where, within a timely framework, case management is still the key to survival (Bhutta *et al.*, 2011). The severity of sepsis among children is compounded by the high incidence of overprescription of inappropriate antibiotics that fuel antimicrobial resistance and increase healthcare costs (Barbieri *et al.*, 2020). As pediatrics continues to improve, there is still an urgent call for efficient protocols that center around sepsis prevention and management. These interventions, in addition to requesting more knowledge regarding the pediatric sepsis epidemiology, highlight the necessity for antimicrobial stewardship programs that are capable of making efforts toward improved health outcomes and reduced mortality rates in PICUs worldwide.

10.1. Understanding Infectious Diseases in Pediatrics

Learning Outcome

1. Common Infectious Diseases in Children.
2. Modes of Transmission.
3. Risk Factors for Infections in Pediatric Patients.
4. Symptoms and Clinical Presentation.
5. Diagnostic Methods for Pediatric Infections.
6. Treatment Options for Infectious Diseases.
7. Role of Vaccinations in Prevention.
8. Impact of Infectious Diseases on Pediatric Health.
9. Emerging Infectious Diseases in Children.

The pediatric infectious diseases have a high degree of complexity when it comes to comprehending the unique presentation and impact on this vulnerable group. Children exhibit diverse immunologic responses compared to adults, making diagnosis and treatment complicated. Sepsis, a state of systemic inflammatory response syndrome to infection, is highly dangerous in the pediatric intensive care unit. Evidence suggests that pediatric antimicrobial stewardship programs (ASPs) are of fundamental importance in stemming the threats posed by antibiotic overuse, which is a widespread condition in hospital and community health environments. ASPs have proved to decrease unnecessary antibiotic use substantially, leading to enhanced patient care and reduced healthcare costs (Barbieri *et al.*, 2020). Organizational funding, like that of the Wellcome Trust, is making it possible to conduct more research on such infectious diseases and how care methodologies can be optimized (King *et al.*, 2017). Hence, building an equilibrium understanding of childhood infections is essential to improving end outcomes and optimizing healthcare resources (Figure 10.1).

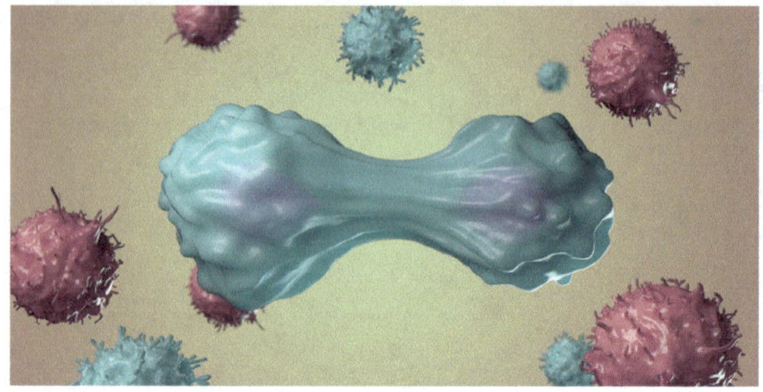

Figure 10.1. Children exhibit different immunological responses compared to adults, which can complicate both diagnosis and treatment.

Source: https://www.mdanderson.org/images/publications/cancerwise/Generics/T-cell-division.jpg.

10.1.1. Common Infectious Diseases in Children

Infectious diseases among children are a significant challenge to pediatrics, often causing serious complications such as sepsis. Particularly, conditions such as pneumonia, diarrhea, and measles have a high potential for progression, particularly in vulnerable individuals. For instance, studies indicate that sepsis death rates among children remain far greater than those of other common diseases, like pneumonia and measles, indicating the need for intervention in the management of such conditions (Andrade *et al.*, 2011). In addition, the availability of improved medical care programs, funded by agencies like the Wellcome Trust and MRC Centre for Medical Mycology, has shown promise in lowering children's sepsis rates (King *et al.*, 2017). However, despite the ongoing improvement in the healthcare system, sepsis continues to be a significant cause of morbidity, and this underscores the imperative for ongoing research and the realization of certain health policies to shield pediatric populations from such infectious insults.

10.1.2. Modes of Transmission

Modes of transmission for infectious diseases in children's intensive care settings are multifaceted and dependent on both environmental and patient demographics. Of interest, pathogens such as *Candida spp.* are capable of inducing nosocomial-acquired bloodstream infections with significant implications for mortality and morbidity in critically ill children. Studies show that such infections are prevalent among patients with underlying illness in intensive care units, where the risk of severe sepsis and septic shock is high, particularly when the systemic inflammatory response is intense (Edmond *et al.*, 2006). In addition, infections like Group B streptococcus pose threats for late-onset disease in neonates, where transmission may be either perinatally or postpartum, pointing towards the significance of environmental exposure and maternal colonization (Berardi *et al.*, 2022). Understanding such modes of transmission is significant in planning effective prevention strategies, thereby reducing the incidence of sepsis and improving outcomes in the pediatric intensive care unit (Figure 10.2).

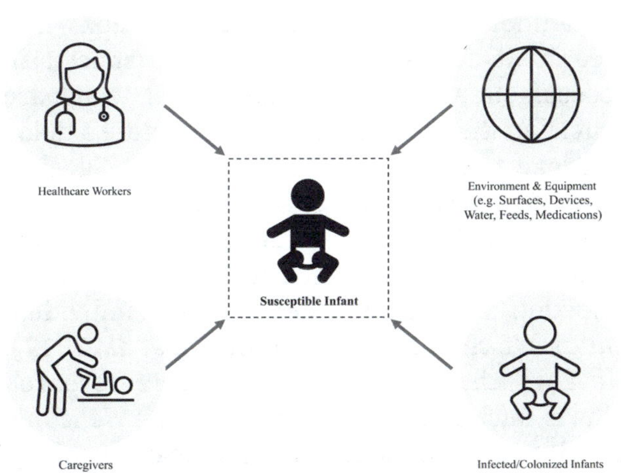

Figure 10.2. The modes of transmission for infectious diseases in pediatric intensive care settings are multifaceted, often influenced by environmental factors and patient demographics.

Source: https://www.clinicalmicrobiologyandinfection.com/cms/10.1016/j.cmi.2022.11.007/asset/d5f05ede-4665-4290-92e2-29e30a4e7b71/main.assets/gr1_lrg.jpg.

10.1.3. Risk Factors for Infections in Pediatric Patients

In children, a number of risk factors are the cause of the heightened vulnerability to infection, particularly in the intensive care unit. One of the problems of initial concern is their immature immune response, which compromises their ability to effectively repel pathogens. Other medical conditions, such as congenital cardiac anomalies or tumors, also serve to enhance these risks further by providing a terrain for infection. Prolonged hospital stay and the use of invasive medical devices still put patients at risk of nosocomial infections, with high-level infection control measures needed. Evidence-based guidelines emphasize the importance of early detection and management of intra-abdominal infections (IAI) in children since they have a tendency to become sepsis if not managed on time (Chang *et al.*, 2017). In addition, ongoing research emphasizes the role of individually tailored antimicrobial therapy and aggressive Source control to minimize risks secondary to infection, paving the way for improved outcomes in critically ill children (King *et al.*, 2017).

10.1.4. Signs and Clinical Presentation

The clinical presentation of pediatric intensive care unit infectious diseases is apt to be a syndrome of symptoms whose characterization may shift profoundly depending on the pathogen causing the disease. The symptoms might encompass fever, altered mental status, respiratory distress, and signs of hemodynamic instability such as hypotension and tachycardia. These are the clinical signs that make the diagnosis of sepsis possible, an often-lethal condition that comprises a dysregulated host response to infection. For instance, EURECA recognizes that systematic determination and description of clinical management and outcomes of infections, particularly those related to carbapenem-resistant Enterobacteriaceae, is a challenge in the pediatric setting in particular (Ferrer *et al.*, 2017). Furthermore, early recognition of signs and timely clinical intervention are paramount as rates of mortality may escalate alarmingly. Delayed diagnosis and therapy (King *et al.*, 2017). Therefore, a good understanding of these symptoms will enhance diagnostic accuracy and patient outcomes in critical care (Figure 10.3).

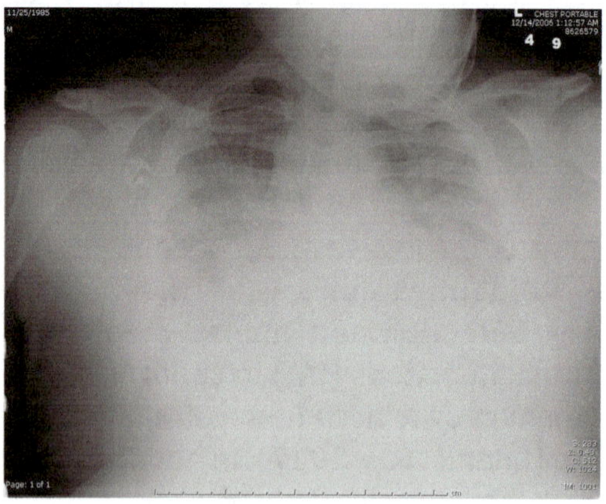

Figure 10.3. Common symptoms include fever, altered mental status, respiratory distress, and signs of hemodynamic instability such as tachycardia and hypotension.

Source: https://www.cancertherapyadvisor.com/wp-content/uploads/sites/12/2019/01/ch412.fig1_.jpg.

10.1.5. Diagnostic Methods for Pediatric Infections

In the context of pediatric infections, especially within intensive care units, rapid and precise diagnostic approaches are critical to effective management. Traditional methods such as culture and polymerase chain reaction (PCR) have remained the cornerstone for pathogen identification, but their limitations, especially with regard to speed and sensitivity, can potentially be restrictive to early decision-making. More recent technologies, such as cell-free plasma next-generation sequencing (CFPNGS), have now emerged as good alternatives with much higher detection rates. For cases of hospitalized children presenting with community-acquired pneumonia (CAP), CFPNGS identified pathogens in 86% of the cases, in contrast to the 47% identification rate of conventional methods (Bradley *et al.*, 2019). Also, inclusion of guidelines like the Japanese Clinical Practice Guidelines for Management of Sepsis and Septic Shock enhances the diagnostic strategy by combining evidence-based guidelines for pediatric patients, which highlights the necessity for continuous development in diagnostic practice for optimal patient outcomes in pediatric intensive care (Kazuyoshi *et al.*, 2018).

10.1.6. Infectious Disease Treatment Options

Strong treatment modalities are required in pediatric intensive care management of infectious diseases to improve patient outcomes. Guidelines for intra-abdominal infection (IAI) treatment, for instance, emphasize strict risk assessment and early Source control, which are crucial in the pediatric age group, where a delay can lead to severe complications. The Surgical Infection Society (SIS) guidelines lay significant stress on the usage of an individualized approach in antimicrobial therapy, in terms of timing, selection, and duration, depending on individual children's clinical situation (Chang *et al.*, 2017). Notably, the efforts of mega-scale research efforts, such as those supported by the Wellcome Trust and MRC Centre for Medical Mycology, indicate sustained attention to demarcating the complexity of pediatric infections and refining treatment models (King *et al.*, 2017). Ultimately, routine revision and evidence-based practice are needed to maintain momentum with shifting infectious threats in critical pediatric populations (Figure 10.4).

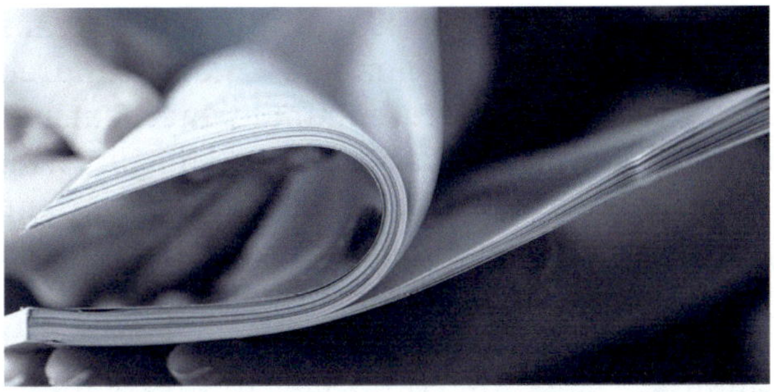

Figure 10.4. Recommendations for treating intra-abdominal infections (IAI), for instance, emphasize the importance of rigorous risk assessment and timely *Source* control, which are critical in the pediatric population where delay can lead to severe complications.

Source: https://www.facs.org/media/vgthf513/acs-store-journalperiodical.jpg?rnd=133917256252030000.

10.1.7. Role of Vaccinations in Prevention

Vaccines play a critical role in preventing infectious disease, working significantly to enhance child health and reduce the incidence of disease that may progress to sepsis. By stimulating the immune system so that it will recognize and combat pathogens, vaccines are actually reducing the threat of serious viral and bacterial infections in children, a group highly vulnerable to sepsis. Incorporation of vaccination programs in pediatric intensive care strategies fulfills comprehensive public health efforts aimed at alleviating the healthcare burden associated with infectious diseases. As indicated in the imperative global response to sepsis cited in recent reports, such as demands for setting up national action plans against sepsis (Jakob *et al.*, 2023), it is more critical now to emphasize that robust vaccination efforts form a front-line defense. These interventions not only protect individual children but also contribute to establishing community immunity, which is critical in the prevention of outbreaks among vulnerable communities (Meduri *et al.*, 2016).

10.1.8. Effects of Infectious Diseases on Child Health

The impact of infectious diseases on children's health is profound, particularly in vulnerable populations such as neonates and early childhood. Almost one million newborn infants die from infection annually, the majority occurring in low-income countries, where case management in a timely manner remains a persistent challenge. Implementation of community-based interventions, such as oral and injectable antibiotics, has been shown to have the promise to greatly reduce neonatal mortality due to sepsis and pneumonia, with estimated up to 80% reductions in some inpatient institutions by expert opinion (Bhutta *et al.*, 2011). Additionally, the use of antibiotics on a large scale, although necessary, is also accompanied by risks of resistance due to inappropriate application, with the need for the institution of pediatric antimicrobial stewardship programs (ASPs).

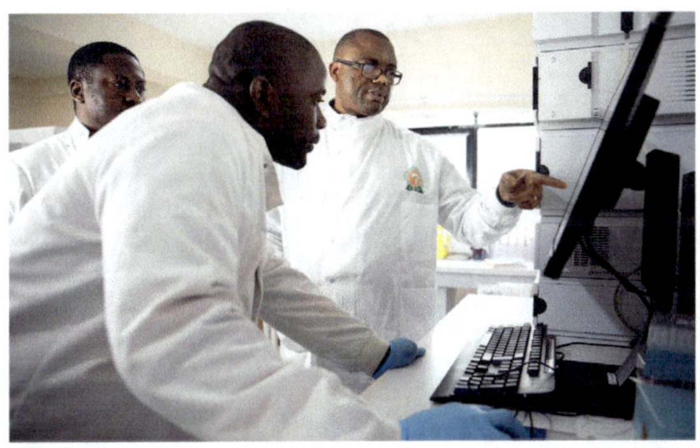

Figure 10.5. Annually, almost one million newborns succumb to infections, predominantly in low-income countries, where timely case management remains a critical challenge.

Source: https://images.gatesnotes.com/12514eb8-7b51-008e-41a9-512542cf683b/7c5c194c-b9f2-4434-a0b8-7f0debc41b0a/Charles-Wondji-malaria-research-2400px_by_1500px-001.jpg?w=1400&h=900&fit=clip&fm=jpg&q=75.

Such interventions have also been successful in reducing unwarranted prescriptions and healthcare spending, ultimately leading to improved antibiotic effectiveness and patient outcomes (Barbieri *et al.*, 2020). Treating infectious diseases with appropriate interventions is thus essential to enhancing the health outcomes and mortality of pediatric intensive care patients (Bohm *et al.*, 2020) (Figure 10.5).

10.1.9. Emerging Infectious Diseases in Children

Pediatric infectious disease epidemiology continues to evolve, particularly with the emergence of new pathogens posing significant challenges in the clinical context. Increased worldwide travel, urbanization, and climate change have favored the spread of infectious agents, which produce outbreaks in disproportionate numbers among children owing to their immature immune mechanisms. Of particular interest is bacterial meningitis with its dynamic epidemiology because of vaccine policies against common pathogens. Research advances on the human microbiome further highlight the complex interactions between host immunity and infection, possibly explaining mechanisms of increased susceptibility in children (Janowski *et al.*, 2017). Moreover, intra-abdominal infections commonly result in sepsis and thus require appropriate management planned with children in mind. The development of updated evidence-based guidelines serves to identify a need for action to treat these newly found infectious diseases in pediatric populations to improve outcomes and reduce morbidity in the pediatric intensive care unit (Chang *et al.*, 2017).

Test Your Knowledge

1. What is the clinical significance of community-acquired versus hospital-acquired infections in children?
2. How is meningitis diagnosed and managed in pediatric patients in the ICU?

10.2. Sepsis: Definition, Causes, and Risk Factors

Learning Outcome

1. Definition of Sepsis in Pediatric Patients.
2. Pathophysiology of Sepsis.
3. Common Causes of Sepsis in Children.
4. Risk Factors Specific to Pediatric Populations.
5. Early Signs and Symptoms of Sepsis.
6. Diagnostic Criteria for Sepsis.
7. Importance of Early Recognition and Intervention.
8. Differences in Sepsis Presentation between Adults and Children.
9. Long-term Effects of Sepsis in Pediatric Patients.

Sepsis is a dangerous, systemic response to an infection that can lead to failure of multiple organs as well as death, particularly in vulnerable populations such as children. Sepsis is a multifactorial process whose pathogenesis involves an uncontrolled immune response of the body, resulting in widespread inflammation and potential damage to organ systems. Age, status of health, and timing of treatment are determinants of sepsis development in children. Younger patients, especially those younger than 18 months, are at greater risk, and respiratory infection is one of the most significant precipitating causes (Hadzhieva-Hristova *et al.*, 2025). Additionally, the frequency of such diseases as multisystem inflammatory syndrome in children (MIS-C) makes the clinical scenario even harder, requiring timely diagnosis and treatment (Abramova *et al.*, 2025). Understanding the definition, etiology, and pathophysiology of the risk factors of sepsis is essential to optimize the outcome in the pediatric intensive care unit (Figure 10.6).

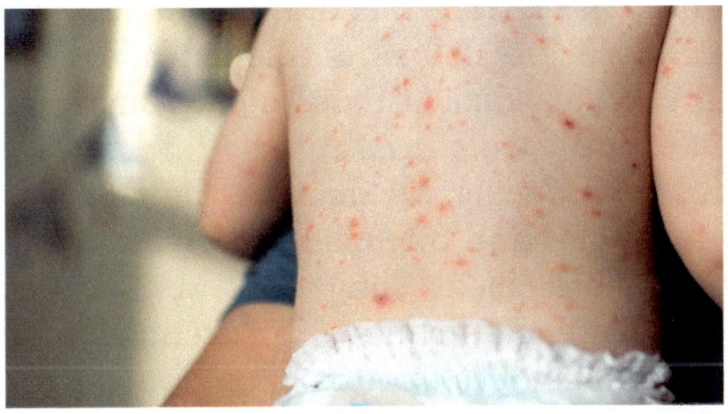

Figure 10.6. Sepsis represents a critical, systemic response to infection that can lead to multi-organ failure and death, particularly in vulnerable populations such as children.

Source: https://images.ctfassets.net/4f3rgqwzdznj/6xIV49MlD4g7H1SPrkGZR4/4656a882ed488b41ce315256df3b8a48/closeup_child_in_diaper_with_chicken_pox_1478102344.jpg.

10.2.1. Definition of Sepsis in Pediatric Patients

The definition of pediatric sepsis has progressed significantly to emphasize the complexity of the lethal condition. Sepsis is a dysregulated host response to infection, and if not treated promptly, this can result in organ dysfunction. Clinical presentation in the pediatric population, particularly in intensive care units, can be less overt and more variable compared to adults and hence warrants strict guidelines for management. The Japanese Clinical Practice Guidelines for the Management of Sepsis and Septic Shock 2016 provide vital information on this complexity by encompassing pediatric-specific factors, which correct for unique physiological and immunological variation in children (Kazuyoshi *et al.*, 2018). Moreover, existing literature highlights early recognition and treatment because delayed sepsis detection is responsible for additional morbidity and mortality among children (Chang *et al.*, 2017). Thus, a precise and brief definition of sepsis in this population is essential for maximizing outcomes and guiding clinical practice.

10.2.2. Pathophysiology of Sepsis

The pathophysiology of sepsis is a complex interaction between the host's immune response and that of the invading organism, particularly in the pediatric age group. In children and neonates, the immaturity of the immune system typically translates into an inadequate response to infection, which contributes to the morbidities and mortalities associated with septic diseases.

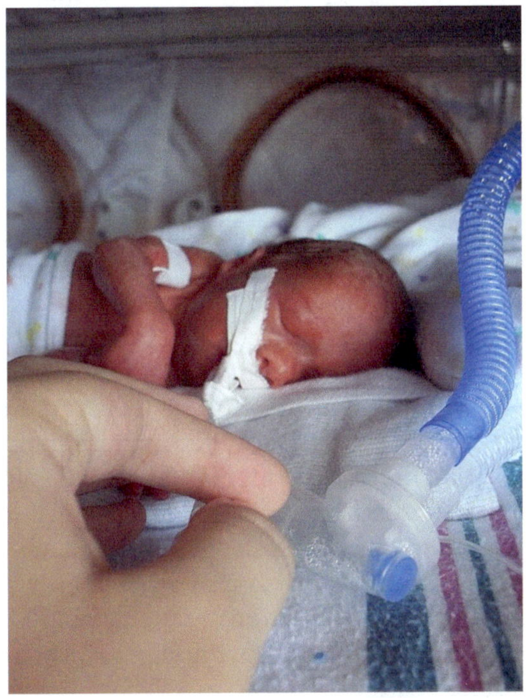

Figure 10.7. In children, particularly neonates, the immature immune system often leads to an inadequate response to infection, contributing to the high rates of morbidity and mortality associated with septic conditions.

Source: https://upload.wikimedia.org/wikipedia/commons/thumb/3/3e/Premature_infant_with_ventilator.jpg/640px-Premature_infant_with_ventilator.jpg.

A major factor in this dysregulated response is the production of pro-inflammatory cytokines, such as interleukins –6 and –8. However, a study shows that in neonates with evidence of early infection, low concentrations of such cytokines may not be useful indicators of systemic bacterial infection, and therefore make diagnosis and management cumbersome (Bezrukov *et al.*, 2018). Additionally, the development of extreme inflammatory responses may lead to problems such as acute respiratory distress syndrome (ARDS), and thus, the need to regulate systemic inflammation to improve outcomes. Prolonged therapy with glucocorticoids has also been successful in suppressing this inflammatory reaction without further risk of secondary infection (Meduri *et al.*, 2016) (Figure 10.7).

10.2.3. Common Causes of Sepsis in Children

Childhood sepsis is typically caused by several infectious causes, of which infection from bacteria is the most common. *Streptococcus pneumoniae, Escherichia coli*, and *Staphylococcus aureus* are some common pathogens that are highly virulent in children. Based on a retrospective analysis of pediatric sepsis in Brazil, the mortality rate for bacterial sepsis in children remained disproportionately high among other conditions, such as pneumonia and diarrhea (Andrade *et al.*, 2011). Sepsis is also aggravated by malnutrition and delayed medical intervention, which are common in lower socio-economic strata.

The persistence of high death rates despite improvements in healthcare suggests that the underlying susceptibilities of the health system are continuing to fuel this crisis (King *et al.*, 2017). It is necessary to overcome these common causes by targeted healthcare intervention in order to decrease the incidence and mortality of sepsis among children globally.

10.2.4. Pediatric Population-Specific Risk Factors

Children are particularly vulnerable to infections and sepsis due to a variety of intrinsic and extrinsic risk factors. Immature immune systems in children are not as developed as those of adults, which makes them highly susceptible to infections, which can rapidly lead to severe illness or sepsis. Premature delivery, low birth weight, and ongoing underlying medical conditions such as congenital abnormalities also predispose children. Vaccination and antimicrobial development have greatly altered the landscape of infectious disease; however, the epidemiology of bacterial meningitis and other infections is still an issue with newly emerging pathogens and effects of antibiotic prophylaxis at birth (Janowski *et al.*, 2017). In addition, exposure to pathogens, crowding, and restricted healthcare access in settings only exacerbates these risks as they increase treatment difficulties for these patients in intensive care units (King *et al.*, 2017). Knowledge of these particular risk factors is critical to enhancing results in pediatric patients confronted with severe infections (Figure 10.8).

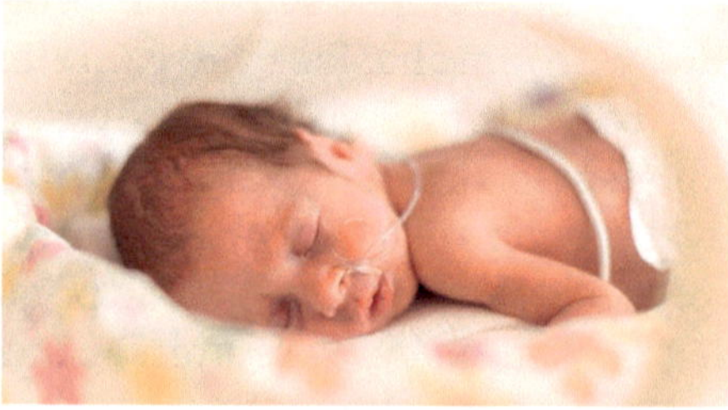

Figure 10.8. Children's developing immune systems lack the maturity seen in adults, making them more susceptible to infections, which can escalate rapidly into severe illness or sepsis.

Source: https://s3-publishing-cmn-svc-prd.s3.ap-southeast-1.amazonaws.com/article/ThF6-tybag0vHEKikhsp9/original/005393700_1635751567-Fakta-Sepsis-Neonatorum-Infeksi-Darah-pada-Bayi-Baru-Lahir.jpg.

10.2.5. Early Signs and Symptoms of Sepsis

Recognition of the early signs and symptoms of sepsis in critically ill children is vital for prompt intervention and better outcomes in the intensive care unit. Presentation may be fever, tachypnea, and a change in heart rate or blood pressure, signifying the body's systemic response to infection. Altered mental status or lethargy may also occur in younger children, which, in the chaotic clinical environment, may be overlooked. Of note, early recognition of these symptoms can be an important factor in survival, as timely treatment is essential to minimize mortality in severe cases (King *et al.*, 2017). As per current literature, sepsis-related infections tend to be due to resistant pathogens, emphasizing the necessity of strict surveillance for infection risk factors such as carbapenem-resistant Enterobacteriaceae in this high-risk population (Ferrer *et al.*, 2017). Through the advocacy for recognizing these early warning signs, doctors can enhance diagnostic specificity and initiate appropriate treatment programs, thereby improving outcomes in child care.

10.2.6. Diagnostic Criteria for Sepsis

Sepsis, an acute illness caused by a hyperactive immune response to infection, is a significant enemy in the intensive care unit in children. The establishment of criteria for the diagnosis of sepsis in neonates is particularly difficult due to their insidious presentation and immature immune system. Key markers are elevated concentrations of C-reactive protein in conjunction with clinical evaluations of organ dysfunction, which may be very early in life. Studies have determined that despite having low levels in neonatal infection, interleukins –6 and –8 remain significant in elevating C-reactive protein, which normally becomes a more effective discriminator for infectious processes in the newborn (Bezrukov *et al.*, 2018). Second, antimicrobial resistance in developing nations complicates treatment and underscores the need for vigilant diagnosis protocols that can keep up with the mutating resistant disease pathogens and guide appropriate management interventions among children (India clen *et al.*, 2017) (Figure 10.9).

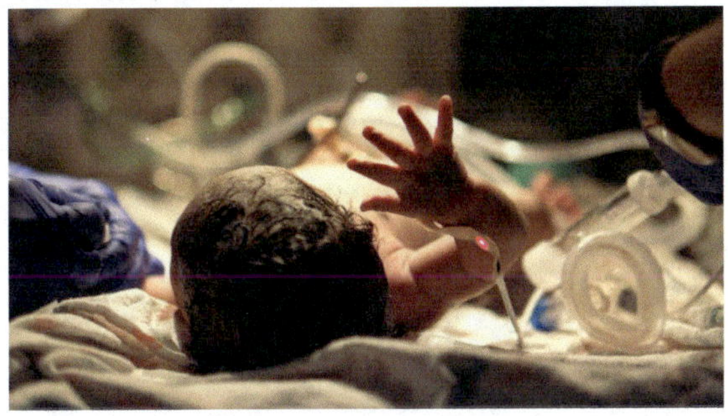

Figure 10.9. Sepsis, a critical condition stemming from an overwhelming immune response to infection, poses a significant challenge in the pediatric intensive care setting.

Source: https://images.onlymyhealth.com/only-my-health-english/images/2024/12/20/article/image/mn-neonatal-sepsis-1734671188322.jpg.

10.2.7. Importance of Early Recognition and Intervention

Early detection and intervention are essential in improving the outcome of pediatric patients who present with infectious diseases and sepsis in intensive care settings. The capacity to identify essential symptoms promptly has the potential to make a huge difference in the prognosis, bearing in mind that sepsis is associated with high mortality levels in children, particularly if late diagnosis is made. Research accentuates the importance of early management practices involving fluid resuscitation and antimicrobial therapy, resulting in strong recommendations from expert panels for early care practices (Alhazzani *et al.*, 2017). Additionally, the understanding of child-specific issues, such as processes involved in immune development and the impact of primary immune deficiencies, is critical in the successful tailoring of interventions (McCulloh *et al.*, 2014). Hence, the combination of rapid assessment tools and heightened awareness among healthcare providers can facilitate early interventions, eventually enhancing survival rates and reducing the long-term health effects of severe infections in children.

10.2.8. Differences in Sepsis Presentation Between Adults and Children

It is critical to understand the difference in the presentation of sepsis between children and adults to optimize management in the pediatric intensive care unit (PICU). In contrast to adults, children can present with atypical signs and symptoms of sepsis, such as altered consciousness, irritability, and a change in feeding behavior, instead of the usual signs and symptoms like fever and respiratory impairment.

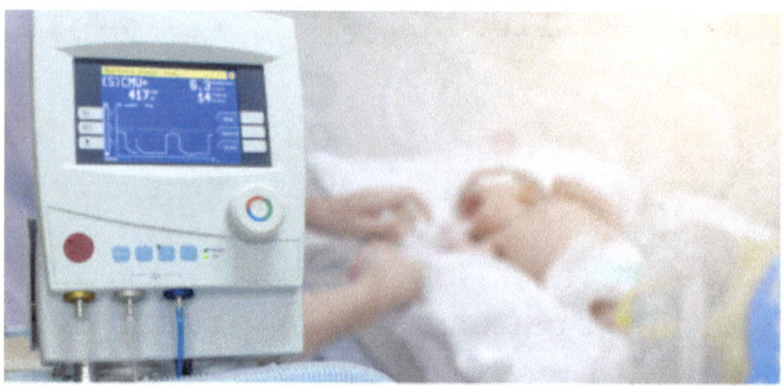

Figure 10.10. Understanding the differences in sepsis presentation between adults and children is crucial in optimizing care within pediatric intensive care units (PICUs).

Source: https://www.sriramakrishnahospital.com/wp-content/uploads/2024/02/Mask-group-73.png.

This disparity in presentation renders early diagnosis and treatment challenging, ultimately impacting outcomes. Furthermore, underdeveloped immune systems in children also lead to response differences against infecting agents, making it hard to measure the severity (Lara *et al.*, 2020). For example, while adults would present with more apparent systemic inflammatory responses to comorbidities, children will have less apparent clinical presentations, which can result in sepsis underdiagnosis (Ma *et al.*, 2020). Such nuances demand heightened vigilance on the part of the medical practitioner to the need for early intervention to avoid morbidity and mortality of children afflicted with sepsis (Figure 10.10).

10.2.9. Long-Term Effects of Sepsis in Pediatric Patients

Childhood sepsis may lead to a myriad of long-term effects with far-reaching impacts on their health status and quality of life. Survivors will also have cognitive impairments, such as difficulty in concentrating, recalling information, and carrying out decisions, which may compromise school performance as well as interpersonal interactions. Such children will also develop physical impairments, such as muscle weakness and decreased mobility, thus requiring ongoing rehabilitation interventions.

The prolonged nature of systemic inflammation, as reported in adults, also may serve as a determinative factor in the development of chronic conditions, including respiratory complications that are similar to those seen in patients with acute respiratory distress syndrome (ARDS), where the long-term use of glucocorticoids has proven to be effective in reducing morbidity and enhancing recovery (Meduri *et al.*, 2016). Furthermore, the risk of secondary complications, e.g., acute kidney injury from the septic process as well as from interventions provided later on, justifies long-term observation of these patients (Benoit *et al.*, 2016).

Test Your Knowledge

1. What host factors increase the risk of sepsis in neonates and young children?
2. How does the immune response in children differ from that of adults in the context of sepsis?

10.3. Management of Sepsis in Pediatric Intensive Care

Learning Outcome

1. Initial Assessment and Stabilization.
2. Fluid Resuscitation Protocols.
3. Antibiotic Therapy and Its Importance.
4. Use of Vasopressors in Treatment.
5. Monitoring and Supportive Care in PICU.
6. Multidisciplinary Approach to Sepsis Management.
7. Role of Technology in Monitoring Sepsis.
8. Challenges in Managing Sepsis in Children.

Optimal management of sepsis in the pediatric intensive care unit is crucial due to the unique physiological considerations and frailties of the neonate and child. Prompt identification and management are absolutely essential for improved outcomes, often involving the urgent application of broad-spectrum antibiotics along with supportive therapies matched to the condition of the child. Research suggests that injectable antibiotic management programs at community levels may be efficient in reducing neonatal mortality from sepsis and pneumonia, highlighting the importance of immediate medical interventions in emergencies (Bhutta *et al.*, 2011). Moreover, the inclusion of comprehensive care guidelines in intensive care settings may also enhance survival rates and general quality of recovery, further highlighting the need for systemic redevelopment of healthcare centers (King *et al.*, 2017). The subtleties of sepsis care demand an interprofessional approach with urgent diagnostic and therapeutic management to ensure that the pediatric patient receives what he or she needs in a timely manner to overcome the life-threatening disease (Figure 10.11).

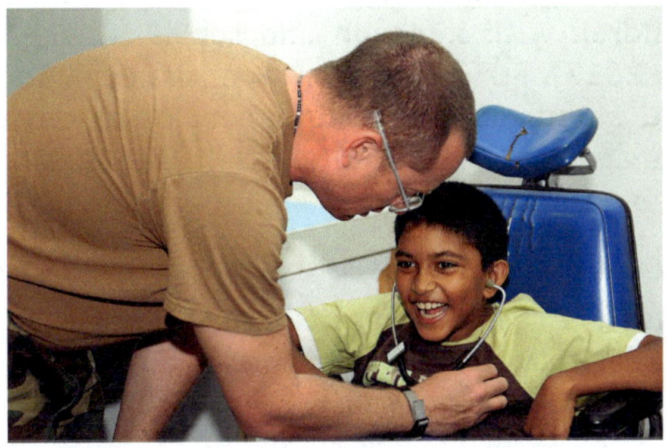

Figure 10.11. Early recognition and intervention play a pivotal role in improving outcomes, often necessitating the rapid administration of broad-spectrum antibiotics alongside supportive therapies tailored to the child's condition.

Source: https://upload.wikimedia.org/wikipedia/commons/thumb/7/7c/USS_Kearsarge_medical_team_treat_patients_at_Arima_District_Health_Facility_DVIDS126489.jpg/1200px-USS_Kearsarge_medical_team_treat_patients_at_Arima_District_Health_Facility_DVIDS126489.jp.

10.3.1. Initial Assessment and Stabilization

In pediatric intensive care, early diagnosis and stabilization of sepsis patients are important in optimizing outcomes. It is achieved by a step-by-step process to evaluate hemodynamic stability, closely monitor vital signs, and find the presence of infectious foci. The Surviving Sepsis Campaign requires immediate interventions, such as intravenous fluid administration and administration of broad-spectrum antibiotics, to reduce the septic shock risks (Alhazzani *et al.*, 2017). The assessment also needs to be performed taking into account the patient's unique physiological and pathologic factors. Through the practice of evidence-based guidelines, in which timely intervention is stressed, medical professionals can ensure greater effectiveness in treatment regimens and eventually lead to higher survival rates among children with infection and sepsis (Chang *et al.*, 2017). Strict attention to initial evaluation and stabilization is one aspect of extensive management of critically ill child patients.

10.3.2. Fluid Resuscitation Protocols

Effective fluid resuscitation interventions are critical to the treatment of pediatric sepsis patients because they play a crucial role in restoring hemodynamic stability and improving overall therapy. Early aggressive fluid resuscitation is a foundational therapeutic strategy for sepsis and septic shock per the Surviving Sepsis Campaign Guidelines, calling for isotonic crystalloids initially as a method of increasing blood volume and cardiac output (Alhazzani *et al.*, 2017).

For the child patient, the Japanese Clinical Practice Guidelines further extend in their formation of these measures by taking into consideration the unique physiological responses among children and tailoring the recommendations to ensure these are catered to, thus offering improved-quality care to such vulnerable children (Kazuyoshi *et al.*, 2018). Not only do these guidelines assist in minimizing the risk of organ dysfunction, but they also assist in minimizing mortality rates among critically ill children. Thus, adherence to evidence-based fluid resuscitation practice remains critical in the intensive care of children in order to counteract the dangers posed by infectious disease and sepsis (Figure 10.12).

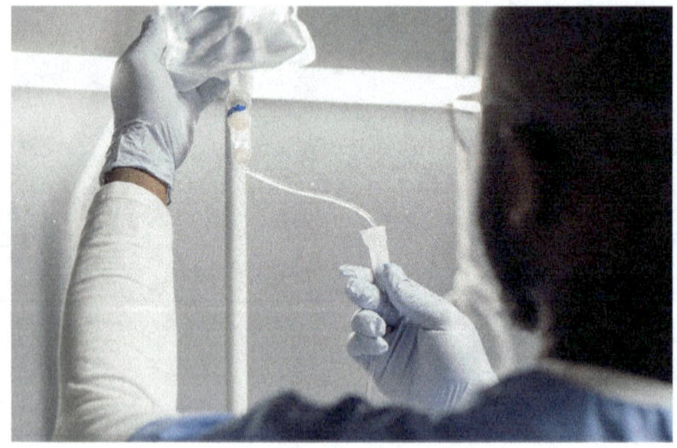

Figure 10.12. Effective fluid resuscitation protocols are paramount in managing pediatric patients with sepsis, as they are critical for restoring hemodynamic stability and improving overall outcomes.

Source: https://lotustotalcare.com/wp-content/uploads/2023/11/anesthesiologist-working-with-infusion-drip.jpg.

10.3.3. Antibiotic Therapy and Its Importance

The critical role played by antibiotic treatment in the management of infectious disease and sepsis in pediatric intensive care must not be overlooked. Early treatment with appropriate antibiotics dramatically improves outcome by means of effective antibacterial action and prevention of further dissemination of the infection. In pediatric patients, this is particularly significant since they may be challenging to diagnose because of the atypical presentation of the disease. Current guidelines call for tailoring antibiotic selection based on both pathogens' susceptibility patterns and the clinical context of the infection, e.g., intra-abdominal infections that typically require special treatment (Chang *et al.*, 2017). Moreover, frequent use of antibiotics can also lead to dysbiosis of the gut microbiota, potentially exacerbating nosocomial infections and complications such as sepsis (Knight *et al.*, 2016). Thus, while antibiotic therapy remains a cornerstone of therapy, careful attention must be given to its effect on the microbiome and patient outcomes in the pediatric intensive care unit.

10.3.4. Use of Vasopressors in Treatment

The management of sepsis in pediatric intensive care also frequently necessitates the use of vasopressors to support hemodynamics and ensure adequate perfusion to vital organs. The use of vasopressors such as norepinephrine and epinephrine in septic shock in children is perhaps pivotal in combating hypotension due to systemic vasodilation and septic capillary leak. Specifically, prompt vasopressor intervention has been found to be beneficial, highlighting the value of expedient assessment and treatment initiation in this at-risk group (Hadzhieva-Hristova *et al.*, 2025).

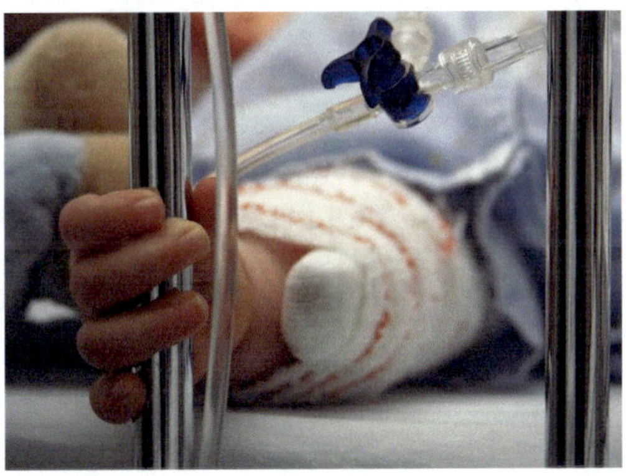

Figure 10.13. In children affected by septic shock, the administration of vasopressors such as norepinephrine and epinephrine can be critical in countering hypotension that arises from systemic vasodilation and capillary leak associated with septic processes.

Source: https://d148x66490prkv.cloudfront.net/hmp_ln/styles/max_1300x1300/s3/2021-11/2112%20Pediatric%20sepsis%20PALS%20guidelines%20EMS%20emergency%20medical%20services_0.jpg.

In addition, titration of these drugs must be carefully managed since aggressive administration may result in unwanted effects like end-organ ischemia. Increased awareness about sources of infection, especially in regard to the possibility of nosocomial infections like those from opportunistic pathogens like *Pluralibacter gergoviae*, highlights the importance of strict compliance with infection control practices in addition to pharmacological management in intensive care units (Abdulrahman Özel *et al.*, 2024) (Figure 10.13).

10.3.5. Monitoring and Supportive Care in PICU

Efficient supportive care and surveillance in the Pediatric Intensive Care Unit (PICU) is paramount for the treatment of sepsis and infectious diseases in children, given the unique problems associated with this high-risk group. Continued vigilance of such vital signs as heart rate, blood pressure, and oxygen saturation facilitates early recognition of the deterioration of a patient's condition. In particular, the use of early warning scores, such as the Oncological Pediatric Early Warning Score (O-PEWS), aids in identifying vulnerable patients by medical professionals, thereby enabling early intervention to decrease mortality and morbidity (Boscato *et al.*, 2023).

Besides, supportive therapy interventions, including resuscitation of fluids, nutrition therapy, and support ventilation by a number of different forms of ventilation, are central aspects of treatment for children with severe infections (Nielsen *et al.*, 2019). Consequently, the interaction of intensive monitoring and multimodal supportive management is of extreme significance in enhancing clinical outcomes and reducing PICU mortality rates for child patients with severe infectious illness.

10.3.6. Multidisciplinary Sepsis Management

The management of pediatric intensive care sepsis needs a multidisciplinary team to ensure the best outcome for the children affected. The collaboration of different healthcare providers like pediatric intensivists, infectious disease doctors, pharmacists, and microbiologists ensures a comprehensive approach in diagnosis and treatment. For example, the pharmacokinetics of antibiotics occurring in neonates and infants uniquely determine their effective use, requiring careful monitoring and customized dosing regimens (John *et al.*, 2018). In addition, recent emerging instances, such as Pediatric Inflammatory Multisystem Syndrome with COVID-19, highlight the need for cross-disciplinary agreement in clinical practices. Swiss pediatric specialists established best practice recommendations by consensus with the need for multidisciplinary input in delivering effective care in the various clinical presentations of sepsis (Aebi *et al.*, 2021).

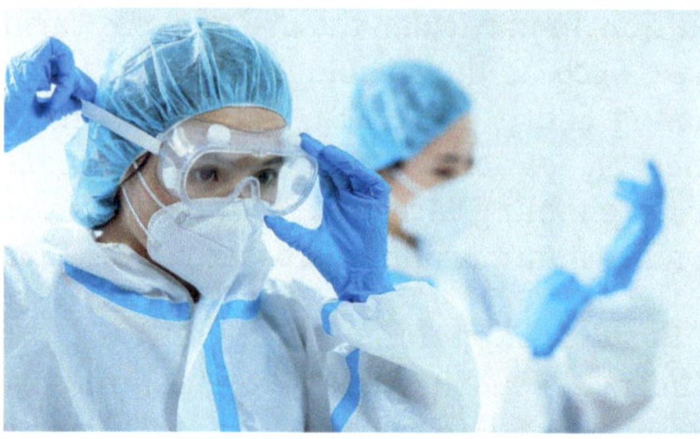

Figure 10.14. The collaboration of diverse healthcare professionals—including pediatric intensivists, infectious disease specialists, pharmacists, and microbiologists—ensures a comprehensive strategy for diagnosis and treatment.

Source: https://assets.isu.pub/document-structure/250523085243-23224b50443f7bb57835285882c9d57c/v1/3fa290b6d83bfcafaaf2db64fbb3a892.jpeg.

Shared knowledge not only enhances treatment outcomes but also facilitates continuous learning and adjustment to evolving evidence-based practices in the management of pediatric sepsis (Figure 10.14).

10.3.7. Role of Technology in Monitoring Sepsis

The use of technology in monitoring sepsis in pediatric intensive care units significantly enhances patient outcomes through timely interventions. Advanced monitoring systems, including continuous observation of vital signs and sophisticated diagnostic tools, enable early identification of sepsis symptoms, thus enabling early clinical response. For instance, the use of electronic health records and alert tools improves healthcare professionals' capacity to recognize deteriorating patient conditions through the delivery of real-time data and alerts upon attainment of critical thresholds. These technologies are also synergistic with Surviving Sepsis Campaign guidelines, which emphasize early detection and intervention in the management of severe sepsis, as delineated in many expert consensus guidelines. In addition, studies continue to support further development of such technologies to improve their efficacy and reliability and ultimately aid in the quality of treatment for vulnerable children patients battling infections (Antonelli *et al.*, 2013).

10.3.8. Challenges in Treating Sepsis in Children

Management of sepsis in children is faced with peculiar challenges that complicate care algorithms and outcomes. Children present with atypical presentations and abrupt clinical progression of disease that compromises early diagnosis, leading to late intervention. Children also come in a range of age groups with varied physiological responses to infection, necessitating tailored approaches in care and management. Current guidelines, such as those of the Surviving Sepsis Campaign, also place significant importance on early detection and treatment. Application in children, however, requires caution because the majority of the recommendations are primarily grounded on adult literature (Alhazzani *et al.*, 2017). In addition, advances in the management of intra-abdominal infections, as underscored by the Surgical Infection Society, highlight optimizing antimicrobial therapies and Source control among children (Chang *et al.*, 2017). Therefore, such advanced solutions are critical to improve sepsis outcomes in the pediatric intensive care setting among children (Figure 10.15).

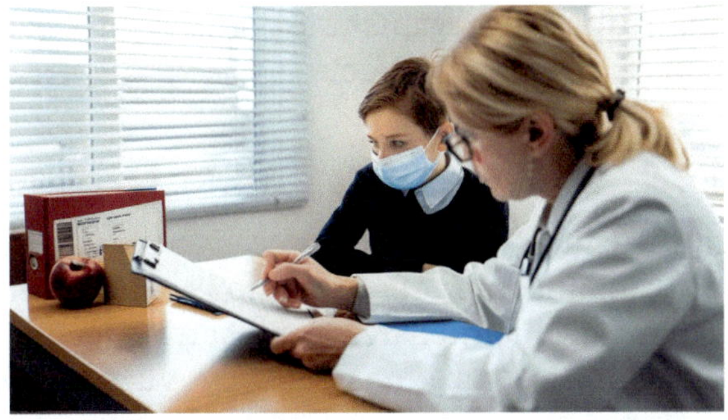

Figure 10.15. Pediatric patients often exhibit atypical symptoms and swift disease progression that can obscure initial diagnosis, leading to delays in appropriate intervention.

Source: https://davis-adams.com/wp-content/uploads/2025/01/Pediatric-Sepsis-Misdiagnosis.png.

Test Your Knowledge

1. What are the most appropriate empiric antibiotics for neonatal versus older pediatric septic patients?
2. What role do corticosteroids play in refractory pediatric septic shock?

10.4. Prevention Strategies for Infectious Diseases and Sepsis

Learning Outcome

1. Importance of Hand Hygiene.
2. Vaccination Programs and Their Impact.
3. Education for Healthcare Providers and Families.
4. Infection Control Measures in PICU.
5. Role of Nutrition in Preventing Infections.
6. Surveillance and Reporting of Infectious Diseases.
7. Community Health Initiatives.
8. Research and Development of New Vaccines.
9. Future Directions in Prevention Strategies.

Effective prevention measures of infectious illness and sepsis are particularly critical within pediatric intensive care units, particularly in light of the exceptional vulnerability of neonates and early children. Oral antibiotics were highly effective in reducing neonatal pneumonia mortality, as a meta-analysis showed reduced all-cause neonatal mortality (RR 0.75) when administered in community conditions (Bhutta *et al.*, 2011). Further, specialist advice is that injectable antibiotics, administered either at home or in the community, could potentially have even higher sepsis-specific reductions in mortality, at a conservatively estimated 65% when administered in the community (Bhutta *et al.*, 2011). Parallel to this, the use of vaccines, particularly those targeted against meningitic pathogens, has transformed bacterial meningitis epidemiology, sharply reducing incidence and improving clinical outcomes. The interplay of these intricate prevention measures underscores the importance of proper and timely interventions in the safeguarding of pediatric patients against the perils of infectious diseases and sepsis effects.

10.4.1. Importance of Hand Hygiene

Hand washing is a critical factor in preventing the transmission of contagious infections, particularly in intensive care settings where child patients are particularly vulnerable. Adherence to strict measures of hand washing can considerably lower the incidence of hospital-acquired infections, including those resulting from severe sepsis, which is a common and dangerous affliction among this population. There has been evidence that strict adherence to hand hygiene procedures on a regular basis significantly decreases the rates of infection, thereby improving patients' outcomes and reducing healthcare costs. In addition, ingraining a culture of safety into healthcare institutions fosters high compliance with such basic practices that prevention of infection becomes a priority goal of healthcare providers in their work.

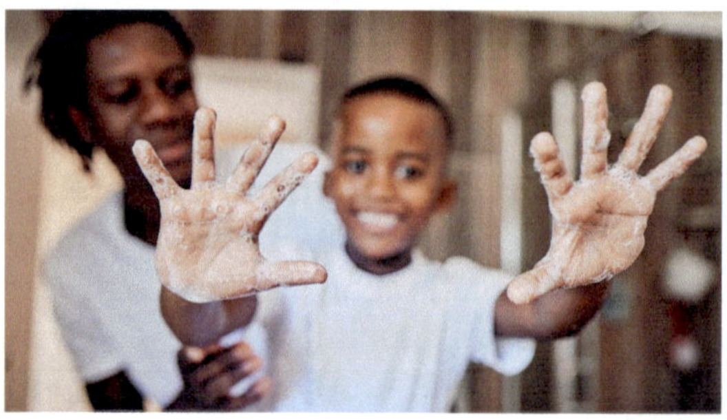

Figure 10.16. Hand hygiene is a critical component in preventing the transmission of infectious diseases, particularly in pediatric intensive care settings where patients are particularly vulnerable.

Source: https://www.cdc.gov/clean-hands/media/images/Untitleddesign2.png.

Through the enforcement of rigorous hygiene practices of hands, as proposed by the European Federation of Nurses Associations, clinicians can extend effective intervention in preventing vulnerable pediatric patients, as well as mitigating the impact of infectious diseases within intensive care units (Burke *et al.*, 2008) (Figure 10.16).

10.4.2. Vaccination Programs and Their Impact

The role of vaccine programs in reducing the transmission of infectious diseases, such as sepsis, in children cannot be exaggerated. The programs provide robust herd immunity, which has a significant impact of reducing the prevalence of preventable illnesses such as pneumonia and measles, which can lead to acute complications like sepsis. For instance, a trial in Brazil revealed that the establishment of universal primary care programs was associated with a considerable decrease in the incidence of sepsis, even though hospital sepsis mortality rates remained unacceptably high (Andrade *et al.*, 2011). This shows that while vaccination reduces infectious disease incidence as a whole, other health interventions must be pursued in order to lower mortality due to sepsis. In addition, as highlighted in the European experience, coordination in addressing awareness, prevention, and sepsis treatment is essential towards improving outcomes in pediatric patients (Jakob *et al.*, 2023).

10.4.3. Education for Healthcare Providers and Families

Proper education of healthcare workers and families is imperative in infectious disease control, and by extension, sepsis, in pediatric intensive care units. Due to the multisystemic presentation of sepsis, there has to be a proper understanding of recognition, response, and intervention strategies among health professionals. Training efforts must be focused on creating training on early detection and treatment guidelines for sepsis as recommended by the consensus recommendations of a Swiss policy workshop, which confirms the need for increased healthcare human resource training on sepsis care (Jakob *et al.*, 2023). Moreover, families also have a central role to play in the continuum of care and must therefore receive specialized educational resources that help them recognize early signs of infection and obtain proper medical attention. Both of these education strategies for both health providers and families result in a comprehensive framework for addressing the devastating impact of sepsis, ultimately reducing morbidity and mortality rates for vulnerable pediatric patients (Figure 10.17).

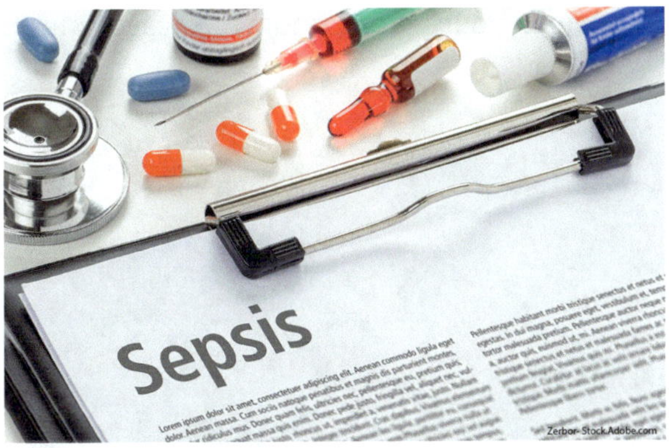

Figure 10.17. Effective education for healthcare providers and families is essential in the management of infectious diseases, particularly sepsis, within pediatric intensive care settings.

Source: https://www.the-hospitalist.org/wp-content/uploads/2024/08/AdobeStock_110860650-Zerbor_WEB.jpg.

10.4.4. Infection Control Measures in PICU

Infection control measures within the Pediatric Intensive Care Unit (PICU) are important in avoiding the development of sepsis and other infectious diseases among vulnerable pediatric patients. Some of these practices involve rigorous hand washing techniques, the use of personal protective gear, and rigorous methods of sterilizing medical equipment. Effective prevention of infection also depends on the use of evidence-based guidelines recognized for their significant function in standardizing care and enhancing patient outcomes. The Surgical Infection Society guidelines, for instance, emphasize the significance of Source control and early antimicrobial therapy in the treatment of intra-abdominal infections, elements of crucial significance in pediatric patients in an intensive care environment (Chang *et al.*, 2017). In addition, a qualitative Indian review cites shocking degrees of antimicrobial resistance, highlighting the necessity of strict antibiotic stewardship and infection control policies to tackle these problems effectively (India clen *et al.*, 2017). It is important to strengthen these guidelines for improved overall patient safety in the PICU.

10.4.5. Role of Nutrition in Preventing Infections

The role of nutrition in preventing infection among pediatric intensive care patients cannot be overestimated, as nutrition at optimal levels is essential to maintain immune status. Malnutrition in the critically ill child is prevalent and has been associated with risk of infection and sepsis, enormously complicating the recovery process. Evidence indicates that an optimal macronutrient and micronutrient intake not only maintains health-promoting gut microbiota growth but can also augment the immune status of the host, thereby reducing nosocomial infection rates (Knight *et al.*, 2016). Moreover, guidelines formulated for managing severe sepsis emphasize the importance of nutritional support and infection control as integral components of managing severe sepsis, highlighting the interplay between nutrition and overall patient outcome. Hence, inclusion of meticulous nutritional analysis and care in intensive care practice is pivotal to the minimization of infection hazards and optimization of recovery trajectories in children's intensive care units (Figure 10.18).

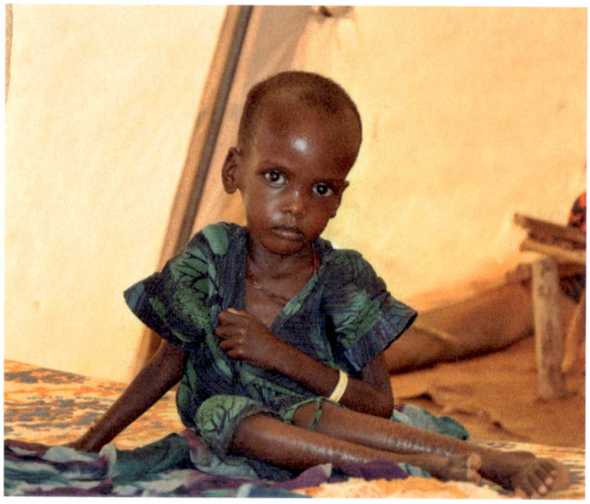

Figure 10.18. Malnutrition is prevalent in critically ill children and is associated with an increased risk of infections and sepsis, considerably complicating recovery strategies.

Source: https://upload.wikimedia.org/wikipedia/commons/3/39/A_malnourished_child_in_an_MSF_treatment_tent_in_Dolo_Ado.jpgs.

10.4.6. Surveillance and Reporting of Infectious Diseases

Effective surveillance and reporting of infectious diseases are important components in the administration of pediatric sepsis in intensive care unit settings. Monitoring patterns of antimicrobial resistance is particularly vital in light of the staggering rates noted in many populations. For example, research has indicated that overwhelmingly high resistance levels among common Gram-negative bacteria, that is, *Klebsiella pneumoniae* and *Escherichia coli*, are of grave concern for pediatric patients, with first-line therapy-resistant strains such as ampicillin being up to 95.9% for K pneumoniae (India clen *et al.*, 2017). Moreover, the occurrence of nosocomial infection in intensive care units is a testament to how much surveillance systems are needed, as seen through studies conducted in regions like Fiji, testifying to Gram-negative dominance as pathogens in such settings (Bissell *et al.*, 2016). This comprehensive monitoring not only informs treatment protocols but also assists antibiotic stewardship and infection control practices crucial for improving patient outcomes in pediatric intensive care units.

10.4.7. Community Health Initiatives

Community health programs play a crucial role in the prevention and control of infectious diseases and sepsis among pediatric populations, particularly in intensive care unit settings. These programs are focused on increasing public awareness, motivating preventive measures, and ensuring early access to healthcare centers.

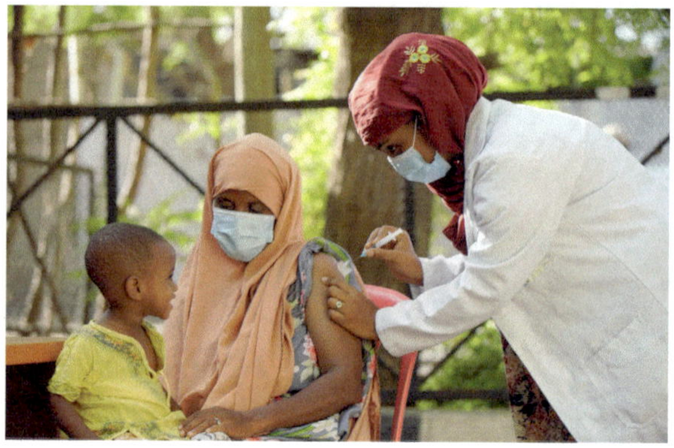

Figure 10.19. Community health initiatives play a pivotal role in addressing infectious diseases and sepsis within pediatric populations, particularly in intensive care settings.

Source: https://www.unicef.org/sites/default/files/styles/hero_extended/public/UN0446643.jpg.webp?itok=Tkas8cQl.

Through education and community involvement, these programs can tremendously reduce the number of severe infections among children, who are extremely vulnerable due to their underdeveloped immune systems. Epidemiological research indicates that sepsis is the most prevailing cause of death among children worldwide, which highlights the importance of specific interventions in pediatric settings in sepsis epidemiology and management

(McCulloh *et al.*, 2014). Apart from that, antimicrobial stewardship programs are integral components of community health initiatives that promote prudent use of antibiotics and evidence-based clinical behavior (Albrecht *et al.*, 2024). Therefore, collaborative action at the community level is needed to improve outcomes and resilience against infectious diseases in children (Figure 10.19).

10.4.8. Research and Development of New Vaccines

Ongoing research and development of new vaccines play a central role in the battle against infectious disease and sepsis, particularly in the pediatric intensive care unit. It is essential to combat the evolving nature of pathogens disproportionately affecting children, with recent vaccines playing a profound role in the disease epidemiology of conditions such as bacterial meningitis. For instance, the introduction of vaccines against common meningitic etiologic agents has led to dramatic declines in incidence rates, pointing towards the potential of emerging immunization technologies to enhance children's health outcomes (Janowski *et al.*, 2017). Furthermore, since children have a unique immunological profile, vaccine design should be modified to consider their age and health vulnerabilities (McCulloh *et al.*, 2014). By placing research on novel vaccine formulations at the top priority, the medical community promotes a proactive approach towards preventing infections and thereby reducing the sepsis burden as well as increasing survival rates among children.

10.4.9. Future Directions in Prevention Strategies

As pediatric intensive care becomes more advanced, prevention of infectious disease and sepsis in the future must aim for a multidisciplinary approach that encompasses early detection, targeted interventions, and enhanced patient care. Grounded on technological advancements in microbiological diagnostics, it will be possible to identify the pathogens at an early stage so that etiological therapy, which is usually superior to empirical therapy, can be established. This is crucial as most pediatric sepsis is caused by respiratory infections, as highlighted in recent studies (Hadzhieva-Hristova A *et al.*, 2025). Furthermore, continuous education and training of healthcare professionals on the new risk factors and clinical presentation are required to maximize outcomes in critically ill children. Implementation of new monitoring technologies can also facilitate early detection of sepsis and organ dysfunction, especially in high-risk populations such as acute liver failure, where etiology is often still multifactorial and complex (Georgy *et al.*, 2025).

Test Your Knowledge

1. What are the best practices for central line insertion and maintenance to prevent CLABSIs?
2. How can antibiotic stewardship reduce the risk of antimicrobial resistance in PICU settings?

SUMMARY

The potentially lethal problems infectious diseases and sepsis cause in intensive care units for children necessitate a long-term emphasis on research and improved clinical practice. The findings point to a disconcerting rate of infection in the hospital setting, which underscores the urgent need for effective infection control measures, especially considering that respiratory and bloodstream infections remain endemic in children (Bissell *et al.*, 2016). Further, the sudden emergence of carbapenem-resistant Enterobacteriaceae (CRE) poses an emergent public health threat that could potentially amplify infection severity described in intensive care units. Outcomes from complete cohorts, such as the EURECA study, will be imperative to develop risk factors and clinical outcomes related to these infections, thus guiding interventions as well as policy recommendations (Ferrer *et al.*, 2017). Treating these complex problems will far better the outcomes of pediatric patients, highlighting the necessity of multidisciplinary practices in today's medical practice.

In examining the complexities of sepsis and sepsis-like infectious diseases in pediatric intensive care, several pertinent observations emerge from recent investigations. Special challenges have been introduced during the COVID-19 pandemic, particularly regarding the presentation of severe acute respiratory syndrome coronavirus 2 (SARS-CoV-2) infection in children. While infections are normally mild or even asymptomatic, a more severe complication, multisystem inflammatory syndrome in children (MIS-C), can arise weeks later, with characteristics of high fever and extreme inflammation, somewhat comparable to Kawasaki disease (Consiglio *et al.*, 2020). This condition is a cause for vigilant follow-up of pediatric patients, as well as an examination of the distinctive immune responses at play. Additionally, the pediatric intensive care units (PICUs) have brought into perspective a relatively lower burden of COVID-19 in children compared to adults and emphasized the importance of customized treatment and care approaches in this susceptible group (Lara *et al.*, 2020). These findings are significant in the ongoing quest for enhanced outcomes in the context of pediatric critical care.

KEY TERMS FROM THIS CHAPTER

- Antimicrobial stewardship programs
- Infection
- Measles
- Postpartum
- Pathogens
- Tumors
- Hypotension
- Enterobacteriaceae
- Polymerase chain reaction (PCR)
- Sepsis
- Diarrhea
- Neonates
- Immune response
- Cardiac anomalies
- Intra-abdominal infections (IAI)
- Tachycardia
- Culture

CRITICAL THINKING QUESTIONS

1. **What is the most common cause of sepsis in neonates?**
   a. *Streptococcus pneumoniae*
   b. Group B Streptococcus
   c. *Neisseria meningitidis*
   d. *Escherichia coli*
2. **Which of the following is a key indicator of septic shock in pediatric patients?**
   a. High blood pressure
   b. Slow capillary refill time
   c. Normal lactate level
   d. Hypothermia only
3. **What is the first-line treatment for septic shock in a child?**
   a. Vasopressors
   b. Corticosteroids
   c. Broad-spectrum antibiotics and fluid resuscitation
   d. Mechanical ventilation
4. **Which of the following organisms is commonly associated with healthcare-associated infections in PICU?**
   a. *Haemophilus influenzae*
   b. *Pseudomonas aeruginosa*
   c. *Staphylococcus epidermidis*
   d. Enterovirus
5. **What is the most common site of infection leading to sepsis in children?**
   a. Gastrointestinal tract
   b. Skin and soft tissues
   c. Urinary tract
   d. Respiratory tract

Short Answer Questions

1. What are the most common infectious diseases leading to PICU admission in children?
2. How do viral and bacterial pneumonias differ in clinical presentation in pediatric patients?
3. What is the current pediatric definition of sepsis and septic shock?
4. What are the most common pathogens responsible for pediatric sepsis across different age groups?
5. What are the initial steps in the management of pediatric sepsis according to the Surviving Sepsis Campaign?
6. How is fluid resuscitation tailored in children with septic shock?
7. What vaccination strategies are essential for preventing severe infections in children?
8. How can hospital-acquired infections be reduced in the PICU?

Answers to Critical Thinking Questions

1. (b); 2. (b); 3. (c); 4. (b); 5. (d)

REFERENCES

1. Abramova, N., Avrusin, I., Kozlova, O., Firsova, L. A., Kuleshova, A. G., Kondratyev, G. V., Aleksandrovich, Y., *et al.* (2025). Analysis of risk factors for lethal outcome in patients of pediatric intensive care units with immuno-inflammatory diseases. *Messenger of Anesthesiology and Resuscitation*. https://www.semanticscholar.org/paper/3dbc80bca8f542b8eb3db8482aca2c4cc0508a90 (accessed on 30th June 2025).
2. Aebi, C., Agyeman, P., Albisetti, M., Andre, M., *et al.* (2021). Best practice recommendations for the diagnosis and management of children with pediatric inflammatory multisystem syndrome temporally associated with SARS-CoV-2 (PIMS-TS; multisystem inflammatory syndrome in children, MIS-C) in Switzerland. https://core.ac.uk/download/479290768.pdf (accessed on 30th June 2025).
3. Albrecht, B., Barber, K. E., Barfield, R. K., Bland, C., *et al.* (2024). A baker's dozen of top antimicrobial stewardship intervention publications in 2022. https://core.ac.uk/download/616959302.pdf (accessed on 30th June 2025).
4. Alhazzani, W., Angus, D. C., Annane, D., Antonelli, M., *et al.* (2017). Surviving Sepsis Campaign: International guidelines for management of sepsis and septic shock: 2016. https://core.ac.uk/download/286716214.pdf (accessed on 30th June 2025).
5. Andrade, M. C., Branchini, O. A., Carcillo, J., Kissoon, N., *et al.* (2011). Bacterial sepsis in Brazilian children: A trend analysis from 1992 to 2006. https://core.ac.uk/download/12212371.pdf (accessed on 30th June 2025).
6. Antonelli, M., Bonten, M., Cecconi, M., Chastre, J., *et al.* (2013). Year in review in intensive care medicine 2012. II: Pneumonia and infection, sepsis, coagulation, hemodynamics, cardiovascular and microcirculation, critical care organization, imaging, ethics and legal issues. https://core.ac.uk/download/29469432.pdf (accessed on 30th June 2025).
7. Aoyama, K., Azuhata, T., Doi, K., Matsuyuki, D., Egi, M., Fujimura, N., Fujishima, S., *et al.* (2018). The Japanese clinical practice guidelines for management of sepsis and septic shock 2016 (J-SSCG 2016). https://core.ac.uk/download/154950014.pdf (accessed on 30th June 2025).
8. Avakyan, G. A., Bykov, Y. V., & Obedin, A. N. (2025). Intensive care for acute liver failure in pediatric practice (Review). *General Reanimatology*. https://www.semanticscholar.org/paper/388a6ddfb4a78e349af5e4df977b4c2c37677177 (accessed on 30th June 2025).
9. Barbieri, E., Daverio, M., Donà, D., Giaquinto, C., *et al.* (2020). Implementation and impact of pediatric antimicrobial stewardship programs: A systematic scoping review. https://core.ac.uk/download/286270886.pdf (accessed on 30th June 2025).
10. Benoit, D., Lameire, N., Van Biesen, W., & Vanholder, R. (2016). Acute kidney injury in critically ill cancer patients: An update. https://core.ac.uk/download/55807820.pdf (accessed on 30th June 2025).
11. Berardi, A., Buttera, M., Di Martino, M., Frabboni, I., Insalaco, A., Lugli, L., Miselli, F., *et al.* (2022). Transmission of group B *Streptococcus* in late-onset neonatal disease: A narrative review of current evidence. https://core.ac.uk/download/566651279.pdf (accessed on 30th June 2025).
12. Bezrukov, L., Koloskova, O., & Vlasova, O. (2018). Diagnostic value parameters of acute phase reactance's of infectious-inflammatory process in diagnostics of early neonatal sepsis. https://core.ac.uk/download/301580762.pdf (accessed on 30th June 2025).

13. Bhutta, Z. A., Black, R., Cousens, S., Ganatra, H. A., *et al.* (2011). Effect of case management on neonatal mortality due to sepsis and pneumonia. https://core.ac.uk/download/13093714.pdf (accessed on 30th June 2025).

14. Bissell, K., Graham, S. M., Nabose, I., Naidu, S., *et al.* (2016). A descriptive study of nosocomial infections in an adult intensive care unit in Fiji: 2011–12. https://core.ac.uk/download/156651817.pdf (accessed on 30th June 2025).

15. Boscato, S. (2023). Risk factors and outcomes of oncohematologic patients admitted to pediatric intensive care unit: ONCOTIPNET, an Italian multicenter study. https://core.ac.uk/download/588606296.pdf (accessed on 30th June 2025).

16. Bradley, J. S., Cannavino, C. R., Coufal, N. G., Farnaes, L., *et al.* (2019). Community-acquired pneumonia in children: Cell-free plasma sequencing for diagnosis and management. https://core.ac.uk/download/323066460.pdf (accessed on 30th June 2025).

17. Ferrer Bravo, J., Gutiérrez Gutiérrez, B., Pascual Hernández, Á. (Coordinador), Rodriguez Baño, J., *et al.* (2017). EUropean prospective cohort study on Enterobacteriaceae showing REsistance to CArbapenems (EURECA): A protocol of a European multicenter observational study. https://core.ac.uk/download/299806525.pdf (accessed on 30th June 2025).

18. Burke, J., Smith, L. N., Sveinsdóttir, H., Willman, M., *et al.* (2008). Patient safety in Europe: Medication errors and hospital-acquired infections. https://core.ac.uk/download/90014.pdf (accessed on 30th June 2025).

19. Chang, P. K., Diaz, J. J., Jr., Huston, J. M., *et al.* (2017). The Surgical Infection Society revised guidelines on the management of intra-abdominal infection. https://core.ac.uk/download/74358329.pdf (accessed on 30th June 2025).

20. Consiglio, C. R., Cotugno, N., Sardh, F., Pou, C., Amodio, D., Rodriguez, L., Tan, Z., *et al.* (2020). The immunology of multisystem inflammatory syndrome in children with COVID-19. *Cell, 183*, 968–981.e7. https://doi.org/10.1016/j.cell.2020.09.016 (accessed on 30th June 2025).

21. Edmond, M. B., Seifert, H., Wenzel, R. P., Wisplinghoff, H., *et al.* (2006). Inflammatory response and clinical course of adult patients with nosocomial bloodstream infections caused by *Candida* spp. https://core.ac.uk/download/pdf/81937318.pdf (accessed on 30th June 2025).

22. Hadzhieva-Hristova, A., Stoeva, T., Niyazi, D., & Iotova, V. (2025). Clinical profile and etiological structure of diseases in children with septic and critical conditions hospitalized in a pediatric intensive care unit in Bulgaria: A single-center study. *Scripta Scientific Medica*. https://www.semanticscholar.org/paper/458bf92b5414976572c892ca536790b238a32f16 (accessed on 30th June 2025).

23. India Clen, Indian Council of Medical Research, INSAR Group, DeNIS Collaboration, National Centre for Disease Control, National Nosocomial Infections Surveillance System, *et al.* (2017). High reported rates of antimicrobial resistance in Indian neonatal and pediatric bloodstream infections. https://core.ac.uk/download/82918917.pdf (accessed on 30th June 2025).

24. Jakob, S. M., Meylan, S., Schlapbach, L. J., Stocker, M., *et al.* (2023). Swiss Sepsis National Action Plan: A coordinated national action plan to stop sepsis-related preventable deaths and to improve the support of people affected by sepsis in Switzerland. https://core.ac.uk/download/597777276.pdf (accessed on 30th June 2025).

25. Janowski, A. B., & Newland, J. G. (2017). From the microbiome to the central nervous system, an update on the epidemiology and pathogenesis of bacterial meningitis in childhood [version

1; referees: 3 approved]. https://core.ac.uk/download/80495074.pdf (accessed on 30th June 2025).

26. King, J., Lehrnbecher, T., Pana, Z. D., Steinbach, W. J., *et al.* (2017). Recognition and clinical presentation of invasive fungal disease in neonates and children. https://core.ac.uk/download/131024549.pdf (accessed on 30th June 2025).

27. Knight, R., McDonald, D., & Wischmeyer, P. E. (2016). Role of the microbiome, probiotics, and 'dysbiosis therapy' in critical illness. https://core.ac.uk/download/323065571.pdf (accessed on 30th June 2025).

28. Ma, X., Zhu, J., & Du, L. (2020). Neonatal management during the coronavirus disease (COVID-19) outbreak: The Chinese experience. *NeoReviews, 21*, e293–e297. https://doi.org/10.1542/neo.21-5-e293 (accessed on 30th June 2025).

29. McCulloh, R. J., & Randolph, A. G. (2014). Pediatric sepsis: Important considerations for diagnosing and managing severe infections in infants, children, and adolescents. https://core.ac.uk/download/28948161.pdf (accessed on 30th June 2025).

30. Meduri, G. U., & Schwingshackl, A. (2016). Rationale for prolonged glucocorticoid use in pediatric ARDS: What the adults can teach us. https://core.ac.uk/download/323079960.pdf (accessed on 30th June 2025).

31. Nielsen, J. S. A., Brierley, J., Dohna-Schwake, C., Krause, M., *et al.* (2019). PICU mortality of children with cancer admitted to pediatric intensive care unit: A systematic review and meta-analysis. https://core.ac.uk/download/227040533.pdf (accessed on 30th June 2025).

32. Özel, A., Kutlu, N. O., Yüce, S., Ozdalgicoglu, C., & Erol, M. (2024). Nosocomial sepsis triggered by *Pluralibacter gergoviae* in a pediatric intensive care unit: A case report and literature review. *Journal of Pediatric Infectious Diseases*. https://www.semanticscholar.org/paper/a0a6f72bc71a5ab903bfde43bf411f41081fbd32 (accessed on 30th June 2025).

33. Shekerdemian, L. S., Mahmood, N., Wolfe, K. K., Riggs, B. J., Ross, C. E., McKiernan, C., Heidemann, S. M., *et al.* (2020). Characteristics and outcomes of children with coronavirus disease 2019 (COVID-19) infection admitted to US and Canadian pediatric intensive care units. *JAMA Pediatrics, 174*, 868–868. https://doi.org/10.1001/jamapediatrics.2020.1948 (accessed on 30th June 2025).

34. van den Anker, J., Bielicki, J. A., Pfister, M., *et al.* (2018). Key components for antibiotic dose optimization of sepsis in neonates and infants. https://core.ac.uk/download/161866644.pdf (accessed on 30th June 2025).

TOXICOLOGY AND POISONING

11

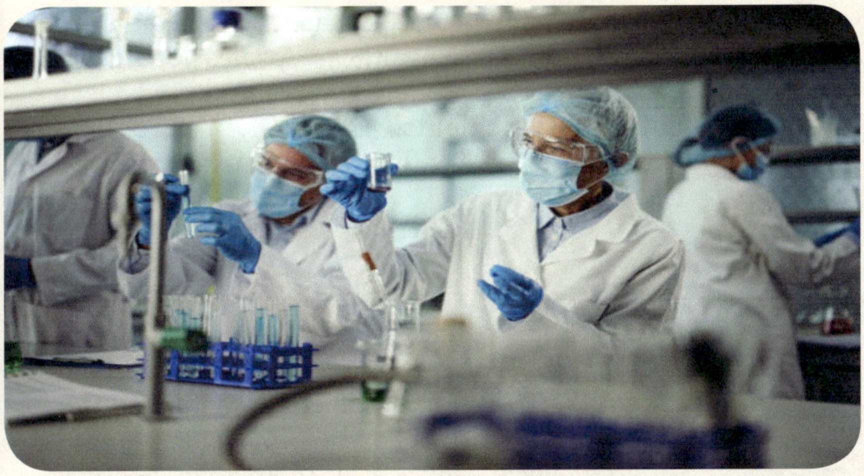

LEARNING OBJECTIVES

After studying this chapter, you will be able to:

1. Understand Types of Poisons and Their Effects.
2. Explain Diagnosis and Assessment in Pediatric Poisoning.
3. Describe Treatment and Management Strategies.
4. Focus on Prevention and Education.

Introduction

The prevalence of toxidromes in children necessitates the in-depth examination of poisoning and intensive care management. Children are particularly prone to poisoning due to their curiosity and the relative toxicity of agents in the smaller size of the child. This heterogeneity requires specialized protocols and treatments, particularly because some antidotes, like fomepizole in the instance of methanol poisoning, have been poorly evaluated for safety and efficacy in children, and especially in diverse populations like those in Taiwan (Chen *et al.*, 2016). Additionally, developments in therapies such as poisoning treatment through extracorporeal interventions continue to reflect the evolving nature of pediatric toxicology; however, evidence continues to be limited for these therapies, usually in the form of case reports rather than robust clinical trials (Anseeuw *et al.*, 2016). Therefore, a detailed analysis of these features becomes necessary for better outcomes and safe practices in the pediatric intensive care unit (Figure 11.1).

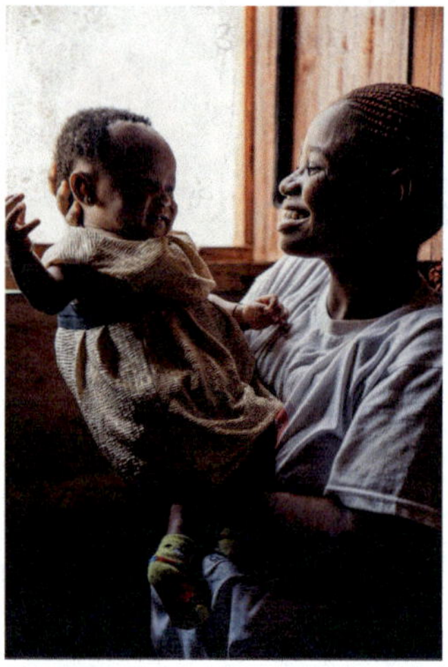

Figure 11.1. Children are uniquely vulnerable to poisoning due to their exploratory behavior and the relative toxicity of various substances in their smaller bodies.

Source: https://ceh.unicef.org/sites/default/files/2025-04/uni767615.jpg.

11.1. Types of Poisons and Their Effects

Learning Outcome

1. Classification of Poisons.
2. Common Household Poisons.
3. Pharmaceutical Overdoses.
4. Environmental Toxins.
5. Heavy Metals and their Impact.
6. Biological Toxins.
7. Chemical Agents in Poisoning.
8. Symptoms Associated with Different Poisons.
9. Long-term Effects of Poisoning.

Knowledge of the various types of poisons and their mechanisms is critical in pediatric intensive care because children are particularly sensitive to toxic exposure. Poisons can be from traditional drugs, such as opioids and cocaine, to newly emerging psychoactive drugs that can significantly alter neurological function. These drugs have a tendency to enhance neurotransmitter release or inhibit reuptake, eliciting severe physiological reactions that need prompt medical attention (Irwin *et al.*, 2013). Additionally, the large number of cases of pediatric poisoning underscores the need for targeted preventive measures and educational programs to protect populations at risk (Karpushkina *et al.*, 2022). The diversity of these cases is also compounded by the heterogeneity of substances with different toxicological profiles and treatment protocols. Identifying all these variables enables healthcare professionals to enact impactful, timely interventions against poisoning incidents, ultimately improving patient outcomes within the pediatric intensive care setting.

11.1.1. Classification of Poisons

Identification of the poison type is critical in pediatric intensive care, particularly with the unique susceptibilities of children to toxins. Poisons can be categorized in a number of different ways, such as by their Source—e.g., natural poisons, synthetic poisons, or industrial poisons—and by their mode of action, including neurotoxins, cytotoxins, and hemotoxins. Practically speaking, awareness of the poison type is crucial to optimal treatment and management.

For example, research indicates that certain drugs, like bath salts, exhibit extreme psychological and physical effects that need immediate medical attention and can lead to fatal outcomes in children (Cook *et al.*, 2015). Moreover, the toxicological profile of each poison assists medical staff in predicting possible complications and creates a treatment strategy on the basis of each individual case (Brophy *et al.*, 2005). A deeper understanding of these categories can enhance the quality of care that is being provided in pediatric intensive care units, ultimately producing better patient outcomes (Figure 11.2).

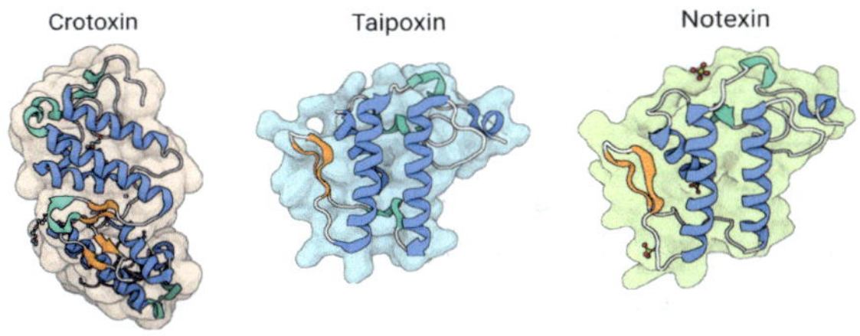

Figure 11.2. Poisons can be classified in various ways, including by their *Source*—such as natural, synthetic, or industrial poisons—and by their mechanism of action, which encompasses neurotoxins, cytotoxins, and hemotoxins.

Source: https://pub.mdpi-res.com/toxins/toxins-16-00012/article_deploy/html/images/toxins-16-00012-g007.png?1703581573.

11.1.2. Common Household Poisons

Household poisons are a serious problem in pediatric toxicology, particularly among the most susceptible age group of children younger than five years, to whom accidental exposure poses immediate dangers. Household poisons consist of ordinary items such as medicines, detergents, and even cigarette tobacco, which, when ingested internally, can be very dangerous. A backward look unveiled that 37.9% of the incidents of poisoning among children were caused by drugs and 32.0% caused by cigarettes, indicating the greatest need for effective preventive strategies (Elisavet *et al.*, 2023). Additionally, the documented increase in poison cases during the COVID-19 pandemic underscores the necessity of enhanced parental monitoring on safe storage of toxic substances within the home (Hampango *et al.*, 2015). Preventing the availability of such products and educating caregivers about the danger involved with household poisons is the most crucial action in preventing the danger involved, ultimately safeguarding children's health in pediatric intensive care units.

11.1.3. Pharmaceutical Overdoses

Pharmacologic overdoses represent a significant issue in pediatric intensive care and most often result from unintentional ingestion of improperly stored medications or confusion of medications with candy by children. Increased use and sophistication of prescription drugs have made such events more likely. Opiates and benzodiazepines, traditionally abused drugs, are most frequently implicated in such events and have produced severe toxicologic responses necessitating prompt medical attention. Notably, new psychoactive drugs, some of which were initially researched as medicines, have emerged as powerful villains, with complex pharmacodynamics that could pose difficulties for management (Abraham, 2013; Irwin *et al.*, 2013). For overdoses of some drugs, including phenytoin, extracorporeal therapies present a valuable option for detoxification despite the low incidence of serious adverse outcomes from these drugs (Anseeuw *et al.*, 2016). Thus, a thorough understanding of such toxicological problems is essential for effective prevention and treatment in pediatric populations (Figure 11.3).

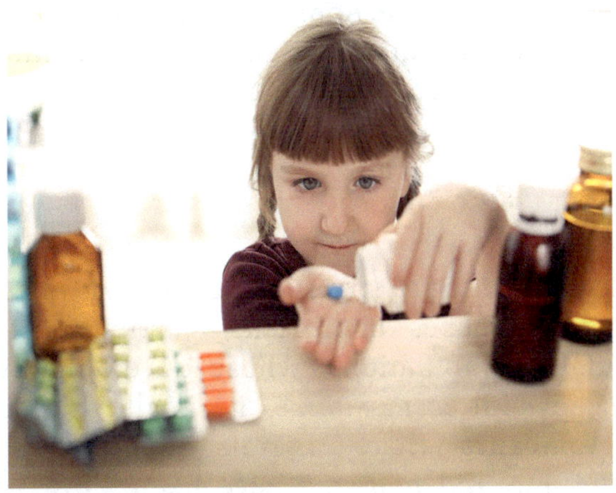

Figure 11.3. Pharmaceutical overdoses present a significant challenge in pediatric intensive care, often resulting from the accidental ingestion of medications that are improperly stored or perceived as candy by children.

Source: https://elitekingwood.com/wp-content/uploads/2022/06/ACCIDE1.jpg.

11.1.4. Environmental Toxins

In pediatric intensive care, increased awareness of environmental toxins poses significant challenges to medical professionals. Young children are particularly vulnerable to contaminants such as heavy metals, pesticides, and etiologic agents that can contaminate food and water supplies. These toxins have been found to cause acute health emergencies, augmenting the necessity of effective toxicological intervention. For instance, as the studies have documented, climatic variations can be the causative factor for the epidemics of waterborne conditions such as cholera and dysentery, particularly in places with no infrastructure to guarantee safe drinking water (Heaviside *et al.*, 2018). These situations once again emphasize the need for real-time monitoring and rapid response to environmentally exacerbated epidemics. Moreover, pediatric caregivers are increasingly needed to address cases of poisoning from both long-term exposure to toxins and acute poisonings, supporting the role of technology, such as the Antidote Application. The application assists with instant treatment recommendations in emergency conditions (Long *et al.*, 2016).

11.1.5. Heavy Metals and Their Impact

The ubiquitous situation of heavy metal exposure poses high risks, particularly to pediatric populations, whose developmental susceptibilities maximize the health impacts of toxicants. Heavy metals such as lead, cadmium, and mercury have been shown to produce various health impairments, including neurotoxicity and cognitive deficiency. These metals have been studied for long-term exposure and resultant DNA damage, additionally maximally contributing to their detrimental effects on human health (Baceva *et al.*, 2016). In pediatric intensive care, early detection and treatment of heavy metal poisoning are important because delayed treatment results in life-threatening complications (Long *et al.*, 2016). Antidote Application is a new technology that aims to improve toxicological emergency outcomes through timely, patient-specific antidote recommendations. This technological advancement is a significant step towards safeguarding vulnerable members of the population from the crafty dangers of heavy metal poisoning, thereby generally enhancing pediatric healthcare measures against cases of poisoning (Figure 11.4).

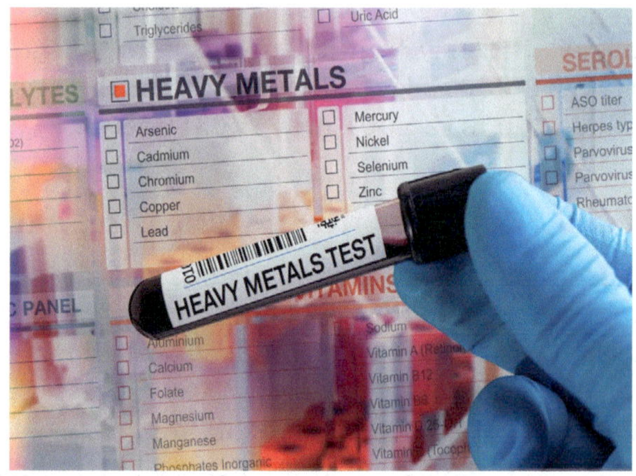

Figure 11.4. Metals such as lead, cadmium, and mercury have been linked to various health complications, including neurotoxicity and impaired cognitive development.

Source: https://www.eatthis.com/wp-content/uploads/sites/4/2022/12/heavy-metal-test.jpg?quality=82&strip=all.

11.1.6. Biological Toxins

Biological toxins are a dangerous risk among children's patients since the physiological characteristics of children amplify the toxic effects of the substances. The usual sources of biological toxins include plant toxins, bacterial toxins, and animal venoms, which are all capable of inducing severe health consequences among vulnerable groups. Prompt identification of toxin exposure is essential since delayed treatment can have life-threatening consequences. There has been the development of novel tools, such as the Antidote Application (AA), to address the urgent need for immediate and accurate therapeutic interventions in toxicological emergencies; the computer application automates patient-specific antidote recommendations and calculation of dose appropriate for various toxins (Long *et al.*, 2016). Moreover, the diagnostic problem presented by toxin-induced acute kidney injury (AKI) is further compounded in children and necessitates biomarkers capable of accurately representing nephrotoxicity as well as guiding effective management (Edelstein *et al.*, 2011). Enhancing such complexities is instrumental to optimizing outcomes in pediatric intensive care.

11.1.7. Chemical Agents in Poisoning

Chemical toxins in poisoning are harmful, especially in children, where exposure is the result of a mistake of ingestion or deliberate harm. Among these toxins, organophosphates (OPs) are a cause for concern as they are widely utilized as pesticides and have potential as chemical warfare agents. Acute OP poisoning can result in rapid and extensive neurological injury, and hence, early treatment is necessary. Studies indicate that despite existing antidotes to counteract acute life-threatening features, they are not effective in the therapeutic management of long-term neurological impairments of OP poisoning, necessitating research into optimal therapeutic regimens (FP *et al.*, 2016). In addition, the emergence of new psychoactive substances introduces the complexity of these agents not being addressed by conventional treatment algorithms and even precipitating acute toxic effects, which might require sophisticated interventions like intravenous lipid emulsion therapy (Irwin *et al.*, 2013). Hence, a pediatric intensive care unit with a multidisciplinary approach is crucial to manage effectively and enhance outcomes (Figure 11.5).

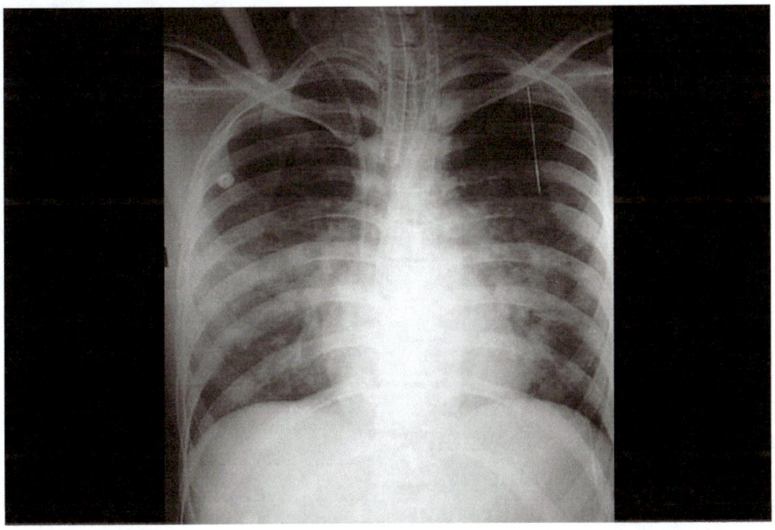

Figure 11.5. Chemical agents in poisoning pose significant risks, especially in the pediatric population, where exposure can result from both accidental ingestion and intentional harm.

Source: https://img.medscapestatic.com/pi/features/slideshow-slide/common-ingestions-6015019/fig%201.jpg.

11.1.8. Symptoms Associated with Different Poisons

Symptoms of different poisons in pediatric poisoning are likely to be varied and have a significant impact on patient outcomes when they are admitted to intensive care units. For instance, inhalation injury, which is likely to be caused by substances such as carbon monoxide and cyanide, is likely to cause nonspecific clinical presentations such as cardiovascular collapse, which needs instant and specific treatments to improve survival. Such symptoms are due to increased blood flow through the bronchial vessels and attendant airway obstruction, and therefore enhanced respiratory distress in the exposed children. The diagnosis of other toxins, such as heavy metals or organophosphates, presents with neurological impairment, gastrointestinal discomfort, or respiratory failure, and therefore diagnosis and treatment are complicated (Marks *et al.*, 2021). Recognizing such diverse symptoms is also vital for clinicians to administer immediate treatments, reduce morbidity, and address directly the particular issues of poisoning cases in intensive care among children. Because of this, toxicology knowledge not only helps in the identification of symptoms but also outlines particular therapeutic interventions.

11.1.9. Long-Term Effects of Poisoning

The long-term effects of poisoning among children can be serious, not only to their physical health but also to their psychological and developmental health. Tests have indicated that exposure to toxic substances could cause irreparable neurological deficits, learning disabilities, and behavioral disorders, which may need ongoing medical and psychological intervention (McCarthy *et al.*, 2004). Apart from that, the effects of such toxic exposure can not only be within the individual but also extend to family dynamics as well as to outcomes of community health, particularly in vulnerable populations (McDonald *et al.*, 2025). Early intervention and multidisciplinary care approaches are important in minimizing these effects; however, the heterogeneity of toxicant responses requires personalized therapeutic modalities and ongoing monitoring. With the advances of pediatric intensive care, emphasis should also be given to the integration of protocols addressing the long-term follow-up of poisoned children, proving the necessity for continuous research and collaboration between the medical staff. An improved outcome depends on recognizing the deep impact of poisoning and fostering resilience among poisoned children (Figure 11.6).

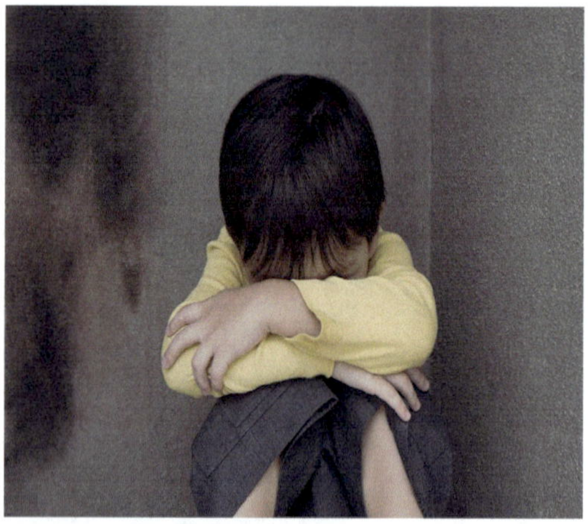

Figure 11.6. The long-term effects of poisoning in children can be profound, impacting not only their physical health but also their developmental and psychological well-being.

Source: https://www.verywellmind.com/thmb/B2PdzhetjgkgKV2rgffty2GfJRk=/1500x0/filters:no_upscale():max_bytes(150000):strip_icc()/GettyImages-80487462-59833fb6d088c000112fcc2c.jpg.

Test Your Knowledge

1. What clinical signs are associated with organophosphate (cholinergic) poisoning?
2. How does hydrocarbon ingestion (e.g., lamp oil, gasoline) typically present in children?

11.2. Diagnosis and Assessment in Pediatric Poisoning

Learning Outcome

1. Initial Assessment Protocols.
2. Importance of History-taking.
3. Physical Examination Techniques.
4. Laboratory Tests for Toxicology.
5. Imaging Studies in Poisoning Cases.
6. Role of Toxicology Screens.
7. Use of Clinical Scoring Systems.
8. Challenges in Diagnosing Pediatric Poisoning.

Accurate diagnosis and assessment of pediatric poisoning are critical components of the treatment of poisoned children who present to pediatric intensive care units (PICUs). Because of the unique physiological differences between children and adults, the diagnostic process should be carefully charted in consideration of age-specific signs and symptoms. Symptoms tend to be nonspecific in a majority of cases, and in some may aggravate the clinical picture, thus necessitating appropriate history-taking and examination as mandatory. Monitoring is imperative because the progression of poisoning can be unanticipated, leading to unavoidable complications that will prolong hospitalization and have a negative impact on outcomes (Ciomaga *et al.*, 2019). Moreover, extensive examination of toxic plasma levels can enhance diagnostic accuracy, providing information on the severity of intoxication and informing treatment decisions (Andresen *et al.*, 2012). Hence, a multidisciplinary strategy involving both clinical expertise and sophisticated diagnostic resources is needed to maximize treatment and enhance prognoses in pediatric patients experiencing bouts of poisoning.

11.2.1. Initial Assessment Protocols

The first assessment criteria in the pediatric case of poisoning are critical to ensuring prompt and effective intervention in the pediatric intensive care unit. Presentation in the pediatric patient should have an extensive history obtained in the form of the drug taken, the dose, and the time of intake. This enables clinicians to establish an immediate plan with a focus on stabilizing critical functions as well as controlling any life-threatening complications. As explained in existing literature, the unpredictable nature of poisoning necessitates constant monitoring to detect and address potential declines in a timely fashion (Ciomaga *et al.*, 2019). Furthermore, high levels of emergency department service quality will likely make a significant difference to patient satisfaction, which means that these first impressions should also concentrate on communication and responsiveness to family concerns (Baqir *et al.*, 2014). Ultimately, a rigorous initial evaluation process not only enhances clinical outcomes but also generates confidence and reassurance in concerned caregivers and parents (Figure 11.7).

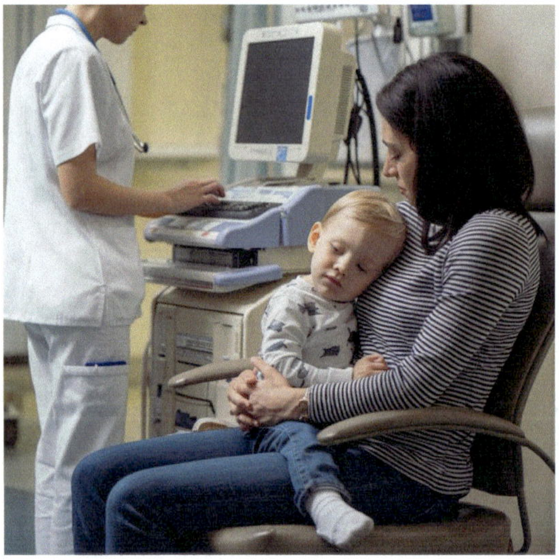

Figure 11.7. The initial assessment protocols in the context of pediatric poisoning are critical for ensuring timely and effective intervention in the pediatric intensive care setting.

Source: https://i0.wp.com/iem-student.org/wp-content/uploads/2024/12/a-photo-of-a-1-and-a-half-year-old-boy-the-immage-was-produced-by-using-ideogram-2.0.jpeg?fit=656%2C656&ssl=1.

11.2.2. Importance of History-Taking

Proper history-taking is a critical component of the pediatric patient's treatment process when they present with toxicology or poisoning due to its foundation for the clinicians. The history obtained in depth unravels significant information such as the type of substance, exposure time, and any pre-existing medical condition that influences treatment choice. Clarification of the above factors is important, particularly in cases where immediate intervention is required, for example, in severe phenytoin toxicity, which is surprisingly responsive to extracorporeal removal methods, irrespective of the interference that high protein binding has (Anseeuw *et al.*, 2016). Also, taking history aids in the identification of potential electrolyte imbalances that can exacerbate complications, for example, seizures, which are classically related to sodium disturbances, hypocalcemia, and hypomagnesemia (Badshah *et al.*, 2015). Thus, meticulous history-taking not only guides timely clinical intervention but also facilitates long-term care of children in pediatric intensive care units.

11.2.3. Techniques of Physical Examination

In pediatric intensive care, the application of whole physical examination techniques is most crucial in toxicology and poisoning cases. The procedure of examination not only assists in on-spot evaluation of the status of the child but also serves as a foundation for planning further interventions. Clinicians apply an organized sequence, beginning with a screening for vital signs and responsiveness, followed by a detailed examination for signs such as altered consciousness, respiratory distress, or gastrointestinal symptoms that indicate poisoning episodes.

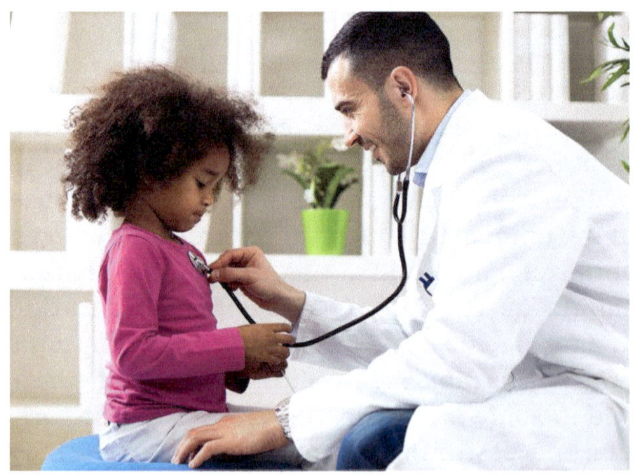

Figure 11.8. In pediatric intensive care, the application of thorough physical examination techniques is paramount when evaluating cases of toxicology and poisoning.

Source: https://media.post.rvohealth.io/wp-content/uploads/2020/08/physical-examination_thumb-1-732x549.jpg.

According to recent literature, physical examination findings guide the classification of poisonings, varying significantly from accidental ingestion to complex, purposeful exposures (Ciomaga *et al.*, 2019). Furthermore, the skillset required to appreciate pediatric patients' clinical presentations is nuanced, and therefore, there exists an imperative for practitioners to be proficient in these approaches for optimizing patient outcomes in the high-stakes PICU setting (University VC, 2018) (Figure 11.8).

11.2.4. Laboratory Tests for Toxicology

In pediatric intensive care, toxicology laboratory tests are central to the diagnosis and treatment of cases of poisoning. Such tests, especially in the form of rapid urinary drug screens, have a significant impact on patient management, especially in emergency situations where speed in decision-making is paramount. Research highlighted that targeted urinary drug testing in patients presenting with specific high-risk conditions, such as acute respiratory failure and severe overdose of opioids, improved the therapeutic intervention in a high percentage of cases, leading to improved patient outcomes (Erdmann *et al.*, 2015).

Furthermore, the unpredictability of poisoning development in children necessitates careful monitoring and rapid intervention, which highlights the importance of these laboratory investigations within a pediatric intensive care unit (PICU) environment (Ciomaga *et al.*, 2019). Consequently, the implementation of toxicological testing not only facilitates the identification of substances involved but also enables more effective management plans directed towards stabilizing and preserving damaged younger patients.

11.2.5. Imaging Studies in Poisoning Cases

Imaging studies play an important role in pediatric poisoning cases for the diagnosis and management of toxicological emergencies. X-rays and CT scans are valuable radiographic techniques to detect foreign bodies, ascertain the grade of internal injury, and search for the impact of specific toxic substances. For instance, certain drugs like opioids induce respiratory depression, which may need emergency treatment based on imaging findings in many cases (Ebrahimi *et al.*, 2015). In addition, in cases of severe drug toxicity, for example, lidocaine, imaging allows for the evaluation of cardiac function and enhances decisions in intensive care in the case of complications, for example, seizures (Elmi *et al.*, 2018).

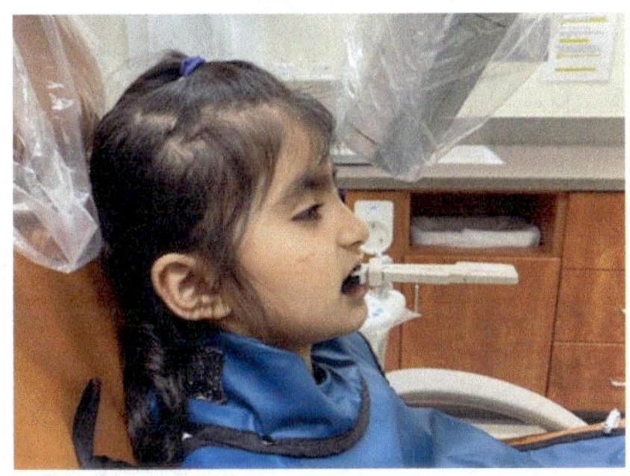

Figure 11.9. Radiographic techniques, including X-rays and computed tomography (CT) scans, are invaluable for identifying foreign bodies, assessing the extent of internal damage, and detecting specific toxic agents' effects.

Source: https://images.ctfassets.net/u2qv1tdtdbbu/2AarOKI90UxNchIZPAWOr6/4e17eb9f5f2129e91412b4a62bd3edb6/ce63-fig-9_png.jpg.

Because the child patient is prone to the toxic effects of poisoning, the use of advanced imaging modalities enhances the accuracy of diagnosis and treatment and ultimately enhances patient outcomes in intensive care. Emphasis on the integration of imaging into the management plans would further increase the effectiveness of toxicology interventions in such emergent cases (Figure 11.9).

11.2.6. Role of Toxicology Screens

Toxicology screens are of critical value in pediatric intensive care, particularly when handling potential drug overdoses or toxic exposures. Toxicology screens provide expedient and useful information that has the potential to affect medical decision-making and treatment plans. In an emergency department setting, for example, with approximately 40,000 annual admissions, studies demonstrated that targeted use of urinary drug screens could be extremely influential in inpatient care, with over one-third of tests influencing therapeutic management, diagnostic workup, or monitoring (Erdmann *et al.*, 2015). Such findings are especially relevant in the case of acute respiratory distress or altered mental status, typically seen in severe presentations of pediatric illness. Moreover, awareness of the determinants of pediatric fatal trauma and toxicology factors can also aid in the development of prevention strategies. Inferences of such research may also guide care pathways and promote proactive care in the prevention of trauma, with major importance laid upon toxicology screens for the optimization of pediatric care outcomes (Ellingsen *et al.*, 2009).

11.2.7. Clinical Scoring Systems Use

The use of clinical scoring systems in pediatric intensive care units (PICUs) plays a key role in the management of toxicological emergencies, mostly in the instance of poisoning. The scoring systems facilitate the identification and evaluation of a patient's clinical status at an early stage in order to enable medical professionals to categorize severity and determine the treatments. As referred in the literature, the unpredictability of poisoning evolution renders necessary monitoring and treatment in a timely fashion, thereby rendering scoring essential (Ciomaga *et al.*, 2019). Furthermore, among disproportionately affected populations, the systems have the ability to identify patients who could potentially be at higher risk according to determinants that are environmental and social, thus the need to target healthcare resources and interventions appropriately (Hynes *et al.*, 2012). By applying clinical scoring systems to daily practice, PICUs can maximize patient care on an individual basis as well as reduce systemic inequalities in healthcare access and response, thus maximizing overall efficacy of toxicological management (Figure 11.10).

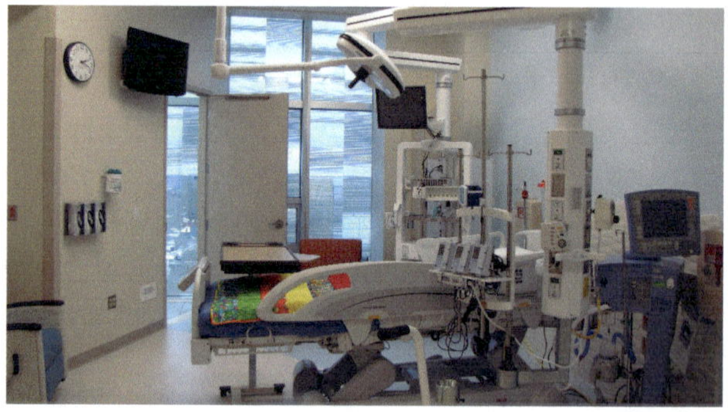

Figure 11.10. The use of clinical scoring systems in pediatric intensive care units (PICUs) plays a crucial role in the management of toxicological emergencies, especially concerning poisoning cases.

Source: https://upload.wikimedia.org/wikipedia/commons/7/7c/Helen_DeVos_Children%27s_IMG_0454_%285246843158%29.jpg.

11.2.8. Challenges in Diagnosing Pediatric Poisoning

Diagnosis of child poisoning is fraught with numerous difficulties that can complicate clinical management and outcomes. The differential nature of children, particularly their metabolic processes and body responses, can lead to an uncharacteristic presentation of the toxic effect in comparison to adults. For example, cannabinoids possess variable pharmacokinetics among children due to the immaturity of gastrointestinal and metabolic systems of their bodies, which affects bioavailability and symptom intensity upon ingestion (Brancato *et al.*, 2025). Furthermore, the spontaneity and variability of the episodes of poisoning, like accidental ingestion of drugs, demand a strong level of suspicion from clinicians. The diagnostic process is also likely to be hampered by symptom heterogeneity and the need for confirmatory testing, such as in the case of bath salt psychosis, where confirmation via lab tests is not always feasible (Cook *et al.*, 2015). These conditions thus put emphasis on highly skilled practitioners capable of addressing such complexities in pediatric critical care.

Test Your Knowledge

1. How can toxidromes be used to narrow the differential diagnosis in poisoned children?
2. What role do serum drug levels play in diagnosing acetaminophen or salicylate poisoning?

11.3. Treatment and Management Strategies

Learning Outcome

1. Immediate Care Protocols.
2. Decontamination Methods.
3. Antidotes and their Applications.
4. Supportive Care in Intensive Care.
5. Role of Activated Charcoal.
6. Use of Intravenous Fluids.
7. Monitoring and Follow-up Care.
8. Multidisciplinary Approach to Treatment.
9. Ethical Considerations in Treatment.

Successful treatment and management of pediatric intensive care toxicological conditions rely on an interconnected system based on the individual needs of each child. One of the most important factors is the selection of appropriate pharmacological interventions, which can have a dramatic effect on outcomes. For instance, recent studies have established that levetiracetam (LEV) yields positive results as an alternative to phenobarbital (PB) in neonatal seizures, an indicator that the trend is leaning towards the use of newer and more effective drugs in high-risk patients (Barbagallo *et al.*, 2019). Furthermore, the use of multidisciplinary teams provides end-to-end care that takes into account not only the physiological but also the psychological well-being of the child. With the employment of advanced monitoring techniques and patient-specific treatment protocols, clinicians are well-equipped to deal with the complexity of pediatric toxicity. Such interventions are not only important for acute clinical stabilization but also for long-term developmental outcomes, thus highlighting the imperatives of continuous evaluation and adjustment of treatment protocols for pediatric intensive care (Aristarán *et al.*, 2016).

11.3.1. Immediate Care Protocols

In poisoning and toxicology, the immediate care protocols are crucial in the Pediatric Intensive Care Unit (PICU). The protocols are intended for the timely stabilization, evaluation, and monitoring of poisoned patients due to the challenges posed by pediatric cases of poisoning. Staff knowledge and high-tech medicine are essential in optimizing patient outcomes by the early detection of complications and timely interventions (Ciomaga *et al.*, 2019). Rodenticide intoxications, for example, present certain challenges, as evidenced by inconclusive findings regarding compounds such as brodifacoum and bromadiolone. It has been observed that early referral and care plans tailored to the individual needs of the patient significantly improve survival rates and prognosis (Weng *et al.*, 2013). Therefore, effective immediate care protocols must incorporate continuous training of care providers and attending physicians and organizational strategies aimed at life support and vigilant monitoring of vital signs in poisoned children (Figure 11.11).

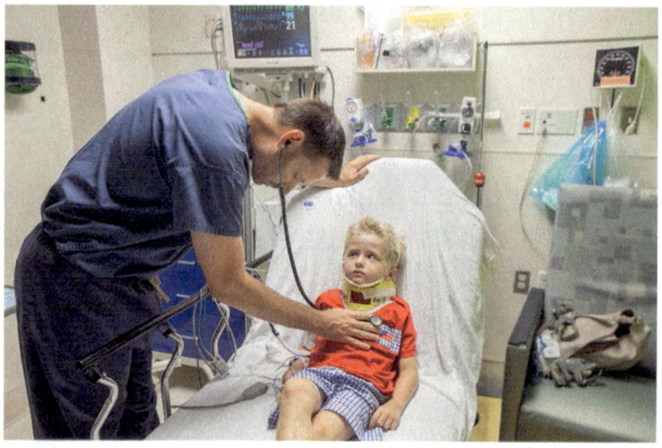

Figure 11.11. Immediate care protocols are critical in the Pediatric Intensive Care Unit (PICU).

Source: https://musckids.org/-/sm/news-center-media/news-center-images/2019-images/08/pruitt.jpg?h=666&w=1000&la=en&hash=95EF5FFC6D28929CC0B02B40F0C0548F.

11.3.2. Decontamination Methods

In pediatric intensive care, effective decontamination processes are instrumental in the management of toxic exposures in children. Decontamination planning varies significantly with the type of toxin; for instance, in phenytoin poisoning, extracorporeal modalities such as intermittent hemodialysis can be utilized based on the moderate dialyzability of the drug and potential severe toxicity, particularly in comatose states of prolonged duration (Anseeuw *et al.*, 2016). In addition, the spectrum of rodenticides is diverse, the two being frequently used in clinical practice being brodifacoum and bromadiolone, which require special decontamination protocols. The presentation of patients with brodifacoum poisoning will typically be severe coagulopathy and can be managed with vitamin K, while bromadiolone poisoning can be managed with earlier referral to avoid complications (Weng *et al.*, 2013). Thus, awareness of the nuances is essential to facilitating the betterment of such pediatric poisoning outcomes.

11.3.3. Antidotes and Their Uses

Antidote usage in pediatric intensive care is a critical branch of toxicology, particularly in the initial management of poisoning. Because of the inherent vulnerability of children, efficacy and timely application of antidotes can significantly alleviate life-threatening outcomes.

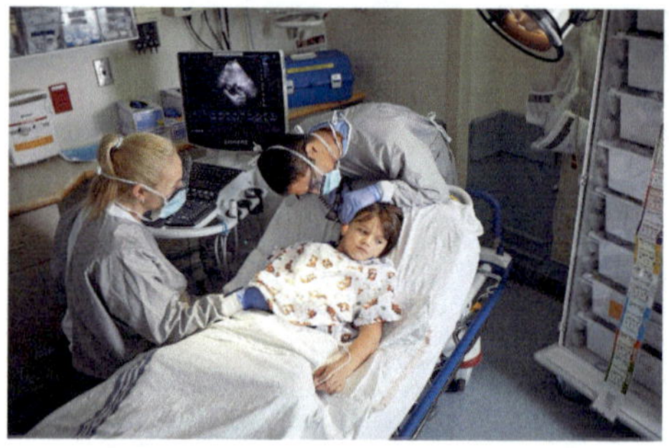

Figure 11.12. The application of antidotes in pediatric intensive care units is a critical aspect of toxicology, particularly in the timely treatment of poisoning.

Source: https://news.christianacare.org/wp-content/uploads/2018/12/pediatric-emergency.181112CC-0405.jpg.

For instance, during organophosphate poisonings, the use of established antidotes stabilizes patients and reduces neurological damage that may arise following exposure (FP *et al.*, 2016). Besides, enhanced technology has seen the establishment of resources like the Antidote Application (AA), which supports clinical decision-making through rapid antidote recommendations and correct dosing calculations for individual patients (Long *et al.*, 2016).

These innovations point not just to having accessible and effective antidotes but to being able to readily access the proper information so that healthcare providers can offer timely interventions. Thus, these devices plug the key gaps in the treatment process and increase survival rates in cases of pediatric toxicology (Figure 11.12).

11.3.4. Supportive Care in Intensive Care

In pediatric intensive care units (PICUs), supportive therapy is the key to the management of cases of toxicology and poisoning, maximizing recovery and reducing the risk of long-term complications. The treatment protocol is too complex for it to require a single approach, requiring instead a multidisciplinary approach by combining pharmacological treatment with round-the-clock medical support.

For instance, the creation of new formulations for opioid addiction treatment, such as the sublingual film version of buprenorphine + naloxone (Suboxone®), highlights the importance of effective and timely treatment while guaranteeing safety in children (Ling *et al.*, 2011). Additionally, advancements in technology, such as the Antidote Application (AA), facilitate rapid decision-making through the provision of tailored antidote recommendations and dose calculations, which are crucial in toxicological emergencies where time is of the essence (Long *et al.*, 2016). Thus, the interaction of novel treatment modalities and supportive care interventions is crucial in determining outcomes of children with poisonings.

11.3.5. Activated Charcoal Role

Activated charcoal is at the core of the management of toxic ingestions in pediatric intensive care units (PICUs) and is a key intervention for preventing the absorption of most poisonings. This is due to its vast surface area and porosity, whereby it is able to adsorb a wide variety of toxic substances and thereby lower their bioavailability. With the seriousness of child poisonings, which is usually progressive and acute with clinical deterioration, the timely administration of activated charcoal may be lifesaving by preventing further systemic absorption of the toxins. Of particular note is its administration in the setting of certain drugs, where standard treatment measures may fall short (Ciomaga *et al.*, 2019). Although its use is to be applauded, that of activated charcoal must also be reserved, since it is contraindicated in some circumstances, such as a change in level of consciousness or ingestion of caustic substances (Anseeuw *et al.*, 2016). Thus, whereas activated charcoal remains a pillar of toxicology, usage within pediatric practice must have the appropriate balancing of clinical conditions (Figure 11.13).

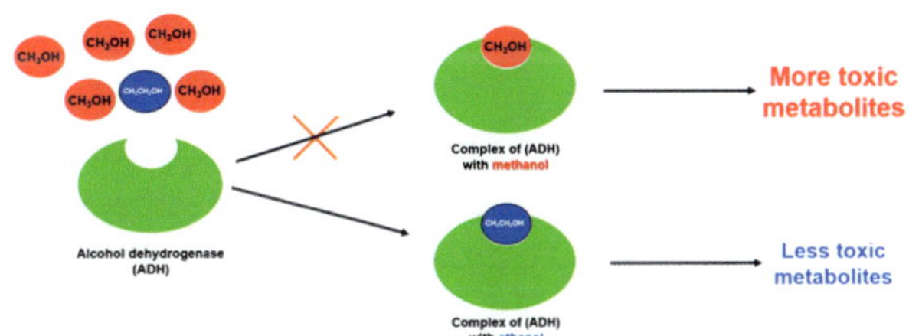

Figure 11.13. Activated charcoal plays a pivotal role in the management of toxic ingestions in pediatric intensive care units (PICUs), serving as a critical intervention for mitigating the absorption of various poisons.

Source: https://pub.mdpi-res.com/toxics/toxics-11-00723/article_deploy/html/images/toxics-11-00723-g001.png?1692794121.

11.3.6. Use of Intravenous Fluids

In pediatric emergency situations of toxidromes, IV fluids are equally important in stabilization as well as treatment. IV fluids play a vital role in correcting disturbances of electrolytes, maintaining hydration, and preserving renal function during episodes of poisoning, particularly in the context of the pediatric intensive care unit (PICU). Provision of the appropriate fluids has the ability to reverse the adverse impacts of toxins, enhance clearance, and ultimately improve patient outcomes. As a case point, in cases of severe phenytoin intoxication, prudent administration of IV fluids and fluidics has been found to be critical in placing the patient on the nod for extracorporeal therapies, as noted in the recommendation of intermittent hemodialysis to provide toxin clearance (Anseeuw *et al.*, 2016). In addition, ongoing monitoring in the PICU is critical, as it enables the healthcare team to rapidly evaluate the efficacy of fluid therapy and make necessary adjustments, thus recognizing complications that might occur throughout the treatment (Ciomaga *et al.*, 2019).

11.3.7. Monitoring and Follow-up Care

Tracking and follow-up in pediatric intensive care are critical components in the successful management of toxic exposure. The reasons for this are that poisoning cases are volatile and prone to unexpected complications, necessitating immediate action. Advanced monitoring technology, in combination with the medical staff's experience, offers a method of continuous monitoring of essential functions, which directly influences the outcome of the patient. For instance, in methanol poisoning, although it is uncommon among children, it can result in complicated outcomes when diagnosed late; therefore, initiating therapies such as fomepizole plays an essential role in inhibiting the production of toxic metabolites (Chen *et al.*, 2016). Moreover, effective monitoring processes are also essential to ensure prompt identification of complications, thereby reducing hospital stay and improving survival rates (Ciomaga *et al.*, 2019). Thus, the proper systematic monitoring and follow-up treatment process does make a big difference in managing poisoned children in intensive care units (Figure 11.14).

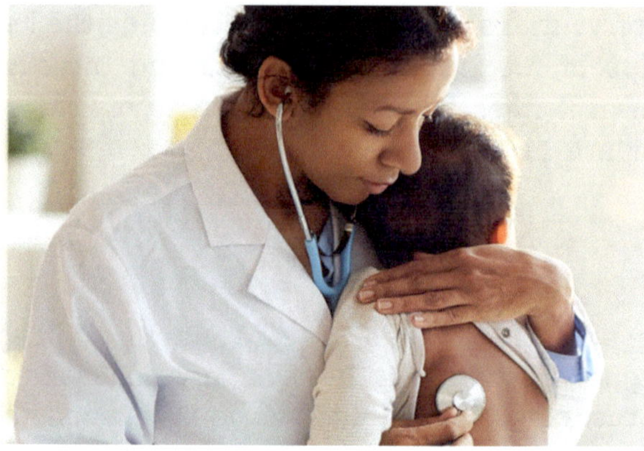

Figure 11.14. Close vigilance is necessary due to the unpredictable nature of poisoning cases, which can lead to sudden complications, necessitating prompt intervention.

Source: https://www.ucsfbenioffchildrens.org/-/media/project/ucsf/ucsf-bch/images/clinic/hero/pediatric-intensive-care-unit-2x.jpg?rev=38d1afce020b46c98601f75382afd152.

11.3.8. Multidisciplinary Approach to Treatment

In pediatric intensive care, particularly where toxicology and poisoning are concerned, a multidisciplinary approach is critical in achieving maximum patient outcomes. This model brings together the expertise of emergency physicians, medical toxicologists, nurses, and other experts to deal with the complexity of children's toxic exposure in a holistic manner. For instance, the sentinel roles of emergency medicine and medical toxicology are exemplified in cases of overdose, where prompt identification and treatment can make a significant difference in outcomes. In one such case, timely antidote therapy and vigorous supportive management were most critical in preparing for potential organ donation in a dual diagnosis involving a gunshot wound and an acetaminophen overdose (Albertson *et al.*, 2010). Furthermore, the use of advanced interventions like extracorporeal membrane oxygenation (ECMO) in life-threatening drug intoxications, such as bupropion overdose, shows the necessity of adopting a team approach while treating life-threatening ailments effectively (Awuah *et al.*, 2024).

11.3.9. Ethical Considerations in Treatment

In pediatric intensive care, particularly when referring to toxicology and poisoning cases, ethical problems emerge when formulating treatment. Doctors need to navigate intricacies in problems, where the equilibrium between coercive intervention and the quality of life of the abused child is strained. Such circumstances call for a delicate appreciation of patient autonomy, parents' rights, and the impacts of treatment at the end of life. Experts are now advocating more interdisciplinary interventions that ensure ethics and social responsibility in treatment processes, as argued in recent research emphasizing such a move in medical training (Tyler *et al.*, 2008). Moreover, care for vulnerable patients, such as infants with life-limiting illnesses, emphasizes the importance of compassionate care and ethical sensitivity. The delivery of palliative interventions, in an ethical manner, guarantees that both the physical and emotional needs of the family and child are well met (Ryskamp *et al.*, 2010) (Figure 11.15).

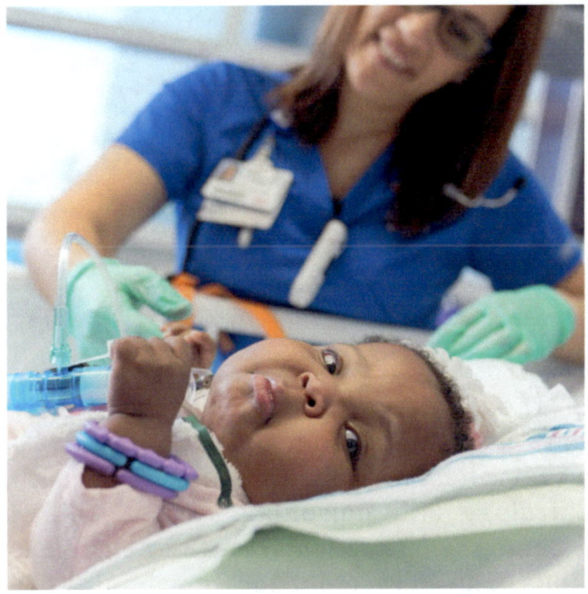

Figure 11.15. Medical professionals must navigate complex dilemmas, where the balance between aggressive intervention and the quality of life for the affected child is often precarious.

Source: https://res.cloudinary.com/baptisthealth/image/upload/ar_1:1,c_fill,f_auto,q_auto,f_webp,fl_lossy/WolfsonChildrens/SupportingServices/20171106_ss_picu-porthole.jpg.

Test Your Knowledge

1. What is the role of naloxone in managing opioid poisoning in children?
2. When should hemodialysis be considered in a poisoned pediatric patient?

11.4. Prevention and Education

Learning Outcome

1. Importance of Public Awareness.
2. Strategies for Poison Prevention.
3. Role of Healthcare Providers in Education.
4. Community Resources and Support.
5. Parental Education on Poison Safety.
6. School-based Prevention Programs.
7. Legislative Measures for Toxin Regulation.
8. Impact of social media on Awareness.
9. Future Directions in Prevention Efforts.

In the context of pediatric intensive care, prevention and education must be overemphasized, particularly regarding toxicology and poisoning. Acute pediatric poisoning being a common cause for emergency admissions, targeted educational initiatives must be implemented in families and caregivers. Studies have proven that most cases of poisoning involve easily accessible items at home, and thus the application of appropriate measures of prevention, tailored to specific categories, that is, the 2-5 years age group, which is extremely vulnerable to such accidents (Ebrahimi *et al.*, 2015). Furthermore, widespread educational campaigns are required to promote the health risks of chemical poisoning because this has the potential to lead to a wealth of serious developmental issues, including learning disability and respiratory disease (Hitchcock *et al.*, 2011). This way, communities will be able to mitigate the occurrence of poisoning and optimize children's overall safety.

11.4.1. Importance of Public Awareness

Public health plays a crucial role in preventing and managing pediatric poisoning, a critical public health problem in intensive care unit settings. Children are particularly vulnerable as nearly half of poison exposures occur among children below six years of age, which underlines the importance of effective public education concerning harmful substances and storage (Basilicata *et al.*, 2024).

Additionally, knowledge of symptoms and the potential for severe exposure can prompt earlier medical attention, which is essential in these emergent conditions where time is critical. In response to rising numbers of adolescent self-poisoning, knowledge of the dangers of medication, such as bupropion and its increased morbidity compared with other antidepressants, is necessary (Froberg *et al.*, 2019). By giving parents and caregivers information regarding potential poisons and what to do, we can make the whole setting safer for kids, ultimately reducing morbidity and mortality rates of toxic exposures in the pediatric intensive care unit (Figure 11.16).

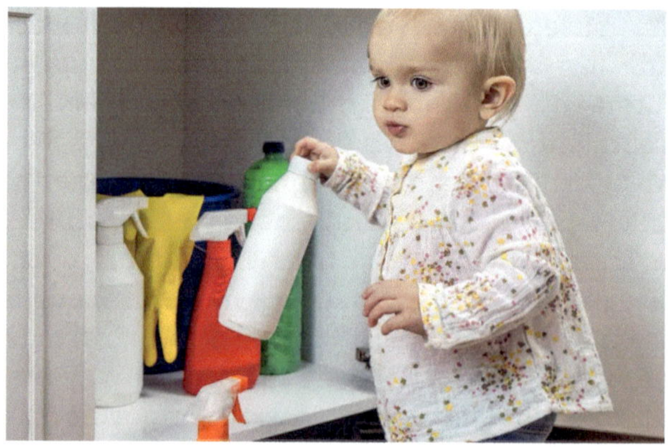

Figure 11.16. Public awareness plays a crucial role in preventing and managing pediatric poisoning, which remains a significant health concern in intensive care settings.

Source: https://img.lb.wbmdstatic.com/vim/live/webmd/consumer_assets/site_images/article_thumbnails/BigBead/child_poisoning_bigbead/1800x1200_children_poisoning_bigbead.jpg?resize=750px:*&output-quality=75.

11.4.2. Strategies for Poison Prevention

Effective poison prevention strategies are needed in pediatric practice, particularly in view of the alarming figures of accidental child poisoning. Education and awareness campaigns within families are necessary, as the majority of poisonings occur at home and from easily accessible household chemicals. For instance, a report noted that 23% of the reported cases of poisoning were caused by household chemicals, and at the top of the list were corrosives and organic solvents. Besides, preventive measures such as the application of child-resistant packaging for domestic products and medications can simply reduce the risk of accidental ingestion. Besides these precautions, physicians need to advise parents to keep in close contact with Poison Control Centers, especially in cases of suspected exposure. Contact with such centers can help in assessing the situation and suitable actions (Ebrahimi *et al.*, 2015). Ultimately, the solution requires an interdisciplinary strategy involving education, regulation, and support systems in safeguarding children's populations from the risk of poisoning.

11.4.3. Role of Healthcare Providers in Education

In pediatric intensive care, the educational function of healthcare professionals extends outside the clinical setup, with a significant influence on the outcome of cases of poisoning and toxicology. It is the mandate of healthcare workers, nurses, and physicians to provide necessary information on the prevention and management of exposure to poison to parents and guardians. Through the provision of information to families about home poisons and appropriate medication practices, physicians are central in mitigating risk from child poisoning. Furthermore, educational interventions can potentially increase public awareness and preparedness, particularly during disasters as emphasized in the present consensus conferences of experts targeting this all-encompassing issue (Garrett *et al.*, 2009). The incorporation of strict education measures in pediatrics not only provides a team-based pattern of handling health but also empowers families, ultimately leading to the prevention of toxicological emergencies (Figure 11.17).

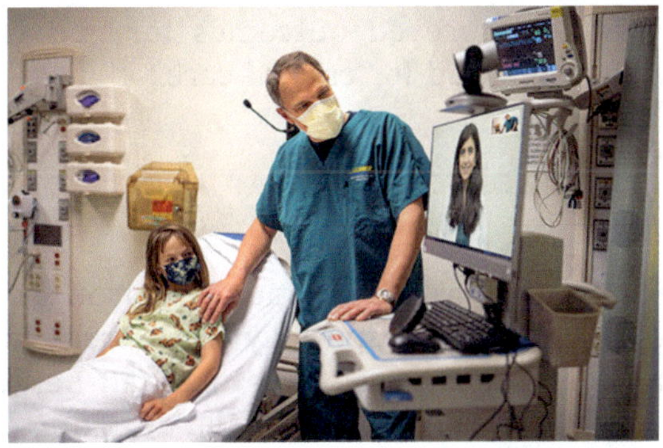

Figure 11.17. Healthcare professionals, including nurses and physicians, are responsible for disseminating critical information about the prevention and management of poison exposure to parents and caregivers.

Source: https://health.ucdavis.edu/media-resources/children/images/Promo/PICU_Telehealth.jpg.

11.4.4. Community Resources and Support

Effective pediatric cases of toxicology in intensive care settings are often reliant on strong community support systems and resources. These are very important in lessening the effects of toxic exposure, particularly among underprivileged communities that could be disproportionately affected. Societies that have social inequalities and restricted access to medical care tend to show increased susceptibility to poisoning episodes, for the most part as a result of factors like poor preparedness and diminished recovery capacity (Hynes *et al.*, 2012). These gaps should be filled through efforts directed at strengthening local healthcare infrastructure. Integrative initiatives, such as designing tools like the Antidote Application, are capable of making toxicologic emergency response more effective by providing quick, personalized treatment recommendations to reduce treatment delays (Long *et al.*, 2016). By strengthening support systems within the community, clinicians can render the toxic exposure response more efficient, ultimately leading to improved outcomes for pediatric patients admitted for critical care.

11.4.5. Parental Education on Poison Safety

The parent education function in poison safety is very important, especially in the reduction of risk from toxic exposures that can be very dramatic to the child's health and development. Parents need to be well-versed in recognizing potential hazards and the correct actions to take during emergencies. Research indicates that exposure to toxicity could be responsible for various health issues, including learning disorders and behavioral disorders, thus calling for effective education programs for caregivers (Hitchcock *et al.*, 2011).

Moreover, uncomplicated approaches, such as the use of pictograms to relay medication information, can enhance understanding and compliance among parents even if the existing evidence about their impact is limited (Chan *et al.*, 2016). Through the encouragement of an informed reaction to poison safety, parents are able to improve the safety of environments, eventually reducing the incidence of poisoning among children and improving pediatric intensive care outcomes. This kind of education forms a significant component of ongoing preventive measures in health care (Figure 11.18).

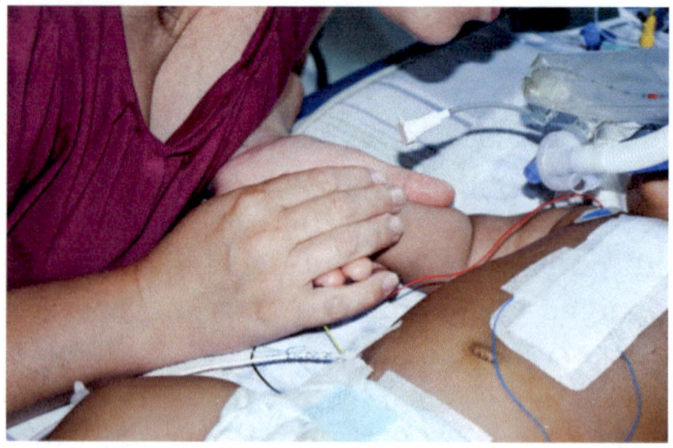

Figure 11.18. The role of parental education in poison safety is paramount, especially in mitigating risks associated with toxic exposures that can severely impact children's health and development.

Source: https://prakashhospitalgn.com/wp-content/uploads/2024/09/Paediatric-Intensive-Care-1.png.

11.4.6. School-Based Prevention Programs

The use of school-based prevention programs is an emergent measure in the management of toxic exposure and episodes of poisoning among children, particularly in pediatric intensive care. These programs not only seek to educate students on safety issues regarding toxic substances but also promote healthier environments that lower risk. By promoting awareness of risks such as exposure to lead, schools are able to prepare a preventive approach beforehand. Centers for Disease Control and Prevention puts special importance on primary prevention in their lead poisoning guidelines, advocating for collaboration between educational and healthcare sectors. Besides, an attention to environmental justice, as noted by Hynes *et al.* (2012), further underscores the importance of intersectoral community-based prevention that engages schools in affected communities. Such combined efforts can significantly reinforce protective factors, ultimately putting a cap on the frequency of tox-related emergencies among children's populations.

11.4.7. Legislative Measures for Toxin Regulation

In intensive care among children, the necessity for tight legislative controls over toxin regulation cannot be overstated. Children being very vulnerable to the adverse effects of toxins, policies for the regulation of hazardous substances are essential in maintaining their well-being. Regulation of the sale and distribution of hazardous substances has become a pressing need to reduce the risk of exposure. For example, legalizing adult marijuana use, as captured in Colorado's Amendment 64, has brought along both public health benefits and risks, including increased health visits and poison center calls following commercialization (Chilukuri *et al.*, 2017). Further, integrating poison center data with syndromic surveillance systems facilitates early detection of possible public health threats, thereby informing timely intervention (Law *et al.*, 2016). In the end, successful legislative efforts need to ensure the health and welfare of at-risk populations, and especially children, so that the problems caused by toxic environmental agents in pediatrics are reduced (Figure 11.19).

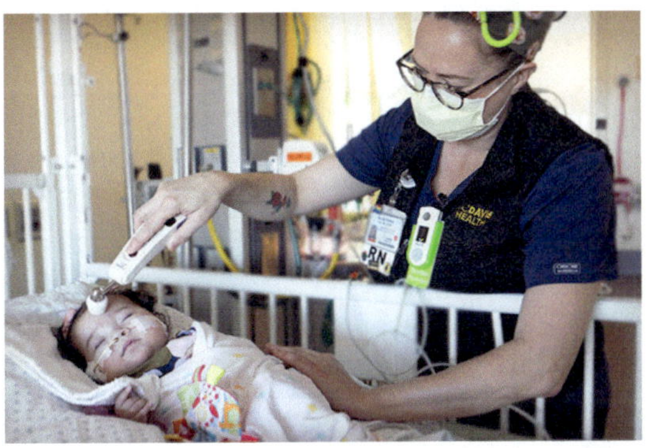

Figure 11.19. As children are particularly vulnerable to the adverse effects of toxins, policies aimed at regulating hazardous substances play a crucial role in safeguarding their health.

Source: https://health.ucdavis.edu/media-resources/children/images/Marquee/PICU-nurse-with-infant.jpg.

11.4.8. Impact of Social Media on Awareness

The extensive coverage of social media has made a significant contribution to the public awareness profile for pediatric toxicology and poisoning. Social media platforms like Twitter and Facebook offer critical channels for the sharing of information on the risks posed by materials present within homes, thereby creating enhanced levels of awareness for caregivers and parents. Such initiatives are significant as they can be used to achieve a reduction in the incidence of accidental poisoning cases.

For instance, campaigns initiated on social media can reach a large audience effectively, allowing rapid communication of important information about prevention and first-response in cases of pediatric poisoning. It is evident that more interaction with social media correlates to greater awareness and learning about important health matters, including toxic exposures (Chilukuri *et al.*, 2017). Also, social media can become a valuable means of bridging families with care structures and resources and building well-informed communities that can respond efficiently to crises.

11.4.9. Future Directions in Prevention Efforts

With pediatric intensive care increasingly confronted by the complexities of toxicology and poisoning, future prevention efforts need a multidisciplinary approach that combines technology, education, and healthcare policy reform. Simulation techniques, as referred to by Katsaliaki and Mustafee, offer possible alternatives for educating healthcare professionals in the detection and handling of cases of poisoning (Amoako-Gympah *et al.*, 2011). Also, consistent focus on mental health programs is required, especially in the context of the state of self-harm behavior among young people, which entails high risks for poisoning.

By keeping direct observation and anticipatory interventions as the priority, healthcare systems can develop robust structures that not only address immediate cases but also develop resilience in vulnerable populations (Luster *et al.*, 2017). Finally, the implementation of these strategies in practice can create a more preventive and responsive pediatric intensive care environment that considerably minimizes the risks of toxic exposures.

Test Your Knowledge

1. How can child-resistant packaging reduce the incidence of pediatric poisonings?
2. What are the most effective educational strategies to prevent medication errors in children?

SUMMARY

The complexity of poisoning and toxicology in pediatric intensive care demands a complete understanding of both acute and chronic consequences following exposure. The need for targeted therapy approaches is emphasized by recent evidence that conditions such as phenytoin poisoning require careful assessment of extracorporeal therapy modalities, as evidenced by the outcomes of the EXTRIP Workgroup showing that phenytoin is dialyzable to a moderate extent and should inform clinical advice in severe cases (Anseeuw *et al.*, 2016). Further, the long-term neurologic effects of organophosphate poisoning highlight the necessity for ongoing research on effective treatments to reverse the sustained increase in calcium and prevent neurologic impairment, as established by recent survival studies in rat models (FP *et al.*, 2016). Thus, the development of the pediatric toxicology specialty needs a conceptual framework to integrate short-term care methods with prolonged therapeutic expertise in order to improve aggregate patient outcomes in this high-risk population.

In addressing the basic problems of pediatric intensive care-based toxicology and poisoning, certain noteworthy issues come up that highlight the necessity of rapid intervention and decision-making. Harmful chemical exposure can exert a damaging influence on children's health and development, as well as result in different adversities such as learning disabilities and behavior disorders, for which immediate action by healthcare professionals is needed (Hitchcock *et al.*, 2011). Further, 0.8% of emergency department visits annually due to poisonings necessitate timely intervention measures among the child population (Long *et al.*, 2016). Innovation was involved in the development of new technologies such as the Antidote Application, which is a reflection of an effective response to existing needs through the provision of prompt, patient-specific antidote recommendations and antidote dosing calculation. This application not only hastens the clinical response time in instances of toxicologic emergencies but also helps to minimize medication errors, hence providing improved outcomes for vulnerable pediatric patients.

KEY TERMS FROM THIS CHAPTER

- Poisoning
- Antidotes
- Methanol poisoning
- Opioids
- Natural poisons
- Industrial poisons
- Prescription
- Phenytoin
- Heterogeneity
- Fomepizole
- Pediatric toxicology
- Cocaine
- Synthetic poisons
- Benzodiazepines
- Opiates
- Cholera

CRITICAL THINKING QUESTIONS

1. **What is the most common cause of pediatric poisoning requiring ICU admission?**
   a. Iron overdose
   b. Acetaminophen (paracetamol) toxicity
   c. Organophosphate ingestion
   d. Carbon monoxide poisoning
2. **What is the antidote for acetaminophen toxicity?**
   a. Naloxone
   b. Atropine
   c. N-acetylcysteine (NAC)
   d. Flumazenil
3. **A child presents with miosis, bradycardia, and bronchorrhea. What is the most likely cause?**
   a. Anticholinergic poisoning
   b. Opioid overdose
   c. Organophosphate poisoning
   d. Benzodiazepine overdose
4. **What is the most appropriate initial step in the management of a child with suspected poisoning?**
   a. Start antidote therapy
   b. Gastric lavage
   c. Secure airway, breathing, and circulation (ABCs)
   d. Administer activated charcoal immediately
5. **What is the primary clinical concern with iron overdose in children?**
   a. Seizures
   b. Cardiotoxicity
   c. Hepatic necrosis
   d. Renal failure

Short Answer Questions

1. What are the most commonly ingested toxic substances in pediatric patients?
2. How do iron and acetaminophen toxicity differ in onset, symptoms, and systemic effects?
3. What is the initial approach to a child presenting with unknown poisoning?
4. What are the key components of a pediatric toxicology history and physical exam?
5. What are the first steps in stabilizing a child with suspected toxic ingestion?
6. When is activated charcoal indicated, and what are its contraindications?
7. What are the key components of poisoning prevention education for parents and caregivers?
8. How can safe storage practices reduce accidental poisonings at home?

Answers to Critical Thinking Questions

1. (b); 2. (c); 3. (c); 4. (c); 5. (c)

REFERENCES

1. Albertson, T. E., Daily, M. F., Daubert, G. P., Owen, K., *et al.* (2010). Multiple organ transplantation after suicide by acetaminophen and gunshot wound. https://core.ac.uk/download/pdf/8518615.pdf (accessed on 30th June 2025).
2. Amoako-Gympah, K., Dexter, F., England, W., Hay, J. W., Katsaliaki, K., Murphy, K. M., Mustafee, N., *et al.* (2011). Applications of simulation within the healthcare context. https://core.ac.uk/download/12824593.pdf (accessed on 30th June 2025).
3. Anderson, K. R., Ellsworth, M. A., Freese, D. K., Hall, D. E., *et al.* (2014). Acute liver failure secondary to niacin toxicity. https://core.ac.uk/download/206157380.pdf (accessed on 30th June 2025).
4. Andresen, H., Iwersen-Bergmann, S., Schmoldt, A., Schulz, K., *et al.* (2012). Therapeutic and toxic blood concentrations of nearly 1,000 drugs and other xenobiotics. https://core.ac.uk/download/14525457.pdf (accessed on 30th June 2025).
5. Anseeuw, K., Burdmann, E. A., Ghannoum, M., Gosselin, S., *et al.* (2016). Extracorporeal treatment in phenytoin poisoning: Systematic review and recommendations from the EXTRIP workgroup. https://core.ac.uk/download/46963583.pdf (accessed on 30th June 2025).
6. Aristarán, M., Guevara, M. R., Hartmann, D., Hidalgo, C. A., *et al.* (2016). The Research Space: Using the career paths of scholars to predict the evolution of the research output of individuals, institutions, and nations. http://arxiv.org/abs/1602.08409 (accessed on 30th June 2025).
7. Awuah, K. F., Cheema, T., Modugula, S., Patel, S., *et al.* (2024). From crisis to recovery: A case report and literature review of early extracorporeal membrane oxygenation and esophagogastroduodenoscopy intervention in a patient with extended-release bupropion overdose. https://core.ac.uk/download/613230135.pdf (accessed on 30th June 2025).
8. Baceva, K., Gjorgieva Ackova, D., Kadifkova-Panovska, T., Stafilov, T., *et al.* (2016). Approach to detect possible genotoxic effects of metals in plants. https://core.ac.uk/download/45414795.pdf (accessed on 30th June 2025).
9. Badshah, M., Irshad, M., Jamil, U., Janjua, Z., *et al.* (2015). Serum calcium and magnesium abnormalities in patients with status epilepticus: A single center tertiary care experience. https://core.ac.uk/download/47262905.pdf (accessed on 30th June 2025).
10. Baqir, S. M., Fayyaz, J., Feroze, A., Jamil, M., *et al.* (2014). Real-time patient satisfaction of emergency department services in a tertiary-care hospital in Karachi, Pakistan. https://core.ac.uk/download/84856446.pdf (accessed on 30th June 2025).
11. Barbagallo, M., Corsello, G., Falsaperla, R., Mauceri, L., *et al.* (2019). Short-term neurodevelopmental outcome in term neonates treated with phenobarbital versus levetiracetam: A single-center experience. https://core.ac.uk/download/286528674.pdf (accessed on 30th June 2025).
12. Basilicata, P., Guadagni, R., Marisei, M., Niola, R., *et al.* (2024). Pediatric poisoning management: How clinical practice can benefit from forensic approach. https://core.ac.uk/download/636826428.pdf (accessed on 30th June 2025).

13. Battaglia, F. P., Campbell, S., Dingeman, A., Filbert, M., Karki, P., Konradsen, F., Moorcraft, P., *et al.* (2016). Role of the calcium plateau in the neuronal injury and behavioral morbidities following organophosphate intoxication. https://core.ac.uk/download/84402779.pdf (accessed on 30th June 2025).

14. Brancato, A., Argo, A., Cannizzaro, C., Plescia, F., Lavanco, G., Malta, G., Albano, G. D., *et al.* (2025). Acute cannabis intoxication among the pediatric population. https://core.ac.uk/download/655864188.pdf (accessed on 30th June 2025).

15. Brophy, G. M., Erstad, B. L., Haas, C. E., Jacobi, J., *et al.* (2005). Key articles and guidelines relative to intensive care unit pharmacology—2004. https://deepblue.lib.umich.edu/bitstream/2027.42/90189/1/phco.25.4.585.61024.pdf (accessed on 30th June 2025).

16. Chan, H. K. (2016). Assessment of pictogram use in pediatric oral liquid medication labeling at Sultanah Bahiyah Hospital, Alor Setar, Kedah, Malaysia. https://core.ac.uk/download/78390028.pdf (accessed on 30th June 2025).

17. Chen, T. H., Huang, C. T., Kuo, C. H., Wang, M., *et al.* (2016). Use of fomepizole in pediatric methanol exposure: The first case report in Taiwan and a literature review. https://core.ac.uk/download/pdf/82808512.pdf (accessed on 30th June 2025).

18. Chilukuri, S. (2017). The impacts of recreational marijuana legalization on Colorado: Policy analysis on Amendment 64. https://core.ac.uk/download/232580895.pdf (accessed on 30th June 2025).

19. Ciomaga, I. M., Frăsinariu, O., Nistor, N., Rugină, D., *et al.* (2019). Poisoning in the pediatric intensive care unit. https://core.ac.uk/download/322441124.pdf (accessed on 30th June 2025).

20. Cook, C. A., Fish, A. F., Silva, V., Stiles, M., *et al.* (2015). Bath salt-induced psychosis: Nursing assessment, diagnosis, treatment, and outcomes. https://core.ac.uk/download/621678359.pdf (accessed on 30th June 2025).

21. Ebrahimi, M., Mehrpour, O., & Sharifi, M. D. (2015). Pattern of acute pediatric poisonings in Birjand City, East of Iran. https://core.ac.uk/download/483635490.pdf (accessed on 30th June 2025).

22. Edelstein, C. L., Klawitter, J., & Sirota, J. C. (2011). Biomarkers of acute kidney injury. https://core.ac.uk/download/pdf/8636677.pdf (accessed on 30th June 2025).

23. Ellingsen, C. L., Krüger, A. J., Søreide, K., Tjosevik, K., *et al.* (2009). Pediatric trauma deaths are predominated by severe head injuries during spring and summer. https://core.ac.uk/download/pdf/8255920.pdf (accessed on 30th June 2025).

24. Elmi, M., Forouzanfar, R., Hassanian-Moghaddam, H., Rahimi, M., *et al.* (2018). Acute lidocaine toxicity: A case series. https://core.ac.uk/download/483638288.pdf (accessed on 30th June 2025).

25. Erdmann, A., Hugli, O., Werner, D., Yersin, B., *et al.* (2015). Focused use of drug screening in overdose patients increases impact on management. https://core.ac.uk/download/84059359.pdf (accessed on 30th June 2025).

26. Froberg, B., Morton, S., Overberg, A., Wagner, D., *et al.* (2019). Toxicity of bupropion overdose compared with selective serotonin reuptake inhibitors. https://core.ac.uk/download/288117269.pdf (accessed on 30th June 2025).

27. Garrett, A. L., & Redlener, I. E. (2009). Pediatric emergency preparedness for natural disasters, terrorism, and public health emergencies: A national consensus conference: 2009 update. https://core.ac.uk/download/161435134.pdf (accessed on 30th June 2025).

28. Hampango, M. (2015). Prevalence and clinical management of common poisoning in pediatric patients seen at the University Teaching Hospital in Lusaka. https://core.ac.uk/download/618068164.pdf (accessed on 30th June 2025).

29. Heaviside, C., Lake, I., & Nichols, G. (2018). Climate change and water-related infectious diseases. https://core.ac.uk/download/322490318.pdf (accessed on 30th June 2025).

30. Hitchcock, E., & Madsen, T. (2011). *Growing Up Toxic: Chemical Exposures and Increases in Developmental Disease*. https://core.ac.uk/download/71358334.pdf (accessed on 30th June 2025).

31. Hynes, H. P., & Lopez, R. (2012). Cumulative risk and a call for action in environmental justice communities. https://digitalscholarship.unlv.edu/cgi/viewcontent.cgi?article=1111&context=jhdrp (accessed on 30th June 2025).

32. Irwin, M. G., & Wong, G. T. C. (2013). Poisoning with illicit substances: Toxicology for the anesthetist. https://core.ac.uk/download/38010126.pdf (accessed on 30th June 2025).

33. Karpushkina, E. S. (2022). Acute poisoning in children: Etiology, structure, treatment tactics and outcomes. https://core.ac.uk/download/564139965.pdf (accessed on 30th June 2025).

34. Kotsi, E. (2023). Evaluation of acute child poisoning in Greece and the impact of the COVID-19 pandemic. https://core.ac.uk/download/580001917.pdf (accessed on 30th June 2025).

35. Law, K. Y. (2016). Syndromic surveillance using poison center data: An examination of novel approaches. https://core.ac.uk/download/129453090.pdf (accessed on 30th June 2025).

36. Ling, W., Miotto, K., Mooney, L., Nielsen, D., *et al.* (2011). Selective review and commentary on emerging pharmacotherapies for opioid addiction. https://core.ac.uk/download/323076737.pdf (accessed on 30th June 2025).

37. Long, J. B. (2016). A clinical decision support system for the treatment of common toxin overdose. https://open.bu.edu/bitstream/2144/15194/1/Long_bu_0017N_10981.pdf (accessed on 30th June 2025).

38. Luster, J., Marchionni, C., Papadimos, T. J., Seoane, L., *et al.* (2017). Patient self-harm in the emergency department: An evidence-based approach. https://core.ac.uk/download/322431943.pdf (accessed on 30th June 2025).

39. Marks, A. (2021). Intensive insulin therapy for children in early primary school: The narratives of parents, school teachers and diabetes educators. https://core.ac.uk/download/544084292.pdf (accessed on 30th June 2025).

40. McCarthy, D., & Leatherman, S. (2004). *Quality of Health Care for Children and Adolescents: A Chartbook*. https://core.ac.uk/download/71354153.pdf (accessed on 30th June 2025).

41. McDonald, M., Sanjeevan, S., & Moore, T. G. (2025). Evidence-based service modules for a sustained home visiting program. https://core.ac.uk/download/pdf/30672643.pdf (accessed on 30th June 2025).

42. Ryskamp, J. L. (2010). Anencephaly: Concepts of personhood, ethical questions, and nursing care. https://core.ac.uk/download/58823336.pdf (accessed on 30th June 2025).

43. Tyler, E. T. (2008). Allies not adversaries: Teaching collaboration to the next generation of doctors and lawyers to address social inequality. https://core.ac.uk/download/56703780.pdf (accessed on 30th June 2025).
44. Virginia Commonwealth University. (2018). *Virginia Commonwealth University Professional Bulletin*. https://core.ac.uk/download/215485746.pdf (accessed on 30th June 2025).
45. Weng, C. H., Hsu, C. W., Yu, H. Y., Lin, J. L., Fu, J. F., Lin, J. H., Chen, K. H., *et al.* (2013). Outcomes of patients with rodenticide poisoning at a Far East poison center. https://core.ac.uk/download/pdf/81796755.pdf (accessed on 30th June 2025).

TRAUMA AND BURNS

12

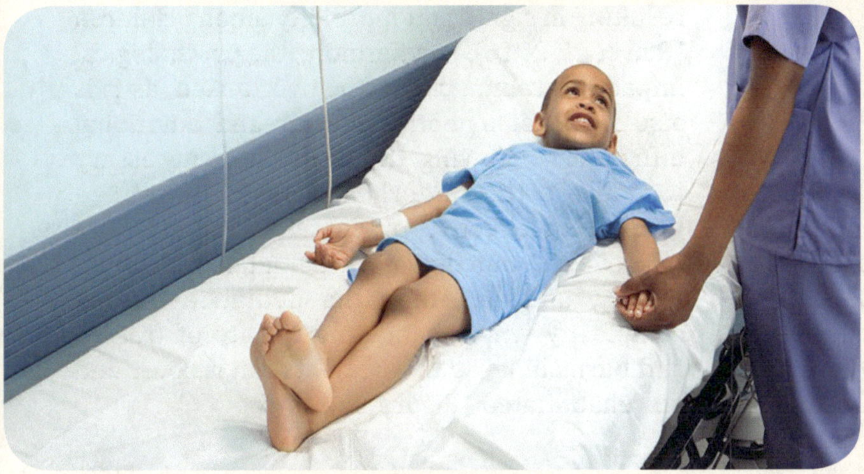

LEARNING OBJECTIVES

After studying this chapter, you will be able to:

1. Understand Types of Trauma in Pediatric Patients.
2. Explain Burns in Pediatric Patients.
3. Describe Management of Trauma and Burns in Pediatric Intensive Care.
4. Focus on Psychological and Emotional Support for Pediatric Patients.

Introduction

Burns and trauma management in pediatric intensive care is a critical nexus of medical sophistication that carries far-reaching implications for the young patient. Burn injuries remain a frequent occurrence, particularly in low- and middle-income countries, where conditions such as a lack of proper safety measures during cooking by fire continue to escalate the risk of severe complications (Ismail *et al.*, 2013). In such settings, young children are disproportionately represented in both morbidity and mortality and, as such, require targeted prevention programs based on local environmental determinants. Moreover, the integration of advanced methodologies, such as artificial intelligence and machine learning, has the potential to enhance the early detection of complications such as acute kidney injury in trauma patients (Blackmon *et al.*, 2020). Awareness of the unique dynamics of pediatric trauma and burn patients is essential in creating effective treatment regimens and prevention methods, leading the way for continued refinement of results in this vulnerable group.

12.1. Types of Trauma in Pediatric Patients

Learning Outcome

1. Common Causes of Trauma in Children.
2. Types of Injuries Sustained.
3. Psychological Impact of Trauma on Children.
4. Role of Caregivers in Trauma Situations.
5. Assessment and Diagnosis of Pediatric Trauma.
6. Treatment Protocols for Traumatic Injuries.
7. Long-term Effects of Trauma on Development.
8. Importance of Prevention Strategies.

The type of trauma experienced by children is diverse and tends to have significant psychological and physical impacts. Amongst these, burns are a prevalent form of trauma, particularly in low- and middle-income countries where the risk factors for them are extremely dissimilar from those in high-income settings. For instance, young children and infants, especially those aged one to three years, are particularly vulnerable, often suffering from burns caused by household cooking fires, a significant source of morbidity within these regions (Ismail *et al.*, 2013). In addition, underlying illnesses, such as epilepsy, can increase the risk of burns when seizures occur. Knowledge of these trends is important as they point to the requirement for focused prevention efforts that take into account local contexts and risk factors. In addition, the effects of trauma cut across immediate treatment, so the treatment and healing process for children in pediatric intensive care units needs a holistic approach (Kellum *et al.*, 2013).

12.1.1. Common Causes of Trauma in Children

The children are particularly vulnerable to various forms of trauma, which could result in severe health complications, especially in a pediatric intensive care unit. Accidental injuries such as falls, burns, and motor vehicle accidents, as well as non-accidental injuries resulting from child abuse, constitute the major causes of trauma in children. Burns, for instance, are a ubiquitous problem, often occurring due to being scalded by liquids, fire, or electricity, and aggressive medical intervention may be necessary. Studies have indicated that injury patterns were varied and tended to involve burn injuries with hot liquids and electricity as the cause of injury, resulting in significant morbidity among children (Ren *et al.*, 2016). Furthermore, the psychological impact of trauma cannot be overlooked, as it is also manifest in both behavior and emotional difficulties following the event. It is necessary to address the underlying causes of trauma to develop effective preventive strategies and improve the outcomes of traumatized children. Finally, understanding the pediatric trauma complexity will enhance the quality of trauma and burns units so that patients can recover and be rehabilitated (Figure 12.1).

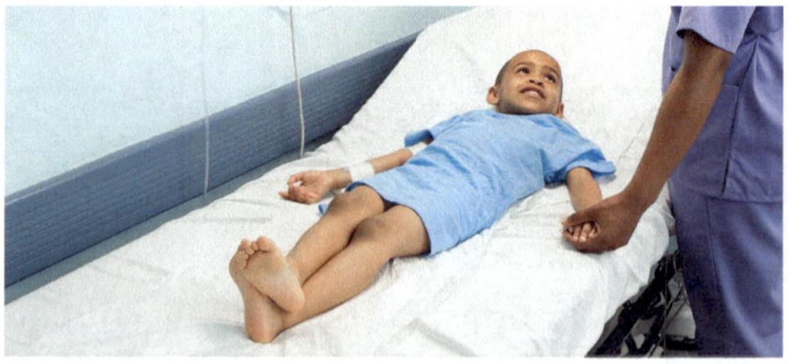

Figure 12.1. Children are particularly vulnerable to various forms of trauma, which can lead to significant health complications, especially within a pediatric intensive care setting.

Source: https://cdn.sanity.io/images/1gm9mx7i/production/bfdad7a668765996b3d51e575c7e8cadc51931ff-1060x424.jpg?w=1920&q=90&fit=max&auto=format.

12.1.2. Types of Injuries Sustained

For the pediatric intensive care setting, it is essential to understand the type of injuries sustained and how they are managed and avoided. Burns are one of the most serious injuries, particularly among younger children whose sensitive skin is in greater jeopardy of being burned by fire and heat. Research indicates that the vast majority of burns occur in low and middle-income economies, predominantly because of inappropriate household circumstances, the majority of which are located around cooking stoves (Ismail *et al.*, 2013). Aside from trauma, additional examples are rib fractures, head injury, and hemothorax, which are prevalent among children. Such types of injuries do not just demand enormous medical intervention but also result in higher morbidity and longer lengths of stay in the hospital. Therefore, it is essential to meet the complicated nature of such injuries with efficient prevention and treatment in optimizing outcomes for children in intensive care.

12.1.3. Psychological Impact of Injury on Children

The psychological effects of trauma in children, particularly those with burn injuries, can be serious and enduring. Trauma can lead to many emotional and behavioral difficulties, such as depression, anxiety, and post-traumatic stress disorder (PTSD) (Drummond *et al.*, 2013). In the case of children in pediatric intensive care, the trauma is often compounded by pain and disfigurement associated with severe burns. Such a dual burden is going to skew conventional development and affect social interactions because the children will show loneliness due to injuries (Ismail *et al.*, 2013).

Moreover, the psychological impact extends to the family and the community relationships, necessitating a comprehensive treatment regimen that will specifically treat emotional as well as psychological healing. By applying focused psychological intervention and support techniques, caregivers are able to enhance recovery more effectively, thus enhancing overall child outcomes in cases of traumatic burn injuries (Figure 12.2).

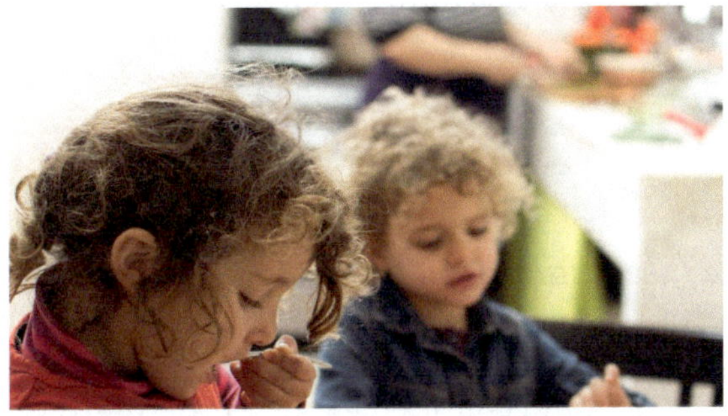

Figure 12.2. The psychological consequences of trauma in children, particularly those who experience burn injuries, can be profound and long-lasting.

Source: https://akm-img-a-in.tosshub.com/indiatoday/images/story/202406/what-are-the-long-term-effects-of-childhood-trauma-on-development-243717466-16x9_0.jpg?VersionId=XXX.Jxh0ZciqfOsTg3i0BOwgdI0KV4y6.

12.1.4. Role of Caregivers in Trauma Situations

Trauma care is mediated by caregivers, specifically, most notably pediatric intensive care, where infant patients' physical and emotional well-being is significantly affected. These caregivers, who encompass nurses, physicians, and family members, form a complete care network with the duty to provide both medical and psychological care to traumatized children. Their practice extends beyond mere clinical intervention; they must establish a climate of open communication and trust, as highlighted by the significance of interdisciplinary practice in critical care settings (Kleinpell *et al.*, 2021). Further, effective caregiving in trauma cases often calls for immediate assessment and intervention, particularly in managing complications of extreme injuries, such as those resulting from burns or esophageal injury (Mircéa Chirica *et al.*, 2019). By intertwining their knowledge and empathy, caregivers not only enhance patient recovery but also cushion the emotional impact on families, underlining their invaluable role in trauma care.

12.1.5. Pediatric Trauma Assessment and Diagnosis

The assessment and diagnosis of pediatric trauma include a multidisciplinary and systematic approach towards offering timely and sufficient intervention. Pediatric patients with trauma have unique challenges in view of the physiological and anatomical differences from adults, and specific evaluation strategies need to be employed. The initial assessments would highlight airway, breathing, and circulation, and a sufficient history of the incident. Health professionals tend to use complex diagnostic tools, including imaging examinations and biomarkers, to enhance the accuracy of their evaluations.

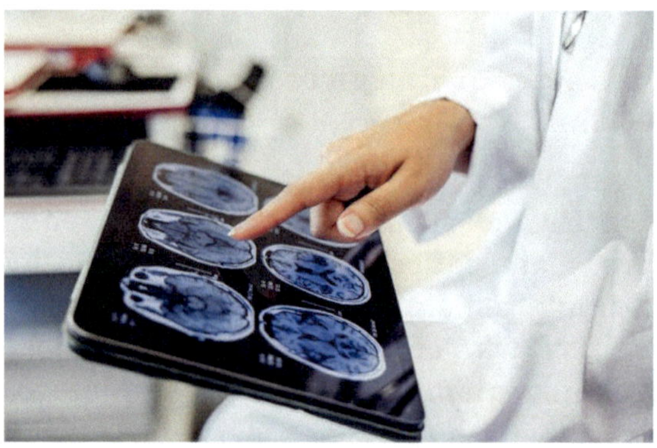

Figure 12.3. Medical professionals frequently employ advanced diagnostic tools, including imaging studies and biomarkers, to enhance the accuracy of their evaluations.

Source: https://imageio.forbes.com/specials-images/imageserve/67c86f60dfc60d1bb54bfea5//960x0.jpg?height=474&width=711&fit=bounds.

Current studies highlight the application of biomarkers such as neutrophil gelatinase-associated lipocalin (NGAL) in the detection of acute kidney injury (AKI) among children trauma patients, with findings outpacing traditional methods such as creatinine testing and urine output (Blackmon *et al*., 2020). Furthermore, the addition of agency recommendations from organizations such as Kidney Disease: Improving Global Outcomes helps keep clinicians current with current evidence-based recommendations for the diagnosis and management of AKI (Kellum *et al*., 2013). Such holistic approaches are instrumental in optimizing outcomes in pediatric trauma care (Figure 12.3).

12.1.6. Treatment Protocols for Traumatic Injuries

In pediatric intensive care, rigid treatment protocols for traumatic injury are essential in the management of the issues entailed in treating children. Such protocols typically comprise a multidisciplinary system, including rapid assessment and stabilization, which is central in the acute phase of managing trauma. This entails doing early interventions such as airway management, optimization of circulation, and fluid resuscitation to reverse shock. Of interest in particular is the evolving evidence on sepsis complications, as outlined in recent studies, to highlight the importance of prompt identification and management of infections likely to follow traumatic injury. As sepsis can have ruinous immune impairment alongside increased mortality, the guidelines are also supposed to address the need for intensive care monitoring and intervention, implementing new advances in critical care medicine to enhance long-term outcomes for children with trauma (Matthew *et al*., 2016; Jeffrey *et al*., 2016).

12.1.7. Long-Term Trauma Effects on Development

Long-term effects of trauma on development are significant, particularly if one takes into account children who have suffered severe injuries, such as burns, found in critical care. Traumatic events may lead to extensive psychological challenges, including post-traumatic stress disorder (PTSD), depression, and anxiety, which may disrupt cognitive and emotional development. Research has indicated that children exposed to acute trauma may experience disruptions of their neurodevelopmental processes, such as learning and social interactions, years following the initial event. In addition, traumatic incidents themselves may be added to by the medical complicating factors of recovery from traumatic injury, such as those seen in the pediatric intensive care environment. In environments in which children are exposed to life-threatening situations, the interaction between trauma at the physical and psychological levels demands care that takes full account of both short-term medical problems and long-term developmental outcomes (Chimbira *et al.*, 2001; Bull *et al.*, 2019) (Figure 12.4).

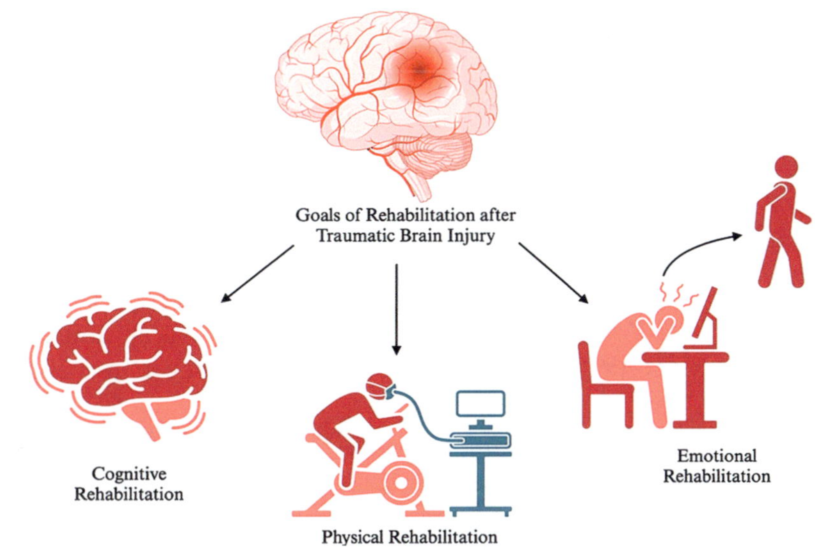

Figure 12.4. The effects of traumatic experiences can be compounded by the medical complexities associated with recovery from traumatic injuries, such as those frequently seen in pediatric intensive care.

Source: https://assets.cureus.com/uploads/figure/file/1039230/article_river_f48affa0192111efa397a9eeefb0c9fa-WhatsApp-Image-2024-05-22-at-9.08.42-PM.png.

12.1.8. Importance of Prevention Strategies

The application of effective prevention methods in pediatric intensive care is important in order to reduce the incidence and severity of trauma and burns in children. By applying adequate educational programs for families and healthcare providers, risk factors can be reduced regarding such injuries. Such efforts can significantly reduce unfamiliarity with critical conditions like intra-abdominal hypertension and acute lung injury, as evidenced by the recognition of consensus definitions and management practices after publication (Keulenaer *et al.*, 2014). Early prevention and treatment can also enhance outcomes for conditions like acute respiratory distress syndrome, where early diagnosis is critical (Chimbira *et al.*, 2001). Always use correct grammar and punctuation. Finally, positioning prevention in the lead not only protects vulnerable children from the physical and psychological consequences of trauma and burns but also relieves the economic load on health systems, reinforcing the value of an active response within pediatric healthcare settings.

Test Your Knowledge

1. What are the typical signs and symptoms of traumatic brain injury in children?
2. How does the anatomy of pediatric patients affect their vulnerability to specific types of trauma?

12.2. Burns in Pediatric Patients

Learning Outcome

1. Classification of Burns.
2. Common Causes of Burns in Children.
3. Assessment of Burn Severity.
4. Immediate First Aid for Burn Injuries.
5. Treatment Options for Pediatric Burns.
6. Psychological Effects of Burns on Children.
7. Rehabilitation and Recovery Processes.
8. Prevention of Burn Injuries in Children.

Burn care in kids is particularly challenging, necessitating specialized care in units such as Pediatric Intensive Care Units (PICUs). Burn injuries are the fifth leading cause of non-fatal morbidity in kids, with flame and scald burns representing the most frequent etiology and being responsible for a high percentage of cases (Rahimpour *et al.*, 2025). Pediatric patients possess distinct physiological characteristics that render them difficult to manage and expose them to a higher level of complications, such as infection and respiratory distress (Benlamkaddem *et al.*, 2023). Moreover, research finds that age, total body surface area affected, and the Source of the burn are significant variables that affect the duration of hospital stay; thus, an extensive evaluation and personalized interventions are necessary (Rahimpour *et al.*, 2025). Effective management planning, in this case, will need to address early identification of high-risk patients and coordination of care in order to optimize outcomes for this at-risk population and reduce the long-term impact of burn injury.

12.2.1. Classification of Burns (Thermal, Chemical, Electrical)

Pediatric burns fall under three broad categories, which include thermal, chemical, and electrical, each with its own intensity of challenges and intensive care management. Thermal burns are the most prevalent and are primarily caused by scalds involving liquids or direct contact with fire, particularly in young children, because of such exposure at home in the presence of parents (Kawalec *et al.*, 2018).

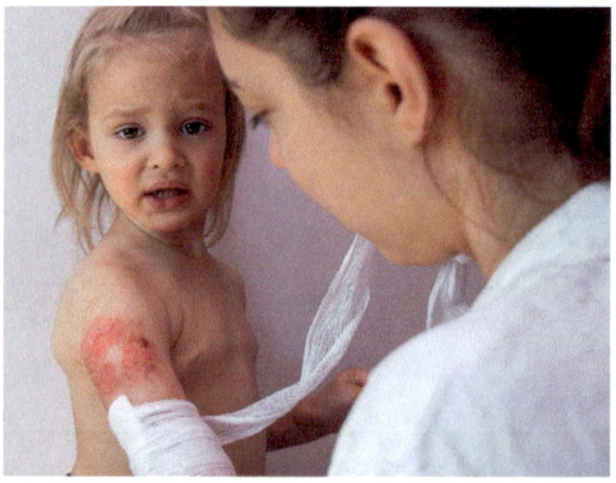

Figure 12.5. Burns in pediatric patients can be classified into three primary categories: thermal, chemical, and electrical, each presenting unique challenges and management protocols in intensive care settings.

Source: https://prodcraftsa01.blob.core.windows.net/assets/articles/no-issue/pediatric-burn-care-strategies-for-identification-and-treatment/_1200x630_crop_center-center_82_none/pediatric-burn_GettyImages-1824231544.jpg?mtime=1737132527.

Chemical burns, due to caustic substances, involve widespread tissue damage and require immediate decontamination and specialty treatment. Electrical burns, although rarer, cause deep tissue and systemic damage that may not be apparent at first. Recognition of these groups is crucial in planning treatment to minimize morbidity and promote improved outcomes for pediatric burn injury. Multidisciplinary and fluid resuscitation-based care plans are critical in the management of the volatilities of burn injuries (Krakowski *et al.*, 2019) (Figure 12.5).

12.2.2. Common Causes of Burns in Children

Understanding the typical etiology of burns in children is crucial in designing effective prevention measures, especially in pediatric intensive care units. Burns occur most frequently among young children, aged between one and three years, with households being high-risk places. Open fire and scalding liquids are a significant risk because children are prone to being burned by open fires and scalding fluids, and vigilant supervision during meal time is a must. In addition, diseases such as epilepsy have the potential to enhance vulnerability, with the individual being particularly vulnerable near causes of fire. The belief that burns are inevitable highlights the importance of education on avoiding burns in communities. Having environment-specific precautions is imperative, given that most instances of burns are preventable by increased awareness and proper measures against injury (Ismail *et al.*, 2013). Preventing these risks can reduce the incidence of burns and improve outcomes among injured children in pediatric hospitals (Kellum *et al.*, 2013).

12.2.3. Assessment of Burn Severity

Assessment of burn severity is a critical component of pediatric intensive care unit management. Burn depth and area significantly influence treatment planning and outcome, and therefore, it becomes imperative to make appropriate and timely assessments.

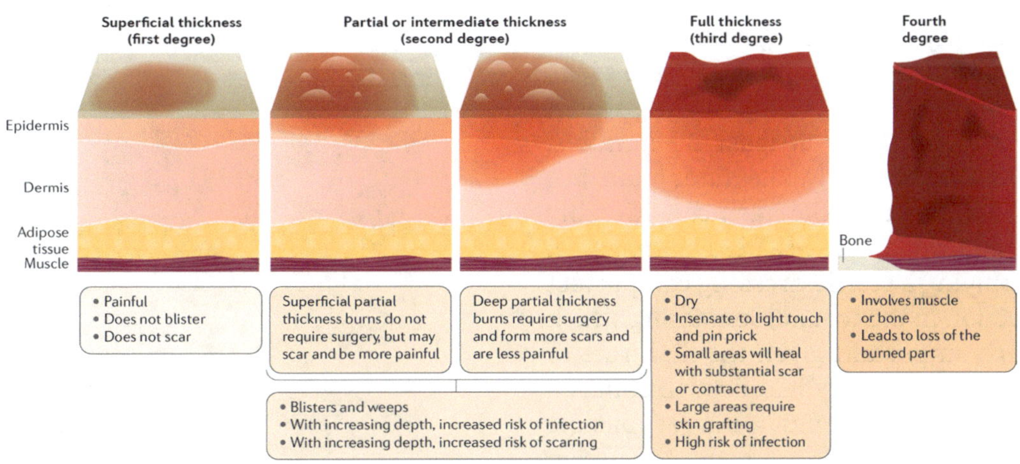

Figure 12.6. Severity is commonly classified based on the percentage of total body surface area (TBSA) affected and the depth of tissue injury, categorized as first, second, or third-degree burns.

Source: https://media.springernature.com/lw1200/springer-static/image/art%3A10.1038%2Fs41572-020-0145-5/MediaObjects/41572_2020_145_Fig1_HTML.png.

Severity can be typically classified on the basis of percentage of total body surface area (TBSA) burned and depth of injury, into first, second, and third-degree burns. Good assessment tools, such as the Lund and Browder chart, allow clinicians to estimate TBSA more precisely, with implications for fluid resuscitation as well as surgical intervention. Moreover, information regarding the patient's clinical status, including potential complications such as acute respiratory distress syndrome (ARDS), adds a further dimension to the assessment. As in pediatric respiratory failure situations with frequent ARDS, assessment of organ function remains the key to anticipating outcomes and guiding treatment decisions (Chimbira *et al.*, 2001). Enhanced burn assessment practice is capable of greatly impacting the quality of care provided to such critically ill patients (José *et al.*, 2025) (Figure 12.6).

12.2.4. Immediate First Aid for Burn Injuries

Early first aid to burn wounds is critical in order to minimize damage and obtain the optimum result, particularly in pediatric patients. The first step is to remove the child from the source of the burn and cool the wound using running water, ideally 15°C to 25°C, for at least 20 minutes. This intervention not only alleviates pain but also reduces the level of the burn considerably by halting additional heat-related damage. In addition, applying a sterile dressing can protect against infection in the wound, something which is particularly important given the high rate of complications associated with burns in children (Dijk *et al.*, 2016). Prompt first aid is responsible for having a major influence on the long-term result, as indicated by research that surrounds the role of proper and timely treatment in severe respiratory complications arising from injuries (Chimbira *et al.*, 2001). Prompt and effective first aid interventions are therefore crucial in the process of treating burn injuries among children in the initial process.

12.2.5. Treatment Options for Pediatric Burns

Best treatment interventions for pediatric burns are crucial in minimizing trauma and maximizing recovery in children. Initially, management of appropriate wound care is required through the use of restrictive dressings with the ability to minimize edema and risk of pressure injury; significantly, the use of tubular elastic bandages has been found useful in both goals within a cost-effective method (Hiller *et al.*, 2025). Addressing the individual psychological needs of pediatric burn injury patients is also important, as studies indicate a high prevalence of posttraumatic stress disorder (PTSD) among this patient population (Graf, 2013). Pain control, family psychotherapy, and establishing a safe and routine environment should be incorporated into multidisciplinary treatment plans to assist both the child and the caregiver in reducing trauma-related stress. Through the combination of these complex strategies, healthcare providers are able to improve recovery benefits and overall health for pediatric burn patients in critical care units (Figure 12.7).

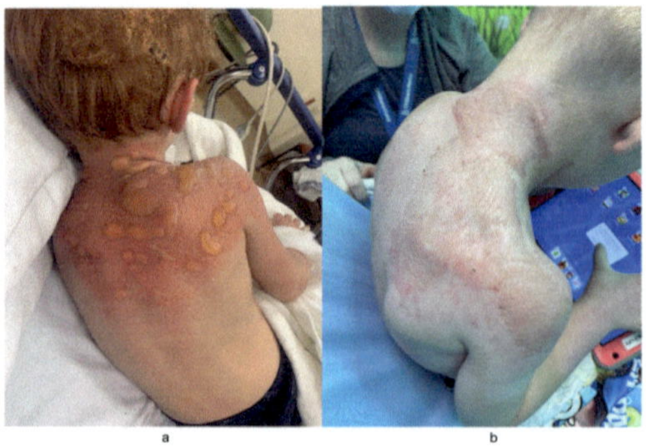

Figure 12.7. Effective treatment options for pediatric burns are crucial in minimizing trauma and ensuring optimal recovery in young patients.

Source: https://ars.els-cdn.com/content/image/1-s2.0-S1055858622000786-gr5.jpg.

12.2.6. Psychological Effects of Burns on Children

The psychological effects of burn injuries on children are profound and far-reaching, more often leading to persistent emotional problems that go far beyond the physical burn scar. Burn injury can act as a precipitant for anxiety, depression, and PTSD, and has a significant influence on a child's self-esteem and social adaptation. As the children deal with their altered appearance and the pain of recovery, they tend to feel alone, separated from their friends by their unique circumstances. Furthermore, the intensive care environment can fuel these psychological needs, as it may introduce fear and uncertainty regarding the future. With all these intricacies, integrating psychological support into the care plan is crucial. Therapeutic interventions, as modified towards the young survivors of burns, and tailored to suit the personal experiences of the youngsters, enhance the resilience and coping capacity that accompanies these individuals throughout navigating the traumatic outcomes, both physical and emotional (Duc *et al.*, 2022).

12.2.7. Rehabilitation and Recovery Processes

Rehabilitation and recovery protocols in the pediatric intensive care environment play a key role in ensuring the optimal healing and long-term outcome for traumatized and burned children. The protocols encompass a multidisciplinary process of physical, occupational, and psychological rehabilitation tailored to address the unique needs of each child. The significance of early intervention cannot be overemphasized, as research has shown the important role of early rehabilitation in reducing complications and maximizing functional recovery. Furthermore, the appropriate management of the psychological impact of trauma, such as post-traumatic stress and anxiety, is significant in overall recovery by offering therapy. It is also crucial to note the economic burden of such injuries; according to *et al.*Sen *et al.* (2019), treatment costs for chronic wounds can total billions of dollars a year, making it imperative to have effective rehabilitation processes. In the end, an inclusive rehabilitation process is essential to regain mobility, independence, and overall quality of life in pediatric patients (Figure 12.8).

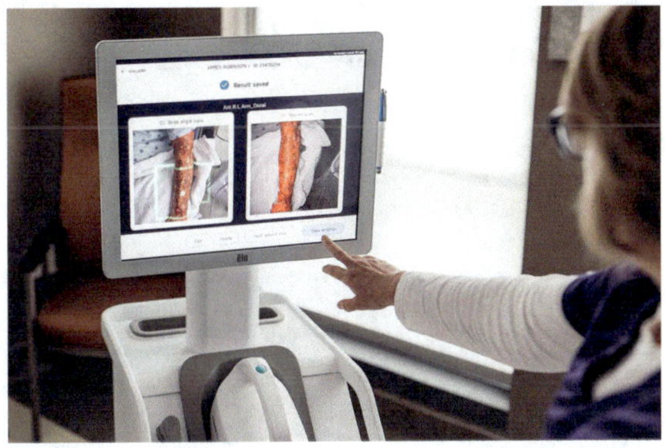

Figure 12.8. In the context of pediatric intensive care, rehabilitation and recovery processes are essential for ensuring optimal healing and long-term outcomes for young patients suffering from trauma and burns.

Source: https://www.spectral-ai.com/wp-content/uploads/2024/08/burns-assessment.jpg.

12.2.8. Prevention of Burn Injuries in Children

Prevention of pediatric intensive care patients' burn injuries is a significant area of consideration because the majority of such injuries occur at home, and they tend to be in close proximity to fire when cooking. Prevention measures in the form of education interventions among children and adults are critical in curbing such risks. Data show that modification of the home setting, for example, excluding children from open flames and closely monitoring individuals with conditions like epilepsy, can possibly reduce risk for burns. (Ismail *et al.*, 2013) highlights that prevention strategies need to be tailored to individual environments in consideration of local risk factors as well as available community resources. Furthermore, the physiological subtleties of burn injuries need to be identified and addressed on an immediate basis to prevent complications such as intra-abdominal hypertension, particularly in the case of extensive severe burns. (Keulenaer *et al.*, 2015) emphasizes the important role that fluid management plays in these risk groups because over-resuscitation in the patient can exacerbate problems. Therefore, a multifaceted approach through education and modification of the environment is essential in effective prevention.

Test Your Knowledge

1. What special considerations are there for fluid resuscitation in pediatric burn patients?
2. What are the common causes of pediatric burns (e.g., scalds, electrical, chemical)?

12.3. Management of Trauma and Burns in Pediatric Intensive Care

Learning Outcome

1. Role of the Pediatric Intensive Care Unit.
2. Multidisciplinary Approach to Care.
3. Pain Management Strategies.
4. Nutritional Considerations for Recovery.
5. Monitoring and Assessment in the PICU.
6. Family Involvement in Care Decisions.
7. Ethical Considerations in Treatment.
8. Transitioning Care from PICU to Home.
9. Innovations in PICU Practices for Trauma and Burns.

Effective management of burns and trauma in pediatric intensive care is a three-dimensional process that revolves around prevention, acute care, and rehabilitation. Since the largest proportion of burn injuries occurs in low and middle-income countries, it is critical to address the environmental and socio-economic determinants that result in these incidents in order to enhance child safety (Ismail *et al.*, 2013). For instance, the prevention of home cooking fires and their risks has proved to be effective in reducing burn incidence in young children. Additionally, the wound burden of pediatric patients indicates the need for tailored treatment protocols that account for hidden risk factors, that is, malnutrition and underlying chronic illness (Sen *et al.*, 2019). Multi-component intervention, including prevention education, early health intervention, and extended family support, can ultimately yield improved outcomes for children with traumatic injury and burns admitted to intensive care units.

12.3.1. Pediatric Intensive Care Unit (PICU) Role

The Pediatric Intensive Care Unit (PICU) plays a crucial role in the management of pediatric patients who are seriously ill, especially traumatized and burned children. The unique physiological and developmental needs of children demand specialized care, which is provided by an interdisciplinary team in the PICU. For instance, the management of pediatric acute respiratory distress syndrome (PARDS) complicating burn injury shows the unit's capacity to deliver interventions of an advanced nature, such as invasive mechanical ventilation and extracorporeal membrane oxygenation (ECMO) (Benlamkaddem *et al.*, 2023). Furthermore, evidence-based pain management strategies are paramount, as demonstrated by the development of a pediatric analgesia support guidance tool to maximize the treatment of burn children with severe total body surface area (TBSA) involvement, emphasizing the importance of precision-tuned analgesic interventions (Wratney *et al.*, 2022). The PICU is finally the key environment to enhance outcomes and reduce mortality in badly injured children (Figure 12.9).

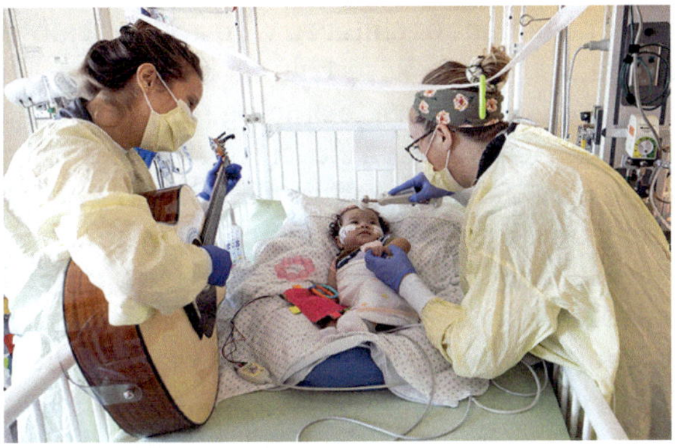

Figure 12.9. The Pediatric Intensive Care Unit (PICU) plays a crucial role in the management of critically ill children, especially those suffering from trauma and burns.

Source: https://health.ucdavis.edu/media-resources/contenthub/health-library/health-topics/pediatric-critical-care-2-column.jpg.

12.3.2. Multidisciplinary Approach to Care

Effective management of trauma and burns in pediatric intensive care is greatly reliant on a multidisciplinary model of care. The model involves collaboration between various healthcare providers, such as intensivists, nurses, pharmacists, and therapists, each with specialized knowledge, to achieve maximal improvement of the patient. In pediatric presentation, where physical as well as psychological subtleties of treatment are more pronounced, uniting diverse skills becomes crucial. As the Society of Critical Care Medicine points out, multidisciplinary rounds foster not only whole-person care discussions but also a culture of collaborative decision-making between family members, thereby, enhance the overall care experience (Kleinpell *et al.*, 2021). Furthermore, the pandemic has illuminated the function of organized multidisciplinary care models that are capable of responding to dynamic health crises, and it is emphasizing the need for cooperative interprofessional teams within surgical and intensive care environments in order to treat patients with prompt, effective interventions (Kjetil Søreide *et al.*, 2020). The interdisciplinary coordination in pediatric intensive care is essential in order to resolve the complicated issues entailed in treating major traumas and burns.

12.3.3. Pain Management Strategies

Highly effective pain management measures in pediatric trauma and burn patients are essential for optimal outcomes and quality of care. Due to the unique developmental characteristics of children, pain assessments should address both physiological and behavioral indicators targeted at age-related manifestations of distress. Multimodal pain management techniques that include the employment of adjuvant therapy, like nerve blocks, in combination with pharmacologic measures like non-steroidal anti-inflammatory drugs or opioids, are increasingly being discovered to be extremely effective in stopping extreme discomfort. Non-pharmacologic methods like distraction interventions, play therapy, and cognitive-behavioral therapies also emerge to effectively counteract perceived amounts of pain in children. Multidisciplinary interventions aim not only to control pain but also to address its psychological impact, especially among at-risk groups for burn injury, according to community education literature on prevention programs (Ismail *et al.*, 2013). These interventions are required to facilitate recovery and minimize trauma and burn sequelae in the long term (Chimbira *et al.*, 2001) (Figure 12.10).

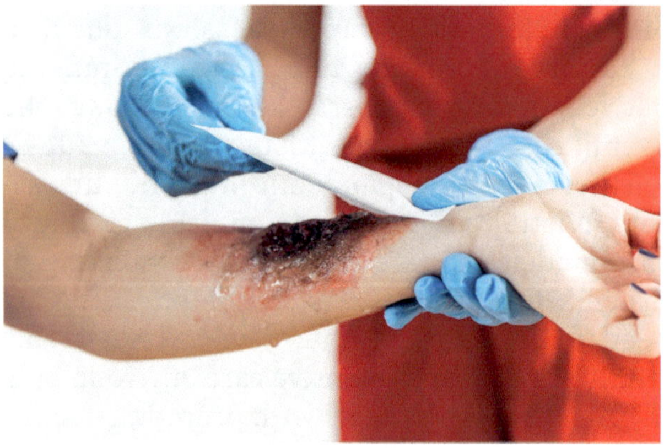

Figure 12.10. Effective pain management strategies for pediatric patients suffering from trauma and burns are crucial for improving outcomes and enhancing the quality of care.

Source: https://www.firstaidpro.com.au/wp-content/uploads/2024/11/first-aid-training-burn-injury-2024-10-18-09-53-32-utc-scaled.jpg.

12.3.4. Nutritional Considerations for Recovery

In the area of intensive care of children for trauma and burn rehabilitation, nutritional considerations move to the forefront in the facilitation of healing and restoration. The physiologic stress of these injuries necessitates increased caloric and protein intake to meet metabolic demands and allow for tissue repair. Special considerations for children involve individualized nutrition regimens sensitive to their own special growth needs and complications of their injuries. Current studies accentuate that the integration of specialist dietary interventions not only optimizes recovery results but also reduces hospital stay time, underlining the importance of a multidisciplinary treatment process. For instance, adequate protein intake has been linked to improved wound healing and immune status in children (Brophy *et al.*, 2005). Moreover, micronutrient supplementation can also contribute towards recovery as deficiency slows down healing and increases susceptibility to infection (Brophy *et al.*, 2009). Thus, proper nutrition is a critical component of the therapeutic care for young trauma and burn patients.

12.3.5. PICU Monitoring and Assessment

Effective monitoring and evaluation in the Pediatric Intensive Care Unit (PICU) are vital for the management of children who are critically ill, particularly those with trauma and burns. The application of modern technology and guidelines assists professionals in closely following the vital signs, fluid balance, and metabolic parameters, which are vital for early interventions. For instance, the implementation of tight glycemic control practices has been shown to improve patient outcomes by reducing the rates of critical illness complications (Ceriello *et al.*, 2010).

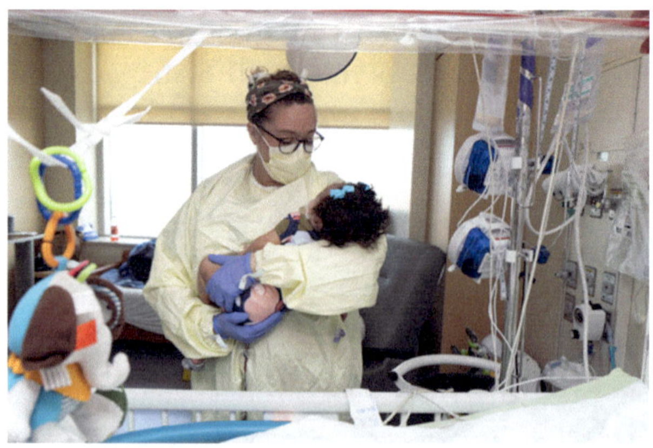

Figure 12.11. In the pediatric intensive care unit (PICU), effective monitoring and assessment are paramount for managing critically ill children, particularly those suffering from trauma and burns.

Source: https://health.ucdavis.edu/media-resources/contenthub/health-library/health-topics/pediatric-critical-care-marquee.jpg.

Additionally, Pediatric Early Warning systems (PEWs) provide early warning of patient deterioration, ultimately resulting in less invasive therapies and shorter PICU length of stay (Carrol *et al.*, 2014). As they develop, these methods emphasize the need for good monitoring and evaluation methods to enhance not only the quality of care provided but also general recovery outcomes for pediatric patients under intensive care (Figure 12.11).

12.3.6. Family Involvement in Care Decisions

Family involvement in the decision-making process is valuable in pediatric intensive care, particularly for trauma and burn patients. Family members as providers of care carry with them unique information about the child's history, the child's preferences, and the child's emotional needs that are valuable in organizing effective therapy. Literature has indicated that effective communication and collaborative decision-making also significantly enhance the quality of care because families are likely to suffer from moral distress when they cannot participate effectively in such decisions (EG *et al.*, 2018). Additionally, literature has delineated five aspects of family involvement as presence, support, communication, decision-making, and contributing to the care (SM *et al.*, 2016). By establishing a scenario in which families are enabled to engage proactively in discussion and decision making about their child's care, healthcare professionals can mitigate feelings of helplessness and strengthen family relationships at times of need. By integrating family feedback, patient care is indeed enhanced, but so is the holistic strategy required for managing complex pediatric cases.

12.3.7. Ethical Considerations in Treatment

In pediatric intensive care trauma and burns, ethical considerations in making decisions regarding treatment arise. Doctors generally encounter dilemmas in matters of resource utilization when there is a mismatch between available resources and the demand for services. This is more evident in pediatric burn treatment, where demand for specialized treatment often exceeds the money allocated for it. Existing studies reinforce the need for undertaking meticulous evaluation of the cost-effectiveness of interventions, with consideration of the provision of ethical rationing of health care systems where burn injuries are considered a public health issue (Dijk *et al.*, 2016). The challenge is not only having equal access to treatment, but also that children receive therapy that will ensure they achieve their best potential of recovery without subjecting families to unnecessary expenses. Balancing these variables necessitates a judicious approach that optimizes both ethical responsibility and therapeutic efficacy (Henderson *et al.*, 2013) (Figure 12.12).

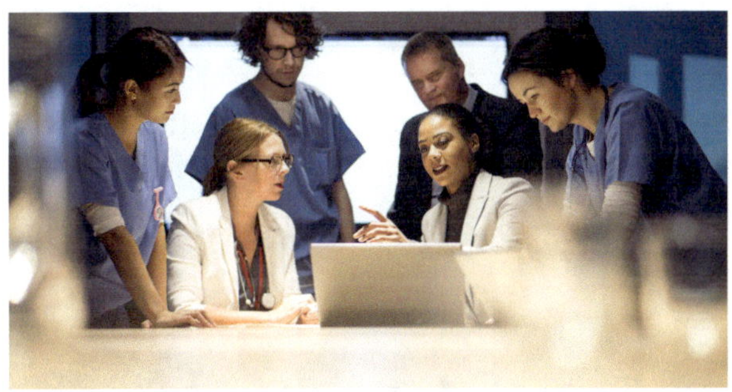

Figure 12.12. Healthcare providers often grapple with dilemmas regarding resource allocation, particularly when the demand for services exceeds available resources.

Source: https://healthcareitsm.com/wp-content/uploads/2023/04/Healthcare_IT-Service_Featured.jpg.

12.3.8. Transitioning Care from PICU to Home

Transition of care from the Pediatric Intensive Care Unit (PICU) to home is a complex problem requiring meticulous planning and support. For recovering children with trauma and burns, such a transition is important because their requirements might extend beyond medical care into emotional and psychological support. Effective communication between healthcare workers, families, and community services is essential in the continuity of care. Per recent research, involving families in the discharge planning process greatly enhances outcomes such that caregivers feel empowered and adequately prepared to take care of the child's ongoing needs at home. In addition, follow-up care, such as outpatient care and home health services, is key to preventing complications and supporting recovery (Hyrkas *et al.*, 2020). By having a strong focus on an inclusive family-centered strategy at the moment of transition, healthcare providers are able to facilitate improved health outcomes and enhance the overall well-being of pediatric patients.

12.3.9. Innovations in PICU Practices for Trauma and Burns

During the last three or four years, tremendous strides have been made in Pediatric Intensive Care Units (PICUs) that have transformed care for trauma and burn patients. Of all the innovations, autologous cultured epidermal grafts, also known as cultured epithelial autografts (CEA), have been a particularly remarkable technique for the management of deep burns. This approach addresses the limitation of limited donor sites by growing the skin cells from the patient's own tissue, thereby reducing complications from standard grafting techniques. Studies have established inconsistent results as far as CEA use is concerned, with survival and healing being contingent on factors of total body surface area (TBSA) participation and the overall condition of the patient's health (Maye *et al.*, 2012). Although the definitive impact of CEA on mortality and hospitalization is uncertain, its potential benefits in some cases emphasize the importance of additional studies and clinical enhancement of new practices in PICUs to enhance recovery in children with traumatic injuries.

Test Your Knowledge

1. How is fluid resuscitation calculated and monitored in pediatric burn patients?
2. What are the indications for blood transfusion in pediatric trauma?

12.4. Psychological and Emotional Support for Pediatric Patients

Learning Outcome

1. Importance of Mental Health in Recovery.
2. Common Psychological Issues Faced by Pediatric Patients.
3. Role of Child Life Specialists in the PICU.
4. Family Dynamics and Support Systems.
5. Coping Strategies for Children and Families.
6. Long-term Psychological Support Options.
7. Impact of Trauma and Burns on Family Relationships.
8. Community Resources for Ongoing Support.
9. Research on Psychological Outcomes in Pediatric Trauma and Burn Patients.

Emotional and psychological care of the children's patients in the case of trauma and burns is highly necessary, particularly in the intensive care unit. The children are likely to be more anxious and fearful due to their illnesses, and a lack of attention to their emotional needs may worsen their suffering and hinder recovery. Giving them a supportive setting that involves therapeutic interventions, including play therapy and counseling, can considerably strengthen their coping skills and reduce feelings of loneliness. Furthermore, the effect of burnout among healthcare professionals should also be recognized, as this emotional depletion can negatively impact patient care (Chemali *et al.*, 2019). Creating assurance that caregivers not only receive training to manage physical traumas but are also empathetic towards the emotional well-being of their pediatric patients is essential for overall care. Thus, including psychological support in the treatment process not only fosters resilience in pediatric patients but also facilitates overall recovery (Kjetil Søreide *et al.*, 2020) (Figure 12.13).

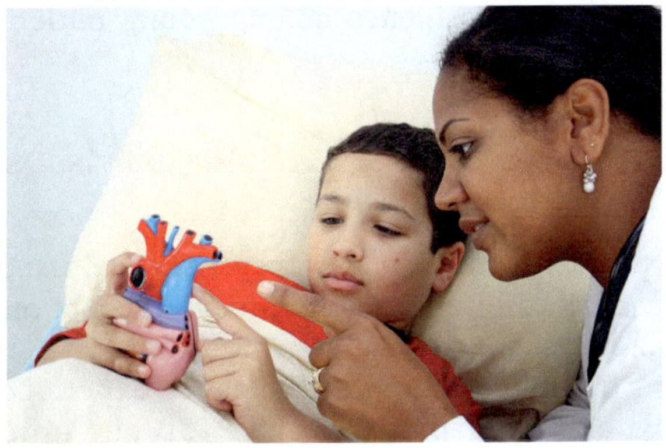

Figure 12.13. The psychological and emotional support for pediatric patients in the context of trauma and burns is critical, particularly within the intensive care setting.

Source: https://www.healthcaretoolbox.org/sites/default/files/inline-images/Doctor_child_w_heart_1.jpg.

12.4.1. Importance of Mental Health in Recovery

The significance of recovery of mental health from traumatic injury and burns in children's intensive care should not be overstressed as it has a direct influence on psychological health and rehabilitation. Following traumatic injury, for example, severe burns, children can experience more emotional distress and posttraumatic stress disorder (PTSD) symptoms, which, if not addressed, can complicate physical recovery. Empirical studies indicate that, left to their own devices, PTSD prevalence can only drop moderately during the initial three to six months after a traumatic event, highlighting the importance of early support and interventions within this key window (Fearon *et al.*, 2016). Secondly, the stress experienced by parents during the treatment of their child contributes to the rehabilitation process, thus providing a need to have well-established mental health care systems dealing with child and caregiver stress (Abidin *et al.*, 2005). Utilization of structured mental health interventions can assist in leading towards better recovery pathways, ultimately establishing resilience among young patients and caregivers.

12.4.2. Common Psychological Issues Faced by Pediatric Patients

In pediatric intensive care, psychological issues faced by children's patients may be acute and complicated, particularly where there is burn and trauma. Children are likely to experience high anxiety, depression, and PTSD due to the traumatic nature of the incidents and injuries. The resulting emotional trauma due to extensive hospital stay, painful procedures, and disruption of their normal lifestyle can be used to reinforce such feelings of loneliness and terror. It has been established by research that children who experience extreme trauma or injury, such as those in intensive care, are likely to exhibit diffuse psychological distress, which needs to be managed through special interventions (Drummond *et al.*, 2013).

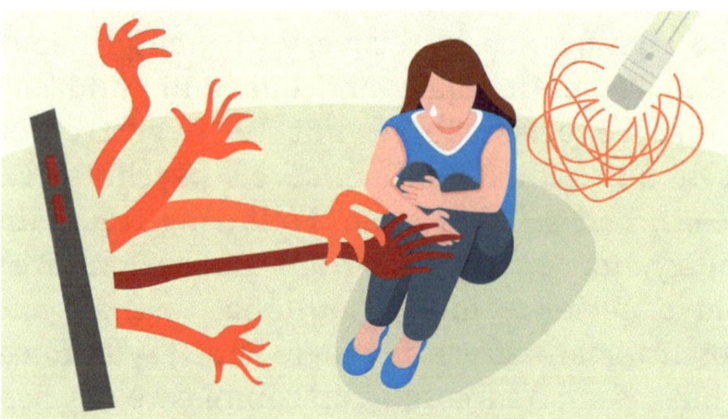

Figure 12.14. Children often experience heightened anxiety, depression, and post-traumatic stress disorder (PTSD) due to the traumatic nature of their experiences and the severity of their injuries.

Source: https://assets.clevelandclinic.org/transform/LargeFeatureImage/0ed1f8ed-c26d-4e24-802d-ab54f9282165/healing-trauma-218622570.

In addition, burns, which are to a great extent preventable, present other psychosocial levels of difficulty, since burned children can have issues with self-perception and social integration as a result of disfigurement (Ismail *et al.*, 2013). These concerns highlight the need for continued psychological care specific to the needs of pediatric patients in intensive care environments (Figure 12.14).

12.4.3. Role of Child Life Specialists in the PICU

In the Pediatric Intensive Care Unit (PICU), child life specialists play a critical role in reducing psychological stress experienced by children undergoing trauma and burn care. They are trained to provide emotional support and to use developmentally appropriate interventions that not only address the child's short-term concerns and fears but also enhance coping skills while hospitalized. By offering a favorable environment, child life specialists help children understand their medical procedures in terms of age-relevant explanations, in addition to play therapy, which may enhance their well-being and faster recovery. Interventions are particularly crucial in cases of polytrauma, in which children may experience more than one injury and thus have high psychological as well as emotional challenges. Staff readiness and far-reaching support measures, as referenced in the literature, take precedence over sound case management of such high-stress clients (As *et al.*, 2014; Henderson *et al.*, 2013).

12.4.4. Support Systems and Family Dynamics

The profound impact of family structure and support systems is starkly demonstrated in pediatric trauma and burns presenting in intensive care units. The evolving healthcare policy context, especially during the COVID-19 pandemic, has similarly highlighted the critical roles family members have to play in the care process. Studies have established that the family caregiver's role is core to patient-centered care as they provide emotional and mental well-being by being present, as well as effective communication and advocacy for the patient's interests (Montesanti *et al.*, 2023). Moreover, the stress healthcare workers harbor in such intense settings can affect family interactions and result in burnout, which compromises care delivery (Buckley *et al.*, 2022). Therefore, identification and encouragement of family participation is essential not just for the recovery of the patient but also to ensure the strength of familial relationships during crises, ultimately strengthening the safety net that is so important during medical crises (Figure 12.15).

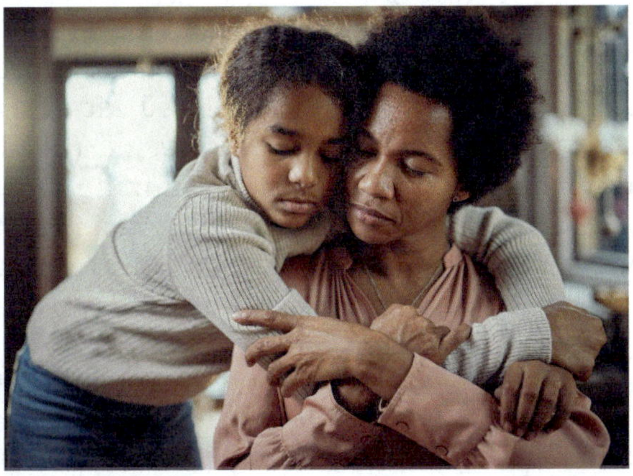

Figure 12.15. The profound impact of family dynamics and support systems is particularly evident in the context of pediatric trauma and burns within intensive care settings.

Source: https://www.health.com/thmb/qpF2JlH_ZXP7Q1DDC_H3w00M_sQ=/5612x0/filters:no_upscale():max_bytes(150000):strip_icc()/generationaltrauma-GettyImages-1445387381-a541781b67aa4f029c68b49071c2791d.jpg.

12.4.5. Coping Strategies for Children and Families

For pediatric intensive care, the application of efficient coping strategies in children and families is crucial for minimizing the psychological impact of burns and trauma. Adaptive coping, such as mindfulness interventions, has been shown to have positive outcomes on stress reduction and symptoms of trauma, hence enhancing well-being (Ortiz *et al.*, 2017). These interventions not only support children's mental and emotional health but also foster resilience within families facing significant challenges. Additionally, addressing factors that contribute to burnout among pediatric nurses is crucial, as their well-being has a direct impact on patient care quality and family support (Buckley *et al.*, 2020). Through a focus on structured programs that promote mindfulness and resiliency in children and healthcare providers, pediatric intensive care units can promote a healing-focused environment, ultimately leading to enhanced outcomes for the young patients and their families as they navigate the intricacies of trauma and recovery.

12.4.6. Long-Term Psychological Support Options

In pediatric critical care, trauma and burns constitute a scenario under which long-term mental health support alternatives need to be addressed to facilitate recovery and overall well-being. Traditional interventions, such as burn camps and peer support groups, provide ample community support; however, such programs lack the therapeutic components necessary to cope with psychological distress holistically. It is suggested by studies that a high-intensity psychosocial guided retreat, performed by experienced mental health professionals, is capable of influencing self-esteem and posttraumatic stress disorder (PTSD) symptoms in teenage burn patients (Sarah *et al.*, 2020). Secondly, the psychological impact of catastrophic injury transcends acute recovery and requires expert interventions for young children, who are often overlooked in trauma research despite being vulnerable (Graf, 2013). Through the utilization of extensive, assessment-driven approaches, medical professionals are better positioned to meet the emotional needs of child patients, fostering resilience and a recovery process that identifies physical, along with psychological healing (Figure 12.16).

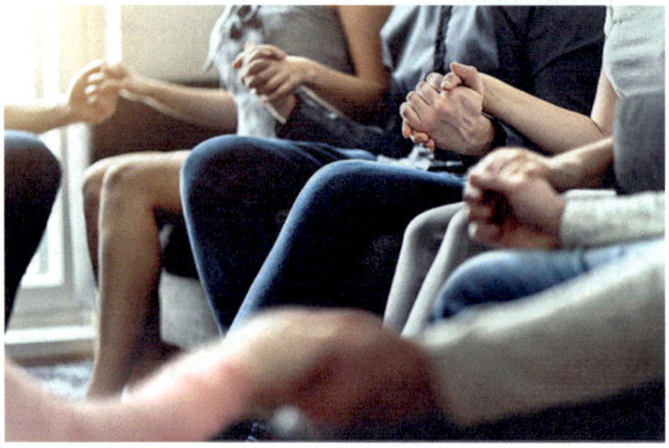

Figure 12.16. Traditional methods, such as burn camps and peer support groups, provide valuable community support; yet, these programs often lack the therapeutic components necessary to address psychological distress adequately.

Source: https://ctb.ku.edu/sites/default/files/chapter_files/group_therapy_holding_hands.jpg.

12.4.7. Impact of Trauma and Burns on Family Relationships

The impact of trauma and burns on family interactions may be remarkable, often inducing severe emotional distress, disruption, and tension. Families frequently experience a jarring transition from routine to acute crisis because the severity of a child's injuries may generate fear, hopelessness, and alienation among members of the same family. These interactions may generate increased caregiver burden and conflict, with members of the family reacting differently to trauma, frequently disrupting communication and support systems. Psychological and physical stress in pediatric intensive care may also contribute to isolation, as families struggle with their own emotional requirements and seek to provide care for the traumatized child. As highlighted by recent guidelines, maximizing family-centered care in the ICU context is important for improving overall outcomes. Interventions to promote family communication, support, and collaboration among healthcare providers can contribute positively to minimizing the adverse effects of trauma on family functioning (Carson *et al.*, 2018; Judy *et al.*, 2016).

12.4.8. Community Resources for Ongoing Support

Extended support in pediatric intensive care is imperative for the provision of community resources, particularly in cases of trauma and burns. They encompass a range of services, which can be psychological support, rehabilitation programs, and educational services to cater to the diverse needs of the affected children and families. For instance, tailored kit design patterns, as explained in Batra *et al.* (2021), have the capability of optimizing local healthcare capacity by preparing facilities to handle pediatric care surges and thus ensure comprehensive support systems.

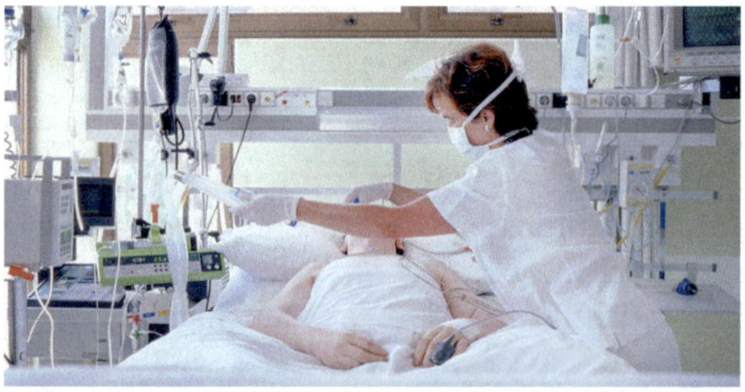

Figure 12.17. The provision of community resources is essential for ongoing support in pediatric intensive care, particularly following trauma and burns.

Source: https://media.post.rvohealth.io/wp-content/uploads/2021/01/INTENSIVE-CARE-UNIT-1200x628-facebook-1200x628.jpg.

In addition, cleft prioritization in the presence of resource constraints suggests the necessity for a well-structured care pathway with immediate and long-term healthcare implications. By creating a network of community-based care, physician providers can not only diminish the physical impact of trauma but also enable the psychological and emotional well-being of child patients and ultimately lead to improved overall health status and quality of life for these vulnerable populations (Figure 12.17).

12.4.9. Research on Psychological Outcomes in Pediatric Trauma and Burn Patients

Psychological outcomes of pediatric trauma and burn injury patients are major factors in recovery and overall health in intensive care units. Psychological disorders like anxiety and post-traumatic stress disorder (PTSD) are prevalent in children following traumatic injuries such as motor vehicle accidents and serious burns. Reports show that the severity of such trauma in most cases is proportional to very high levels of psychological distress, which are further exacerbated by long hospital stays and harsh interventions. A case in point is burned children, who not only endure the direct physical effects of their burns but also the indirect and long-term effects of their experiences of pediatric intensive care unit interventions. This mandates an interdisciplinary treatment plan, with psychological assessment and intervention incorporated into the medical treatment protocols. Further, tailored nutrition after injury has been demonstrated to play a role in better psychological and overall recovery, with implications for holistic care models (Kuok *et al.*, 2022; Bul *et al.*, 2021).

Test Your Knowledge

1. How can child life specialists support children undergoing painful or frightening procedures?
2. What interventions help reduce anxiety and fear in hospitalized children?

SUMMARY

Burn and trauma management in pediatric intensive care is an interdisciplinary approach that involves continuous innovations in clinical practice and research studies. The intricacy of the relationship between trauma severity and heightened susceptibility to secondary infection underscores the necessity for new therapeutic interventions. As stressed by Frieri *et al.* (2016), the urgency for solutions to antimicrobial resistance calls for innovative therapeutic options to conventional antibiotics to manage the complex biofilm-related issues prevalent among pediatric burn patients. Moreover, the implications of sepsis in these vulnerable patients, along with increasing rates of chronic critical illness, accentuate the extreme significance of refining care guidelines as discussed by Jeffrey *et al.* (2016). Pediatric intensive care demands an unyielding commitment to outcome improvement by early diagnosis, augmenting supportive therapy, and a full appreciation for the long-term consequences of trauma and burn injury in children.

In contemplating the pivotal aspects of trauma and burns in pediatric intensive care, it is important to emphasize the subtleties pertaining to the management and outcomes for such susceptible patients. The onset of acute kidney injury (AKI) within such a population has emerged as a significant concern, and thus, there is a necessity to strictly follow guidelines for appropriate risk assessment, prevention, and management measures (Kellum *et al.*, 2013). Moreover, the intricacy of polytrauma in children still underscores the importance of preparedness among physicians and healthcare providers since an adequately prepared emergency room can greatly improve the survival and recovery chances of pediatric polytrauma patients (PPPs) (As *et al.*, 2014). Combined, these considerations not only emphasize the multifaceted difficulties faced in pediatric critical care but also continue to support the imperative for universal, evidence-based approaches that address acute medical concerns and promote optimal recovery in children with trauma and burns.

KEY TERMS FROM THIS CHAPTER

- Burns
- Fire
- Machine learning
- Falls
- Non-accidental injuries
- Electricity
- Head injury
- Post-traumatic stress disorder (PTSD)
- Trauma management
- Artificial intelligence
- Trauma
- Motor vehicle accidents
- Child abuse
- Rib fractures
- Hemothorax
- Emotional well-being

CRITICAL THINKING QUESTIONS

1. **What is the most common cause of traumatic injury requiring PICU admission in children?**
   a. Falls
   b. Motor vehicle accidents
   c. Sports injuries
   d. Animal bites
2. **Which of the following is the primary concern in the initial management of a child with major burns?**
   a. Pain control
   b. Fluid resuscitation
   c. Infection prevention
   d. Nutritional support
3. **The Parkland formula for fluid resuscitation in burns recommends:**
   a. 4 mL × body weight (kg) × %TBSA burned over 24 hours
   b. 2 mL × body weight (kg) × %TBSA burned over 48 hours
   c. 10 mL × body weight (kg) × %TBSA burned over 12 hours
   d. 3 mL × body weight (kg) × %TBSA burned over 24 hours
4. **Which burn depth involves damage to the epidermis and part of the dermis, often presenting with blistering and pain?**
   a. Superficial (1st degree)
   b. Superficial partial-thickness (2nd degree)
   c. Deep partial-thickness (3rd degree)
   d. Full-thickness (4th degree)
5. **Which of the following is NOT a common complication of severe pediatric trauma?**
   a. Traumatic brain injury
   b. Hypothermia
   c. Hyperkalemia
   d. Compartment syndrome

Short Answer Questions

1. What are the most common mechanisms of trauma in infants versus older children?
2. How do patterns of injury differ between accidental trauma and non-accidental trauma (child abuse)?
3. What are the differences between superficial, partial-thickness, and full-thickness burns in children?
4. How does the total body surface area (TBSA) burned affect prognosis in pediatric burn patients?
5. What are the initial priorities in the management of a child with multi-system trauma?
6. How is airway management handled in pediatric trauma with facial burns or inhalation injury?
7. What are the common psychological effects of trauma and burns in children?
8. How can healthcare providers identify signs of post-traumatic stress disorder (PTSD) in pediatric patients?

Answers to Critical Thinking Questions

1. (b); 2. (b); 3. (a); 4. (b); 5. (c)

REFERENCES

1. Abidin, Å., Åkerlund, C., Andersson, B., Andersson, C., Bakker, J., Brusselaers, N., Cohen, M., *et al.* (2005). Internet-based information and self-help program for parents of children with burns: Study protocol for a randomized controlled trial. https://core.ac.uk/download/pdf/82749357.pdf (accessed on 30th June 2025).
2. Auerbach, S. M., Bottorff, J., Collins, S., Edwards, P. M., Fallis, W. M., Friedson, E., Institute of Medicine, *et al.* (2016). Patient and family involvement in adult critical and intensive care settings: A scoping review. https://core.ac.uk/download/74395959.pdf (accessed on 30th June 2025).
3. Batra, P., Galwankar, S., Shah, D., Gist, R. E., Shah, A. P., Krishnan, S., Arquilla, B., *et al.* (2021). The 2021 toolkit for emergency preparedness and mitigation to combat surge of pediatric COVID-19 patients in India: The World Health Organization Collaborating Center for Emergency and Trauma in South East Asia recommendations. *Journal of Emergencies, Trauma, and Shock, 14*, 153–172. https://www.semanticscholar.org/paper/7e5367a1075f271831187e51e11208 54c3435f37 (accessed on 30th June 2025).
4. Benlamkaddem, S., Bouyerman, F., Berdai, M., & Harandou, M. (2023). Pediatric acute respiratory distress syndrome in a Moroccan intensive care unit: A retrospective observational study of 23 cases. *The Pan African Medical Journal, 44.* https://www.semanticscholar.org/paper/69c 476896846faeb159110e0a9c4be1e329c08f8 (accessed on 30th June 2025).
5. Blackmon, T., Palmieri, T. L., Rashidi, H. H., Sen, S., *et al.* (2020). Early recognition of burn- and trauma-related acute kidney injury: A pilot comparison of machine learning techniques. https://core.ac.uk/download/323069263.pdf (accessed on 30th June 2025).
6. Brophy, G. M., Dager, W. E., Devlin, J. W., Erstad, B., *et al.* (2009). Key articles and guidelines relative to intensive care unit pharmacotherapy: 2009 update. https://deepblue.lib.umich.edu/bitstream/2027.42/90162/1/phco.29.10.1228.pdf (accessed on 30th June 2025).
7. Buckley, L., Berta, W., Cleverley, K., & Widger, K. (2022). Exploring pediatric nurses' perspectives on their work environment, work attitudes, and experience of burnout: What really matters? *Frontiers in Pediatrics, 10.* https://doi.org/10.3389/fped.2022.851001 (accessed on 30th June 2025).
8. Buckley, L., Berta, W., Cleverley, K., Medeiros, C., & Widger, K. (2020). What is known about pediatric nurse burnout: A scoping review. *Human Resources for Health, 18.* https://doi.org/10.1186/s12960-020-0451-8 (accessed on 30th June 2025).
9. Bul, C. (2021). Nutrition treatment in pediatric burns patients. *Clinical Science of Nutrition.* https://www.semanticscholar.org/paper/03e147d57f51c49d99e10160eb0e63e25d6c2469 (accessed on 30th June 2025).
10. Bull, A., Mayhew, E., Milwood Hargrave, J., Pearce, R., *et al.* (2019). Blast injuries in children: A mixed-methods narrative review. https://core.ac.uk/download/227470209.pdf (accessed on 30th June 2025).
11. Burns, C. S., Burns, R., Sanseau, E., Mazor, S., Reid, J., Stone, K., & Thomas, A. (2018). Pediatric emergency medicine simulation curriculum: Marijuana ingestion. *MedEdPORTAL.* https://doi.org/10.15766/mep_2374-8265.10780 (accessed on 30th June 2025).
12. Carrol, E. D., Lane, S., Lisboa, P. J. G., McGrath, C., *et al.* (2014). What impact did a pediatric

early warning system have on emergency admissions to the pediatric intensive care unit? An observational cohort study. https://core.ac.uk/download/42136646.pdf (accessed on 30th June 2025).

13. Ceriello, A., Ceriello, A., Ceriello, A., Chiaretti, A., Rovlias, A., Russo, A., Russo, A., *et al.* (2010). Control of hyperglycemia in pediatric intensive care (CHiP): Study protocol. https://core.ac.uk/download/20330333.pdf (accessed on 30th June 2025).

14. Chemali, Z., Ezzeddine, F. L., Gelaye, B., Dossett, M. L., Salameh, J., Bizri, M., Dubale, B. W., *et al.* (2019). Burnout among healthcare providers in the complex environment of the Middle East: A systematic review. *BMC Public Health, 19.* https://doi.org/10.1186/s12889-019-7713-1 (accessed on 30th June 2025).

15. Chimbira, W., Crawford, H., Gupta, S., Legg, C., *et al.* (2001). Acute lung injury in pediatric intensive care: Course and outcome. https://core.ac.uk/download/pdf/8715345.pdf (accessed on 30th June 2025).

16. Chirica, M., Kelly, M. D., Siboni, S., Aiolfi, A., Riva, C. G., Asti, E., Ferrari, D., *et al.* (2019). Esophageal emergencies: WSES guidelines. *World Journal of Emergency Surgery, 14.* https://doi.org/10.1186/s13017-019-0245-2 (accessed on 30th June 2025).

17. Davidson, J. E., Aslakson, R. A., Long, A. C., Puntillo, K., Kross, E. K., Hart, J. L., Cox, C. E., *et al.* (2016). Guidelines for family-centered care in the neonatal, pediatric, and adult ICU. *Critical Care Medicine, 45*, 103–128. https://doi.org/10.1097/ccm.0000000000002169 (accessed on 30th June 2025).

18. Keulenaer De , B. L., De Laet, I., De Waele, J., Debergh, D., *et al.* (2014). Awareness and knowledge of intra-abdominal hypertension and abdominal compartment syndrome: Results of an international survey. https://core.ac.uk/download/55846801.pdf (accessed on 30th June 2025).

19. Keulenaer De , B. L., De Laet, I., De Waele, J., Ejike, J., *et al.* (2015). Intra-abdominal hypertension and abdominal compartment syndrome in pancreatitis, pediatrics, and trauma. https://core.ac.uk/download/55855279.pdf (accessed on 30th June 2025).

20. Delano, M. J., & Ward, P. A. (2016). The immune system's role in sepsis progression, resolution, and long-term outcome. *Immunological Reviews, 274*, 330–353. https://doi.org/10.1111/imr.12499 (accessed on 30th June 2025).

21. Docking, R., Kinsella, J., Moss, L., Sim, R., *et al.* (2012). An investigation into the effects of commencing hemodialysis in the critically ill. https://core.ac.uk/download/1439066.pdf (accessed on 30th June 2025).

22. Drummond, P. D., & Kemp, M. (2013). Sample representation in a psychological treatment study after single event pediatric trauma. https://core.ac.uk/download/11237927.pdf (accessed on 30th June 2025).

23. Epstein, E. G., Falcó-Pegueroles, A., Jameton, A., Leske, J., Schroeter, K., Meyers, L. S., *et al.* (2018). Moral distress in critical care nursing: The state of the science. https://core.ac.uk/download/213088610.pdf (accessed on 30th June 2025).

24. Escarce, J. J., & Kapur, K. (2025). Do patients bypass rural hospitals? Determinants of inpatient hospital choice in rural California. https://core.ac.uk/download/pdf/6401717.pdf (accessed on 30th June 2025).

25. Fearon, P., Fraser, A., Halligan, S. L., Hiller, R., *et al.* (2016). Research review: Changes in the prevalence and symptom severity of child posttraumatic stress disorder in the year following trauma–A meta-analytic study. https://core.ac.uk/download/41993811.pdf (accessed on 30th June 2025).

26. Frieri, M., Kumar, K., & Boutin, A. (2016). Antibiotic resistance. *Journal of Infection and Public Health, 10*, 369–378. https://doi.org/10.1016/j.jiph.2016.08.007 (accessed on 30th June 2025).

27. Gotts, J. E., & Matthay, M. A. (2016). Sepsis: Pathophysiology and clinical management. *BMJ*. https://doi.org/10.1136/bmj.i1585 (accessed on 30th June 2025).

28. Graf, A. (2013). Posttraumatic stress and behavior in injured and severely ill infants and preschoolers. https://www.semanticscholar.org/paper/36ec78d86eca48cdc80ab7d8fe7b25670705d93e (accessed on 30th June 2025).

29. Henderson, T. (2013). Pediatric consultation-liaison psychiatry: A description of the consultation-liaison service offered by a tertiary level children's hospital in Cape Town, South Africa. https://core.ac.uk/download/185391899.pdf (accessed on 30th June 2025).

30. Hiller, J., Moran, C., & Newton, K. (2025). 627 Use of tubular elastic bandage to reduce device related PI (PI) in burn patients. *Journal of Burn Care & Research: Official Publication of the American Burn Association, 46*, S197–S197. https://www.semanticscholar.org/paper/8b622680677e1023418edb45035df9cff9029ed3 (accessed on 30th June 2025).

31. Hoang, D. M., Pham, P. T., Bach, T. Q., Ngo, A. T., Nguyen, Q. T., Phan, T. K. T., Giang, N. H., *et al.* (2022). Stem cell-based therapy for human diseases. *Signal Transduction and Targeted Therapy, 7*. https://doi.org/10.1038/s41392-022-01134-4 (accessed on 30th June 2025).

32. Hyrkas, K., & LaFlamme, J. (2020). The Center for Nursing Research and Quality Outcomes. https://core.ac.uk/download/352343815.pdf (accessed on 30th June 2025).

33. Ismail, H., Temu, J., Mary, M., Mbembati, N. A., Mgalilwa, H., *et al.* (2013). Burns in Tanzania: Morbidity and mortality, causes and risk factors: A review. https://core.ac.uk/download/pdf/16666898.pdf (accessed on 30th June 2025).

34. Kawalec, A. M. (2018). Problem of burns in children: Opportunities for health improvement. https://core.ac.uk/download/322435472.pdf (accessed on 30th June 2025).

35. Kellum, J. A., & Lameire, N. (2013). Diagnosis, evaluation, and management of acute kidney injury: A KDIGO summary (part 1). https://core.ac.uk/download/55846642.pdf (accessed on 30th June 2025).

36. Kleinpell, R., Grabenkort, W. R., Boyle, W. A., Vines, D., & Olsen, K. M. (2021). The Society of Critical Care Medicine at 50 years: Interprofessional practice in critical care: Looking back and forging ahead. *Critical Care Medicine, 49*, 2017–2032. https://doi.org/10.1097/ccm.0000000000005276 (accessed on 30th June 2025).

37. Kotovich, D., Sarna Cahan, S., Ohana Sarna Cahan, L., Ben Hamo, M., Hashavya, S., & Gross, M. (2025). 585 Minimizing unnecessary procedures: Revisiting fiberoptic laryngoscopy protocols for pediatric burn patients in the emergency department. *Journal of Burn Care & Research: Official Publication of the American Burn Association, 46*, S168–S168. https://www.semanticscholar.org/paper/c13de8ed4986be6e3c9243ea239078f7f227d058 (accessed on 30th June 2025).

38. Krakowski, A. C., Sojka, J., & Stawicki, S. P. (2019). Burn shock and resuscitation: Many priorities, one goal. https://core.ac.uk/download/322442935.pdf (accessed on 30th June 2025).

39. Kuok, C., & Chan, W. (2022). Motor vehicle collision and acute kidney injury in children. *Pediatric Emergency Care, 38*, 545–549. https://www.semanticscholar.org/paper/7dec0d0dc465b4291182683b2c12b1dbfdb32280 (accessed on 30th June 2025).

40. Madokoro, S., Hirano, Y., Kondo, Y., & Okamoto, K. (2024). Epidemiology and outcome analysis of blast injury patients in Japan: An analysis of the nationwide trauma registry database. *Medicine, 103*. https://www.semanticscholar.org/paper/a9420832f088e197f19921509b267e7f35b379b0 (accessed on 30th June 2025).

41. Maye, H. (2012). Cultured epithelial autografts in the management of burn injuries: A review of the literature. https://core.ac.uk/download/77162775.pdf (accessed on 30th June 2025).

42. Montesanti, S., MacKean, G., Fitzpatrick, K., & Fancott, C. (2023). Family caregivers as essential partners in care: Examining the impact/s of restrictive acute care visiting policies during the COVID-19 pandemic in Canada. *BMC Health Services Research, 23*. https://doi.org/10.1186/s12913-023-09248-3 (accessed on 30th June 2025).

43. Ortiz, R., & Sibinga, E. (2017). The role of mindfulness in reducing the adverse effects of childhood stress and trauma. *Children, 4*, 16–16. https://doi.org/10.3390/children4030016 (accessed on 30th June 2025).

44. Rahimpour, A., Saurborn, E., Fox, N., Giangrosso, G. V., Denning, D. A., Harrison, C. W., Bown, P., *et al.* (2025). Predictors of prolonged hospitalization in pediatric burn patients: Insights from a rural burn intensive care unit (BICU) in Appalachia. *Cureus, 17*. https://www.semanticscholar.org/paper/47e405ae417507f85435bf4f000da8052b62be66 (accessed on 30th June 2025).

45. Ren, Y. (2016). Negative pressure wound therapy is useful in pediatric burn patients: A retrospective review. https://open.bu.edu/bitstream/2144/16825/1/Ren_bu_0017N_11860.pdf (accessed on 30th June 2025).

46. Sen, C. K. (2019). Human wounds and its burden: An updated compendium of estimates. https://core.ac.uk/download/299809006.pdf (accessed on 30th June 2025).

47. Søreide, K., Hallet, J., Matthews, J. B., Schnitzbauer, A. A., Line, P.-D., Lai, P. B. S., Gestal Otero, J. J., *et al.* (2020). Immediate and long-term impact of the COVID-19 pandemic on delivery of surgical services. *British Journal of Surgery, 107*, 1250–1261. https://doi.org/10.1002/bjs.11670 (accessed on 30th June 2025).

48. Stoycos, S. A., Sammons, A. J., Cartelli, L., & Price, L. A. (2020). 766 Clinical outcome assessment of a psychosocial intensive retreat for girls with severe burns. *Journal of Burn Care & Research, 41*. https://www.semanticscholar.org/paper/a8361b1ac5752a8aa5db057345f8a82967493cab (accessed on 30th June 2025).

49. van As, A. B., van Dijk, M., Mevius, H., Numanoglu, A., *et al.* (2014). The management of pediatric polytrauma: Review. https://core.ac.uk/download/43313566.pdf (accessed on 30th June 2025).

50. van Dijk, M., ter Meulen, E. W., Poley, M. J., Rode, H., *et al.* (2016). The hospital costs associated with acute pediatric burn injuries. https://core.ac.uk/download/154418031.pdf (accessed on 30th June 2025).

POST-OPERATIVE AND TRANSPLANT CRITICAL CARE

13

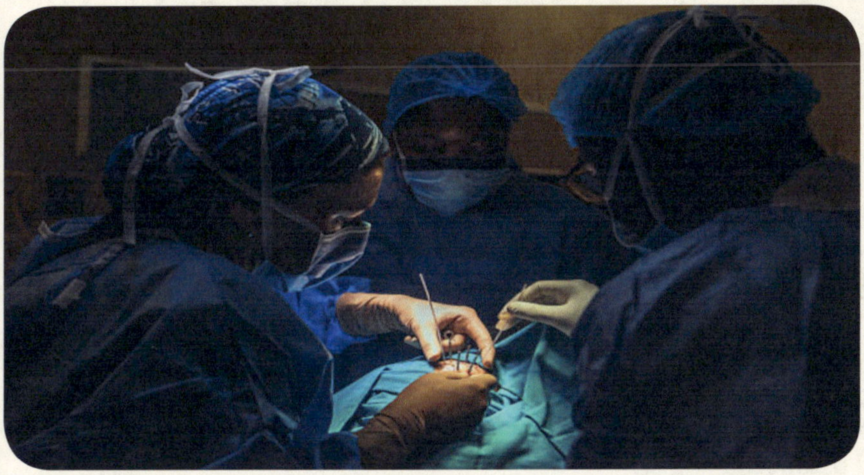

LEARNING OBJECTIVES

After studying this chapter, you will be able to:

1. Understand Post-operative Care in Pediatric Patients.
2. Explain Transplant Procedures in Pediatric Patients.
3. Describe Critical Care Management in Pediatric Intensive Care.

Introduction

The intricacies of transplant and post-operative critical care in pediatric intensive care units (PICUs) pose one of the biggest challenges for healthcare practitioners, as they navigate the intricate needs of vulnerable patient groups. Under such circumstances, knowledge of the poliomyelitis of care—from the surgical operation to the process of recovery in a specialist environment—assumes greater significance. The importance of multidisciplinary practice is highlighted by the evolving nature of conditions in children, calling for timely and effective intervention to improve outcomes. Recent trends recognize augmented vulnerability among children, particularly to global health crises, with care pathways being adaptive enough to respond to emergent incidents, like the COVID-19 pandemic, that have influenced therapeutic practice (Sullivan *et al.*, 2020). With growth in pediatric critical care comes adherence to suggested guidelines and their standards as well, having an imperative role in securing optimal quality of care, with standards keeping up with the particular needs of this group (Stout *et al.*, 2018).

13.1. Post-Operative Care in Pediatric Patients

Learning Outcome

1. Immediate Post-operative Monitoring Requirements.
2. Pain Management Strategies for Children.
3. Nutritional Considerations after Surgery.
4. Infection Prevention Protocols.
5. Psychological Support for Pediatric Patients.
6. Family Involvement in Post-operative Care.
7. Transitioning from ICU to General Ward.
8. Long-term Follow-up Care Post-surgery.

In pediatric post-operative management, particularly following complex surgery such as liver transplant, attention to strict observation and early intervention cannot be stressed sufficiently. PICU children are particularly prone to the development of a range of complications from a few hours after surgery, and thus, close monitoring of the vital parameters, fluid balance, and neurological status becomes imperative.

As reinforced in the literature, every organ system may be involved with the procedure and medications themselves, thus highlighting the need for individualized care strategies to achieve optimal recovery with minimal risk of morbidity and mortality. Specifically, early extubation and hemodynamic monitoring are proposed to optimize oxygenation and perfusion to facilitate transition to recovery. Besides, the inclusion of infection control practices and early nutritional therapy is essential to ensure acceptance of the graft and overall patient well-being, as addressed in recent guidelines (Scott *et al.*, 2021; Pudjiadi, 2020) (Figure 13.1).

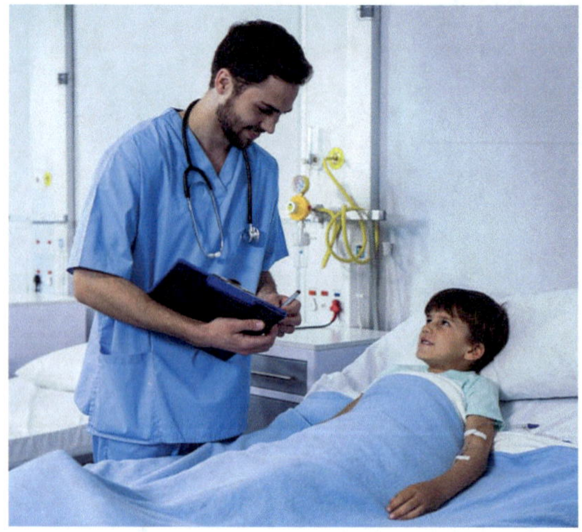

Figure 13.1. Children in the Pediatric Intensive Care Unit (PICU) are particularly vulnerable to a range of complications that can arise shortly after surgery, necessitating vigilant observation of vital signs, fluid balance, and neurological status.

Source: https://suryahospitals.com/speciality/6561bf8febe98Expertise---Pediatric-Intensive-Care-(PICU).jpg.

13.1.1. Immediate Post-Operative Monitoring Requirements

In the early post-operative period, it is necessary to observe pediatric patients to obtain physiological stability following surgery, particularly in transplant cases where there is a high risk of complications. Ongoing observation of vital signs, including heart rate, blood pressure, and oxygen saturation, is vital in the early identification of hemodynamic instability or respiratory compromise. Special attention is required with fluid management in that children are highly sensitive to electrolyte disturbances and renal problems due to their lower body stores and ongoing growth. Moreover, according to guidelines given in the recent past, post-operative monitoring strategies following surgery should be thorough and should look for infection, bleeding, and organ function immediately after surgery, particularly in patients with comorbidities like liver disease or those undergoing complex procedures, according to the suggestions in (Scott *et al.*, 2021) and (Steven *et al.*, 2020). Coordination of an effective monitoring plan is thus essential in enabling recovery and minimizing post-operative complications in this high-risk group.

13.1.2. Pain Management Strategies for Children

Efficient management of pediatric post-surgical and transplant pain is a multifaceted problem that requires tailored approaches to accommodate the differences in children's development. Both pharmacologic and non-pharmacologic measures must be used in conjunction to achieve optimal outcomes. For instance, analgesics like opioids and NSAIDs may be titrated based on the individual child's status and response to treatment.

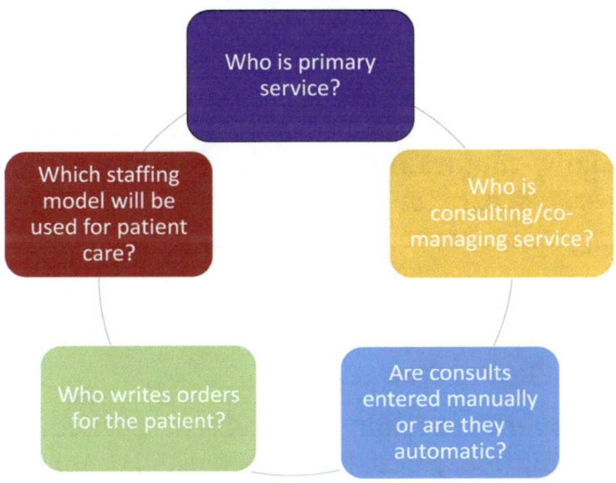

Figure 13.2. Effective pain management in pediatric post-operative and transplant care is a multifaceted challenge that requires tailored strategies to accommodate the developmental variances among children.

Source: https://www.advancesinpediatrics.org/cms/10.1016/j.yapd.2021.05.010/asset/642574c1-3f55-4e4a-8e6c-4321a20d36ef/main.assets/gr2_lrg.jpg.

In addition, adjuvant treatments such as cognitive-behavioral interventions, distraction techniques, and involvement of family members can significantly enhance pain control and reduce anxiety in the recovery process. Personalized protocols, underscored by existing recommendations, emphasize the need for team-based care strategies with multidisciplinary experts to establish holistic pain management for conditions like Morquio A syndrome and postoperative recovery (Akyol *et al.*, 2019). Moreover, in some operative environments, advances in dynamic monitoring clarify the role of anticipatory fluid management in preventing pain and complications (Gutierrez *et al.*, 2013) (Figure 13.2).

13.1.3. Nutritional Considerations After Surgery

Pediatric post-operative rehabilitation involves a thorough assessment of nutritional needs to facilitate healing and minimize complications. A healthy diet is critical not only to support healing but to prevent complications of malnutrition, particularly in the case of children in whom major surgical interventions are done, such as organ transplants. Studies highlight that intensive nutrition therapy can significantly enhance development and decrease hospitalization time, with a clear correlation being observable between tailored nutritional treatment and improved clinical outcomes in this patient population (Bavetta *et al.*, 2013). Further, in transplant surgery, there have been reported instances where alterations in immunosuppression protocols have minimized complications and improved patient health, thus indirectly emphasizing the importance of appropriate nutrition to aid in recovery from the surgery (Abu-Elmagd *et al.*, 2005). Therefore, placing nutritional requirements at the center of post-surgical care assists in aiding recovery and enhancing the overall prognosis for pediatric patients who are undergoing critical care.

13.1.4. Infection Prevention Protocols

Infection control policies are critical elements of post-transplant and post-operative care in pediatric patients because they directly impact recovery outcomes and overall patient safety. Proper policies must involve strict sanitation procedures, vigilant monitoring for signs of infection, and the administration of prophylactic antibiotics at the correct time, all tailored to the unique needs of high-risk pediatric patients. A stepwise infection control strategy is important, particularly in cases like transfusion-dependent thalassemia, where there's an elevated risk of healthcare-associated infections due to frequent invasive procedures and compromised immunity (Farmakis *et al.*, 2022). Furthermore, adherence to set standards, such as the KDIGO, ensures that health care professionals assess all the infection risk factors to ensure a stringent system of evaluation that puts the highest consideration on the safety of patients during transplantation (Steven *et al.*, 2020). Overall, adherence to these infection control practices is key to maximizing clinical outcomes in pediatric intensive care units (Figure 13.3).

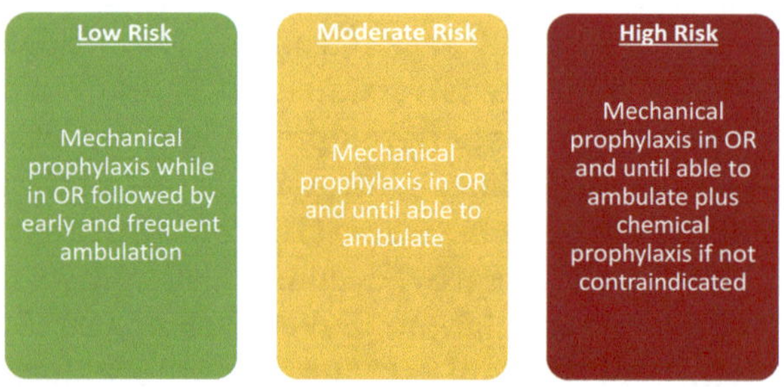

Figure 13.3. Infection prevention protocols are critical components of post-operative and transplant care for pediatric patients, as they significantly influence recovery outcomes and overall patient safety.

Source: https://www.advancesinpediatrics.org/cms/10.1016/j.yapd.2021.05.010/asset/52a2b3f3-fe54-4605-aab5-85407677183f/main.assets/gr4_lrg.jpg.

13.1.5. Psychological Support for Pediatric Patients

In the complex realm of post-operative and transplant recovery, the psychological care of the pediatric patient is most crucial in the enhancement of overall recovery and well-being. Children who are awaiting surgery or transplants often battle anxiety, fear, and a lack of understanding, which subsequently exacerbate their physical distress and disrupt healing. Mental health intervention and child life intervention can greatly mitigate these psychological burdens, inducing feelings of safety and understanding. In addition, research reveals that intensive psychological intervention not only enhances the emotional resilience of child patients but also is linked with enhanced medical outcomes, enabling a vital interaction between physical and psychological well-being within pediatric intensive care settings (Argent *et al.*, 2017). As is highlighted, psychological problems must be resolved, particularly in more complex cases where the risk of complications is so great that it can have lasting impacts on patients and caregivers alike (Barr *et al.*, 2009). Finally, maintaining mental health in post-operative care for children is key to augmenting long-term recovery trajectories.

13.1.6. Family Involvement in Post-Operative Care

Post-operative family involvement, particularly in pediatric critical care, is crucial for the recovery of the child and the health of family members. Studies indicate that active involvement of families in care has a significant impact on improved health outcomes, where the child's recovery process is fostered in an environment. The movement towards family-centered care models is highlighted by collaboration between healthcare providers and families to enable individually focused care plans taking into account familial environment and culture (Kristina *et al.*, 2019). Additionally, the management of various risk factors and co-morbid conditions with regard to the patient's suitability for procedures, that is, kidney transplantation, demands that family members be educated and active participants in decision-making processes (Steven *et al.*, 2020). This partnership not only improves the delivery of care but also reduces the emotional burden on families and results in an overall method for pediatric post-surgical recovery in intensive care units (Figure 13.4).

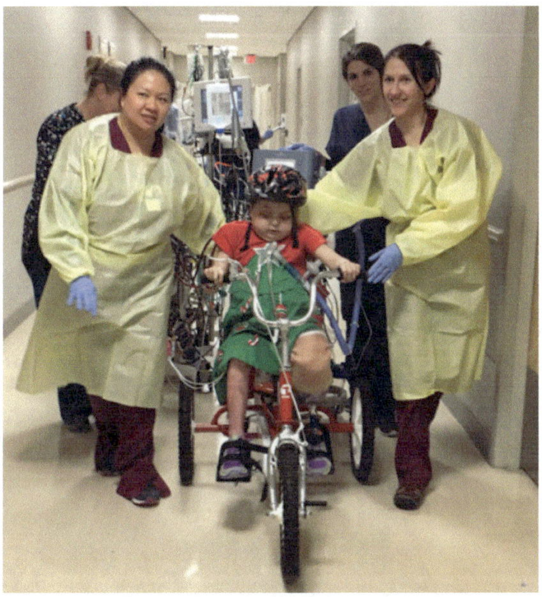

Figure 13.4. In the context of post-operative care, particularly in pediatric intensive care, family involvement is crucial for both the child's recovery and the well-being of family members themselves.

Source: https://www.thelancet.com/cms/asset/a1c56d7d-2b96-460b-9e35-1b496a5cdb43/fx1.jpg.

13.1.7. Transitioning from ICU to General Ward

Transition from the intensive care unit (ICU) to the general ward is a phase that is essential in the recovery process of pediatric patients following post-operative and transplant surgery. The phase requires comprehensive coordination and overall assessment to ensure that the patient's condition is stable and his/her needs are appropriately addressed. With the patient being transferred to a less regulated environment, medical practitioners must consider many aspects, such as how probable complications will be managed and care continuity, which is critical in preventing readmission or prolonged hospitalization. To ensure maximum effectiveness while undertaking this, hospitals can implement standardized pathways that provide for seamless transition, using proven practices highlighted in current literature (Stone *et al.*, 2022). Moreover, the importance of judicious usage of antibiotics at this stage cannot be overstated because misuse is likely to lead to resistance and complications, supporting the need for adherence to guidelines for the use of antibiotics (Sartelli *et al.*, 2023).

13.1.8. Long-Term Follow-up Care Post-surgery

The significance of long-term follow-up after surgery cannot be overemphasized, particularly in pediatric intensive care for transplant surgery. Since children generally have complex recovery and complication trajectories, comprehensive follow-up models are required to evaluate for chronic health issues arising from surgery. For instance, studies indicate that children who underwent transplant and were in need of intensive care had a large incidence of complications, such as new dialysis-dependent renal failure and hospital readmissions, that negatively impacted post-discharge long-term survival rates (Zinter *et al.*, 2023). Along with this, increasing trends in lung transplantation for severe respiratory disease like COVID-19-associated ARDS make it crucial to be aware of long-term survival for such recipients, since survival following lung transplant is excellent despite the presence of complex preoperative problems (Kurihara *et al.*, 2022). Thus, individualized and regular follow-up becomes imperative to achieve the best possible quality of life as well as optimize long-term prognosis in such vulnerable pediatric recipients (Figure 13.5).

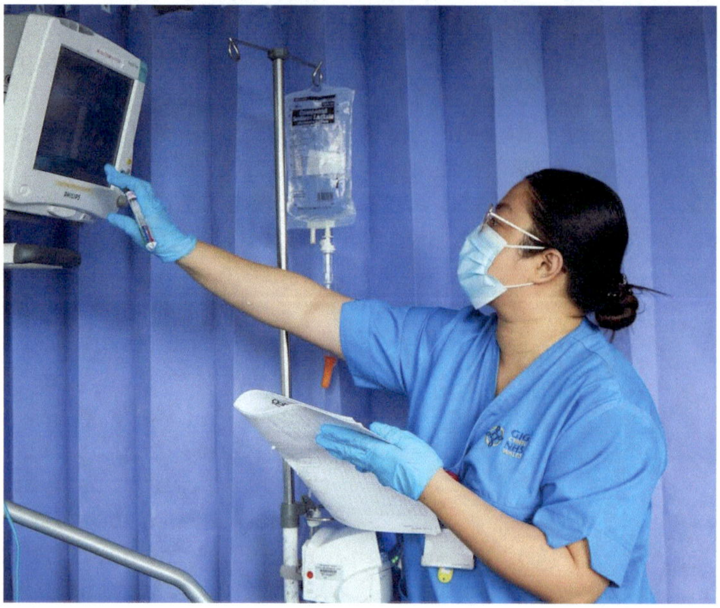

Figure 13.5. As children often experience unique complications and recoveries, comprehensive follow-up strategies are essential to monitor ongoing health issues stemming from surgical interventions.

Source: https://ugc.futurelearn.com/uploads/images/73/8f/header_738fe230-df86-4e9e-94e7-57797226694d.jpg.

Test Your Knowledge

1. How is respiratory function monitored and supported post-operatively in high-risk pediatric patients?
2. What role does early enteral nutrition play in post-surgical recovery in PICU?

13.2. Transplant Procedures in Pediatric Patients

Learning Outcome

1. Types of Transplants Performed in Pediatrics.
2. Indications for Pediatric Organ Transplantation.
3. Pre-operative Assessment and Preparation.
4. Surgical Techniques Specific to Pediatric Transplants.
5. Post-operative Care Specific to Transplant Patients.
6. Immunosuppressive Therapy Management.
7. Complications Associated with Pediatric Transplants.
8. Ethical Considerations in Pediatric Transplantation.
9. Success Rates and Outcomes in Pediatric Transplant Cases.

Children's transplant surgery is a focal point of intersection between technological innovation and ethical responsibility, necessitating the specialized provision of care within post-operative settings. Sophistication in the care of pediatric transplant patients stems from their particular physiological responses and the particular demands of growth and development, as well as enduring comorbidities that exist before transplant. With advancing postoperative management, vigilant monitoring for complications such as rejection, infection, and organ failure must be ensured to ensure optimal survival and long-term organ viability. Children typically require customized immunosuppression regimens to prevent rejection without compromising their future growth potential and overall health. In addition, psychological counseling of both the patients and families is a vital component to assist them in their recovery, particularly for Chronic Liver Disease, which may need transplantation due to chronic complications like ascites and hepatic encephalopathy, highlighting its complexity as identified by current guidelines of the medical society (Scott *et al.*, 2021). Furthermore, the dynamics of care delivery are also increased in pandemics, as seen in the rapid changes that occurred in pediatric hospitals (Stylianos *et al.*, 2020).

13.2.1. Types of Transplants Performed in Pediatrics

Pediatric transplants involve a variety of procedures intended for the management of severe organ dysfunction or failure in kids, of which the most prevalent are hematopoietic cell transplants and solid organ transplants. Hematopoietic cell transplantation (HCT) is particularly known for curing different types of malignant and non-malignant disorders, but in most instances, it normally necessitates intensive post-surgical care due to the complex complications of the recovery process, including respiratory and renal support requirements (Amanda *et al.*, 2024).

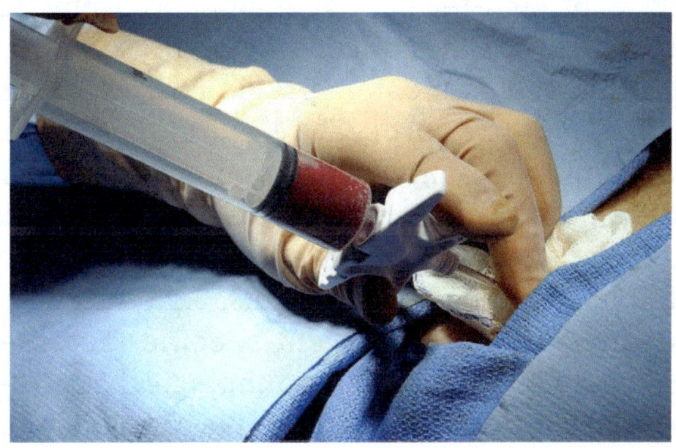

Figure 13.6. Pediatric transplants encompass a variety of procedures designed to treat severe organ dysfunction or failure in children, with hematopoietic cell transplants and solid organ transplants being the most prevalent types.

Source: https://pharmaceutical-journal.com/wp-content/uploads/2021/01/Haematopoietic-stem-cell-transplant-in-children--scaled.jpg.

Also, solid organ transplantation, such as kidney, liver, and heart transplantation, has become more prominent, enabling children with end-stage organ disease to regain organ function and quality of life. However, these interventions present grand challenges in the context of critical care, including co-morbid management and integrating multidisciplinary teams to address special physiological characteristics of children (Isacksson *et al.*, 2024). Optimization of transplant results is dependent on appropriate management in the Pediatric Intensive Care Unit (Figure 13.6).

13.2.2. Indications for Pediatric Organ Transplantation

In children, indications for organ transplantation are often set by catastrophic, irreversible organ failure that considerably diminishes quality of life and threatens survival. Cleft heart disease, cystic fibrosis, and end-stage renal disease are common precursors that necessitate transplantation in children. Particularly, the advent of high-technology medical therapy has augmented the list of candidates by rendering treatment feasible for previously incurable disorders. The procedure is multi-faceted and demands a multi-disciplinary team with assessment of not only the medical illness but also the psychosocial factors of compliance with post-transplant protocols. As outlined in current guidelines, patient-specific factors—age, comorbidities, and immunological status—are most crucial in determining candidacy for transplant (Scott *et al.*, 2021). Further, it offers timely and appropriate referral for transplant, and the outcomes are improved because delays in access to transplant service can increase complications and the risk of mortality (Steven *et al.*, 2020).

13.2.3. Pre-Operative Assessment and Preparation

Good pre-operative assessment and preparation are crucial parameters in obtaining good post-operative outcomes, particularly in pediatric patients with complex surgeries. Pre-operative assessment includes careful examination of the child's medical history, nutritional level, and physiological status, which significantly influence their coping capacity during and after the operation. For instance, studies indicate a high rate of malnutrition among children with congenital heart disease, leading to post-operative complications like extended length of stay and infection (Sameh *et al.*, 2021).

Further, the use of standardized protocols can enhance pediatric operating room to intensive care unit transitions of care, thereby minimizing the risk of information loss and maximizing coordination among teams (Weigl *et al.*, 2023). Therefore, an effective pre-operative strategy not only enhances patient readiness but also forms the beginning of improved care pathways and enhanced clinical results in the context of pediatric critical care facilities (Figure 13.7).

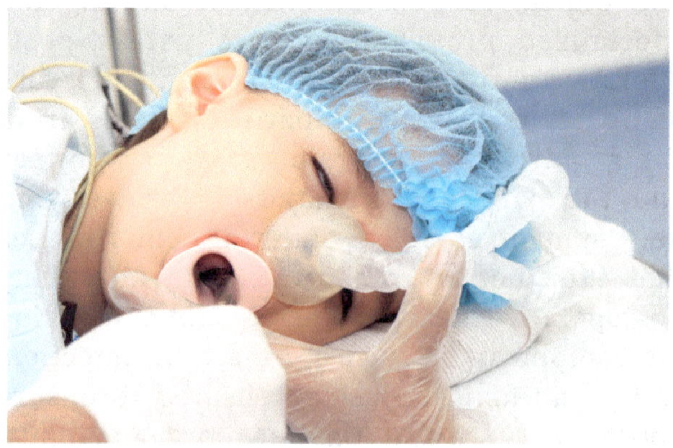

Figure 13.7. Effective pre-operative assessment and preparation are critical components in ensuring positive post-operative outcomes, particularly in pediatric patients undergoing complex procedures.

Source: https://decisionsindentistry.com/wp-content/uploads/2016/01/ThinkstockPhotos-464675964.jpg.

13.2.4. Surgical Techniques Specific to Pediatric Transplants

The surgical techniques utilized in pediatric transplants are specially adapted to accommodate the anatomical and physiological differences of children compared to adults. Pediatric transplant surgeons must cleverly navigate these challenges, employing methodologies that both minimize trauma and facilitate optimal graft function. One of the more frequent techniques is the use of laparoscopic techniques, which have gained popularity due to their benefits of reduced postoperative pain and reduced recovery times. Moreover, the methods in vascular anastomosis during kidney or liver transplantation involve precision in handling thin vessels since there is a reduction in vessel size and variability in children. Doctors should also be cautious of complications that could occur, such as rejection and infection, which are potentially higher among children. Care coordination, including multi-dimensional pre-surgery evaluation and post-surgery care, emphasized by the new guidelines, is critical in achieving successful outcomes in such multi-dimensional surgical interventions (Scott *et al.*, 2021; Steven *et al.*, 2020).

13.2.5. Post-Operative Care Specific to Transplant Patients

Postoperative care in transplant patients is particularly critical, as transplant patients are at heightened risk of infection and operative complications. In pediatric intensive care units (PICUs), intense monitoring is imperative to identify early signs of graft-versus-host disease (GVHD), which is possible in recipients of hematopoietic stem cell transplants and affects almost half of them. Also, fluid and electrolyte balance should be given due attention since acute kidney injury is present in a high percentage of children and will influence global recovery (Jan *et al.*, 2025). Standardized protocols ensure that early intervention is made with scope to reduce the risk of prolonged PICU course and related death (Jan *et al.*, 2025). Moreover, post-surgery practice needs to entail stringent infection control and individualized rehabilitation protocols as preventive care is associated with improved outcomes in this high-risk population (Jan *et al.*, 2025). Overall, post-operative care is important to make healing possible and achieve the highest survival rates among children receiving transplants (Figure 13.8).

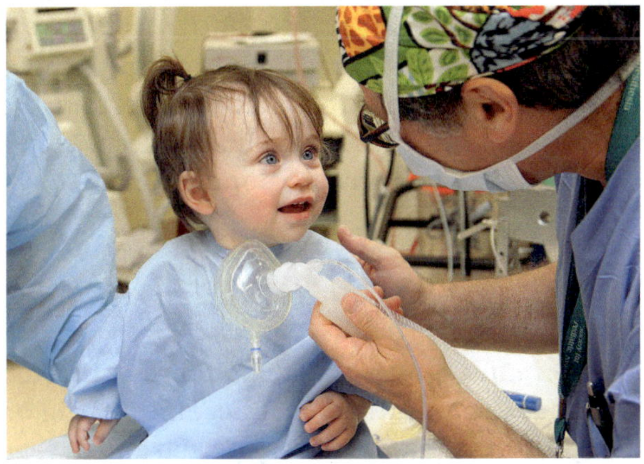

Figure 13.8. In pediatric intensive care units (PICUs), robust monitoring is essential to identify early signs of graft-versus-host disease (GVHD), which can arise in hematopoietic stem cell transplant recipients, affecting nearly half of such patients.

Source: https://pbs.twimg.com/media/DjA2WybUwAE9gr1.jpg.

13.2.6. Immunosuppressive Therapy Management

The management of immunosuppressive treatment is central to post-operative and transplant critical care in the pediatric intensive care unit because it directly influences patient survival and long-term graft outcome. Due to variability in pharmacokinetics and pharmacodynamics, including differences between children and adults, customized immunosuppressive regimens have to be optimized for effectiveness with decreased risks of infection and drug toxicity. There are also detailed guidelines to help healthcare practitioners make decisions for transplantation that consider both immunologic and psychosocial problems that could affect therapeutic decisions (Steven *et al.*, 2020). Besides, the evolving landscape of healthcare in times of crises such as the COVID-19 crisis demands practical flexibility in responding to the need to adapt immunosuppressive regimens to lower threats from viral infections in immunocompromised children (Moulik *et al.*, 2020). Thus, an interdisciplinary approach that brings all these aspects together is important to ascertain the effective and safe use of immunosuppressive therapy in this vulnerable population.

13.2.7. Pediatric Transplant Complications

Children undergoing transplants are subjected to various complications that become a drain on their post-transplant recovery period and overall quality of life. The most direct of these is the rise in serum lactate, which has been reported to correlate with complications following surgery, including biliary and neurological complications, graft dysfunction, and mortality among children receiving liver transplants. Specifically, a serum lactate level >3.0 mmol/L on admission to the PICU indicates elevated risk for the development of such complications (Fern Jópez-Sarmiento *et al.*, 2022). The management of ascites and hepatorenal syndrome (HRS) is also problematic within this group, especially in light of the extreme morbidity associated with both of these diseases (Scott *et al.*, 2021). The interplay between these complications is reflective of the necessity of close observation and tailored interventions in pediatric transplant care, its high-stakes environment highlighting the need for post-operative and transplant critical care in the attainment of optimal results among these vulnerable patients (Figure 13.9).

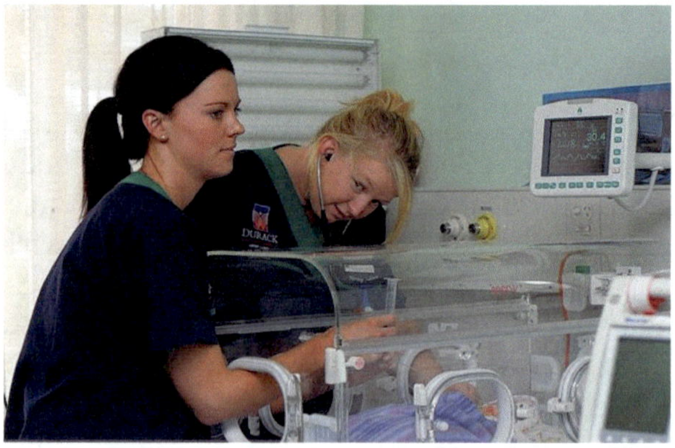

Figure 13.9. Pediatric transplant recipients face a myriad of complications that can significantly impact their recovery and quality of life.

Source: https://upload.wikimedia.org/wikipedia/commons/thumb/6/63/Student_enrolled_nurses.jpg/640px-Student_enrolled_nurses.jpg.

13.2.8. Ethical Considerations in Pediatric Transplantation

The ethical considerations in pediatric transplantation extend beyond the clinical domain into decision-making for critically ill children. Central to these considerations is the notion of justice, in which healthcare workers must ensure equitable access to transplant resources, particularly in pediatric intensive care units. Since donor organs are scarce, ethical considerations arise when deciding on priorities for allocation and candidate selection criteria, including increasing questions on issues of age, medical history, and expectations. Moreover, the ethical responsibility to balance patient autonomy against parent rights complicates consent issues, which require open communication of risks and benefits. Technologies such as 3D printing technology have a crucial role in pre-operative planning, providing more surgical precision and potentially improved outcomes (Jarosław Meyer-Szary *et al.*, 2022). Similarly, the use of Surgical Data Science is transforming the discipline by facilitating smooth data management and analytics in pediatric surgery, providing valuable insights while taking responsible stewardship in the handling of patient data (Maier *et al.*, 2021).

13.2.9. Success Rates and Outcomes in Pediatric Transplant Cases

Success rates and outcomes of children's transplant surgeries significantly depend on advances in medical technologies and data-driven methods. Improved pre-surgery planning, facilitated by developments such as 3D printing, has significantly improved surgical outcomes by allowing improved visualization and understanding of unique patient anatomy, which translates to tailored surgery plans and better patient-specific implants (Jarosław Meyer-Szary *et al.*, 2022). Besides, the use of Surgical Data Science (SDS) in pediatric medicine demonstrates data analysis capacities to enhance transplant surgery and predict outcomes. With the ability to capture data and model, medical professionals can gain insights critical to the optimization of surgical procedures and subsequent treatments (Maier *et al.*, 2021). Thus, these technologies not only enhance procedural accuracy but also introduce increased understanding of long-term patient management, ultimately providing improved success rates in pediatric transplantation. As these fields advance further, implications for maximizing outcomes in pediatric intensive care remain far-reaching.

Test Your Knowledge

1. What are the key components of a pediatric immunosuppression regimen post-transplant?
2. What are the common infectious complications in immunosuppressed pediatric transplant patients?

13.3. Critical Care Management in Pediatric Intensive Care

Learning Outcome

1. Role of the Multidisciplinary Team in Critical Care.
2. Advanced Monitoring Technologies in PICU.
3. Ventilation Strategies for Pediatric Patients.
4. Fluid and Electrolyte Management.
5. Management of Pediatric Sepsis.
6. End-of-life Care Considerations in Critical Situations.
7. Family-centered Care in the PICU.
8. Training and Education for PICU Staff.
9. Research and Advancements in Pediatric Critical Care.

Effective management of pediatric critical care in PICUs needs to have a clear vision of the unique challenges presented by post-operative and transplant children. They, often having pre-existing vulnerabilities, are at higher risk for issues such as postoperative pain and invasive fungal infections (IFIs). Postoperative pain management is particularly trying as the majority of pediatric patients are usually on opioid therapy, and therefore, a cautious re-evaluation and re-adjustment of the analgesic regimen needs to be undertaken to avoid tolerance and ensure proper pain control (Iaco *et al.*, 2022). Additionally, the rate of IFIs has also appreciably increased in this population due to the administration of prolonged antibiotics and invasive procedures, and therefore, early diagnosis and treatment are a priority (AR MB, 2022). The collaboration between pain management and infection prevention is critical, as both directly affect recovery. A multidisciplinary strategy with a specific focus on understanding the distinct requirements of pediatric patients is ideal for optimal critical care management in the PICU (Figure 13.10).

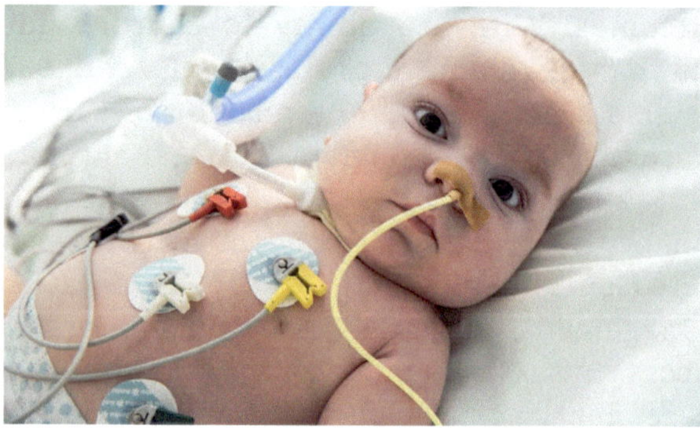

Figure 13.10. Effective management of critical care in pediatric intensive care units (PICUs) necessitates a comprehensive understanding of the unique challenges posed by post-operative and transplant patients.

Source: https://www.sjdhospitalbarcelona.org/sites/default/files/styles/image_1600/public/content/image/2022/05/16/1/cuidados-intensivos-nino-cables-hospital-sant-joan-deu-barcelona-min.jpg.webp.

13.3.1. Role of the Multidisciplinary Team in Critical Care

In pediatric intensive care unit post-operative and transplant critical care, the role of a multidisciplinary team lies at the core of best patient outcomes. It usually consists of pediatric intensivists, surgeons, nurses, pharmacists, dietitians, and social workers who possess unique expertise to address complicated problems of critically ill children. Effective collaboration between these specialists ensures exhaustive patient assessments, personalized treatment modalities, and immediate interventions, all of which are essential in managing the complexities emanating from post-operative and transplant complications. For instance, a coordinated care framework can allow for faster recovery times as well as avoid complications such as infection or rejection of the organ, as recognized in contemporary studies on coordinated care models among children (Scott *et al.*, 2021). Also, rapid protocol adjustment by multidisciplinary teams, including that observed in the COVID-19 pandemic, underlines their central role in maintaining continuity of care even in the most critical situations, having a direct influence on survival rates and quality of life in high-risk patients (Stylianos *et al.*, 2020).

13.3.2. Advanced Monitoring Technologies in PICU

The incorporation of state-of-the-art monitoring technology in the Pediatric Intensive Care Unit (PICU) is pivotal for enhancing post-operative and transplant care for children. The technologies facilitate continuous, real-time monitoring of important vital signs and other parameters around the clock, which is paramount given the multidimensional medical needs of pediatric patients.

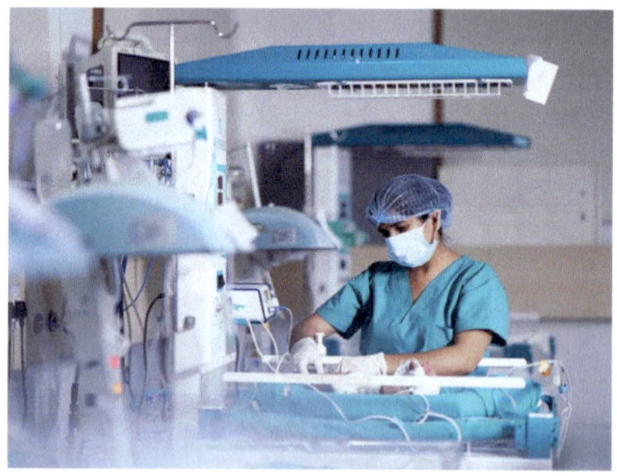

Figure 13.11. The integration of advanced monitoring technologies in the Pediatric Intensive Care Unit (PICU) is pivotal for enhancing post-operative and transplant care in children.

Source: https://www.mgmch.org/images/Pediatrics-one.webp.

Through the utilization of advanced monitoring equipment, clinicians stand to pick up minor changes in the status of a child and therefore have a greater opportunity to intervene in time. For instance, machine learning algorithms are increasingly being employed to review cumulative data sets, detecting trends that may point to a deterioration in status or the onset of complications like infections or organ failure (Maier *et al.*, 2021). Moreover, the technologies facilitate improved decision-making through the provision of comprehensive information, which is crucial in a high-risk environment like PICU (Markiewicz-Gospodarek *et al.*, 2022). Installation of these sophisticated systems is a vital move towards maximizing outcomes for vulnerable children receiving critical interventions (Figure 13.11).

13.3.3. Ventilation Strategies for Pediatric Patients

In the context of transplant and post-operative critical care, ideal ventilation strategies in pediatric patients are pivotal to maximizing respiratory function and minimizing complications. Utilization of individualized mechanical ventilation practices, such as, pressure-controlled ventilation or volume-targeted ventilatory modes, allows for better tailoring to the particular physiological demands of this patient group. Recent pilot experiments have demonstrated the possibility of optimized fluid management algorithms that are correlated with better pulmonary outcomes in children who are critically ill; among them, a reduction in the use of oxygen therapy and mechanical ventilation in patients adhering to minimal fluid management guidelines (Vincent *et al.*, 2023). Moreover, secondary complication surveillance, such as VAP, demands vigilant inspection of ventilation and infection control processes (Nisar *et al.*, 2023). Thus, the primary care strategy should be a multidisciplinary one with special emphasis on individualized ventilation strategies in designing pediatric intensive care recovery pathways.

13.3.4. Fluid and Electrolyte Management

Effective fluid and electrolyte management is central to post-operative and transplant critical care in pediatric intensive care units (PICUs), where the subtle balance of these elements can directly impact recovery outcomes. Children, often quite unlike adults in physiology and metabolic demand, are held in close observation and have their intravenous fluid and electrolyte status manipulated. Recent studies have shown that isotonic crystalloid solutions like 0.9% saline can cause adverse effects, including increased mortality and acute kidney injury due to their excessive chloride load, prompting consideration for the use of balanced solutions like Plasma Lyte as safer alternatives (Hayes *et al.*, 2018). In addition, in critical episodes such as acute lung injury or respiratory failure, infants and children exhibit typical responses that require individualized management with fluid resuscitation and correction of electrolytes (Chimbira *et al.*, 2001). Therefore, a reasoned and evidence-based strategy for fluid and electrolyte management is essential to optimize outcome in this vulnerable group (Figure 13.12).

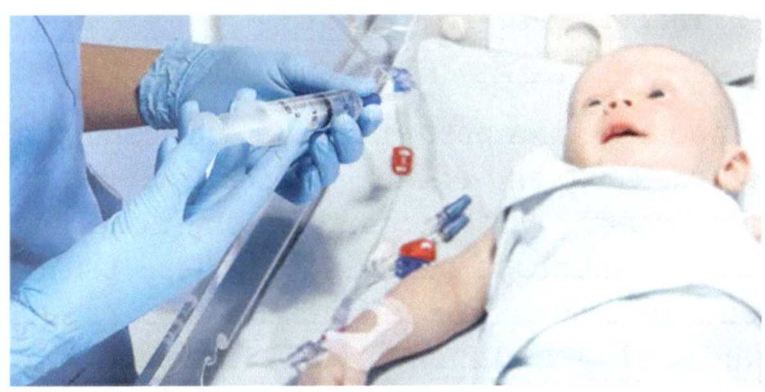

Figure 13.12. Effective fluid and electrolyte management is crucial in post-operative and transplant critical care within pediatric intensive care units (PICUs), where the delicate balance of these elements can significantly impact recovery outcomes.

Source: https://www.icumed.com/media/og5gvhth/hero_nicu-picu_4557_mobile.jpg?format=webp.

13.3.5. Management of Pediatric Sepsis

Successful management of pediatric sepsis is very important in the setting of pediatric critical care, particularly in post-surgical and transplant cases where children become increasingly prone to infection. Sepsis in such patients can develop rapidly and may be further hastened by surgical intervention or immunosuppression from transplant protocols. Prompt response is possible only if signs like tachycardia, altered mental status, and hypotension are recognized early. Diagnostic procedures most often include blood cultures, radiological investigations, and clinical examinations to identify the Source of infection. Treatment involves the immediate infusion of broad-spectrum antibiotics and, in some cases, fluid resuscitation to restore normal hemodynamics. Adherence to sepsis protocols can improve outcomes, decreasing mortality and LOS (Markiewicz-Gospodarek *et al.*, 2022). In addition, an interdisciplinary group of surgeons, intensivists, and infectious disease specialists is required to optimize the treatment of these vulnerable patients (Scott *et al.*, 2021).

13.3.6. End-of-Life Care Considerations in Critical Situations

In pediatric and post-operative and transplant critical care, end-of-life issues are of utmost significance given the complex emotional and ethical landscape surrounding these critical conditions. Pediatric patients undergoing such life-altering treatment expose themselves to severe complications, triggering discussion about the potential of palliative care and advance directives. While parents handle the emotional weight of medical decisions, the medical staff must ensure open communication and support throughout the process. This aligns with recommendations for multidisciplinary care, particularly where most families can barely reconcile hope for recovery with the awareness of diminishing health (Scott *et al.*, 2021). In addition, as noted by the International Society for Pediatric Oncology, the COVID-19 pandemic reiterated existing challenges in ensuring equal treatment, which has seen cries for adaptive strategies that emphasize end-of-life discussions and compassionate treatment (Sullivan *et al.*, 2020). An understanding of these dynamics enables an all-rounded approach towards managing end-of-life scenarios in a pediatric intensive care setting (Figure 13.13).

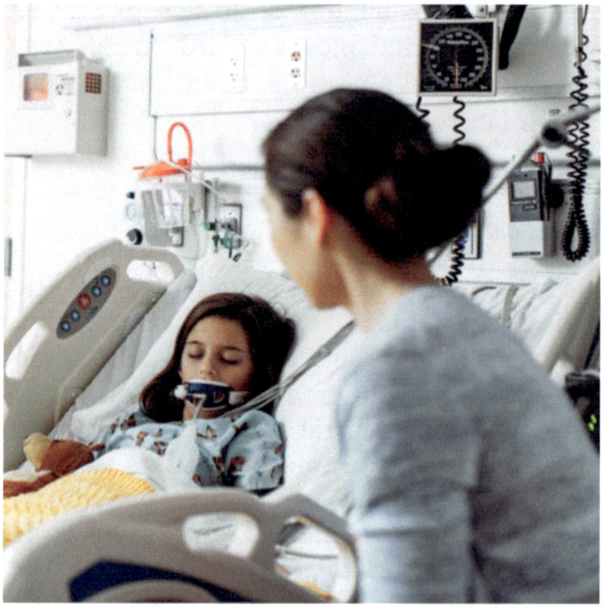

Figure 13.13. Pediatric patients undergoing such life-altering interventions may face significant complications, necessitating discussions around the potential for palliative care and advance directives.

Source: https://clinicalnutrition.baxterhealthcare.co.uk/sites/g/files/ebysai3546/files/2021-08/Challenge-image_1.jpg.

13.3.7. Family-Centered Care in the PICU

In the Pediatric Intensive Care Unit (PICU), family-centered care is of paramount significance to enhance the critically ill children's recovery environment. Family-centered care focuses on cooperation among healthcare professionals and families, recognizing the family member as a vital component of the child's recovery process. By involving parents and guardians actively in decision-making, daily care, and care planning, the PICU not only addresses the child's physiological needs but also preserves the psychological and emotional state of the family. Evidence indicates that family-centered practice is linked to improved health outcomes, reduced parental anxiety, and satisfaction with care. Moreover, identification of family relationships may be particularly important in post-operative and transplant cases, where emotional support greatly characterizes recovery profiles. Last but not least, establishing an intimate partnership with families contributes to the creation of a more holistic, compassionate, and functional model of care in the PICU, as supported by recent studies (Scott *et al.*, 2021; Stylianos *et al.*, 2020).

13.3.8. PICU Staff Training and Education

The need for thorough training and education among PICU staff cannot be overemphasized, especially for post-operative and transplant critical care. As pediatric cases, and indeed cardiac intervention cases in particular, become increasingly complex, it is critical to have a well-trained team to guarantee positive patient outcomes. Curricula for advanced training must encompass sophisticated clinical competencies, critical thinking, and application of frontier technologies that pertain to child care. The constant evolution of treatments and interventions within domains such as Pediatric Cardiac Critical Care (PCCC) requires professional development and updating to keep pace with such innovations. Ensuring that PICU staff are trained in these areas, including the pharmacological and technical innovations outlined in current literature, will definitely enhance the overall competency of care received by high-risk pediatric populations (Pollak *et al.*, 2022; King, 2019) (Figure 13.14).

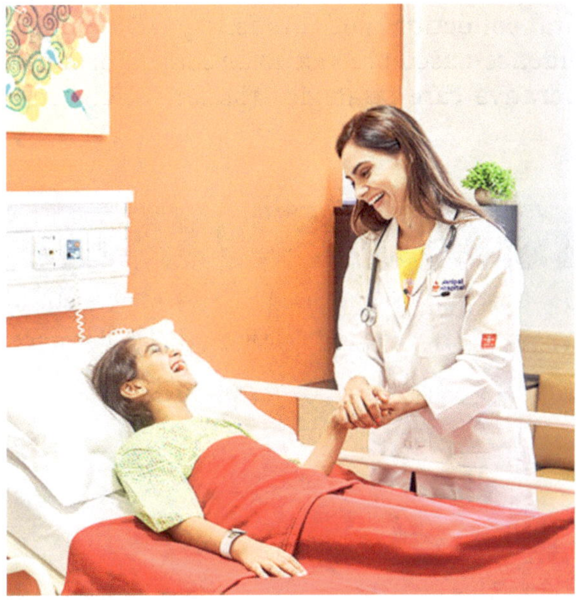

Figure 13.14. The importance of comprehensive training and education for staff in the Pediatric Intensive Care Unit (PICU) cannot be overstated, particularly in the context of post-operative and transplant critical care.

Source: https://www.manipalhospitals.com/bhubaneswar/uploads/specialities/content_photo/paediatric-specialities-in-old-airport-road-bhubaneswar.jpg.

13.3.9. Research and Advancements in Pediatric Critical Care

In recent years, pediatric intensive care has seen dramatic advancements, which have revolutionized care for transplant and post-operative patients within the ICU. Integration of Explainable Artificial Intelligence (XAI) in multiple clinical applications has emerged as a landmark advancement that enables clinicians to better understand reasoning within complex predictive models and improve decision-making in sensitive cases (Martino *et al.*, 2022). Secondly, the establishment of Surgical Data Science (SDS) reveals a growing appreciation of the need to use sophisticated data analysis techniques in an effort to enhance surgical outcomes as well as the safety of patients. By systematic data collection and modeling, SDS enables evidence-based practice to directly inform post-operative care strategies (Maier L-Hein *et al.*, 2021). Combined, these developments represent an era of astute, evidence-based actions that respect the unique needs of pediatric patients, supporting improved recovery trajectories and overall health outcomes in the critical care environment.

Test Your Knowledge

1. What strategies are used for preventing ventilator-associated complications in pediatric patients?
2. How is sedation and delirium monitored and managed in the PICU?

SUMMARY

Effective postoperative and transplant critical care within pediatric intensive care units (PICUs) is critical to ensure optimal results from such advanced surgical procedures. Findings of studies affirm that such complications as pleural effusions can arise after liver transplantation and necessitate interventions such as chest drainage, which represents a notable reduction in complications if performed in the operating room compared to the ICU (Aigner *et al.*, 2020). Similarly, the heterogeneity observed in pediatric kidney transplantation intraoperative management protocols reflects the need for standardized protocols in an effort to achieve maximum uniformity of care across facilities (Abu-Sultaneh *et al.*, 2017). Having brief guidelines will not only minimize complications but also maximize overall recovery trajectories for pediatric patients. Lastly, ongoing discussions to achieve consensus regarding post-operative protocol will further advance the discipline, as long as the unique needs of pediatric patients are met in the critical care environments.

Effective post-transplant and post-operative care plays a vital role in the success of surgical interventions and organ transplants, particularly in children. Such an extensive strategy involves continuous monitoring, immediate interventions, and extensive management interventions that address the unique physiological and development-related conditions of children. For instance, managing potential complications such as infection or rejection during the post-operative stages is crucial since these may have a significant impact on recovery and long-term outcomes. As highlighted in the 2020 Kidney Disease: Improving Global Outcomes (KDIGO) Clinical Practice Guideline, thorough evaluations of individual risk factors and health status are a prerequisite in personalizing post-transplant management for patient safety and transplant success (Steven *et al.*, 2020). Moreover, dedication to successful post-operative care varies from pain management to rehabilitation and ultimately forms a conducive platform for healing and growth (Markiewicz-Gospodarek *et al.*, 2022). Hence, a collaborative post-operative and transplant care strategy is crucial in improving survival and quality of life in children.

KEY TERMS FROM THIS CHAPTER

- Knowledge
- Vital parameters
- Neurological status
- Hemodynamic monitoring
- Perfusion
- Heart rate
- Oxygen saturation
- Analgesics
- Poliomyelitis
- Fluid balance
- Extubation
- Oxygenation
- Nutritional therapy
- Blood pressure
- Surgery
- Pain management

CRITICAL THINKING QUESTIONS

1. **What is the most common early complication following pediatric cardiac surgery?**
   a. Wound infection
   b. Renal failure
   c. Arrhythmias
   d. Neurological deficits
2. **Which of the following is a critical goal in the immediate post-operative period after pediatric liver transplantation?**
   a. High-dose corticosteroids
   b. Strict fluid restriction
   c. Graft perfusion monitoring
   d. Broad-spectrum antivirals
3. **What is the most common immunosuppressive drug used after pediatric solid organ transplantation?**
   a. Methotrexate
   b. Cyclosporine
   c. Tacrolimus
   d. Prednisolone
4. **Which of the following lab values is most indicative of acute renal transplant rejection?**
   a. Decreased serum sodium
   b. Increased serum creatinine
   c. Elevated bilirubin
   d. Decreased white blood cell count
5. **In the PICU, what is a key sign of post-operative bleeding in a pediatric patient?**
   a. Hyperthermia
   b. Increased urine output
   c. Hypotension and tachycardia
   d. Elevated glucose levels

Short Answer Questions

1. What are the immediate post-operative priorities for a child following major surgery?
2. How do post-operative pain management strategies differ between neonates and older children?
3. What are the most commonly performed organ transplants in children?
4. What is the role of HLA matching in pediatric kidney and liver transplantation?
5. What are the fundamental principles of hemodynamic monitoring in critically ill children?
6. How is mechanical ventilation customized for pediatric patients with varying lung compliance?

Answers to Critical Thinking Questions

1. (c); 2. (c); 3. (c); 4. (b); 5. (c)

REFERENCES

1. Abu-Elmagd, K., Bond, G. J., Macedo, C., Mazariegos, G., *et al.* (2005). Intestinal transplantation under tacrolimus monotherapy after perioperative lymphoid depletion with rabbit anti-thymocyte globulin (thymoglobulin®). https://core.ac.uk/download/12205620.pdf (accessed on 30th June 2025).
2. Abu-Sultaneh, S., Goggins, W. C., Hobson, M. J., Lutfi, R., *et al.* (2017). Practice variation in the immediate postoperative care of pediatric kidney transplantation: A national survey. https://core.ac.uk/download/158967822.pdf (accessed on 30th June 2025).
3. Aigner, F., Brandl, A., Dargie, R., Dziodzio, J., *et al.* (2020). Perioperative pleural drainage in liver transplantation: A retrospective analysis from a high-volume liver transplant center. https://core.ac.uk/download/286567879.pdf (accessed on 30th June 2025).
4. Akyol, M. U., Alden, T. D., Amartino, H., Ashworth, J., *et al.* (2019). Recommendations for the management of MPS IVA: Systematic evidence- and consensus-based guidance. https://core.ac.uk/download/323075225.pdf (accessed on 30th June 2025).
5. AlAbdullah, H., Alanzi, F., Alhuthil, R., Alshaibani, T., AlBeeshi, N., Alqahtani, A., Alabdulsalam, M., *et al.* (2024). Post hematopoietic stem cell transplant (HSCT) outcomes in pediatric intensive care unit, experience from a referral center for cellular therapy and hematopoietic stem cell transplantation. *Hematology/Oncology and Stem Cell Therapy, 17*(4), 227–232. https://www.semanticscholar.org/paper/6079cd195a35b7ff0d6e6fdbbd099ab78bb4a2f8 (accessed on 30th June 2025).
6. Argent, A., Festa, M., Lacroix, J., Leteurtre, S., *et al.* (2017). The intensive care medicine clinical research agenda in pediatrics. https://core.ac.uk/download/158171535.pdf (accessed on 30th June 2025).
7. Baalaaji, M. A. R. (2022). Invasive candidiasis in children: Challenges remain. *Indian Journal of Critical Care Medicine*. https://www.semanticscholar.org/paper/1a7c51d7fa56d355b8028d8078e6104f079c7ac9 (accessed on 30th June 2025).
8. Baddour, L. M., Wilson, W. R., Bayer, A. S., Fowler, V. G., Tleyjeh, I. M., Rybak, M. J., Baršić, B., *et al.* (2015). Infective endocarditis in adults: Diagnosis, antimicrobial therapy, and management of complications. *Circulation, 132*, 1435–1486. https://doi.org/10.1161/cir.0000000000000296 (accessed on 30th June 2025).
9. Barr, M., Bogin, V., Broelsch, C., Bronsther, O., Campsen, J., Chan, S., Chan, A., *et al.* (2009). Complications of right lobe living donor liver transplantation. https://core.ac.uk/download/12205665.pdf (accessed on 30th June 2025).
10. Bavetta, S., Di Majo, D., Giammanco, M., Greco, A., *et al.* (2013). Therapeutic effectiveness of nutrition therapy in pediatric patients with chronic liver diseases awaiting liver transplantation. https://core.ac.uk/download/53279313.pdf (accessed on 30th June 2025).
11. Biggins, S. W., Angeli, P., García-Tsao, G., Ginès, P., Ling, S. C., Nadim, M. K., Wong, F., *et al.* (2021). Diagnosis, evaluation, and management of ascites, spontaneous bacterial peritonitis and hepatorenal syndrome: 2021 practice guidance by the American Association for the Study of Liver Diseases. *Hepatology, 74*, 1014–1048. https://doi.org/10.1002/hep.31884 (accessed on 30th June 2025).

12. Chadban, S. J., Ahn, C., Axelrod, D. A., Foster, B. J., Kasiske, B. L., Kher, V., Kumar, D., *et al.* (2020). KDIGO clinical practice guideline on the evaluation and management of candidates for kidney transplantation. *Transplantation, 104*, S11–S103. https://doi.org/10.1097/tp.0000000000003136 (accessed on 30th June 2025).

13. Chimbira, W., Crawford, H., Gupta, S., Legg, J., *et al.* (2001). Acute lung injury in pediatric intensive care: Course and outcome. https://core.ac.uk/download/pdf/8715345.pdf (accessed on 30th June 2025).

14. Chong, S. O. K., Pedron, S., Abdelmalak, N., Laxy, M., & Stephan, A. J. (2023). An umbrella review of effectiveness and efficacy trials for app-based health interventions. *npj Digital Medicine, 6*. https://doi.org/10.1038/s41746-023-00981-x (accessed on 30th June 2025).

15. De Iaco, F., Mannaioni, G., Serra, S., Finco, G., Sartori, S., Gandolfo, E., Sansone, P., *et al.* (2022). Equianalgesic, opioid switch and opioid association in different clinical settings: A narrative review. *European Review for Medical and Pharmacological Sciences, 26*(6), 2000–2017. https://www.semanticscholar.org/paper/8adc7017c36b4b47bf4a3f2a64f5c59d7fd31702 (accessed on 30th June 2025).

16. Di Martino, F., & Delmastro, F. (2022). Explainable AI for clinical and remote health applications: A survey on tabular and time series data. *Artificial Intelligence Review, 56*, 5261–5315. https://doi.org/10.1007/s10462-022-10304-3 (accessed on 30th June 2025).

17. Dreyling, M., André, M., Gökbuget, N., Tilly, H., Jerkeman, M., Gribben, J. G., Ferreri, A. J. M., *et al.* (2022). The EHA research roadmap: Malignant lymphoid diseases. *Hemisphere, 6*, e726–e726. https://doi.org/10.1097/hs9.0000000000000726 (accessed on 30th June 2025).

18. Duron, V. P., Ichinose, R., Stewart, L., Porigow, C., Fan, W., Rubsam, J., Stylianos, S., *et al.* (2023). Pilot randomized controlled trial of restricted versus liberal crystalloid fluid management in pediatric post-operative and trauma patients. *Pilot and Feasibility Studies, 9*. https://www.semanticscholar.org/paper/0e71515945d9b8fa7305da80fb4da484b2057c1f (accessed on 30th June 2025).

19. Farmakis, D., Porter, J. B., Taher, A., Cappellini, M. D., Angastiniotis, M., & Eleftheriou, A. (2022). 2021 Thalassemia International Federation guidelines for the management of transfusion-dependent thalassemia. *Hemisphere, 6*, e732–e732. https://doi.org/10.1097/hs9.0000000000000732 (accessed on 30th June 2025).

20. Fernández-Sarmiento, J., Wilches-Cuadros, M. Á., Hernández-Sarmiento, R., Mulett, H., Moreno, K., Molano, N., Palomar Dominguez, J. A., *et al.* (2022). Association between serum lactate and unsatisfactory outcomes in critically ill children in the immediate post-operative period of liver transplantation. *Frontiers in Pediatrics, 9*. https://doi.org/10.3389/fped.2021.796504 (accessed on 30th June 2025).

21. Gutierrez, M. C., Liu, H., & Moore, P. G. (2013). Goal-directed therapy in intraoperative fluid and hemodynamic management. https://core.ac.uk/download/323069925.pdf (accessed on 30th June 2025).

22. Hayes, W. (2018). Ab-normal saline in abnormal kidney function: Risks and alternatives. https://core.ac.uk/download/195307878.pdf (accessed on 30th June 2025).

23. Isacksson, G. L. T., da Luz de Almeida, L. A., Damasceno, M. X. A., Costa, M. R. C., Ferreira, J. F., Néri, J. dos S. V., & Dantas, J. (2024). The role of the dental surgeon in the pediatric

intensive care unit. *Journal of Health Sciences*. https://www.semanticscholar.org/paper/83237fc5b51b00a4d01fc48762c5b8e664758c77 (accessed on 30th June 2025).

24. Ismail, S. R., Mehmood, A., Rabiah, N., Abu-Sulaiman, R., & Kabbani, M. (2021). Impact of the nutritional status of children with congenital heart diseases on the early post-operative outcome. *Egyptian Pediatric Association Gazette, 69*. https://www.semanticscholar.org/paper/36692b3d3eda549a894d77f2b6cea755e686755c (accessed on 30th June 2025).

25. Jan, I., Nagel, J., Tribble, A., Riggsbee, D., & Davidge, K. N. (2025). P-1149. Short versus long duration of antibiotic therapy in pediatric intensive care unit patients with uncomplicated community acquired pneumonia: Impact of an institutional guideline update. *Open Forum Infectious Diseases, 12*. https://www.semanticscholar.org/paper/c5710e1bf14203b1ec20ebe2afba61316ef941b0 (accessed on 30th June 2025).

26. Johnson, A. K., Cornea, S., Goldfarb, S., Cao, Q., Heneghan, J., & Gupta, A. O. (2024). Risk factors predicting need for the pediatric intensive care unit (PICU) post-hematopoietic cell transplant, PICU utilization, and outcomes following HCT: A single center retrospective analysis. *Frontiers in Pediatrics, 12*, 1385153. https://www.semanticscholar.org/paper/28f23aaee89ca3c07e2109289b45706377bf9ca8 (accessed on 30th June 2025).

27. King, L. (2019). Abstracts for the 43rd Human Genetics Society of Australasia Annual Scientific Meeting. *Twin Research and Human Genetics, 22*, 330–370. https://doi.org/10.1017/thg.2019.80 (accessed on 30th June 2025).

28. Kokorelias, K. M., Gignac, M. A. M., Naglie, G., & Cameron, J. I. (2019). Towards a universal model of family centered care: A scoping review. *BMC Health Services Research, 19*. https://doi.org/10.1186/s12913-019-4394-5 (accessed on 30th June 2025).

29. Kurihara, C., Manerikar, A., Querrey, M., Felicelli, C., Yeldandi, A., Garza-Castillon, R., Lung, K., *et al.* (2022). Clinical characteristics and outcomes of patients with COVID-19-associated acute respiratory distress syndrome who underwent lung transplant. *JAMA*. https://www.semanticscholar.org/paper/4c91e5d68e8834029efbafd9d2625b71fea307c7 (accessed on 30th June 2025).

30. Lasso-Palomino, R. E., Medina, D., Franco, A., Soto-Aparicio, M. J., Tarapues, E. M., Muñoz, D. M., Salazar, E., *et al.* (2024). Outcomes within 100 days of hematopoietic cell transplantation in pediatric patients: Insights from an intensive care unit in Colombia. *Frontiers in Pediatrics, 12*. https://www.semanticscholar.org/paper/e09b014a08089a541c490b6b7477570824860e15 (accessed on 30th June 2025).

31. Liang, W., Zhou, C., Bai, J., Zhang, H., Jiang, B., Wang, J., Fu, L., *et al.* (2024). Current advancements in therapeutic approaches in orthopedic surgery: A review of recent trends. *Frontiers in Bioengineering and Biotechnology, 12*. https://doi.org/10.3389/fbioe.2024.1328997 (accessed on 30th June 2025).

32. Maier-Hein, L., Eisenmann, M., Sarıkaya, D., März, K., Collins, T., Malpani, A., Fallert, J., *et al.* (2021). Surgical data science–From concepts toward clinical translation. *Medical Image Analysis, 76*, 102306–102306. https://doi.org/10.1016/j.media.2021.102306 (accessed on 30th June 2025).

33. Markiewicz-Gospodarek, A., Kozioł, M., Tobiasz, M., Baj, J., Radzikowska-Büchner, E., & Przekora, A. (2022). Burn wound healing: Clinical complications, medical care, treatment, and dressing types: The current state of knowledge for clinical practice. *International Journal*

of Environmental Research and Public Health, 19, 1338–1338. https://doi.org/10.3390/ijerph19031338 (accessed on 30th June 2025).

34. Meyer-Szary, J., Luis, M. S., Mikulski, S., Patel, A., Schulz, F., Tretiakow, D., Fercho, J., *et al.* (2022). The role of 3D printing in planning complex medical procedures and training of medical professionals—Cross-sectional multispecialty review. *International Journal of Environmental Research and Public Health, 19*, 3331–3331. https://doi.org/10.3390/ijerph19063331 (accessed on 30th June 2025).

35. Miller, J. M., Binnicker, M. J., Campbell, S., Carroll, K. C., Chapin, K. C., Gonzalez, M. D., Harrington, A., *et al.* (2024). Guide to utilization of the microbiology laboratory for diagnosis of infectious diseases: 2024 update by the Infectious Diseases Society of America (IDSA) and the American Society for Microbiology (ASM). *Clinical Infectious Diseases*. https://doi.org/10.1093/cid/ciae104 (accessed on 30th June 2025).

36. Moulik, N. R., & Saroha, M. (2020). COPING with CORONA: A developing country perspective on managing children with cancer during COVID-19 pandemic. *Cancer Research Statistics and Treatment, 3*, 97–97. https://doi.org/10.4103/crst.crst_131_20 (accessed on 30th June 2025).

37. Nisar, O., Nisar, S., Khattak, S., Rashid, H. U., Jaffari, S. M. I. A., Haider, Z., Fatima, F., Zahra, S. e., *et al.* (2023). Clinical and etiological exploration of ventilator-associated pneumonia in the intensive care unit of a developing country. *Cureus, 15*. https://www.semanticscholar.org/paper/7f86bf2c39f54fb775947cffac6ca9ea8559a5a5 (accessed on 30th June 2025).

38. Pollak, U., Feinstein, Y., Mannarino, C., McBride, M. E., Mendonca, M., Keizman, E., Mishaly, D., *et al.* (2022). The horizon of pediatric cardiac critical care. *Frontiers in Pediatrics, 10*. https://doi.org/10.3389/fped.2022.863868 (accessed on 30th June 2025).

39. Pudjiadi, A. H. (2020). Intensive care management to reduce morbidities following pediatric liver transplantation in Indonesia. *Transplantation Reports, 5*, 100064–100064. https://doi.org/10.1016/j.tpr.2020.100064 (accessed on 30th June 2025).

40. Racine-Brzostek, S., Cushing, M. M., Gareis, M., Heger, A., Shah, T. M., & Scully, M. (2024). Thirty years of experience with solvent/detergent-treated plasma for transfusion medicine. *Transfusion, 64*, 1132–1153. https://doi.org/10.1111/trf.17836 (accessed on 30th June 2025).

41. Sartelli, M., Barie, P. S., Coccolini, F., Abbas, M., Abbo, L. M., Abdukhalilova, G. K., Abraham, Y., *et al.* (2023). Ten golden rules for optimal antibiotic use in hospital settings: The WARNING call to action. *World Journal of Emergency Surgery, 18*. https://doi.org/10.1186/s13017-023-00518-3 (accessed on 30th June 2025).

42. Scheper-Hughes, N. (2020). *The Global Traffic in Human Organs*. Routledge eBooks. https://doi.org/10.4324/9781003060338-34 (accessed on 30th June 2025).

43. Stone, K., Zwiggelaar, R., Jones, P. D., & Mac Parthaláin, N. (2022). A systematic review of the prediction of hospital length of stay: Towards a unified framework. *PLOS Digital Health, 1*, e0000017–e0000017. https://doi.org/10.1371/journal.pdig.0000017 (accessed on 30th June 2025).

44. Stout, K., Daniels, C. J., Aboulhosn, J., Bozkurt, B., Broberg, C. S., Colman, J. M., Crumb, S. R., *et al.* (2018). 2018 AHA/ACC guideline for the management of adults with congenital heart disease: A report of the American College of Cardiology/American Heart Association Task Force on Clinical Practice Guidelines. *Circulation, 139*. https://doi.org/10.1161/cir.0000000000000603 (accessed on 30th June 2025).

45. Stylianos, S., Mesa-Jonassen, A. E., Albanese, C. T., Bacha, E., Stark, N., Guida, S. J., Goffman, D., *et al.* (2020). The perioperative services response at a major children's hospital during the peak of the COVID-19 pandemic in New York City. *Annals of Surgery, 272*, e199–e203. https://doi.org/10.1097/sla.0000000000004104 (accessed on 30th June 2025).

46. Sullivan, M., Bouffet, É., Rodríguez-Galindo, C., Luna-Fineman, S., Khan, M. S., Kearns, P., Hawkins, D. S., *et al.* (2020). The COVID-19 pandemic: A rapid global response for children with cancer from SIOP, COG, SIOP-E, SIOP-PODC, IPSO, PROS, CCI, and St Jude Global. *Pediatric Blood & Cancer, 67*. https://doi.org/10.1002/pbc.28409 (accessed on 30th June 2025).

47. Troschke, T., Wieczorek, A., Kulinski, K., Ociepa, T., Zielezińska, K., Lode, H. N., & Urasiński, T. (2023). Pediatric hematology and oncology center integrated by telemedicine: Experience, challenges and first results of a cross-border network. *Healthcare, 11*, 1431–1431. https://doi.org/10.3390/healthcare11101431 (accessed on 30th June 2025).

48. Weigl, M., Heinrich, M., Rivas, J., Bergmann, F., Kurz, M., Silbereisen, C., Dieterich, H. J., *et al.* (2023). Teamwork and mental workload in postsurgical pediatric patient handovers: Prospective effect evaluation of an improvement intervention for OR-PICU patient transitions. *European Journal of Pediatrics, 182*, 5637–5647. https://www.semanticscholar.org/paper/bc44e1d75121be8690bb326003afc100d2e5588d (accessed on 30th June 2025).

49. Zinter, M., Brazauskas, R., Strom, J., Chen, S., Bo-Subait, S., Sharma, A., Beitinjaneh, A., *et al.* (2023). Critical illness risk and long-term outcomes following intensive care in pediatric hematopoietic cell transplant recipients. *medRxiv*. https://www.semanticscholar.org/paper/4d58105aba90ef2a3f9e8d79518023b1759dd270 (accessed on 30th June 2025).

ETHICAL AND LEGAL ISSUES

14

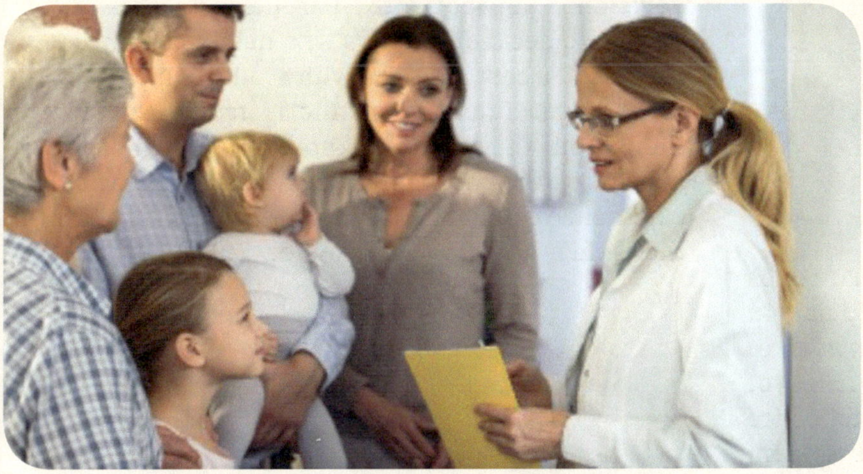

LEARNING OBJECTIVES

After studying this chapter, you will be able to:

1. Understand Ethical Principles in Pediatric Intensive Care.
2. Explain Legal Frameworks Governing Pediatric Care.
3. Describe Ethical Dilemmas in Treatment Decisions.
4. Focus on The Role of Healthcare Professionals in Ethical and Legal Issues.

Introduction

Pediatric intensive care presents a complex landscape of ethical and legal dilemmas specific to the medical treatment of children. Unlike patients over the age of majority, children are generally incapable of articulating their needs, which places a greater onus upon healthcare workers to expertly navigate informed consent and advocacy. This dilemma is additionally heightened in cases involving terminal conditions, where decisions must be made under pressure without a great deal of information. The pandemic of COVID-19 has brought many of these issues to light, as healthcare systems have reacted to novel situations, placing the importance of ethical principles in resource and treatment allocation at the forefront (Somekh *et al.*, 2020). Such events call for a close examination of legal frameworks that govern clinical practice in pediatric intensive care units, as they must weigh patient well-being against the final end of public health (Versporten *et al.*, 2018). Making sense of these issues is essential to creating ethical decision-making procedures in this delicate field of medicine.

14.1. Ethical Principles in Pediatric Intensive Care

Learning Outcome

1. Autonomy and Informed Consent.
2. Beneficence and Nonmaleficence.
3. Justice in Resource Allocation.
4. The Role of Parental Authority.
5. Pediatric Patient Advocacy.
6. Cultural Competence in Ethical Decision-Making.
7. The Impact of Pediatric Palliative Care.
8. Ethical Challenges in End-of-Life Decisions.
9. Balancing Risks and Benefits.

In pediatric intensive care, ethical principles regulating clinical practice are crucial in promoting care that is in the interests of the child but also addresses the wishes of family members. The principle of beneficence is also at the forefront of this ethics system and emphasizes the duty of the health care professional to perform activities that will be helpful for their pediatric patients. Such a principle is likely to get mixed reactions with regard to respect for autonomy, particularly where parents or guardians consider decisions on behalf of the children, calling for a proper balancing act between medical opinion and family values.

Ethical issues are likely to arise in such a scenario, primarily in end-of-life care decisions and organ donation discussions, where emotional pain by family members may disrupt the decision-making process (Sam *et al.*, 2017). Ensuring transparency and tact in such discourse can lead to informed choices that both honor the patients' desires and the moral obligations of the medical team (Eldridge *et al.*, 2016).

14.1.1. Autonomy and Informed Consent

Informed consent is a hallmark of ethical medical practice, particularly in the sensitive setting of pediatric intensive care, where patient autonomy is often complicatedly entwined with parental decision-making. Children, due to the level of their cognitive and affective development, might not possess the capacity to fully understand the meaning of their treatment decisions. Consequently, parents are usually surrogate decision-makers who need to balance their child's best interests with available medical knowledge. Such a dynamic is troublesome, though, as there lies the possibility of moral distress on the part of medical professionals who experience conflict between parental wishes and the child's welfare (Christopher, 2014).

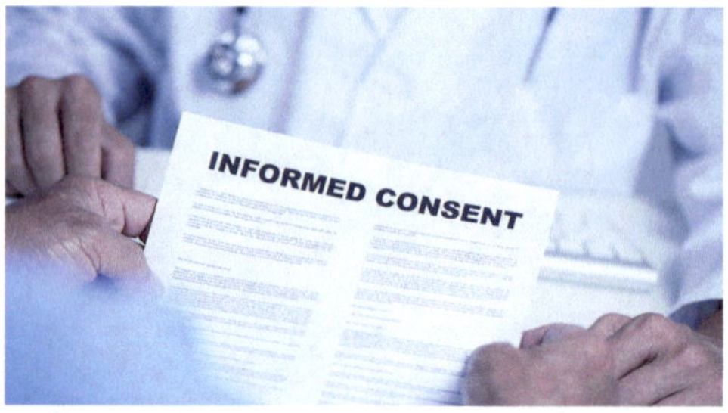

Figure 14.1. Informed consent is a cornerstone of ethical medical practice, particularly in the sensitive context of pediatric intensive care, where patient autonomy is often complexly intertwined with parental decision-making.

Source: https://www.aamc.org/sites/default/files/d/1/9-informed_consent_redboxxmain.jpg__992x558_q85_crop_subsampling-2_upscale.jpg.

Moreover, because the ground that medical interventions cover is growing wide—often including new but unproven therapies—doctors and nurses must enhance communication skills so that families are able to comprehend the risks and benefits of every choice while being mindful of the child's increasing autonomy (Scott, 2014).

Hence, fostering a culture marked by dialogue is of utmost importance in an effort to elicit honest informed consent (Figure 14.1).

14.1.2. Beneficence and Nonmaleficence

The virtues of beneficence and nonmaleficence are crucial in navigating the tricky landscape of pediatric critical care, where health is maximized with a minimization of harm. With an environment of high medical technologies, the potential for saving the critically ill neonate poses the problematic ethical challenges of the propriety of aggressive therapy. As Mills *et al.* (2020) observe, moral distress can occur from the decision of the medical team on end-of-life care and on the balancing of patient autonomy. Balancing the best interests of a child with those of his or her family makes it even more difficult. Vaccination policy also presents us with the tension between parental autonomy and community health, as presented in Kristin *et al.* (2015). Finally, resolving the ethical dilemmas of beneficence and nonmaleficence requires collaborative actions that facilitate open communication between families, patients, and clinicians to ensure compassionate care that is ethically founded.

14.1.3. Justice in Resource Allocation

To ensure justice in the allocation of resources in pediatric intensive care, sensitive attention to both ethical principles and the practical implications of decision-making must be exercised. Within a healthcare setting increasingly influenced by advanced technologies, including artificial intelligence, unequal access to care becomes a possibility. Ethical values demand equitable distribution of resources, but the world at times has variations based on socioeconomic status, geographical context, and availability of advanced medical treatment. As in recent debates regarding genome-wide sequencing, ethical dilemmas frequently arise when the values of beneficence and justice are in conflict, particularly in regard to unsolicited information flooding patients and clinicians alike (Gordon *et al.*, 2024). In addressing such ethical dilemmas, there is a need for the medical community to unite in establishing appropriate guidelines that balance both patient care and equitable resource allocation, thereby preventing the risks of vulnerable populations being devastated by imbalances in access to health care (Eichinger *et al.*, 2021) (Figure 14.2).

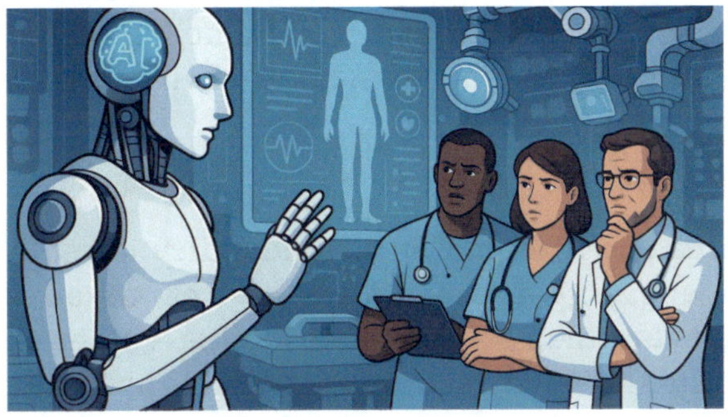

Figure 14.2. In a healthcare landscape increasingly influenced by advanced technologies, such as artificial intelligence, the potential for unequal access to care becomes pronounced.

Source: https://media.licdn.com/dms/image/v2/D5612AQEALHWIuzqvnA/article-cover_image-shrink_720_1280/B56ZaeQbWvHUAI-/0/1746411831164?e=2147483647&v=beta&t=im5yAJY2hZT1_gVj6VNUtHgU8KhRSJjePSn-3Bq8PUo.

14.1.4. The Role of Parental Authority

Parental authority is critical in the pediatric intensive care environment when it comes to decision-making regarding the treatment of their children. Parents are typically sucked into hard situations where not only is their authority legal but ethical as well, because they are torn between medical advice and their personal conscience. As explained in studies, the application of family-centered care relies heavily on the comprehension of power dynamics of imbalance in these situations, where healthcare professionals need to measure their professionalism against parental wishes (Mirlashari *et al.*, 2019). Furthermore, as recommended by ethics guidelines, parental involvement is also essential, particularly in issues of limiting or suspending therapies, where open communication and cultural humility are good practices (Kirsch *et al.*, 2018). Finally, an allowance for parents' power of attorney ensures a working platform that is essential to the provision of empathetic and holistic care in extremely challenging medical environments.

14.1.5. Pediatric Patient Advocacy

In pediatric intensive care, advocacy is central in engaging the complicated web of ethics and law that converges to define vulnerable patients. Pediatric patient advocates are tasked with the duty of ensuring that children's and their families' concerns are voiced within the process of medical decision-making, especially where the stakes are terribly high in critical care scenarios. While families wrestle with difficult choices, effective advocacy can assist in achieving a better understanding of treatment options and outcomes, thereby empowering caregivers to make informed decisions. Moreover, as observed during the COVID-19 pandemic, increased utilization of telemedicine has introduced opportunities as well as challenges in maintaining continuity of care for pediatric patients. This shift of focus underscores the importance of robust advocacy measures that are not just a reaction to immediate health problems but also seek equitable access to care and support systems, thereby exhibiting the quintessential importance of advocacy in the larger picture of pediatric medicine (Bhaskar *et al.*, 2020; Harris *et al.*, 2019) (Figure 14.3).

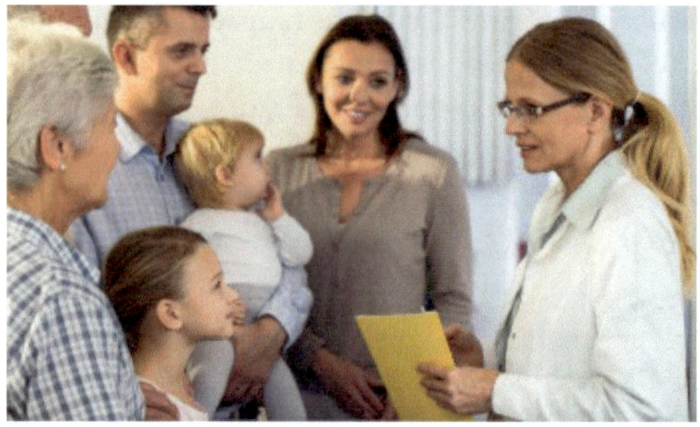

Figure 14.3. Pediatric patient advocates are tasked with ensuring that the voices of children and their families are heard within the medical decision-making process, especially during critical care scenarios where the stakes are particularly high.

Source: https://www.healthychildren.org/SiteCollectionImagesArticleImages/SDM_family_Doc.jpg.

14.1.6. Cultural Competence in Ethical Decision-Making

Cultural competence becomes a critical determinant of ethical decision-making in pediatric intensive care, particularly when navigating through the diverse backgrounds of patients and their families. Familiarity with local cultural determinants of what is known about health, illness, and care has a dramatic effect on the ethical issues in healthcare providers. For instance, with technologies such as virtual simulation (VS) becoming increasingly popular in health training, pedagogy-sensitive cultural awareness remains important, considering that 98% of recent studies on VS come from Europe, North America, and Asia, which reflects potential disparities in the dissemination of digital medical education (Wu *et al.*, 2022). Besides, as pediatric palliative care policies evolve to address international diversity in healthcare settings, utilization of cultural competence is required to recognize and respect the moral and spiritual needs of the families (Benini *et al.*, 2022). Ultimately, cultural sensitivity in decision-making facilitates trust and collaboration between healthcare providers and the populations they serve.

14.1.7. The Impact of Pediatric Palliative Care

Integration of pediatric palliative care (PPC) in pediatric intensive care units (PICUs) has a significant influence on both ethical and legal problems in treatment decision-making. As highlighted in the recent updates of international PPC standards, high-quality palliative care addresses not only clinical requirements but also developmental, psychological, social, ethical, and spiritual requirements of patients and families (Benini *et al.*, 2022).

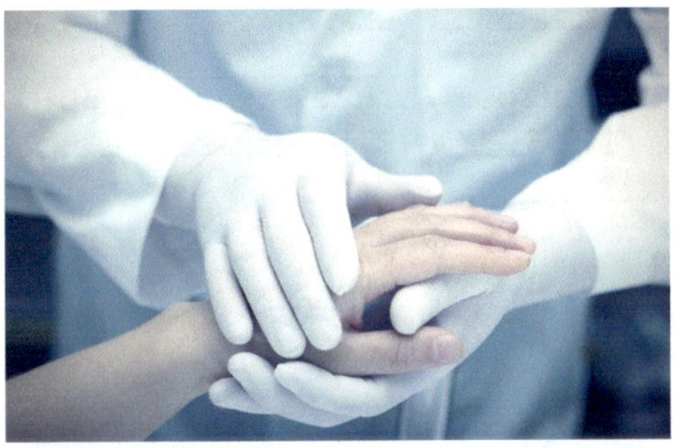

Figure 14.4. Ethical dilemmas frequently arise in PICUs, particularly regarding the balance of interventions aimed at prolonging life versus enhancing comfort, necessitating an informed consent process that involves both parents and healthcare providers.

Source: https://media.licdn.com/dms/image/v2/D5612AQF1YzyKzqjgIg/article-cover_image-shrink_720_1280/article-cover_image-shrink_720_1280/0/1721181413318?e=2147483647&v=beta&t=4YHSdmbAIxNKyUU6GL23MrU6WexRJ-DgQYB7LVpQd-o.

This blended strategy becomes crucial in scenarios where curative treatments become limited or ineffective, making quality of life a priority. Ethical dilemmas tend to occur within PICUs, particularly when it comes to balancing interventions that prolong life with interventions that relieve suffering, necessitating an informed consent process between parents and doctors (Farsi, 2021). By creating definitive standards and transparent communication, pediatric palliative care can reduce such ethical challenges as a means of guaranteeing that care is always consistent with both the patients' best interests and legal obligations in healthcare environments (Figure 14.4).

14.1.8. Ethical Challenges in End-of-Life Decisions

End-of-life care decision-making in pediatric intensive care is a profoundly difficult ethical dilemma, particularly the dilemma of balance between advances in medicine and the dignity of patients and families. With the increase in technology, the provision of life-supporting therapies has a tendency to extend suffering in cases with little hope of recovery. This raises very serious ethical concerns, with clinicians having to respect the declared wishes of families but also consider the ethics of continued aggressive intervention that might lead to prolonged suffering.

As envisaged in discourse on organ donation policy, family discussions must be approached with sensitivity and empathy to optimize decision-making in these highly charged emotional states (Inoue *et al.*, 2019). Moreover, the intricate dynamics between family members blur these decisions even more, calling for a delicate weighing of cultural, religious, and personal values that are not necessarily in accordance with medical recommendations (Sam *et al.*, 2017). Thus, formulating ethical principles that respect the needs and sovereignty of pediatric patients and families is paramount in this situation.

14.1.9. Balancing Risks and Benefits

Administration of the complexity of pediatric intensive care demands a delicate understanding of risk-benefit trade-off, most specifically regarding life-sustaining medical treatment (LSMT). Under conditions of urgency, physicians must gauge the morality of prolonging or withdrawing LSMT by considering the best interests of the child, along with the psychological and emotional weights of families. Being involved in collaborative dialogue among medical staff, families, and ethics advisors is of the greatest importance; open communication strengthens trust and determines goals of care, thus easing the decision-making process (Kathryn *et al.*, 2017). Moreover, the complicated mechanism of drug intake by pregnant women emphasizes the necessity of universal screening and multidisciplinary management of care, with priority on evaluating both infant and maternal outcomes. This holistic strategy guarantees that ethical issues are responsive to the realities of pediatric practice, allowing practitioners to make reflective decisions that are both health- and dignity-oriented (Figure 14.5).

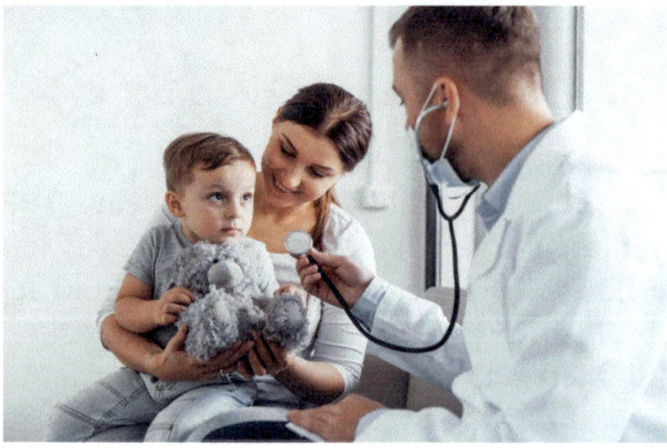

Figure 14.5. Navigating the complexities of pediatric intensive care demands a nuanced understanding of balancing risks and benefits, particularly when it comes to life-sustaining medical treatment (LSMT).

Source: https://brhealthcare.in/uploads/blogs/1715716190_health-care-scaled-1-2048x1365.jpg.

Test Your Knowledge

1. In what situations might non-maleficence conflict with parental wishes in the PICU?
2. How is justice applied when allocating limited PICU resources?

14.2. Legal Frameworks Governing Pediatric Care

Learning Outcome

1. Overview of Relevant Laws and Regulations.
2. The Role of Child Protection Services.
3. Legal Standards for Informed Consent.
4. Medical Malpractice and Liability Issues.
5. Confidentiality and Privacy Laws.
6. The Impact of State versus Federal Laws.
7. Legal Rights of Minors.
8. The Role of Institutional Review Boards.
9. Legal Implications of Research Involving Children.

Legal structures of pediatric care are crucial to the resolution of the complexities of ethical dilemmas that arise in pediatric intensive care units. Legal structures are likely to guide healthcare providers regarding their functions and patients' rights, especially concerning crucial end-of-life choices. For instance, findings indicate extreme diversity in the attitudes and experiences of healthcare professionals towards end-of-life care, reflecting a pressing necessity for clear legal frameworks to facilitate decision-making in pediatric intensive care units (Ćurković *et al.*, 2024).

Additionally, the application of shared decision-making (SDM) models varies within various cultural settings, further complicating the legal framework; parents' attitudes and experience of being involved in end-of-life decisions are highly varied in North America and Europe, necessitating adaptable legal standards in the care of children (Schouten *et al.*, 2021). Therefore, it is critical to create strong legal frameworks in order to promote ethical practice, while considering the different needs of families and healthcare professionals.

14.2.1. Overview of Relevant Laws and Regulations

In pediatric intensive care, the relevant laws and regulations are distinguished by a broad set of legal and ethical concerns. Basic regulations, such as the Health Insurance Portability and Accountability Act (HIPAA), govern confidentiality and patient data security and lay down guidelines for the protection of sensitive information. Additionally, state and federal legislation dictate the consent requirements, particularly with minors, which usually makes it difficult to make decisions in emergency care circumstances. With technology in healthcare moving forward, particularly with digital platforms, the need for a guideline becomes much more crucial. The Vw et al. (2024) report indicates a dire lack of harmonized data protection law, which tends to hinder the ethical handling of pediatric patient data. Besides, conclusions from FRSC MIA (2024) point to the importance of international cooperation to harmonize disparity in the regulation of advanced medical technology while upholding the rights and welfare of children as patients with advancing practices (Figure 14.6).

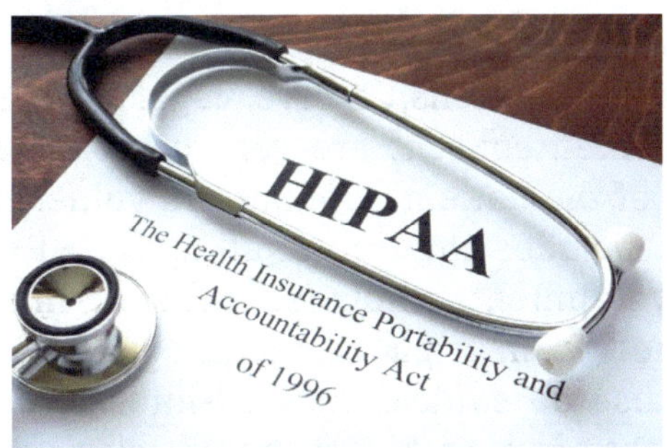

Figure 14.6. Essential regulations, such as the Health Insurance Portability and Accountability Act (HIPAA), govern the confidentiality and security of patient information, providing a framework for protecting sensitive data.

Source: https://www.seasiainfotech.com/blog/wp-content/uploads/2024/01/HIPAA.webp.

14.2.2. The Role of Child Protection Services

In Pediatric Intensive Care, the role of Child Protection Services (CPS) is critical in the defense of vulnerable children who may be at risk of child abuse or neglect. The meeting of ethical and legal challenges in the care of children necessitates interprofessional cooperation between healthcare workers and CPS in safeguarding children's well-being. Such collaboration not only enables communication but also enhances understanding of family relationships and social determinants of health, thereby enabling care teams to effectively address underlying causes. Additionally, where artificial intelligence is used to identify patient data, ethical concerns regarding privacy and data protection arise, as explained in the broader context of health care technology (Wang *et al.*, 2023) and (Sharma *et al.*, 2022). By these complexities, CPS is instrumental in advocating for children's rights and interests and ensuring that medical care is guided by ethical standards and legal regulations.

14.2.3. Legal Requirements for Informed Consent

In pediatric intensive care, legal obligations of informed consent are very complicated by virtue of the patient population's vulnerability, which includes children of all ages and stages of development. Informed consent must be obtained from a guardian or a parent, who must also be sufficiently well-informed about the treatments involved, potential risks, and alternatives. Legal systems stress that consent not just be voluntary but also grounded in a comprehensive understanding of the information provided, which is paramount in high-risk settings such as intensive care units, where decisions can have a direct influence on outcomes. Moreover, courts have traditionally appreciated that informed consent is not a mere ritual but an ethical imperative that reflects the respect for the patient's autonomy even in children. Also, the rules offered in systematic reviews, for example, as discussed worldwide (Versporten *et al.*, 2018), emphasize the need for culturally tailored communication approaches that adapt to populations and offer insight at every care level (Susan, 2022) (Figure 14.7).

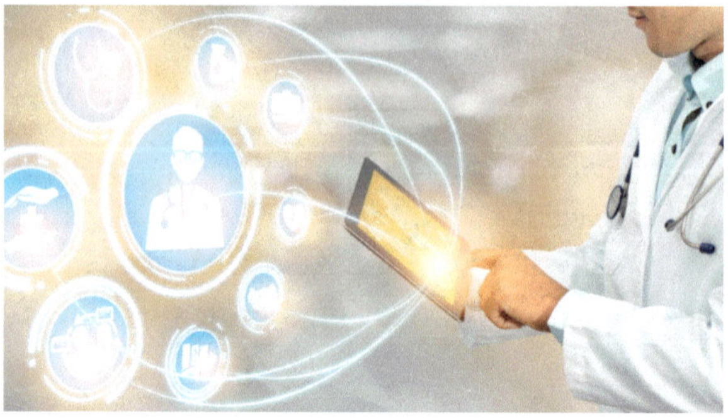

Figure 14.7. Informed consent must be obtained from a parent or guardian, who must be adequately informed about the proposed treatments, potential risks, and alternatives.

Source: https://corporate.cyrilamarchandblogs.com/wp-content/uploads/sites/857/2022/05/Consent-in-Healthcare.png.

14.2.4. Medical Malpractice and Liability Issues

Traveling the landscape of medical malpractice and liability issues in the pediatric intensive care environment is riddled with unique challenges that require close attention to ethical and legal doctrine. Since pediatric patients' ability to understand their health status and treatment can vary, professionals must practice at a high level while grappling with the complexity of informed consent. Increased reliance on technology, and particularly artificial intelligence, can enhance diagnostic accuracy and treatment efficiency but presents certain possible hazards in terms of data accuracy, product liability, and privacy that must be appropriately resolved (Karalis, 2024). Besides, low- and middle-income countries face poor access to healthcare, which aggravates the risks of malpractice and highlights the imperative importance of comprehensive methods of improving health literacy and the healthcare system (Wang *et al.*, 2023). Finally, the intersection of legal responsibility and ethical duty in pediatric intensive care highlights the importance of effective guidelines prioritizing patient safety and well-being.

14.2.5. Laws of Confidentiality and Privacy

In pediatric intensive care, patient confidentiality and adherence to privacy law are absolute legal and ethical imperatives. Beyond ensuring that sensitive health information is kept confidential, such laws ensure trust between healthcare providers and families.

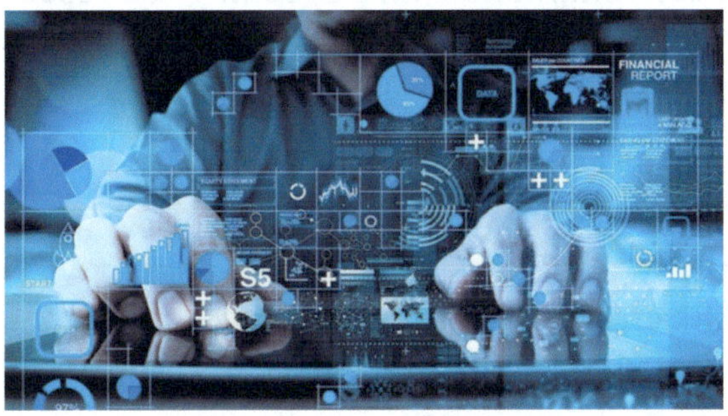

Figure 14.8. As healthcare increasingly integrates advanced technologies, including Artificial Intelligence (AI) tools, the need for transparency in data use becomes critical; a lack of clarity can undermine patient trust and care efficacy.

Source: https://www.hindustantimes.com/ht-img/img/2024/10/16/550x309/0ed45db8-4470-11ec-bd68-b2b71042cab0_1636801007972_1729083157675.jpg.

The Health Insurance Portability and Accountability Act (HIPAA) provides the basis for the protection of patient records and confidentiality, particularly for children whose guardians regularly make tough healthcare decisions on their behalf. Furthermore, with medicine increasingly being modernized through the incorporation of advanced technologies like Artificial Intelligence (AI) devices, transparency in data use is paramount to avoid allowing uncertainty to undermine patient trust and the efficacy of care (Zhang *et al.*, 2022). Maintaining robust data management practices to satisfy both ethical and legal requirements will be important going forward, as pediatric treatment becomes increasingly complicated and reliant upon data-driven decisions (Maier *et al.*, 2021) (Figure 14.8).

14.2.6. The Impact of State Versus Federal Laws

The tension between state and federal regulation has profound effects on pediatric intensive care, extending to practices involving patient treatment, consent, and the delivery of healthcare services. In this case, state legislation generally regulates key aspects of parental consent and addresses certain medical conditions, resulting in a patchwork of laws that can be quite different from one jurisdiction to the next. This disparity can generate ethical dilemmas, particularly when federal laws try to harmonize care practices to mitigate important issues of public health. For instance, the operation of social determinants of health (SDH) is crucial in pediatrics, but disparities in state law could hinder the implementation of effective screening and support measures for vulnerable groups, as noted by Lelinneth *et al.* (2023). In addition, federal laws for new treatments, such as bacteriophage therapy for antibiotic-resistant infections, can make it difficult for state-level policy and become barriers to timely treatment, making the need to integrate policy approaches in pediatric intensive care even more pertinent (Hitchcock *et al.*, 2023).

14.2.7. Legal Rights of Minors

In pediatric intensive care, it is essential to understand the legal rights of children in order to navigate the complex ethical landscape. Children possess certain rights distinct from their role in medical decision-making processes. Of special interest is the right not to know that seeks to uphold a child's autonomy, particularly in cases such as genetic testing. When a child is tested irrespective of their perspective, then such a right is forfeited, and they can be deprived of the ability to participate in making health care decisions about themselves, as highlighted by the increased prevalence of genetic technologies (Borry *et al.*, 2014). In addition to this, moral dilemmas in the case of children are generally resolved within a context of bioethical rules that guarantee disputes between healthcare providers, parents, and caregivers are resolved in favor of the child (Dubler *et al.*, 1994). Awareness and facilitation of such rights are crucial towards ensuring ethical practice among pediatric medicine (Figure 14.9).

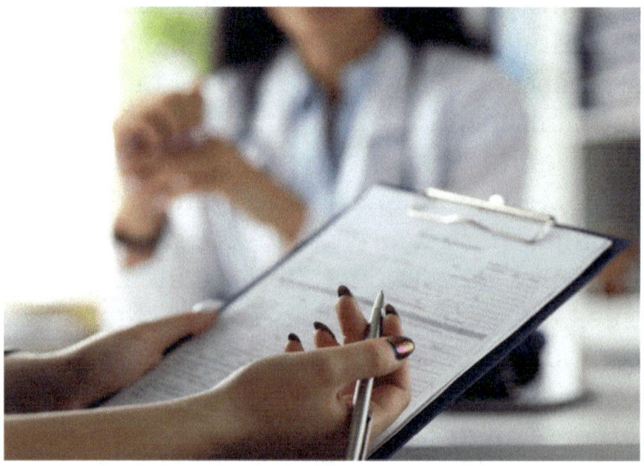

Figure 14.9. Minors possess specific rights that reflect their unique position within medical decision-making processes.

Source: https://hospitalprocedures.org/wp-content/uploads/2024/12/consent-for-health-care-of-a-minor.jpg.

14.2.8. The Role of Institutional Review Boards

Institutional Review Boards (IRBs) play a very important role in safeguarding the ethical integrity of research, particularly in sensitive environments such as pediatric intensive care. IRBs are tasked with the oversight of research proposals to ensure the rights and welfare of child participants are adequately safeguarded, the vulnerabilities in the population notwithstanding. Since research increasingly involves community interaction and participatory approaches, IRBs need to evolve to support ethics standards while promoting stakeholder collaboration (Stephanie *et al.*, 2022). Additionally, the use of high-level data analytics and machine learning in clinical research poses substantial regulatory issues that IRBs will need to navigate (Maier *et al.*, 2021). Secured by innovative research against strict compliance with ethical standards, IRBs are required to be watchful over active investigations. Their role is thus pivotal in patient protection, ethical compliance, and speeding up research advances in pediatric care within legislatively approved protection for children.

14.2.9. Legal Consequences of Research with Children

Children's research, particularly in pediatric intensive care, has grave legal concerns that must be tackled with the utmost precaution. The ethical concern of this group is compounded by the imperative of protecting children who might lack the capacity to provide informed consent. This necessitates creating legally sound frameworks that are child-friendly but facilitate scientific advancement. As part of medical ethical issues discussions, having a code of conduct that balances patient interests with wider healthcare resource issues is essential (Montalto *et al.*, 2014). Further, the need for careful monitoring is echoed in studies attempting to quantify the impacts of PICU admission, where ethical consent and parental consent become necessary components in participants' protection (Coad *et al.*, 2020). Hence, it is the responsibility of researchers to be vigilant in meeting legal standards to uphold the integrity of their research and the rights of young participants.

Test Your Knowledge

1. What are the legal implications of refusing treatment for a critically ill child?
2. What legal protections exist for healthcare providers when acting in the child's best interest against parental wishes?

14.3. Ethical Dilemmas in Treatment Decisions

Learning Outcome

1. Decisions Regarding Life-Sustaining Treatment.
2. The Role of Advanced Directives.
3. Ethical Issues in Experimental Treatments.
4. Conflicts Between Parental Wishes and Medical Advice.
5. Resource Allocation in Critical Care.
6. The Impact of Socioeconomic Status on Treatment Options.
7. Ethical Considerations in Transplantation.
8. The Role of Multidisciplinary Teams in Decision-Making.

In pediatric intensive care, ethical dilemmas in treatment decision-making are more likely to occur within the framework of complex family and medical contexts. Providers must tread on the thin line of withdrawal or withholding life-sustaining treatment, and this can cause significant moral distress in clinicians as well as in families. This fine distinction between these actions is needed since miscomprehension can exacerbate deepening conflicts, depleting the trust of families and the healthcare team. Besides, the absence of clear-cut national guidelines increases these concerns, particularly when clinicians feel pressured to maintain treatments when chances are bleak, as in critically brain-damaged infants (Pant, 2021). A team-based approach with family engagement in decision-making not only facilitates open communication but also respects the unique emotional subtleties of navigating end-of-life care (Gutiez *et al.*, 2023). Thus, a robust framework of ethics is needed to inform treatment decisions in pediatric intensive care units.

14.3.1. Decisions Regarding Life-Sustaining Treatment

As with the complex pediatric intensive care world comes that of life-sustaining treatment decisions, which raise critical ethical and legal challenges. Physicians then have to tread through patient autonomy, parental rights, and the best interest of the child, often in high-pressure situations where emotions are intense. The increased emphasis on pediatric palliative care (PPC) has called for reflection regarding the provision of life-sustaining therapies, particularly for kids with chronic or end-stage illness (Benini *et al.*, 2022).

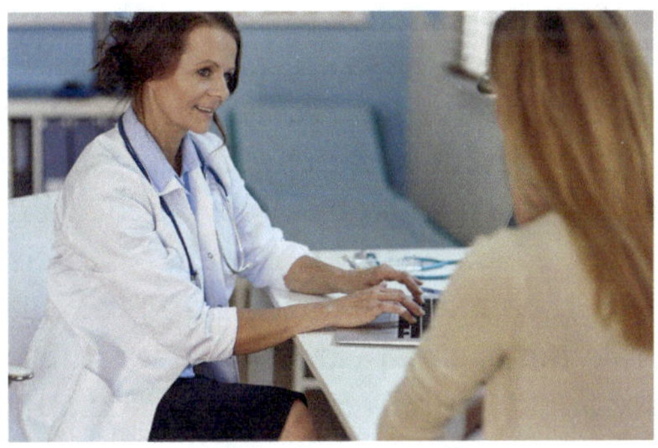

Figure 14.10. Healthcare providers must navigate the intricacies of patient autonomy, parental rights, and the best interests of the child, often in high-stress environments where emotions run deep.

Source: https://domf5oio6qrcr.cloudfront.net/medialibrary/9451/iStock_78445461_MEDIUM.jpg.

As clinicians aim to incorporate high-level medical technology and families' emotional well-being, education, and communication take center stage. Besides, in a world with the overwhelming use of digital platforms, healthcare professionals must remain vigilant when it comes to maintaining ethical values online while taking part in treatment choices and issues of patient care (Farsi, 2021). Lastly, there must be a respectful dialogue between caregivers, families, and medical teams in making decisions that are in line with the ethical principles and legal laws (Figure 14.10).

14.3.2. The Role of Advanced Directives

Advanced directives play a vital role in addressing the ethical and legal problems associated with pediatric intensive care units. Advanced directives are formal documents that express a patient's preferences regarding healthcare so their treatment is aligned with their values and what they want, particularly when they cannot communicate.

Respecting a child's autonomy becomes particularly challenging when legal guardians are involved, emphasizing the role of advance directives as tools for respecting the evolving thoughts of pediatric patients. A comprehensive, interdisciplinary model, as advocated by Schwartz *et al.* (2021), enhances decision-making through the integration of family, cultural, and societal values into consideration for treatment. Moreover, the policy formulation of end-of-life care, as cited in Myatra *et al.* (2014), emphasizes creating guidelines to limit unsuitable interventions while continuing to observe ethical considerations and patient-centered practice. Thus, advance directives become potential tools to impart dignity and respect in making key medical decisions in children.

14.3.3. Ethical Issues in Experimental Treatments

Application of experimental therapy in pediatric intensive care raises an array of ethical considerations that require prudent thinking. Since children are vulnerable, the ethical rule of beneficence—doing what is in the patient's best interest—may be complicated by balancing potential benefit against risk of untested intervention. Informed consent is another vital ethical concern, since the necessity of obtaining informed consent from patients who are incapable of understanding complex medical information poses a dilemma for doctors. Cultural and socio-economic factors may also influence parents' decision-making regarding experimental therapies, with possible variations in access and outcome. As demonstrated in shared decision-making strategies discussions, the level of differing opinions among parents can influence their engagement in the most important health decisions, especially those that involve life-sustaining treatments, reflecting the need for thorough knowledge of ethical models (Ranjith *et al.*, 2023; Schouten *et al.*, 2021) (Figure 14.11).

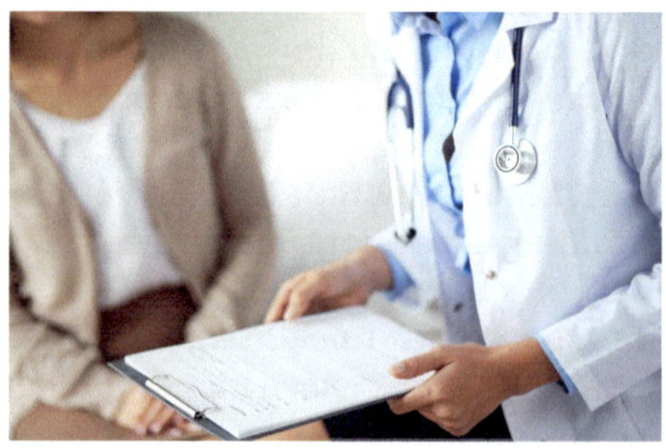

Figure 14.11. Informed consent is another significant ethical concern, as obtaining explicit permission from patients who may lack the capacity to understand complex medical information poses a dilemma for healthcare providers.

Source: https://www.news-medical.net/images/Article_Images/ImageForArticle_24607_17086988947716561.jpg.

14.3.4. Conflicts Between Parental Wishes and Medical Advice

Disagreements between medical advice and parental preferences are the rule in pediatric intensive care, so the ethical framework of treatment decisions becomes even more complicated. Parents will usually champion that which they believe is in their children's best interest, influenced by love and personal values. Providers are forced to navigate these desires through the structures of medical ethics and clinical practice guidelines. The use of shared decision-making strategies might be helpful, as they promote a dialogue of mutual exchange on the part of families and the healthcare team in the hope of finding a resolution of conflicting beliefs about a child's quality of life, especially in complex treatment futility cases. These conflicts can lead to moral distress among healthcare professionals, as parental requests and clinical recommendations stand at odds. This requires a consideration of the impact on the provision of care of various perspectives, in which elaborate discussion of consequence and patient self-determination are central to conflict resolution and ultimately syncing treatment with best medical practice (Mills *et al.*, 2020; Wiener *et al.*, 2015).

14.3.5. Resource Allocation in Critical Care

Within the high-stakes pediatric intensive care setting, resource distribution takes on heightened ethical significance, particularly when faced with shortages in a time of crisis, such as a pandemic. Allocation decisions regarding who receives what of the limited resources at hand—such as ventilators and specially trained staff—need to be filtered through ethical considerations that maximize benefit for the most critically in-need patients. Ethical frameworks call for open triage protocols to guide healthcare workers in such challenging situations, balancing the imperative to save life with the need to uphold standards of care that are equitable (Chopra *et al.*, 2020). These kinds of frameworks are not only required in conventional settings but also when dealing with emergent crises, like the COVID-19 pandemic, where hospitals have to redistribute resources quickly to manage an influx of extremely ill patients. Moreover, how such policies are communicated to employees and families is critical, promoting comprehension and confidence during periods of upheaval (Shokri *et al.*, 2020) (Figure 14.12).

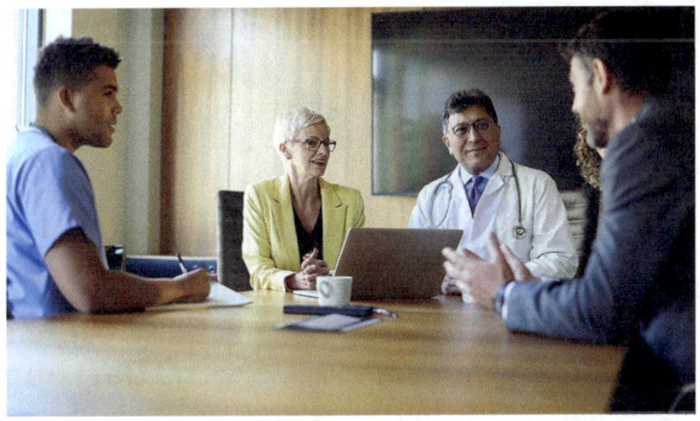

Figure 14.12. Ethical frameworks assert the necessity for transparent triage protocols to guide healthcare providers in these challenging situations, balancing the imperative to save lives against the need to uphold equitable standards of care.

Source: https://www.philips.com/c-dam/corporate/innovation-and-you/global/dec-2023/gettyimages-masthead.jpg.

14.3.6. The Impact of Socioeconomic Status on Treatment Options

Socioeconomic status (SES) is an important factor in decision-making in children's intensive care, controlling both access and the quality of treatment. Improved SES households have more fiscal resources and insurance coverage available, allowing them to receive more costly therapies and specialist assessments that are beyond the means of the financially limited households. Such a differential outcome is ethically objectionable with regard to promoting equity of access to healthcare. Furthermore, as the medical environment evolves with the integration of digital media and social media, as has been documented in recent studies, healthcare workers face additional ethical dilemmas in reaching all socioeconomic strata and informing them well regarding treatment options (Farsi, 2021). Besides, variations in clinical practice at the regional level, particularly in the treatment of diseases like oropharyngeal dysphagia in children, also further support the strong role of SES to influence access and effectiveness of care (Laura *et al.*, 2020).

14.3.7. Ethical Considerations in Transplantation

The ethical landscape of transplantation, particularly in the intensive care of children, demands a fair interpretation of equity, consent, and distribution of resources. Decisions regarding organ donation and transplantation should maintain fairness and the principles of distributive justice to ensure equal access to life-supporting therapy for all patients, regardless of socio-economic status. Moreover, informed consent is further problematic when minors are involved; guardians need to walk the thin line between doing what is best for the child and respecting the family's wishes.

As emphasized by the current debate in global nephrology guidelines, a strong need exists to integrate ethical values into health policy, particularly transplantation planning (Harris *et al.*, 2019). In addition, the allocation of scarce resources, such as organs, in emergencies complicates these ethical issues further because hospitals strive to make life-sustaining interventions when they are under great emotional and moral distress (Chopra *et al.*, 2020) (Figure 14.13).

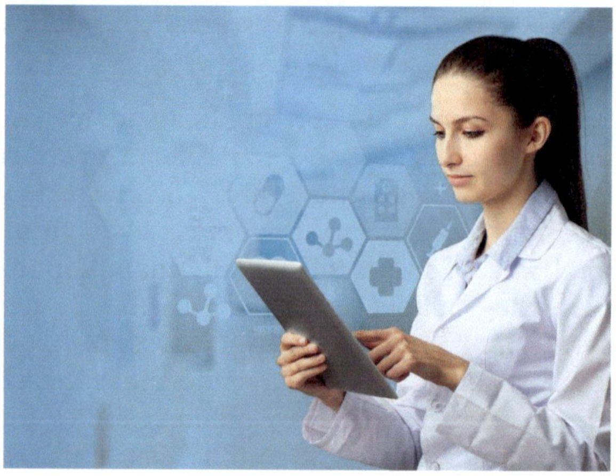

Figure 14.13. Decisions regarding organ donation and transplantation must prioritize the principles of fairness and distributive justice to ensure that all patients, regardless of socioeconomic background, have equitable access to life-saving treatments.

Source: https://assets.isu.pub/document-structure/240514101326-198a546519f39be9f3ba714717484a79/v1/881a19940973ce8ca5912e19ccda6261.jpeg.

14.3.8. The Role of Multidisciplinary Teams in Decision-Making

In pediatric intensive care units, the critical nature of the cases necessitates the involvement of multidisciplinary teams that are a key factor in enriching decision-making strategies. Members' diversity—like physicians, nurses, social workers, and ethicists—offers unique perspectives that guide comprehensive approaches to patient treatment, particularly in cases that pose ethical and legal dilemmas. For instance, active deliberation among team members can clarify complex problems, such as the multifaceted understanding of child maltreatment that can present diagnostic problems in emergency situations, as found in Onyejesi *et al.* (2025). Similarly, opening up inclusive dialogue prior to releasing sensitive information to families, as found in Barnum *et al.* (2023), enforces consistent messaging and permits the identification of parental bereavement, and hence builds trust. Lastly, effective collaboration significantly fortifies clinical judgment and ethical decision-making, enhancing the outcome for at-risk pediatric patients and families in critical care environments.

Test Your Knowledge

1. What ethical concerns surround the use of ECMO or mechanical ventilation in children with poor prognoses?
2. How can healthcare teams manage ethical conflicts when families request treatment that the team believes is futile?

14.4. The Role of Healthcare Professionals in Ethical and Legal Issues

Learning Outcome

1. Responsibilities of Pediatricians.
2. The Role of Nurses in Ethical Decision-Making.
3. Importance of Ethics Committees.
4. Training and Education on Ethical Issues.
5. Communication Skills in Difficult Conversations.
6. The Impact of Burnout on Ethical Decision-Making.
7. Collaboration with Social Workers and Psychologists.
8. Reporting and Addressing Ethical Violations.
9. The Importance of Professional Guidelines.

Health care providers stand squarely in the middle of ethical and legal challenges, particularly in pediatric intensive care, where decisions can seriously impact vulnerable patients. Their work is not merely in the clinical sphere but also in assuming ethical duties such as providing informed consent and ensuring patient care respects the dignity and rights of children and families. With advancing medical technology, experts are faced with complex dilemmas that emerge in conditions like end-of-life care and pediatric palliative care, where ethical guidelines cross over into legal ones. The GO-PPaCS project is a case in point on how pediatric palliative care standards are being enhanced with a priority on the necessity of healthcare professionals to be trained and implement ethical care models that suit the different needs (Benini *et al.*, 2022). Further, in the case of legislation on mandatory vaccination for healthcare workers, experts have to weigh public safety against their ethical responsibility towards patients' well-being, thus highlighting the fine balance they must maintain within the healthcare system (Emanuel *et al.*, 2021).

14.4.1. Responsibilities of Pediatricians

In the intensive care setting for children, the pediatrician's function extends beyond the clinical treatment and diagnosis, broaching a broader ethical and legal obligation. They have an obligation to guarantee that the particular medical, developmental, and emotional requirements of children, particularly those with serious health issues, are addressed in an integral manner. Pediatricians have a mandate to advance their patients' best interests by coordinating with families and multidisciplinary teams to develop appropriate plans of care, providing informed consent, and resolving conflicts that might arise during treatment. Pediatricians are also in an important position to handle the complexities of foster care systems because most children who are given intensive care have adverse histories that complicate their health trajectories. This requirement emphasizes the importance of understanding the ethical aspects of trauma and the impact of social determinants on health outcomes as outlined in current guidelines for pediatric palliative care (Benini *et al.*, 2022; Szilagyi, 2012) (Figure 14.14).

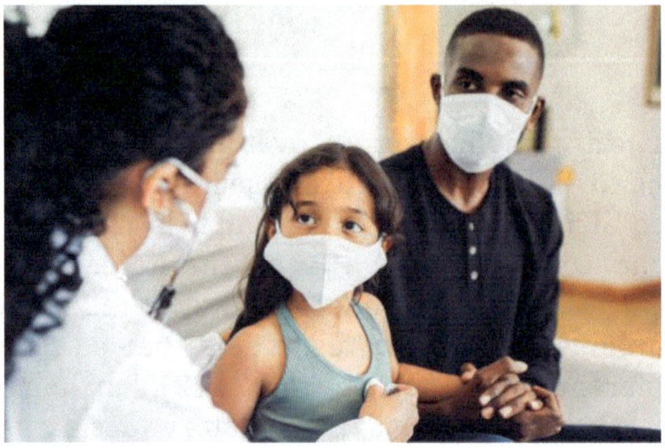

Figure 14.14. Pediatricians must advocate for the best interests of their patients by collaborating with families and interdisciplinary teams to develop appropriate care plans, ensuring informed consent is obtained, and addressing any potential conflicts that may arise during treatment.

Source: https://www.medpro.com/image/image_gallery?uuid=342bf854-1414-485a-ba76-8ef52effb36a&groupId=10502&t=1745821623294.

14.4.2. The Role of Nurses in Ethical Decision-Making

Pediatric intensive care nurses are an essential component of ethical decision-making, serving as representatives for their children and their families. Pediatric cases are frequently so intertwined that nurses must struggle not only with the medical complexity but with families' emotional universes as they make difficult decisions. This dual responsibility increases the call for nurses to be guided by ethical principles, namely, beneficence and non-maleficence, to ensure interventions improve child health. Monitoring of such a kind is crucial in cases like Post-Intensive Care Syndrome (PICS), which could influence long-term outcomes of patients, as outlined in Inoue *et al.* (2019). Moreover, the endemic issue of patient safety in healthcare, where around one in 10 patients experience harm, suggests the need for nurses to be vigilant in ensuring that systems prioritize safety and ethical issues, thereby highlighting the significant economic and human cost entailed by suboptimal quality care, according to Slawomirski *et al.* (2017).

14.4.3. Importance of Ethics Committees

In pediatric intensive care, the significance of ethics committees cannot be overstated, considering the complex ethical issues that medical practitioners typically face. The committees serve as significant resources by providing recommendations on frameworks for decision-making to facilitate respect for the value and rights of both the families and the patients. They facilitate dialogue that explores ethical issues, such as end-of-life decisions or consent to treatment, that help navigate through the emotional landscape that usually defines these. Additionally, ethics committees are pivotal in the facilitation of communication among multidisciplinary teams, and this results in increased understanding of the different perspectives and practices in pediatric care. In addressing such issues, committees also help in adhering to existing legal frameworks, which is an essential step in ensuring continuing trust in the healthcare system (Schmidt *et al.*, 2019; Sam *et al.*, 2017). Thus, inclusion of ethics committees is crucial in promoting ethical deliberation and helping healthcare professionals make ethically appropriate decisions in instances of urgency (Figure 14.15).

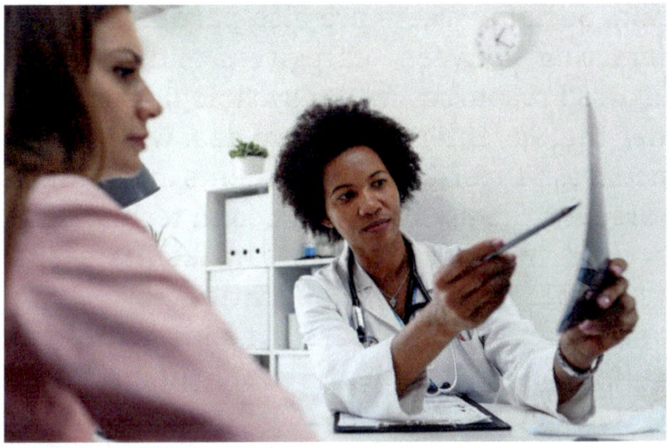

Figure 14.15. In pediatric intensive care, the crucial role of ethics committees cannot be overstated, particularly given the complex ethical dilemmas often faced by healthcare providers.

Source: https://s3.amazonaws.com/utep-uploads/wp-content/uploads/online-regis-college/2021/06/16103028/nurse-and-patient-1.jpg.

14.4.4. Training and Education on Ethical Issues

Training and education on ethics is paramount in the dynamic and trying pediatric intensive care setting among caregivers. Such training equips clinicians with the tools necessary to address dilemmas surrounding patient autonomy, informed consent, and resources, particularly in high-stakes situations where timely, decisive action is demanded. Interdisciplinary models expose caregivers to various perspectives, hence enhancing team-based ethical decision-making among diverse team players. Thus, a solid educational foundation in ethics enhances practitioners' ability to effectively communicate with families about care decisions, which will ultimately lead to improved patient outcomes and patient satisfaction. In addition, insights from contemporary practice, such as those detailed in the adaptations driven by the COVID-19 pandemic, highlight the necessity for clear-cut ethical guidelines in times of healthcare crisis (Shokri *et al.*, 2020; Chopra *et al.*, 2020). Therefore, continuous education in ethics not only makes sense but is necessary for pediatric intensive care teams.

14.4.5. Communication Skills in Difficult Conversations

Effective communication skills are crucial in managing difficult conversations, particularly within the context of pediatric intensive care, where ethical and legal concerns are compounded. Creating an empathic conversation allows healthcare providers to convey hard news regarding the treatment options, likely outcomes, and emotional impacts on families. Active listening and acknowledgment of the worries of parents have the power to make the atmosphere one of cooperation and trust, which enables families to make decisions regarding the care of their child.

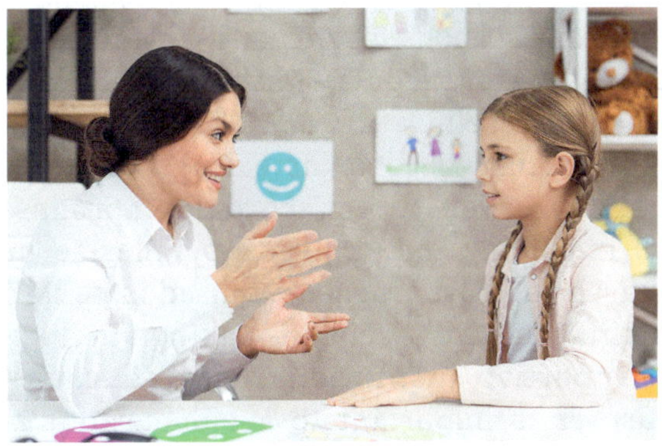

Figure 14.16. Effective communication skills are crucial in navigating difficult conversations, particularly within the realm of pediatric intensive care, where ethical and legal complexities are heightened.

Source: https://vipschool.in/wp-content/uploads/2022/10/How-to-Improve-Childrens-Communication-Skills.jpg.

Besides, good communication can help solve potential misunderstandings or conflicts that may occur, particularly in matters like organ transplant or treatment for severe psychiatric illness in young patients, as underscored in transgender transplant debates (Sarkar *et al.*, 2022). Such debates also present ethical concerns that call for healthcare practitioners to be attentive to the nuances of patient autonomy and consent, thus promoting integrative practice in patient-centered care (Coppola *et al.*, 2021) (Figure 14.16).

14.4.6. The Impact of Burnout on Ethical Decision-Making

In pediatric intensive care, professional burnout in important respects inhibits ethical decision-making, diminishing patient care and the potential for ethical failure. Burnout not only diminishes emotional resilience in managing challenging ethical issues but also instills a disaffection with patient-centered care, something that's especially critical in high-stakes environments. It may contribute to the already complex nature of ethical decisions, particularly in the case of the social determinants of health of vulnerable populations (Lelinneth *et al.*, 2023). Additionally, when clinicians become increasingly consumed, the ability for reflective practice is compromised, thus impacting the ability to synthesize new research and best practice required in pediatric patients' ethical decision-making. Inclusion of supportive institutional and educational measures is important to avoid burnout and optimize the ethical environment in which healthcare professionals work (Xames *et al.*, 2024).

14.4.7. Collaboration with Social Workers and Psychologists

Effective communication with psychologists and social workers is central to addressing the intricate ethical and legal issues encountered in pediatric intensive care units. The emotional and psychological issues encountered by families during critical illness make it essential that mental health professionals be part of the care team. Social workers are also part of the team, mediating between caregivers and providing required resources, with psychologists who can offer therapy interventions to deal with anxiety and stress experienced by patients and families. Moreover, the use of digital health technologies, as cited in most studies, can facilitate such interprofessional collaboration by easing communication and care systems within the healthcare environment (Israel Júnior Borges do Nascimento *et al.*, 2023). Further, pediatric palliative care guidelines emphasize the need for multidisciplinary management taking into account psychological, social, and ethical aspects in order to meet the diverse needs of patients and families to the best possible extent (Benini *et al.*, 2022). Fostering cooperation among these healthcare providers is essential in order to meet the complexities of care in the pediatric intensive care environment (Figure 14.17).

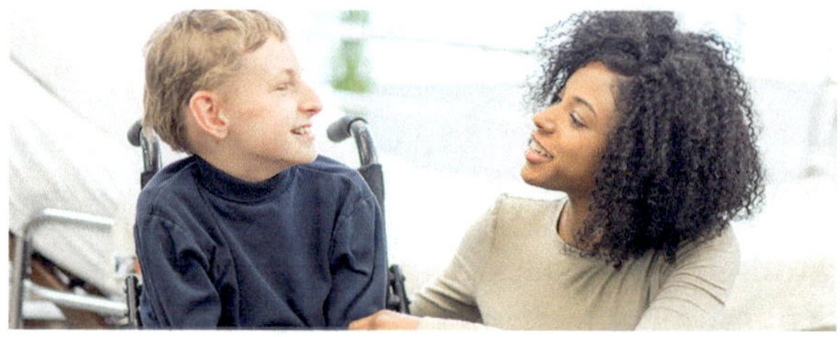

Figure 14.17. Effective collaboration with social workers and psychologists is critical in addressing the multifaceted ethical and legal issues encountered in pediatric intensive care settings.

Source: https://www.onlinemswprograms.com/wp-content/uploads/sites/55/2021/05/pediatric-social-work-in-2020-supporting-children-in-medical-settings_hero.jpg.

14.4.8. Reporting and Addressing Ethical Violations

Reporting and addressing ethical breaches are imperative in pediatric intensive care so that healthcare systems can maintain trustworthiness and integrity. HCPs must deal with highly intricate moral dilemmas wherein ethical breaches occur that undermine patient safety and well-being. Effective reporting mechanisms play a central role; they empower authority staff with the ability to report without the risk of reprisal and ensure openness. Additionally, medical professionals should be properly trained on the ethical concerns of their practices, given that most are not formally taught how to handle such dilemmas, and this can result in less than appropriate responses during critical moments (Harthi *et al.*, 2020). As social media continues to become more embedded in healthcare practice, it also amplifies the ethical duty of professionals when managing them online, demanding care in upholding professional standards (Farsi, 2021). Redress of such violations of ethics not only enhances the quality of care but also entrenches the fundamental tenets of medical ethics in children's settings.

14.4.9. The Importance of Professional Guidelines

In pediatric intensive care, professional standards must be set and observed in order to ensure ethical as well as legal adherence. Guidelines here are not just signs of clinical decision-making paradigms but are also tools of safeguarding vulnerable groups of children. They provide recommendations that are tailored to various circumstances, such as the complex ethics involved in dividing limited medical resources when they are needed, such as during the COVID-19 pandemic. Reports indicate that the development of new habits, backed by updated professional standards, has played a key role in transforming pediatric care, addressing not only immediate medical issues but also previewing long-term effects on the management of patients (Somekh *et al.*, 2020). Besides, transparent protocols ensure standardized care by medical providers and therefore minimize the risk of litigation in case of malpractice or ethical transgression in a healthcare setting (Chopra *et al.*, 2020). The importance of professional guidelines cannot be overstated in guaranteeing high standards of pediatric care.

Test Your Knowledge

1. What are the duties of nurses and allied health professionals when witnessing ethical or legal concerns?
2. How can clinicians ensure culturally sensitive care while upholding ethical standards?

SUMMARY

The multifaceted ethical and legal issues of pediatric intensive care require an approach that is multidimensional and emphasizes both the rights of the patient and the responsibilities of healthcare providers. The increased severity of conditions among children necessitates more in-depth ethical frameworks to guide healthcare decision-making, particularly in at-risk populations. The possibility of post-intensive care syndrome (PICS) highlights the imperative of holistic care interventions that embrace not only the immediate medical needs but also address long-term patient and family wellness (Inoue *et al.*, 2019). Furthermore, the growing pattern of drug use in pregnancy and its implications on neonatal care necessitate a collaborative and compassionate approach that interlinks maternal and child health outcomes within legal frameworks. By carefully moving through these challenges, healthcare professionals can maintain ethical guidelines while providing the optimum care to pediatric patients in critical environments.

In the contemplation of ethical and legal issues in pediatric intensive care, several key points come into consideration that underscore the practice intricacy in this sensitive area. Foremost among them is the general need for informed consent, which must be handled with utmost care in respect to the vulnerable population involved. Physicians are generally confronted with dilemmas when the child's optimal interests intersect with parental autonomy and need a subtle equilibrium of ethical demands and legal requirements. Also, introducing technologies like Artificial Intelligence (AI) into clinical decision-making poses issues about accountability and transparency in treatment. As noted in current literature, it is imperative to learn about the uses of AI in medical education so that professionals can better manage these ethical concerns (Gordon *et al.*, 2024). Furthermore, Explainable Artificial Intelligence (XAI) utilization in pediatrics can help give improved decision-making with confidence that stakeholders understand and believe in the approach employed (Zhang *et al.*, 2022). This intersection of innovation and care necessitates ongoing discussion in ethical and legal arenas.

KEY TERMS FROM THIS CHAPTER

- Informed consent
- Dilemma
- Treatment allocation
- Autonomy
- Medical knowledge
- Communication skills
- Beneficence
- Decision-making
- Advocacy
- Resource
- Ethics
- Discourse
- Moral distress
- Mindful
- Nonmaleficence
- Socioeconomic status

CRITICAL THINKING QUESTIONS

1. **Which of the following is required to obtain informed consent for a medical procedure in a pediatric patient?**
   a. Verbal consent from the child
   b. Consent from a school nurse
   c. Informed consent from a legal guardian
   d. Consent from any adult present
2. **In pediatric intensive care, the best interest standard refers to:**
   a. What the child wants based on their maturity
   b. Decisions based on financial cost
   c. Decisions made solely by medical staff
   d. Choosing interventions that most benefit the child's overall well-being
3. **Which of the following ethical principles is most relevant when withholding or withdrawing life-sustaining treatment?**
   a. Justice
   b. Non-maleficence
   c. Autonomy
   d. Fidelity
4. **Who is legally responsible for making medical decisions for an unconscious pediatric patient without advance directives?**
   a. Attending nurse
   b. Social worker
   c. The attending physician
   d. The child's parent or legal guardian
5. **Which of the following is a legal requirement in cases of suspected child abuse in PICU?**
   a. Inform the media
   b. Notify hospital administration only
   c. Immediate reporting to child protection services
   d. Wait for confirmation before taking action

Short Answer Questions

1. What are the four main ethical principles guiding decision-making in pediatric intensive care?
2. How does the principle of beneficence apply when initiating aggressive life-sustaining therapy in a critically ill child?
3. What are the legal requirements for obtaining informed consent in pediatric intensive care?
4. Under what conditions can a minor legally make their own medical decisions (e.g., mature minor doctrine, emancipation)?
5. What are common ethical dilemmas that arise in decisions about initiating or withdrawing life support?
6. How should clinicians proceed when there is disagreement between parents and the medical team about a child's treatment?

Answers to Critical Thinking Questions

1. (c); 2. (d); 3. (b); 4. (d); 5. (c)

REFERENCES

1. Ahmad, M. I. (2024). Legal challenges in cross-border IVF: The role of bioengineering and bioinformatics. *International Journal of Business Management and Economic Review*. https://www.semanticscholar.org/paper/fb5ac216288e868828ac0964c34ffa3f519c398c (accessed on 30th June 2025).
2. Al Harthi, M., Al Thobaity, A., Al Ahmari, W., & Almalki, M. (2020). Challenges for nurses in disaster management: A scoping review. *Risk Management and Healthcare Policy, 13*, 2627–2634. https://doi.org/10.2147/rmhp.s279513 (accessed on 30th June 2025).
3. Montalto Attard, S. (2014). Ethical principles in pediatric practice. https://core.ac.uk/download/46603075.pdf (accessed on 30th June 2025).
4. Baijens, L. W. J., Walshe, M., Aaltonen, L. M., Arens, C., Cordier, R., Cras, P., Crevier-Buchman, L., *et al.* (2020). European white paper: Oropharyngeal dysphagia in head and neck cancer. *European Archives of Oto-Rhino-Laryngology, 278*, 577–616. https://doi.org/10.1007/s00405-020-06507-5 (accessed on 30th June 2025).
5. Barnum, B., & Derrington, S. (2023). Conflict over death by neurologic criteria: Caution, consent, and nursing considerations. *The American Journal of Bioethics, 23*, 88–90. https://www.semanticscholar.org/paper/831e98196f9a1b969fad3a998c3f55966ccfc9f1 (accessed on 30th June 2025).
6. Benini, F., Papadatou, D., Bernadá, M., Craig, F., De Zen, L., Downing, J., Drake, R., *et al.* (2022). International standards for pediatric palliative care: From IMPaCCT to GO-PPaCS. *Journal of Pain and Symptom Management, 63*, e529–e543. https://doi.org/10.1016/j.jpainsymman.2021.12.031 (accessed on 30th June 2025).
7. Bhaskar, S., Bradley, S., Chattu, V. K., Adisesh, A., Nurtazina, A., Kyrykbayeva, S., Sakhamuri, S., *et al.* (2020). Telemedicine as the new outpatient clinic gone digital: Position paper from the Pandemic Health System REsilience PROGRAM (REPROGRAM) International Consortium (Part 2). *Frontiers in Public Health, 8*. https://doi.org/10.3389/fpubh.2020.00410 (accessed on 30th June 2025).
8. Borges do Nascimento, I. J., Abdulazeem, H. M., Vasanthan, L., Martínez, E. Z., Zucoloto, M. L., Østengaard, L., Azzopardi-Muscat, N., *et al.* (2023). Barriers and facilitators to utilizing digital health technologies by healthcare professionals. *npj Digital Medicine, 6*. https://doi.org/10.1038/s41746-023-00899-4 (accessed on 30th June 2025).
9. Borry, P., Howard, H., & Shabani, M. (2014). Is there a right time to know? The right not to know and genetic testing in children. https://core.ac.uk/download/237011214.pdf (accessed on 30th June 2025).
10. Chopra, V., Toner, E., Waldhorn, R., & Washer, L. (2020). How should U.S. hospitals prepare for Coronavirus Disease 2019 (COVID-19)? *Annals of Internal Medicine, 172*, 621–622. https://doi.org/10.7326/m20-0907 (accessed on 30th June 2025).
11. Coad, J., Colville, G., Curley, M. A. Q., Draper, M., *et al.* (2020). Study protocol for a multicenter longitudinal mixed methods study to explore the outcomes of children and families in the first year after pediatric intensive care: The OCEANIC study. https://core.ac.uk/download/323385694.pdf (accessed on 30th June 2025).

12. Coppola, F., Faggioni, L., Gabelloni, M., De Vietro, F., Mendola, V., Cattabriga, A., Cocozza, M. A., *et al.* (2021). Human, all too human? An all-around appraisal of the "artificial intelligence revolution" in medical imaging. *Frontiers in Psychology, 12*. https://doi.org/10.3389/fpsyg.2021.710982 (accessed on 30th June 2025).
13. Ćurković, M., Rubic, F., Jozepović, A., Novak, M., Filipović-Grčić, B., Meštrović, J., Lah Tomulić, K., *et al.* (2024). Navigating the shadows: Medical professionals' values and perspectives on end-of-life care within pediatric intensive care units in Croatia. *Frontiers in Pediatrics, 12*. https://www.semanticscholar.org/paper/98ec22bb196b7309118afec83c42b4445a8c9e70 (accessed on 30th June 2025).
14. Dubler, N. N. (1994). A "principled resolution": The fulcrum for bioethics mediation. https://core.ac.uk/download/62552950.pdf (accessed on 30th June 2025).
15. Duea, S. R., Zimmerman, E. B., Vaughn, L. M., Dias, S., & Harris, J. (2022). A guide to selecting participatory research methods based on project and partnership goals. *Journal of Participatory Research Methods, 3*. https://doi.org/10.35844/001c.32605 (accessed on 30th June 2025).
16. Eichinger, J., Elger, B. S., Koné, I., Filges, I., Shaw, D., Zimmermann, B., & McLennan, S. (2021). The full spectrum of ethical issues in pediatric genome-wide sequencing: A systematic qualitative review. *BMC Pediatrics, 21*. https://doi.org/10.1186/s12887-021-02830-w (accessed on 30th June 2025).
17. Eldridge, S., Chan, C., Campbell, M. J., Bond, C., Hopewell, S., Thabane, L., & Lancaster, G. (2016). CONSORT 2010 statement: Extension to randomized pilot and feasibility trials. *BMJ*. https://doi.org/10.1136/bmj.i5239 (accessed on 30th June 2025).
18. Emanuel, E., & Skorton, D. J. (2021). Mandating COVID-19 vaccination for health care workers. *Annals of Internal Medicine, 174*, 1308–1310. https://doi.org/10.7326/m21-3150 (accessed on 30th June 2025).
19. Farsi, D. (2021). Social media and health care, Part I: Literature review of social media use by health care providers. *Journal of Medical Internet Research, 23*, e23205–e23205. https://doi.org/10.2196/23205 (accessed on 30th June 2025).
20. Goobie, S. M. (2022). Patient blood management is a new standard of care to optimize blood health. *Anesthesia & Analgesia, 135*, 443–446. https://doi.org/10.1213/ane.0000000000006168 (accessed on 30th June 2025).
21. Gordon, M., Daniel, M., Ajiboye, A., Uraiby, H., Xu, N. Y., Bartlett, R., Hanson, J. L., *et al.* (2024). A scoping review of artificial intelligence in medical education: BEME Guide No. 84. *Medical Teacher, 46*, 446–470. https://doi.org/10.1080/0142159x.2024.2314198 (accessed on 30th June 2025).
22. Harris, D. C. H., Davies, S., Finkelstein, F. O., Jha, V., Donner, J. A., Abraham, G., Bello, A. K., *et al.* (2019). Increasing access to integrated ESKD care as part of universal health coverage. *Kidney International, 95*, S1–S33. https://doi.org/10.1016/j.kint.2018.12.005 (accessed on 30th June 2025).
23. Hendrix, K. S., Sturm, L. A., Zimet, G. D., & Meslin, E. M. (2015). Ethics and childhood vaccination policy in the United States. *American Journal of Public Health, 106*, 273–278. https://doi.org/10.2105/ajph.2015.302952 (accessed on 30th June 2025).

24. Hitchcock, N., Nunes, D. D. G., Shiach, J., Hodel, K. V. S., Barbosa, J. D. V., Rodrigues, L. A. P., Coler, B., *et al.* (2023). Current clinical landscape and global potential of bacteriophage therapy. *Viruses, 15*, 1020–1020. https://doi.org/10.3390/v15041020 (accessed on 30th June 2025).

25. Inoue, S., Hatakeyama, J., Kondo, Y., Hifumi, T., Sakuramoto, H., Kawasaki, T., Taito, S., *et al.* (2019). Post-intensive care syndrome: Its pathophysiology, prevention, and future directions. *Acute Medicine & Surgery, 6*, 233–246. https://doi.org/10.1002/ams2.415 (accessed on 30th June 2025).

26. Karalis, V. (2024). The integration of artificial intelligence into clinical practice. *Applied Biosciences, 3*, 14–44. https://doi.org/10.3390/applbiosci3010002 (accessed on 30th June 2025).

27. Kirsch, R., Balit, C. R., Carnevale, F. A., Latour, J. M., & Larcher, V. (2018). Ethical, cultural, social, and individual considerations prior to transition to limitation or withdrawal of life-sustaining therapies. *Pediatric Critical Care Medicine, 19*, S10–S18. https://doi.org/10.1097/pcc.0000000000001488 (accessed on 30th June 2025).

28. Maier-Hein, L., Eisenmann, M., Sarıkaya, D., März, K., Collins, T., Malpani, A., Fallert, J., *et al.* (2021). Surgical data science–from concepts toward clinical translation. *Medical Image Analysis, 76*, 102306–102306. https://doi.org/10.1016/j.media.2021.102306 (accessed on 30th June 2025).

29. Mills, M., & Cortezzo, D. E. (2020). Moral distress in the neonatal intensive care unit: What is it, why it happens, and how we can address it. *Frontiers in Pediatrics, 8*. https://doi.org/10.3389/fped.2020.00581 (accessed on 30th June 2025).

30. Mirlashari, J., Brown, H. E., Fomani, F. K., de Salaberry, J., Khanmohamad Zadeh, T., & Khoshkhou, F. (2019). The challenges of implementing family-centered care in NICU from the perspectives of physicians and nurses. *Journal of Pediatric Nursing, 50*, e91–e98. https://doi.org/10.1016/j.pedn.2019.06.013 (accessed on 30th June 2025).

31. Myatra, S., Salins, N., Iyer, S., Macaden, S., Divatia, J., Muckaden, M., Kulkarni, P., *et al.* (2014). End-of-life care policy: An integrated care plan for the dying. *Indian Journal of Critical Care Medicine: Peer-reviewed, Official Publication of Indian Society of Critical Care Medicine, 18*, 615–635. https://www.semanticscholar.org/paper/a5994de68348e2d342970499d3409e9cd0846b15 (accessed on 30th June 2025).

32. Novilla, M. L. B., Goates, M. C., Leffler, T., Novilla, N. K. B., Wu, C. Y., Dall, A., & Hansen, C. (2023). Integrating social care into healthcare: A review on applying the social determinants of health in clinical settings. *International Journal of Environmental Research and Public Health, 20*, 6873–6873. https://doi.org/10.3390/ijerph20196873 (accessed on 30th June 2025).

33. O'Connell, C. B. (2014). Gender and the experience of moral distress in critical care nurses. *Nursing Ethics, 22*, 32–42. https://doi.org/10.1177/0969733013513216 (accessed on 30th June 2025).

34. Onyejesi, C. D., Del Castillo Miranda, J. C., Abdelbar, S. M. M. M., Aziz, M. M., Abady, E., Omran, J. A., Zehra, A., *et al.* (2025). Challenges and innovations in diagnosing nonphysical child abuse in pediatric emergency departments. *Pediatric Emergency Medicine Journal*. https://www.semanticscholar.org/paper/918b2e10003782934d1336176955f7e352b4b302 (accessed on 30th June 2025).

35. Pant, S. (2021). Ethical issues around death and withdrawal of life support in neonatal intensive care. *Indian Journal of Pediatrics, 89*, 274–278. https://www.semanticscholar.org/paper/33bb7e31ac51d54b83f6b87301ab6458f49272a4 (accessed on 30th June 2025).

36. Ranjith, S., & Dave, A. (2023). Filling the gaps in oncofertility care by addressing challenges faced by patients and providers. *Cureus, 15*. https://www.semanticscholar.org/paper/264e6b16016c9437019fb571c55bdcbd31fa3996 (accessed on 30th June 2025).

37. Sarkar, S., Grover, S., & Chadda, R. K. (2022). Psychiatric assessment of persons for solid-organ transplant. *Indian Journal of Psychiatry, 64*, S308–S318. https://doi.org/10.4103/indianjpsychiatry.indianjpsychiatry_1015_21 (accessed on 30th June 2025).

38. Schmidt, M., Schmidt, S. A. J., Adelborg, K., Sundbøll, J., Laugesen, K., Ehrenstein, V., & Sørensen, H. T. (2019). The Danish health care system and epidemiological research: From health care contacts to database records. *Clinical Epidemiology, 11*, 563–591. https://doi.org/10.2147/clep.s179083 (accessed on 30th June 2025).

39. Schouten, E., Beyer, M. F., Flemmer, W., Katja, K., Kuehlmeyer, K., Iacovidou, N., Chatziioannidis, I., *et al.* (2021). 4th Congress of Joint European Neonatal Societies: Nursing and healthcare professionals. *Pediatric Research, 90*, 24–26. https://www.semanticscholar.org/paper/6598bfe453c6b896c570e9b57a17bc5e820325ec (accessed on 30th June 2025).

40. Schwartz, D., Barrocas, A., Annetta, M., Stratton, K., McGinnis, C., Hardy, G., Wong, T., *et al.* (2021). Ethical aspects of artificially administered nutrition and hydration: An ASPEN position paper. *Nutrition in Clinical Practice: Official Publication of the American Society for Parenteral and Enteral Nutrition*. https://www.semanticscholar.org/paper/3dc8ff2e0f486f5c935af1ab8d15629db29ec39f (accessed on 30th June 2025).

41. Scott, C. T. (2014). The case for stem cell counselors. *Stem Cell Reports, 4*, 1–6. https://doi.org/10.1016/j.stemcr.2014.10.016 (accessed on 30th June 2025).

42. Sharma, M., Savage, C., Nair, M., Larsson, I., Svedberg, P., & Nygren, J. M. (2022). Artificial intelligence applications in health care practice: Scoping review. *Journal of Medical Internet Research, 24*, e40238–e40238. https://doi.org/10.2196/40238 (accessed on 30th June 2025).

43. Shemie, S. D., Robertson, A., Beitel, J., Chandler, J. A., Ferre, E., Evans, J., Haun, M., *et al.* (2017). End-of-life conversations with families of potential donors. *Transplantation, 101*, S17–S26. https://doi.org/10.1097/tp.0000000000001696 (accessed on 30th June 2025).

44. Shokri, T., & Lighthall, J. G. (2020). Telemedicine in the era of the COVID-19 pandemic: Implications in facial plastic surgery. *Facial Plastic Surgery & Aesthetic Medicine, 22*, 155–156. https://doi.org/10.1089/fpsam.2020.0163 (accessed on 30th June 2025).

45. Slawomirski, L., Auraaen, A., & Klazinga, N. S. (2017). The economics of patient safety. *OECD Health Working Papers*. https://doi.org/10.1787/5a9858cd-en (accessed on 30th June 2025).

46. Somekh, I., Somech, R., Pettoello-Mantovani, M., & Somekh, E. (2020). Changes in routine pediatric practice in light of Coronavirus 2019 (COVID-19). *The Journal of Pediatrics, 224*, 190–193. https://doi.org/10.1016/j.jpeds.2020.05.053 (accessed on 30th June 2025).

47. Szilagyi, M. (2012). The pediatric role in the care of children in foster and kinship care. *Pediatrics in Review, 33*, 496–508. https://doi.org/10.1542/pir.33-11-496 (accessed on 30th June 2025).

48. Tanaka Gutiez, M., Efstathiou, N., Innes, R., & Metaxa, V. (2023). End-of-life care in the intensive care unit. *Anesthesia, 78*. https://www.semanticscholar.org/paper/c938dc8ecd1202ddee599039582ad3206cec2190 (accessed on 30th June 2025).

49. Versporten, A., Zarb, P., Caniaux, I., Gros, M. F., Drapier, N., Miller, M. L., Jarlier, V., *et al.* (2018). Antimicrobial consumption and resistance in adult hospital inpatients in 53 countries: Results of an internet-based global point prevalence survey. *The Lancet Global Health, 6*, e619–e629. https://doi.org/10.1016/s2214-109x(18)30186-4 (accessed on 30th June 2025).

50. Wang, X., Sanders, H. M., Liu, Y., Seang, K., Tran, B. X., Atanasov, A. G., Qiu, Y., *et al.* (2023). ChatGPT: Promise and challenges for deployment in low- and middle-income countries. *The Lancet Regional Health – Western Pacific, 41*, 100905–100905. https://doi.org/10.1016/j.lanwpc.2023.100905 (accessed on 30th June 2025).

51. Wanjihia, V. W., Muriithi, B. K., & Kaneko, S. (2024). A scoping overview of global legislation on data privacy and protection: What are the implications for data use, transfer, and sharing in e-health research? *Austin Public Health*. https://www.semanticscholar.org/paper/83294f08dc1d3d01b50beaa66402938dd956cf4f (accessed on 30th June 2025).

52. Weise, K. L., Okun, A. L., Carter, B. S., Christian, C. W., Katz, A. L., Laventhal, N., Macauley, R., *et al.* (2017). Guidance on forgoing life-sustaining medical treatment. *Pediatrics, 140*. https://doi.org/10.1542/peds.2017-1905 (accessed on 30th June 2025).

53. Wiener, L., Weaver, M. S., Sansom-Daly, U. M., & Bell, C. J. (2015). Threading the cloak: Palliative care education for care providers of adolescents and young adults with cancer. *Clinical Oncology in Adolescents and Young Adults*. https://doi.org/10.2147/coaya.s49176 (accessed on 30th June 2025).

54. Wu, Q., Wang, Y., Lu, L., Chen, Y., Long, H., & Wang, J. (2022). Virtual simulation in undergraduate medical education: A scoping review of recent practice. *Frontiers in Medicine, 9*. https://doi.org/10.3389/fmed.2022.855403 (accessed on 30th June 2025).

55. Xames, M. D., & Topcu, T. G. (2024). A systematic literature review of digital twin research for healthcare systems: Research trends, gaps, and realization challenges. *IEEE Access, 12*, 4099–4126. https://doi.org/10.1109/access.2023.3349379 (accessed on 30th June 2025).

56. Zhang, Z., Al Hamadi, H., Damiani, E., Yeun, C. Y., & Taher, F. (2022). Explainable artificial intelligence applications in cyber security: State-of-the-art in research. *IEEE Access, 10*, 93104–93139. https://doi.org/10.1109/access.2022.3204051 (accessed on 30th June 2025).

QUALITY IMPROVEMENT AND PATIENT SAFETY

15

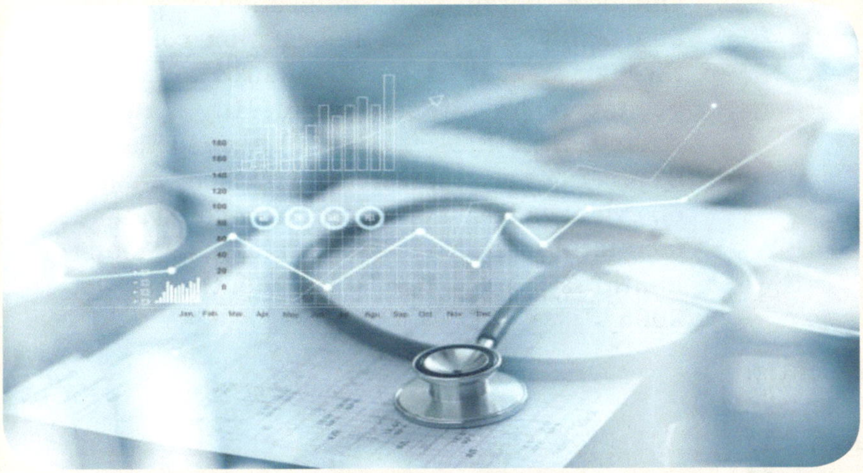

Introduction

The pediatric intensive care unit (PICU) is a high-risk center for offering specialized care to the most fragile patients. It is an environment where there are high stakes and the room for error is very narrow, and this necessitates an uncompromising pursuit of quality improvement and patient safety. The complexity in offering pediatric care, coupled with the rapid pace of change in medical technology, significantly raises the risk of adverse clinical outcomes. As indicated by various studies, it is crucial to tackle complicated matters of care delivery, such as healthcare provider burnout and optimizing the usage of electronic health records (EHRs), to enhance PICU safety measures (Downing *et al.*, 2018). In addition, the establishment of detailed clinical guidelines has become key in harmonizing the procedure of care to ultimately lower risks and improve patient outcomes (Paul *et al.*, 2017). Pursuit of excellence in pediatric intensive care implies that there has to be a collaborative effort to fortify efforts towards quality improvement and robust patient safety infrastructures.

LEARNING OBJECTIVES

After studying this chapter, you will be able to:

1. Understand Key Concepts in Quality Improvement.
2. Explain Patient Safety Strategies in Pediatric Intensive Care.
3. Describe The Impact of Quality Improvement on Patient Outcomes.
4. Focus on Challenges and Barriers to Quality Improvement and Patient Safety.

15.1. Key Concepts in Quality Improvement

Learning Outcome

1. Definition and Principles of Quality Improvement.
2. The Role of Evidence-Based Practice.
3. Quality Improvement Models.
4. Metrics for Measuring Quality in PICUs.
5. Stakeholder Involvement in Quality Improvement.
6. Continuous Quality Improvement (CQI) Framework.
7. Challenges in Implementing Quality Improvement.
8. Case Studies of Successful Quality Improvement Initiatives.
9. Future Directions in Quality Improvement.

Quality improvement (QI) is an essential pediatric intensive care model that entails periodic efforts to enhance patient safety and health outcomes. Key tenets of QI include the identification of particular performance measures, utilization of evidence-based interventions, and regular measurement of outcomes to assess improvement. For example, applying standardized definitions, such as the Berlin definition of acute respiratory distress syndrome, allows clinicians to classify and treat patients more appropriately, which may lead to improved morbidity and mortality rates (Fan *et al.*, 2018). Additionally, the use of multipotential stem cells in therapy puts forward the innovative quality of QI, as the cells have shown promise not only for therapeutic use but also to increase the understanding of children's diseases (Mark *et al.*, 2019). Thus, the implementation of QI in pediatric intensive care is needed to foster a safety culture and ensure that high-quality, patient-centered care is delivered.

15.1.1. Definition and Principles of Quality Improvement

Quality Improvement (QI) in pediatric intensive care is premised on systematic care service development to raise patient outcomes closer to higher and safer levels. The major principles of QI include continuous monitoring and improvement of care processes, with data analysis and collective teamwork between care providers. One of the established methods employed herein is the utilization of patient and family experience information collected through structured questionnaires to enable healthcare practitioners to identify areas of improvement (Hays *et al.*, 2020). Also, successful QI programs are characterized by their reliance on evidence-based practice, safety culture, and facilitating effective communication among multidisciplinary teams (Blumenthal *et al.*, 2006).

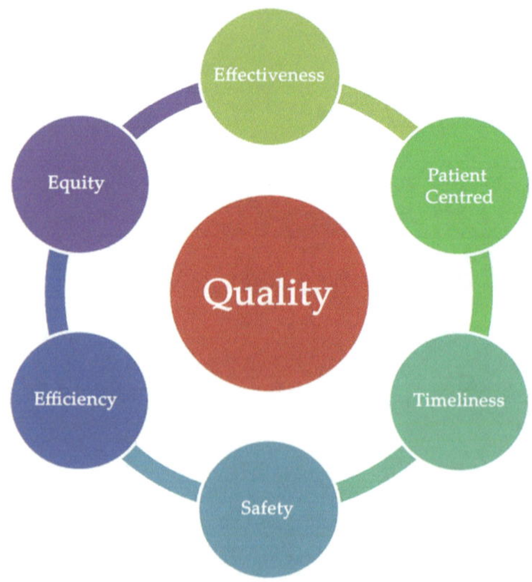

Figure 15.1. Quality Improvement (QI) in pediatric intensive care is rooted in the systematic enhancement of healthcare services, aimed at elevating patient outcomes and ensuring safety.

Source: https://ep.bmj.com/content/edpract/98/5/175/F1.large.jpg.

By combining these principles, healthcare organizations will be able to build a robust

QI infrastructure that not only maximizes the quality of care but also meets the unique needs of pediatric patients and their families, thereby maximizing overall safety in intensive care units (Figure 15.1).

15.1.2. The Role of Evidence-Based Practice

Evidence-based practice (EBP) provides a basis for quality improvement and patient safety within pediatric intensive care. By employing the best current research, along with clinical experience and patient preference, health professionals can implement interventions that optimize care quality. For instance, a systematic review concluded that the implementation of evidence-based practices was the principle to maximizing pediatric patient and family experiences with a high effect on care outcomes and operational efficiency (Hays *et al.*, 2020). Furthermore, interventions like the Skin Champion program reflect how EBP directly reduces hospital-acquired pressure injuries in pediatric patients, with a resounding 85% decrease in severe harm (Gordon *et al.*, 2018). These are but a few of the many examples that not only illustrate the importance of implementing EBP in clinical practice, but also underscore the importance of ongoing education and dedication by health professionals, thus inculcating a culture of safety and continuous improvement in pediatric practice environments.

15.1.3. Quality Improvement Models (e.g., PDSA, Six Sigma)

In pediatric intensive care, the implementation of Quality Improvement (QI) models such as PDSA (Plan-Do-Study-Act) and Six Sigma is instrumental in enhancing patient safety and quality of care. They provide rigorous methods for problem identification, testing interventions experimentally, and outcome evaluation, hence linking evidence-based practice with clinical practice on a daily basis within hospital environments. For instance, PDSA gives priority to iterative testing, which allows healthcare teams to incrementally improve based on real-time feedback, while Six Sigma aims to reduce variation and error in the provision of care through fact-based decision-making. Both models foster a culture of continuous improvement as well as anticipatory problem-solving, which are the pillars of effective healthcare provision. Also, the integration of broader frameworks for understanding and implementing QI can assist in delineating initiatives according to defined patient populations and clinical environments, as seen through research focused on enhancing healthcare-associated infection prevention (Kavita *et al.*, 2023), and prioritizes safety among high-risk specialties like anesthesiology (Abdalla *et al.*, 2022) (Figure 15.2).

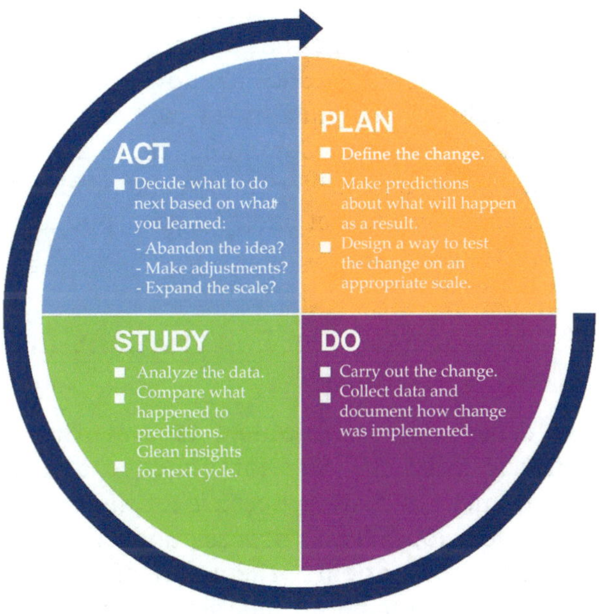

Figure 15.2. PDSA (Plan-Do-Study-Act).

Source: https://i0.wp.com/nycdoeishandbook.org/wp-content/uploads/2021/07/nycdoe_improvement_science_handbook_2018_online_page_083-e1626365630371.jpg?ssl=1.

15.1.4. Metrics for Measuring Quality in PICUs

In pediatric intensive care units (PICUs), measurement of quality plays a central role in ensuring patient safety as well as improving the quality of care. Metrics such as unplanned extubation (UE) rate are tangible measures of the quality of care, reflecting both procedural performance as well as healthcare worker communication patterns. Recent studies indicate that strict adherence to protocolized procedures is able to reduce UE rates significantly, illustrated by the quality improvement program that achieved a 42.7% reduction in the occurrence of events following targeted interventions and staff training (Thabet *et al.*, 2025). Clinical handover process challenges, both at the nurse level and the organizational level, also directly affect continuity of care in PICUs. An in-depth review of these issues is imperative, as it outlines those areas that are required to be optimized that can enhance handover protocols and thereby, overall quality of care delivered (Hamad *et al.*, 2025). Combined, these actions feed into ongoing quality improvement efforts and foster a culture of safety within pediatric intensive care settings.

15.1.5. Stakeholder Engagement in Quality Improvement

Involvement of stakeholders is essential in pediatric intensive care for effective quality improvement initiatives, because it brings value to the decision-making process and enhances the safety of patients. Inclusion of various stakeholders, including healthcare providers, parents, and community organizations, gives a panoramic view to identify as well as address safety issues. For instance, the incorporation of parent findings will elucidate social determinants of health that directly impact pediatric care, building a comprehensive patient need and environment in which children develop and mature. As highlighted in recent literature, the economic and healthcare costs of patient harm in health institutions are high; hence, a culture of partnership-based safety is imperative in minimizing preventable occurrences (Slawomirski *et al.*, 2017). Besides, learning programs, such as medical student training on the issue of advocacy and health inequities, can equip future healthcare providers to appreciate stakeholders' contributions in practice (Melanie *et al.*, 2019). This model of collaboration not only leads to better patient outcomes but also to an organizational commitment to continuous improvement (Figure 15.3).

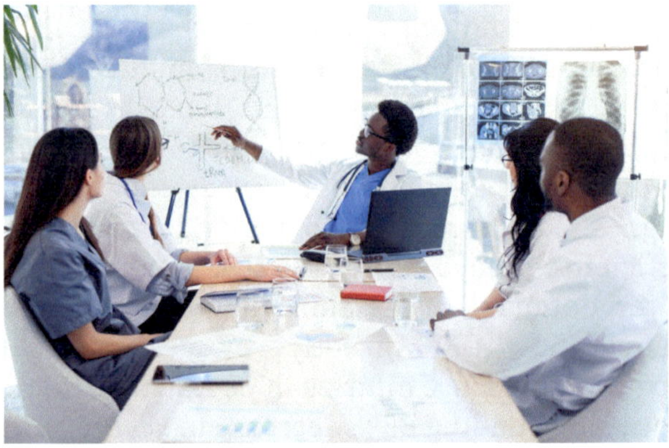

Figure 15.3. Engaging diverse stakeholders, including healthcare providers, parents, and community organizations, allows for a multifaceted approach to identify and address safety challenges.

Source: https://aihcp.net/main/wp-content/uploads/2024/08/Depositphotos_285797620_S.jpg.

15.1.6. Continuous Quality Improvement (CQI) Framework

In pediatric intensive care, the Continuous Quality Improvement (CQI) Framework provides a basis for enhancing patient safety and outcomes of care. The framework is central in fostering a systematic process of health care improvement using an endless loop of continuous planning, implementation, assessment, and adjustment.

Through the application of multidisciplinary practice, CQI programs focus on specific areas of weakness, thereby establishing a culture of responsiveness and accountability in health workers. Particularly, CQI efficiency can be seen when it is applied against operational problems, where techniques such as lean manufacturing are recommended to render processes lean and free from issues like overcrowding and lengthy wait times, particularly in emergency environments (Ortíz-Barrios *et al.*, 2020). Besides, the CQI model supports the community systems of care principles that ensure the utilization of a totalistic strategy considering biopsychosocial factors required by patients, particularly those with behavioral health problems (Larson *et al.*, 2022). By incorporating these practices into pediatric care centers, health care organizations can significantly increase the quality of care delivered to vulnerable groups.

15.1.7. Challenges in Implementing Quality Improvement

The implementation of quality improvement projects in pediatric intensive care units has numerous challenges that can undermine the effectiveness of patient safety programs. Such challenges include resistance from the staff and the complexity of implementing new systems in existing ones. For instance, the development of a universal clinical information system can potentially support continuity and coordination of care in chronic diseases, but is often hindered by inadequate training and staff acceptance (McCarthy *et al.*, 2008). Further, low-income patients' unique needs bring forth innovative care models that increase high-quality service delivery in multiple settings , for example, hospitals and community clinics (Chase, 2010). These barriers highlight the role of strategic planning and robust support structures because overcoming these barriers is to guarantee that quality improvement efforts lead to genuine improvements in patient safety outcomes in pediatric intensive care environments (Figure 15.4).

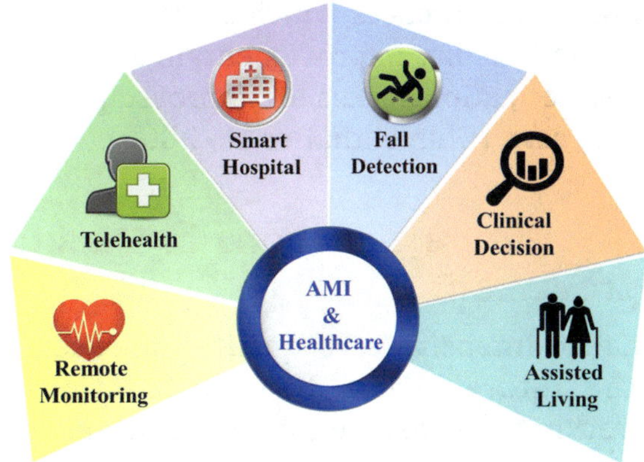

Figure 15.4. The implementation of quality improvement initiatives in pediatric intensive care settings presents a myriad of challenges that can undermine the efficacy of patient safety efforts.

Source: https://www.mdpi.com/electronics/electronics-13-02309/article_deploy/html/images/electronics-13-02309-g006-550.jpg.

15.1.8. Case Studies of Successful Quality Improvement Initiatives

Examining case studies of high-quality improvement initiatives offers significant learning on enhancing patient safety in pediatric intensive care. Such programs typically emerge from collaborative processes in healthcare institutions with innovative practices that reduce major medical mistakes. For instance, various clinical teams have established standardized protocols and checklists, which have proved effective in streamlining procedures and lessening the risks associated with complex pediatric treatment, thereby encouraging a culture of safety. Further, Health Information Technology (HIT) integration has drawn much attention, driving innovation in the management of data and communication between healthcare providers, essential factors in addressing children's health care issues uniquely presented (Simpson *et al.*, 2008). By reviewing the outcomes and learning achieved from such initiatives, medical professionals are able to identify best practices which drive sustainable safety and quality improvement, in accordance with wider national goals for improved pediatric patient care (Blumenthal *et al.*, 2006).

15.1.9. Future Directions in Quality Improvement

Pediatric intensive care quality improvement in the future should be directed towards addressing multistakeholder solutions that present themselves to families experiencing transitions of care complexities. Evidently, parents experience massive emotional trauma when being transitioned from pediatric intensive care units to inpatient wards, thus necessitating tailored support structures to cushion this trauma (Evans *et al.*, 2019). To implement these strategies efficiently, health professionals are able to utilize emerging communication tools, such as e-newsletters, to summarize applicable literature and resources for multidisciplinary teams, thereby enhancing care coordination and understanding of best practices in children's settings (Behere *et al.*, 2017). Additionally, focusing on the coordination of care delivery models in different clinical environments is necessary in order to provide a seamless experience for families. By integrating these components into future quality improvement initiatives, health care providers can significantly improve patient safety and satisfaction within pediatric intensive care units.

Test Your Knowledge

1. What is the role of clinical audits in quality improvement efforts?
2. How are QI projects in the PICU identified, designed, and implemented?

15.2. Patient Safety Strategies in Pediatric Intensive Care

Learning Outcome

1. Identification of Common Safety Risks in PICUs.
2. Implementation of Safety Protocols and Guidelines.
3. Role of Technology in Enhancing Patient Safety.
4. Training and Education for Healthcare Providers.
5. Family Involvement in Safety Practices.
6. Reporting and Learning from Adverse Events.
7. The Importance of a Safety Culture in Healthcare.
8. Strategies for Preventing Medication Errors.
9. Evaluation of Patient Safety Outcomes.

In pediatric intensive care units (PICUs), effective measures of patient safety are vital due to the population being treated. Measures of quality improvement target decreasing the occurrence of events that are related to equipment deficits, which compromise patient safety. A recent study underscored the importance of a multidisciplinary approach to devising an efficient supply chain management (SCM) process map, indicating that adherence to key procedural steps for dealing with missing supplies enormously enhanced operational safety in the PICU (Rice *et al.*, 2022). Additionally, employing rigorous approaches like Failure Modes and Effects Analysis (FMEA) can identify and avert risks associated with interventions such as Early Mobility programs, thus ensuring safer patient outcomes (Gupta *et al.*, 2020). Together, these strategies underscore the requirement for continuous observation and safety procedure adjustment to address the complexities of critical care so that the pediatric patient is provided with the safest environment possible during their most susceptible period.

15.2.1. Identification of Common Safety Risks in PICUs

For better patient safety in Pediatric Intensive Care Units (PICUs), it is crucial to determine and rectify standardized common hazards for safety, which are a threat to the health of vulnerable children. The evidence indicates that healthcare-associated infections (HAIs) are among the leading severe threats, particularly with the complexities involved in the treatment of neonates and infants, such as an imbalanced susceptibility to such risks (Prestel *et al.*, 2023).

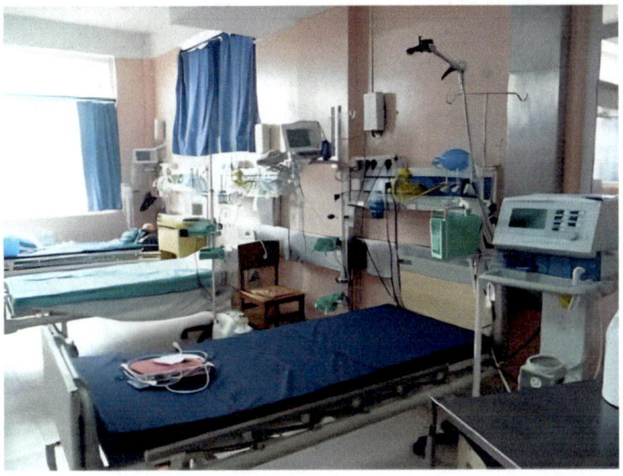

Figure 15.5. In order to enhance patient safety in Pediatric Intensive Care Units (PICUs), it is imperative to systematically identify and address common safety risks that can jeopardize the well-being of vulnerable pediatric patients.

Source: https://pub.mdpi-res.com/children/children-12-00726/article_deploy/html/images/children-12-00726-g003.png?1748684821.

Moreover, the prevalence of severe sepsis within PICUs, as has been observed in recent literature, necessitates a pressing need for increased detection and treatment of this illness, which has a direct impact on mortality rates within admitted children (Elghadban, 2024). By embracing evidence-based infection prevention strategies and safety culture, ensuring early identification and intervention, PICUs can mitigate these risks. Better quality improvement practices in these units are needed not only to minimize complications but also to enhance the overall healthcare experience of patients and their families (Figure 15.5).

15.2.2. Implementation of Safety Protocols and Guidelines

The implementation of safety protocols and processes within institutions is a core factor for fostering quality enhancement and patient security in pediatric intensive care units. Through the use of evidence-based interventions, hospital teams are able to systematically reduce the rate of complications. This goal is achieved through measures that have significantly lowered complication rates among patients who undergo tracheostomy through sharply targeted interventions, such as multidisciplinary rounds and ongoing education for nurses (Anderson *et al.*, 2019). Additionally, patient and family experience data are essential to the identification of areas in which improvement must come, as with tools like the Child Hospital Consumer Assessment of Healthcare Providers and Systems Survey, through which hospital performance can be compared and necessary change implemented (Hays *et al.*, 2020). In the long term, developing rigorous safety protocols not only enhances clinical performance but also sustains a culture of continuous quality improvement, ultimately resulting in safer and more effective care for children.

15.2.3. The Role of Technology in Enhancing Patient Safety

Pediatric intensive care utilizing technology greatly enhances patient safety, primarily by generating standardized practice and improved communication among healthcare professionals. For instance, the implementation of electronic health records (EHR) allows for the monitoring of real-time patient data, reducing the incidence of medical errors. This is emphasized in a study that offers a pre-operative check-off exclusively designed for registered nurses to minimize operating room delays and enhance overall patient outcomes by streamlining processes (Vega *et al.*, 2024). Furthermore, technology facilitates specialized palliative care to be administered in complex cases, addressing the individualized requirements of infants with life-limiting illnesses. With the utilization of sophisticated data analysis and communication tools, healthcare providers can more efficiently coordinate care, ultimately leading to improved patient safety and satisfaction (Iten *et al.*, 2024). Such advancements demonstrate the key role that technological innovation plays in enhancing care provision in pediatric intensive care (Figure 15.6).

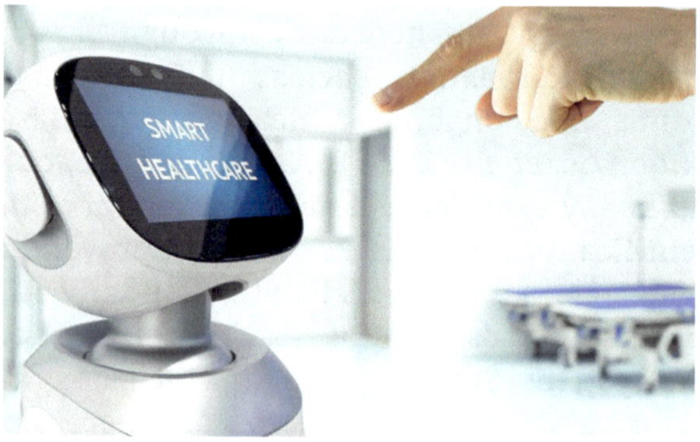

Figure 15.6. The integration of technology in pediatric intensive care significantly enhances patient safety, primarily through the establishment of standardized protocols and improved communication among healthcare professionals.

Source: https://www.obaid.info/wp-content/uploads/2023/07/smart-healthcare-1080x675.jpg.

15.2.4. Training and Education for Healthcare Providers

Appropriate education and training of healthcare providers are essential in enhancing quality and patient safety, particularly in high-complexity environments such as pediatric intensive care units (PICUs). A multidisciplinary approach ensures that every healthcare provider, including nurses, physicians, and pharmacists, receives proper training to handle complex cases proficiently. The example of the implementation of clinical pathways for CAR-T cell therapy illustrates the need for comprehensive training programs. These initiatives involved intensive education in multidisciplinary teams to clarify patient management procedures, ultimately improving safety and the quality of care (Camargo *et al.*, 2023). Similarly, the rapid development of electronic order sets for adult COVID-19 treatment within a pediatric setting illustrates how focused educational interventions can mitigate prospective safety risks while integrating into dominant practices (Gray *et al.*, 2022). These figures underscore that continuous, systematic education sustains the capability of health workers to offer quality, secure patient care in children's high-risk settings.

15.2.5. Involvement of Families with Safety Processes

In pediatric intensive care units, family involvement is crucial in enhancing safety processes and outcomes for the patient. Family participation in the provision of information regarding the child's status can significantly reduce readmission, which is accompanied by the family's understanding of care instructions. The complexity of intensive care cases poses a challenge to achieving such an intervention. Compared to more stable patients in the wards, families of critically ill children may face challenges in receiving continuous education since they stay in hospitals for shorter durations and without continuity in care providers. Some of the possible methods of overcoming the challenges include developing individualized educational tools that are readily available to families and preparing them well so they can monitor their child's needs upon discharge (Mohamed *et al.*, 2025). Besides, integrating a multidisciplinary team approach and the use of technology to provide effective communication can help families adhere to safety protocols, thus improving pediatric intensive care unit quality (Marron *et al.*, 2025) (Figure 15.7).

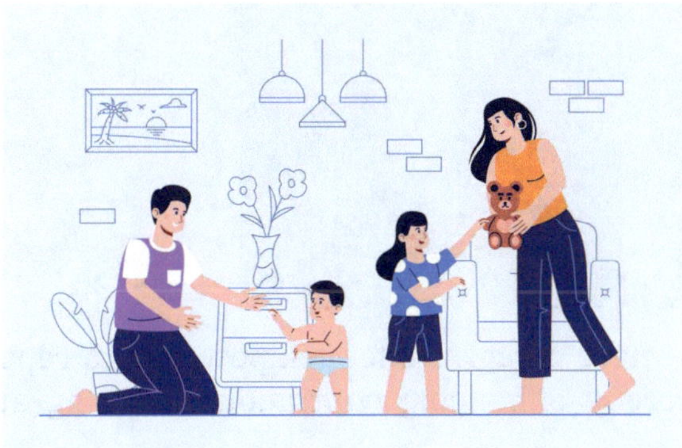

Figure 15.7. Engaging families in providing education about their child's condition can significantly reduce the likelihood of readmissions, which is often tied to the family's understanding of care directives.

Source: https://www.eurokidsindia.com/blog/wp-content/uploads/2024/03/family-importance-in-child-development.jpg.

15.2.6. Reporting and Learning from Adverse Events

In the pursuit of enhancing patient safety within pediatric intensive care units, constructive reporting and learning from adverse events stand as critical components. An effective reporting system not only identifies errors but also develops a culture that is open, where errors are realized that otherwise remain concealed. This cycle of continuous feedback forces healthcare professionals to engage in reflective practices, thereby leading to better clinical outcomes. Also, guidelines set by organizations like the American College of Cardiology (ACC) and American Heart Association (AHA) demonstrate how interventions using evidence-based methods can direct patient safety programs in every field of medicine, even pediatrics (Stout *et al.*, 2018). By implementing standard learning experiences based on such adverse incidents, healthcare providers can establish effective recurrence prevention and best practice promotion mechanisms, thereby enhancing the overall quality of children's care (Paul *et al.*, 2017).

15.2.7. The Importance of a Safety Culture in Healthcare

Ensuring a robust safety culture in healthcare settings, particularly among pediatric intensive care units, is important to ensure high-quality patient outcomes. A safety culture ensures an environment wherein caregivers are convinced that they can report near misses and errors without the risk of recrimination, thereby enhancing continuous learning and improvement. Evidence indicates that incorporating patient and family experience information into quality improvement measures is capable of identifying areas of high priority to be improved. For instance, using experience survey data is now best practice for initiating and evaluating quality improvement initiatives (Hays *et al.*, 2020). Moreover, evidence-based practices and collaborative learning are the pillars of effective safety strategies, allowing clinical teams to share observations and develop new solutions (Blumenthal *et al.*, 2006). Last but not least, prioritizing a culture of safety not only enhances patient safety but also promotes a culture of accountability and trust among pediatric intensive care healthcare practitioners (Figure 15.8).

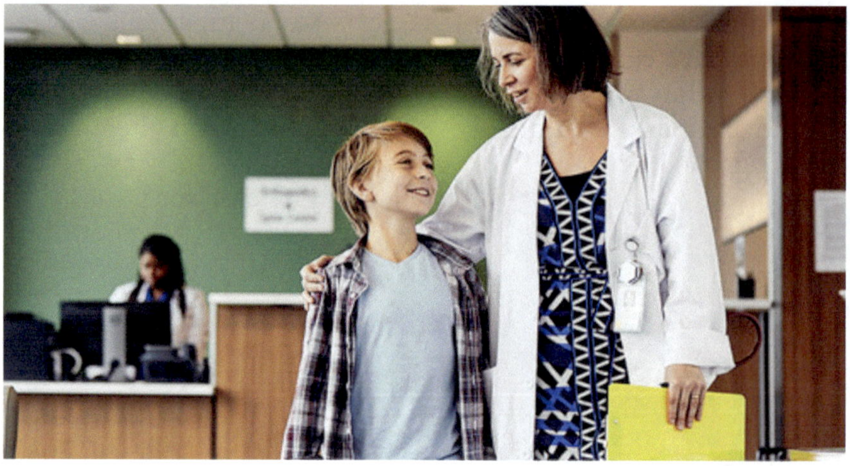

Figure 15.8. A safety culture fosters an environment where caregivers feel empowered to report errors and near misses without fear of reprisal, thereby enhancing continuous learning and improvement.

Source: https://content.cdntwrk.com/mediaproxy?url= https%3A%2F%2Fcontent.cdntwrk.com%2Ffiles%2FaHViPTEyN TczNSZjbWQ 9aXRlbWVkaXRvcmltYWdlJmZpbGVuYW1lPWl0ZW1lZGl0b3JpbWF nZV82MzRk ZDUxMGQwZDRjLmpwZyZ2ZXJzaW9uPTAwMDAmc2 lnPTNjOTI5YWEyMDMxM2JlYzVjMmJjN2FkMjZjMDc0ZThk&size=1&version= 1686162825&sig= 49fc71d3d814a3de5658ea 4d2f7e28c4&default= hubs%2Ftilebg-blogs.jpg.

15.2.8. Strategies for Preventing Medication Errors

In pediatric intensive care, where medication administration is associated with very high stakes, the requirement is to implement strong measures to prevent medication errors. One of the major approaches is the implementation of established guidelines and protocols based on practice evidence. Not only do these assist clinicians in decision-making, but they also reduce the variations that lead to errors. For instance, organizations such as the Infectious Diseases Society of America have developed quick guidelines to maximize treatment practices by systematic reviews of the literature, placing high stakes on evidence in clinical practice (Bhimraj *et al.*, 2020). Besides, we have the American Heart Association and American College of Cardiology emphasizing the use of guideline-directed management and therapy, which enables us to incorporate guidelines into drug interaction assessment and patient safety (Paul *et al.*, 2017). By incorporating such guidelines and strengthening healthcare workers' education, we can greatly enhance the quality and safety of pediatric intensive care unit care.

15.2.9. Patient Safety Outcome Assessment

For pediatric intensive care, patient safety outcomes monitoring is a key area in quality improvement efforts. Monitoring patient and family experience systematically enhances the provision of care as well as identifies where changes are necessary. Through the use of an instrument such as the Child Hospital Consumer Assessment of Healthcare Providers and Systems Survey, medical facilities can benchmark themselves against national standards, generating a culture of excellence and an environment of accountability in pediatric care (Hays *et al.*, 2020). Moreover, the determination of evidence-based practice through the culling of patient feedback lessons enables quality improvement programs to resolve challenges that impede effective care (Hays *et al.*, 2020). Involvement in this intense process of assessment is in line with broader recommendations made for pediatric care, as per sector analyses, which necessitate actionable steps that enable patient safety and optimum outcomes. Thus, a commitment towards measuring patient safety outcomes is critical in the process of advancing quality care for pediatric intensive care (Figure 15.9).

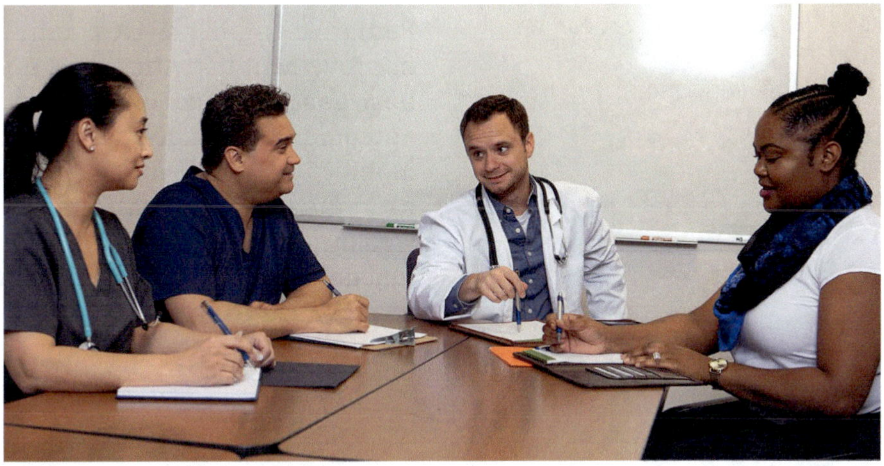

Figure 15.9. The systematic assessment of patient and family experiences not only enhances care delivery but also identifies critical areas for improvement.

Source: https://www.snhu.edu/-/media/images/social/og/quality-improve-healthcare-og.jpg.

Test Your Knowledge

1. How are adverse events reported and analyzed in pediatric critical care?
2. What technologies (e.g., barcode medication administration, EHR alerts) support patient safety?

15.3. The Impact of Quality Improvement on Patient Outcomes

Learning Outcome

1. Relationship Between Quality Improvement and Patient Outcomes.
2. Measuring Patient Outcomes in PICUs.
3. Case Studies Demonstrating Improved Outcomes.
4. The Role of Interdisciplinary Teams in Quality Improvement.
5. Patient and Family Satisfaction as an Outcome Measure.
6. Long-term Effects of Quality Improvement Initiatives.
7. Addressing Health Disparities Through Quality Improvement.
8. Economic Implications of Quality Improvement.
9. Future Research Directions on Patient Outcomes.

In pediatric critical care, quality improvement (QI) interventions have been proven to generate staggering results in patient outcomes, particularly in enhancing safety and quality of care to vulnerable patients. Focusing on evidence-based practice, healthcare organizations have been able to identify and reverse declines in patient care. For instance, intervention deployment of initiatives such as the Skin Champion program led to a staggering 85% reduction in severe hospital-acquired pressure injuries (HAPIs), clearly illustrating how much of an impact concerted QI efforts can have on compliance as well as overall patient safety (Gordon *et al.*, 2018). Likewise, it is important to apply patient and family experience data when quantifying areas for improvement, and this allows hospitals to adjust changes in their strategies accordingly based on real-life feedback from patients (Hays *et al.*, 2020). Lastly, these synergistic QI strategies improve health outcomes while cultivating a culture of continuous learning and adaptability in pediatric care settings.

15.3.1. Relationship Between Quality Improvement and Patient Outcomes

Pediatric intensive care unit (PICU) quality improvement activities have a high correlation between practice change and patient care outcomes. Systematic implementation of early mobility programs, for example, has been linked to reduced complications of PICU-acquired weakness and delirium and improved long-term functional and psychosocial recovery in critically ill pediatric patients.

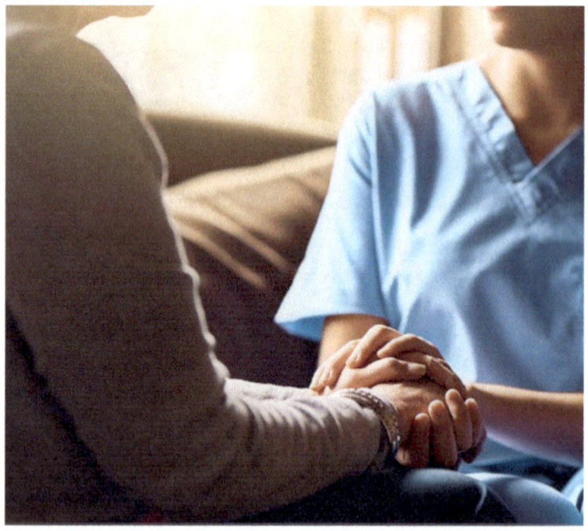

Figure 15.10. The systematic assessment of patient and family experiences not only enhances care delivery but also identifies critical areas for improvement.

Source: https://www.nestlemedicalhub.com/sites/default/files/styles/therapeutic_area_banner/public/2023-09/critical-care.png?itok=ZDJtsboF.

By using an inter-disciplinary collaborative model for quality improvement, not only are the exact mobility goals defined, but also exercise is tailored to the needs of every patient, something which is important in trying to improve recovery

(Morrow, 2021). But though it was designed to enable care, the electronic health record (EHR) system is now a clinician burnout driver that can steal attention away from patient safety and quality efforts (Downing *et al.*, 2018). Thus, such barriers need to be eliminated in order to support productive quality improvement work that has direct effects on the outcomes of PICU patients (Figure 15.10).

15.3.2. Measuring Patient Outcomes in PICUs

In pediatric intensive care units (PICUs), accurate measurement of patient outcomes is crucial to the implementation of successful quality improvement programs and for improving patient safety. One such notable measure is the development of programs for the monitoring and prevention of hospital-acquired pressure injuries (HAPIs). For example, the implementation of a Skin Champion program at one of the large city children's hospitals yielded an astonishing 85% reduction in serious injury associated with HAPIs, with significantly improved nurses' compliance with prevention practices and rates below national averages for pediatric patients (Gordon *et al.*, 2018). Also, by using patient and family survey results, such as the Child Hospital Consumer Assessment of Healthcare Providers and Systems Survey, hospitals are in a position to capture meaningful feedback and benchmark at the national level. The data informs quality improvement by establishing areas that require improvement and creating a culture for continuous care practice improvement (Hays *et al.*, 2020).

15.3.3. Case Studies Demonstrating Enhanced Outcomes

While exploring the field of pediatric intensive care, case studies have emerged as the most valuable tools for the evidence-based demonstration of improved outcomes through quality improvement initiatives. For instance, various healthcare organizations have established considerable patient safety improvements by examining their internal practices and implementing pioneering actions. Through such studies, the mirror is reflected in which the clinical teams can bring important changes by prioritizing evidence-based interventions and nurturing a culture of safety. One stand-out case study is regarding the administration of inhaled nitric oxide (iNO) treatment to preterm infants with pulmonary hypertension (PH). The research highlighted differing approaches among neonatologists, from joint decision-making with parents to prioritizing personal experience and safety over everything else (Dukhovny *et al.*, 2019). This diversity of practice emphasizes the strong imperative for interventions that are specially devised to address patient outcomes, in keeping with the national patient safety initiative's expanded objectives (Blumenthal *et al.*, 2006).

15.3.4. The Role of Interdisciplinary Teams in Quality Improvement

In pediatric intensive care, interprofessional team roles in supporting quality improvement and patient safety cannot be exaggerated. The teams, which include various healthcare professionals like physicians, nurses, pharmacists, and therapists, bring multi-dimensional expertise and experience that are crucial in addressing the complicated issues of critically ill children. By leveraging the unique strengths of each team member, interdisciplinary collaboration produces comprehensive care plans that maximize clinical results as well as communication and productivity within the healthcare environment. This evidence creates a clear correlation between systematized team function and enhanced patient safety metrics with an emphasis on teamwork outcomes and respect for each other (Kleinpell *et al.*, 2021). Moreover, process procedures like the implementation of protocols for in-hospital cardiac arrest interventions are significantly reliant on the active engagement of interdisciplinary teams to ensure effective care delivery and ongoing quality checks in pediatric settings (Paul *et al.*, 2023). To this end, developing teamwork culture remains important to ensure sustained quality improvement activities in pediatric intensive care (Figure 15.11).

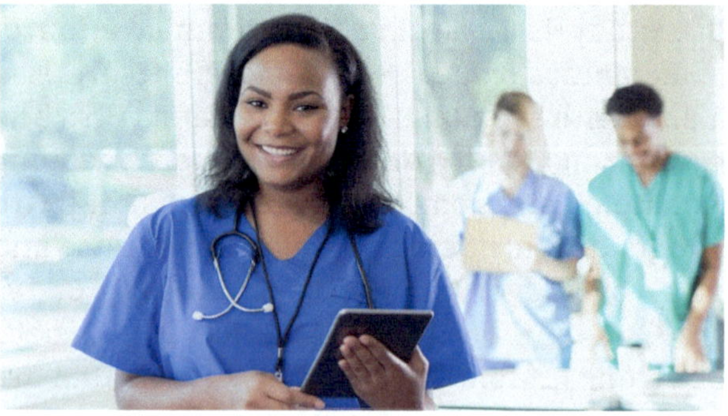

Figure 15.11. In pediatric intensive care, the function of interdisciplinary teams in enhancing quality improvement and patient safety cannot be overstated.

Source: https://www.nurseregistry.com/wp-content/uploads/2024/07/how-to-create-a-positive-work-environment-for-nurses-1200x675.jpg.

15.3.5. Patient and Family Satisfaction as an Outcome Measure

Measuring patient and family satisfaction in pediatric intensive care units (PICUs) is becoming an essential outcome measure that reflects the quality of care. This measure not only addresses the subjective perceptions of families during one of the most traumatic periods but also indirectly measures the safety and effectiveness of clinical practice. When patient and family satisfaction take precedence over healthcare organizations, they are likely to adopt activities that promote communication, openness, and empathy, fundamental elements that aid in the building of a caring environment. Case studies also illustrate how collaboration and implementation of continuous innovations can improve rates of satisfaction as marked by successful strategies presented within various healthcare settings (Blumenthal *et al.*, 2006). Also, with a shared clinical information system, management of chronic diseases and care coordination are made possible in the end, which ultimately leads to more patient and family satisfaction (McCarthy *et al.*, 2008).

15.3.6. Long-Term Effects of Quality Improvement Initiatives

Long-term effects of quality improvement interventions in PICUs are multifaceted and influence clinical practice and institutional culture. In the long term, these interventions foster a safety culture that can profoundly reduce adverse events as well as enhance patient care practices.

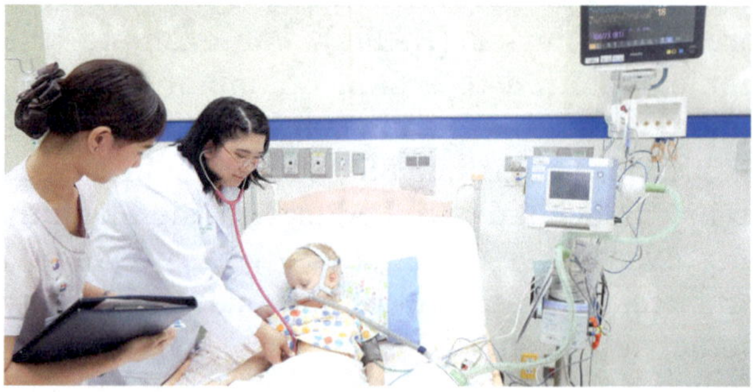

Figure 15.12. The long-term effects of quality improvement initiatives in pediatric intensive care units (PICUs) are multifaceted, influencing both clinical outcomes and institutional practices.

Source: https://mimanihospital.com/wp-content/uploads/2017/02/picu-mimani.jpg.

For instance, systematic use of evidence-based guidelines, such as in interventions that follow (Paul *et al.*, 2017), accelerates the implementation of best practices, leading to long-term reductions in patient rates of morbidity and mortality. In addition, information derived from quality improvement programs can identify persistent gaps in care, which can allow for continuous monitoring and refinement of strategies based on the needs of pediatric populations. Besides, the creation of registries for monitoring outcomes and practices can provide the impetus toward national and global standards that facilitate comparisons and collaborative efforts between health systems. The far-reaching impact of such interventions therefore continues beyond short-term benefits, reshaping the landscape of pediatric care provision to serve future generations (Figure 15.12).

15.3.7. Addressing Health Disparities Through Quality Improvement

Health disparities reduction through addressing quality improvement interventions is of great importance in enhancing patient safety, particularly in pediatric intensive care units. Social determinants are shown to play a central role in generating health inequities, whose disproportional effects predominantly weigh on children of color compared to their White counterparts, as the CDC identifies in operationalizing health disparities as preventable differences in health outcomes experienced by socially disadvantaged populations (John *et al.*, 2022).

By implementing systematic quality improvement practices, health care providers can identify and eliminate biases in care delivery, enhance pain management protocols, and alleviate barriers to access for populations of color. For example, culturally responsive interventions, including workforce diversity representation and culturally competent care, can improve communication and trust with healthcare providers and families. Lastly, highlighting equity in pediatric intensive care not only improves the health outcomes of the high-risk group but also aligns with national health goals aimed at achieving systemic health equity.

15.3.8. Economic Implications of Quality Improvement

The economic consequences of pediatric intensive care quality improvement projects are substantial, both in terms of healthcare cost and patient outcomes. Effective interventions, for example, enhanced hand hygiene protocols, have been shown to have a substantial reduction in healthcare-associated infections (HCAIs), which affect around 1.7 million hospitalized patients annually, resulting in increased morbidity and healthcare costs in healthcare systems (Haque *et al.*, 2018). By committing to quality improvement measures designed to prevent infections, healthcare facilities can minimize adverse events, and with this, the costs of prolonged hospitalization and other treatments. Furthermore, compliance with evidence-based guidelines for sepsis and septic shock management not only ensures alignment with quality care but also has economic advantages, promoting efficient resource utilization and increased patient recovery rates (Rhodes *et al.*, 2017). Ultimately, quality investment itself promotes better health outcomes, as well as a stable financial model for pediatric intensive care units (Figure 15.13).

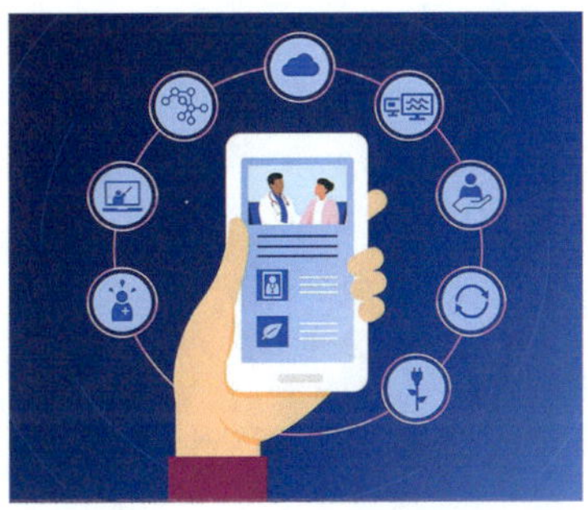

Figure 15.13. The economic implications of quality improvement initiatives within pediatric intensive care are profound, impacting both healthcare costs and patient outcomes.

Source: https://www.philips.com/c-dam/corporate/innovation-and-you/global/dec-2023/hero-2023-healthcare-technology-trends.jpg.

15.3.9. Future Research Directions on Patient Outcomes

Under the evolving paradigm of pediatric intensive care, directions for future research on patient outcomes are imperative in optimizing the potential of quality improvement and safety initiatives. Primary prevention methods are paramount to investigate, particularly with respect to the identification of populations at risk early on and intervention with methods that support mental health and general well-being, much like the shift towards secondary prevention in other health disciplines (Colizzi *et al.*, 2020). Furthermore, expansion of our understanding of chronic diseases that affect children, such as the ongoing studies on the treatment of hepatitis B, may yield some understanding of personalized therapeutic regimens and management strategies (Sarin *et al.*, 2015). Through in-depth research that focuses on clinical practices and patient-reported outcomes, future studies can illuminate the most effective ways for reducing complications and enhancing satisfaction in pediatric intensive care. Ultimately, the acceptance of these lines of research may spark a shift towards more inclusive, patient-centered care within this sensitive area of health.

Test Your Knowledge

1. How do patient and family satisfaction scores reflect the outcomes of QI efforts?
2. How are patient outcome data used to drive QI projects?

SUMMARY

The pursuit of quality enhancement and patient safety in Pediatric Intensive Care Units (PICUs) is a multidimensional approach that entails utilizing both evidence-based practice and the active involvement of patients and families. Successful introduction of quality improvement activities is dependent upon patient-centered experience, as seen through the identification of best practices that include open lines of communication with hospital staff and the utilization of feedback (Hays *et al.*, 2020). Moreover, the complexity of clinical decision-making, particularly in risky cases such as the administration of inhaled nitric oxide therapy, serves to underscore the importance of balancing empirical evidence with clinician judgment and patient values (Dukhovny *et al.*, 2019). Lastly, an organizational culture that prioritizes collaborative learning, multidisciplinary collaboration, and continuous monitoring of performance can greatly improve the safety and quality of care given to children. These programs indicate the commitment to deliver care that not only is effective but also is responsive to vulnerable groups' needs.

In the context of critical aspects of quality improvement and patient safety in pediatric intensive care, several significant issues are raised that need to be borne in mind. Firstly, clinical protocols need to be continuously evaluated for minimizing adverse events and optimizing patient outcomes. Establishing a safety culture in which healthcare workers can freely report mistakes without fear of harassment is equally helpful for this purpose. Moreover, a deeper understanding of family-centered care interventions and the influence they have on improving care coordination can lead to enhancing care coordination significantly, ultimately impacting families and patients positively. Family-centered care interventions, which recognize the significance of patient and family engagement in care decisions, are said to create enhanced satisfaction and outcomes in critical care (Judy *et al.*, 2016). Besides, studies have determined the persistence of SARS-CoV-2 in samples following preliminary negative results, highlighting the importance of proper testing procedures to ensure effective patient protection (Chen *et al.*, 2020). In general, these elements highlight the complex dynamics of practices that define quality improvement in pediatric settings.

KEY TERMS FROM THIS CHAPTER

- Quality improvement
- Electronic health records (ehrs)
- Evidence-based practice (EBP)
- Fact-based decision-making
- Anticipatory problem-solving
- Community organizations
- Patient safety
- Multipotential stem cells
- Six Sigma
- Continuous improvement
- Unplanned extubation (UE) rate
- Continuous Quality Improvement (CQI)

CRITICAL THINKING QUESTIONS

1. **What is the primary goal of quality improvement (QI) initiatives in the PICU?**
   a. Increase the number of admissions
   b. Improve patient outcomes and reduce harm
   c. Train staff in marketing strategies
   d. Reduce the length of PICU shifts
2. **Which of the following is a core principle of patient safety in critical care?**
   a. Competition among staff
   b. Blame-oriented culture
   c. Standardization of care processes
   d. Reducing documentation
3. **Which tool is commonly used to analyze root causes of adverse events in the PICU?**
   a. SWOT analysis
   b. Gantt chart
   c. Root Cause Analysis (RCA)
   d. Business Impact Analysis
4. **What is the primary focus of a morbidity and mortality (M&M) conference in the PICU?**
   a. Assign legal responsibility
   b. Discuss billing errors
   c. Improve clinical outcomes and learning from adverse events
   d. Promote competition among providers
5. **What does the "Plan-Do-Study-Act" (PDSA) cycle refer to in quality improvement?**
   a. A surgical procedure sequence
   b. A disciplinary process for staff
   c. A model for implementing and evaluating changes
   d. A psychological assessment tool

Short Answer Questions

1. What are the foundational principles of quality improvement in healthcare?
2. How does the Plan-Do-Study-Act (PDSA) cycle support continuous improvement in the PICU?
3. What are the most common types of medical errors in the PICU, and how can they be prevented?
4. How do checklists and standardized protocols improve patient safety?
5. What is the evidence for QI initiatives improving ventilator management and weaning protocols?

Answers to Critical Thinking Questions

1. (b); 2. (c); 3. (c); 4. (c); 5. (c)

REFERENCES

1. Abdalla, M. M., Khalil, R. K., Abd Elfattah, M. H., & Fekry, A. N. (2022). Quality improvement in anesthesia practice. *Benha Journal of Applied Sciences, 7*, 35–46. https://doi.org/10.21608/bjas.2022.274272 (accessed on 30th June 2025).
2. Akselsen, P. E., Assmus, J., Harthug, S., Hartveit, *et al.* (2024). Rapid response systems, antibiotic stewardship and medication reconciliation: A scoping review on implementation factors, activities and outcomes. https://core.ac.uk/download/644959221.pdf (accessed on 30th June 2025).
3. Alonso Marron, Totapally, A., Weatherly, A., De, S., Barber, M., Lifsey, A., & Boyle, K. (2025). Pediatric health assessment tracker: A quality improvement initiative to obtain weights consistently and appropriately in a tertiary pediatric intensive care unit. *Pediatric Quality & Safety, 10*. https://www.semanticscholar.org/paper/93b4978be3205825e33d55532275d16d70e7f2bb (accessed on 30th June 2025).
4. Anderson, B., & Samuels, J. (2019). Quality improvement on the long-term care ventilator unit: Interventions to increase patient safety and prevent patient harm. https://core.ac.uk/download/215541262.pdf (accessed on 30th June 2025).
5. Anderson, D. J., Podgorny, K., Berríos-Torres, S. I., Bratzler, D. W., Dellinger, E. P., Greene, L., Nyquist, A. C., *et al.* (2014). Strategies to prevent surgical site infections in acute care hospitals: 2014 update. *Infection Control and Hospital Epidemiology, 35*, 605–627. https://doi.org/10.1086/676022 (accessed on 30th June 2025).
6. Argent, A., & Frey, B. (2018). Safe pediatric intensive care: Part 2: Workplace organization, critical incident monitoring and guidelines. https://core.ac.uk/download/159154992.pdf (accessed on 30th June 2025).
7. Barber, N., Franklin, B. D., Gallivan, S., Taxis, *et al.* (2006). Can the Heinrich ratio be used to predict harm from medication errors? https://core.ac.uk/download/1747122.pdf (accessed on 30th June 2025).
8. Behere, M. D., & Ritz, M. D. (2017). Beat to beat: Implementing a tailored literature review e-newsletter for a multidisciplinary subspecialty group. https://core.ac.uk/download/84904321.pdf (accessed on 30th June 2025).
9. Bhimraj, A., Morgan, R. L., Shumaker, A. H., Lavergne, V., Baden, L. R., Cheng, V. C. C., Edwards, K. M., *et al.* (2020). Infectious Diseases Society of America guidelines on the treatment and management of patients with COVID-19 (April 2020). *Clinical Infectious Diseases, 78*, e83–e102. https://doi.org/10.1093/cid/ciaa478 (accessed on 30th June 2025).
10. Blumenthal, D., & McCarthy, D. (2006). Committed to safety: Ten case studies on reducing harm to patients. https://core.ac.uk/download/71350251.pdf (accessed on 30th June 2025).
11. Branch, C. (2013). Compassion fatigue: Prevalence among nurses at a Midwest pediatric hospital. https://core.ac.uk/download/217321686.pdf (accessed on 30th June 2025).
12. Canonica, G. W., Alacqua, M., Altraja, A., Backer, V., Bel, E. H., Bjermer, L., Björnsdóttir, U. S., *et al.* (2019). International Severe Asthma Registry. *CHEST Journal, 157*, 805–814. https://doi.org/10.1016/j.chest.2019.10.051 (accessed on 30th June 2025).
13. Camargo Carvalho De , M. F. F., DE Brito Santos, F. V., Seber, A., Chiattone, R. R., Bigni, R., Maiolino, Â., Barroso, F., *et al.* (2023). Implementation of clinical pathways for CAR-T cell

therapy in a Brazilian private healthcare organization. *Blood*. https://www.semanticscholar.org/paper/dc2e9e347ecae5dee9bb9854704bdb9a462b0fa2 (accessed on 30th June 2025).

14. Chan, P. S., Greif, R., Anderson, T. D., Atiq, H., Couto, T. B., Considine, J., de Caen, A. R., *et al.* (2023). Ten steps toward improving in-hospital cardiac arrest quality of care and outcomes. *Resuscitation, 193*, 109996–109996. https://doi.org/10.1016/j.resuscitation.2023.109996 (accessed on 30th June 2025).

15. Chen, C., Gao, G., Xu, Y., Pu, L., Wang, Q., Wang, L., Wang, W., *et al.* (2020). SARS-CoV-2–positive sputum and feces after conversion of pharyngeal samples in patients with COVID-19. *Annals of Internal Medicine, 172*, 832–834. https://doi.org/10.7326/m20-0991 (accessed on 30th June 2025).

16. Colizzi, M., Lasalvia, A., & Ruggeri, M. (2020). Prevention and early intervention in youth mental health: Is it time for a multidisciplinary and trans-diagnostic model for care? *International Journal of Mental Health Systems, 14*. https://doi.org/10.1186/s13033-020-00356-9 (accessed on 30th June 2025).

17. Cuevas Guaman, M., Miller, E., Dammann, C., Bishop, C., & Machut, K. Z. (2022). Neonatologist staffing models: urgent change is needed. *Journal of Perinatology, 42*, 1556–1557. https://www.semanticscholar.org/paper/5d76fe358d95f3e01d078027c6de15ec2ac09d6c (accessed on 30th June 2025).

18. Davidson, J. E., Aslakson, R. A., Long, A. C., Puntillo, K., Kross, E. K., Hart, J. L., Cox, C. E., *et al.* (2016). Guidelines for family-centered care in the neonatal, pediatric, and adult ICU. *Critical Care Medicine, 45*, 103–128. https://doi.org/10.1097/ccm.0000000000002169 (accessed on 30th June 2025).

19. Downing, N. L., Bates, D. W., & Longhurst, C. (2018). Physician burnout in the electronic health record era: Are we ignoring the real cause? *Annals of Internal Medicine, 169*, 50–50. https://doi.org/10.7326/m18-0139 (accessed on 30th June 2025).

20. Duffy, S., & Horton-Deutch, T. (2021). The resilience vaccine. https://core.ac.uk/download/534720117.pdf (accessed on 30th June 2025).

21. Dukhovny, D., Guyatt, G., Jack, S., Kirpalani, *et al.* (2019). Factors influencing decision making in neonatology: Inhaled nitric oxide in preterm infants. https://core.ac.uk/download/323069963.pdf (accessed on 30th June 2025).

22. Elghadban, F. (2024). Sepsis epidemiology and outcomes in pediatric intensive care unit of Alkhadra Hospital, Tripoli, Libya. *AlQalam Journal of Medical and Applied Sciences*. https://www.semanticscholar.org/paper/a71bb9031fc306e02baff5f62d1391c00f140247 (accessed on 30th June 2025).

23. Evans, C., Manning, J. C., & Suleman, Z. (2019). Parents' and carers' experiences of transition and aftercare following a child's discharge from a pediatric intensive care unit to an in-patient ward setting: A qualitative systematic review. https://core.ac.uk/download/228155955.pdf (accessed on 30th June 2025).

24. Fan, E., Brodie, D., & Slutsky, A. S. (2018). Acute respiratory distress syndrome. *JAMA, 319*, 698–698. https://doi.org/10.1001/jama.2017.21907 (accessed on 30th June 2025).

25. Gordon, M. D., Hagan, J., *et al.* (2018). Evidence-based skin champion program reduces pressure injuries in a pediatric hospital. https://core.ac.uk/download/212897182.pdf (accessed on 30th June 2025).

26. Gray, S., Silver, S., Seto, W., Pong, S., Theissen, A., Chan, P., Carey, S., *et al.* (2022). PP297 [Quality and safety » data management (EHR, documentation)]: Implementing "Adult COVID-19" electronic order sets in a children's hospital. *Pediatric Critical Care Medicine*. https://www.semanticscholar.org/paper/26ab67a5d80ca6273fc18f9632f0bde49d4fc9f3 (accessed on 30th June 2025).

27. Gupta, N., Sones, A., Powell, M., Robbins, J., Wilson, S., Hill, A., Thomas, C. L., *et al.* (2020). 1263: Quality improvement methodology to optimize safe early mobility in a pediatric intensive care unit. *Critical Care Medicine*. https://www.semanticscholar.org/paper/f9d80b147a8c9c2bac1f456bb70d7a4eb2d36ad2 (accessed on 30th June 2025).

28. Hamad, N., Abdallah, H. M. M., Abdelaliem, S. M. F., & Shaheen, R. S. (2025). Pediatric nurses' challenges in implementing and sustaining clinical handover in intensive care units: Advocating for the safety of critically ill pediatric patients. *Journal of Clinical Nursing*. https://www.semanticscholar.org/paper/109607bb44719d6de3cdfa32543728271cad8df7 (accessed on 30th June 2025).

29. Haque, M., Sartelli, M., McKimm, J., & Abu Bakar, M. (2018). Health care-associated infections–an overview. *Infection and Drug Resistance, 11*, 2321–2333. https://doi.org/10.2147/idr.s177247 (accessed on 30th June 2025).

30. Hays, R. D., Lerner, C., Palimaru, A., Quigley, *et al.* (2020). A review of best practices for monitoring and improving inpatient pediatric patient experiences. https://core.ac.uk/download/287622168.pdf (accessed on 30th June 2025).

31. Iten, R. (2024). Care management trajectories of infants with life-limiting conditions who died before 12 months of age and understanding how we deliver palliative care. https://core.ac.uk/download/621345438.pdf (accessed on 30th June 2025).

32. Kleinpell, R., Grabenkort, W. R., Boyle, W. A., Vines, D., & Olsen, K. M. (2021). The Society of Critical Care Medicine at 50 years: Interprofessional practice in critical care: Looking back and forging ahead. *Critical Care Medicine, 49*, 2017–2032. https://doi.org/10.1097/ccm.0000000000005276 (accessed on 30th June 2025).

33. Lafferty, A., Porteous, K. Y., & Robertson, C. (2024). Perioperative practitioners' experiences of critical incident debriefing: A qualitative explorative study. https://core.ac.uk/download/631304417.pdf (accessed on 30th June 2025).

34. Larson, J., Kazura, A., Fortuna, L. R., French, W. P., Hodas, G. R., Metz, P., McGinty, K. L., *et al.* (2022). Clinical update: Child and adolescent behavioral health care in community systems of care. *Journal of the American Academy of Child & Adolescent Psychiatry, 62*, 367–384. https://doi.org/10.1016/j.jaac.2022.06.001 (accessed on 30th June 2025).

35. Leape, L. L. (2014). Patient safety in the era of healthcare reform. *Clinical Orthopedics and Related Research, 473*, 1568–1573. https://doi.org/10.1007/s11999-014-3598-6 (accessed on 30th June 2025).

36. Marsh, M. C., Supples, S., McLaurin-Jiang, S., Brown, C. L., & Linton, J. M. (2019). Introducing the concepts of advocacy and social determinants of health within the pediatric clerkship. *MedEdPORTAL*. https://doi.org/10.15766/mep_2374-8265.10798 (accessed on 30th June 2025).

37. McCarthy, D., & Leatherman, S. (2004). Quality of health care for children and adolescents: A chartbook. https://core.ac.uk/download/71354153.pdf (accessed on 30th June 2025).

38. McCarthy, D., & Mueller, K. (2008). The New York City Health and Hospitals Corporation: Transforming a public safety net delivery system to achieve higher performance. https://core.ac.uk/download/71353446.pdf (accessed on 30th June 2025).

39. Memon, Z., Memon, Q. Z., Iqbal, H., Haider, S. J., Devi, R., & Maheen, M. (2025). Innovative approaches in pediatric medicine: Emerging trends and future perspectives. *Journal of Medical & Health Sciences Review*. https://www.semanticscholar.org/paper/744e7a451386de5168df76b51c2faf5dc775888b (accessed on 30th June 2025).

40. Mohamed, N. E., Hammoud, E., & Abdelmassih, A. (2025). Barriers to family education, a potential room for improvement of readmission in pediatric intensive care unit. *Journal of Pediatric Critical Care*. https://www.semanticscholar.org/paper/68c214da3427027d8abc2c7e0420e58fe85f2646 (accessed on 30th June 2025).

41. Morrow, B. (2021). Building a culture of early mobilization in the pediatric intensive care unit—a nuts and bolts approach. *Translational Pediatrics, 10*, 2845–2857. https://www.semanticscholar.org/paper/9318773c2ff31c19ca290451a1276ec9bf3ac908 (accessed on 30th June 2025).

42. Omran, D. A. S., Alsayat, J. Y., Kashmiri, M. E., Binmuhareb, A. K., Almutiri, J. M., & Alreshidi, R. E. F. (2024). Comprehensive review of quality improvement strategies in pediatric healthcare. *Journal of Eco Humanism*. https://www.semanticscholar.org/paper/13a3426513c62793297061bfa6ec3a567e7131b8 (accessed on 30th June 2025).

43. Ortíz-Barrios, M., & Alfaro-Saíz, J. J. (2020). Methodological approaches to support process improvement in emergency departments: A systematic review. *International Journal of Environmental Research and Public Health, 17*, 2664. https://doi.org/10.3390/ijerph17082664 (accessed on 30th June 2025).

44. Patton, J. W., Burton, B. N., Milam, A. J., Mariano, E. R., & Gabriel, R. A. (2022). Health disparities in regional anesthesia and analgesia for the management of acute pain in trauma patients. *International Anesthesiology Clinics*. https://doi.org/10.1097/aia.0000000000000382 (accessed on 30th June 2025).

45. Pittenger, M. F., Discher, D. E., Péault, B., Phinney, D. G., Hare, J. M., & Caplan, A. I. (2019). Mesenchymal stem cell perspective: Cell biology to clinical progress. *npj Regenerative Medicine, 4*. https://doi.org/10.1038/s41536-019-0083-6 (accessed on 30th June 2025).

46. Prestel, C., Barnes, L. E. A., Kuhar, D., & Sinkowitz-Cochran, R. (2023). 1707. New directions for infection prevention in the neonatal intensive care unit: A key informant exploration. *Open Forum Infectious Diseases, 10*. https://www.semanticscholar.org/paper/d51c53499329e3a01f0bddfd515bc3bf18d999d3 (accessed on 30th June 2025).

47. Ray-Barruel, G., Silva, T. L., & Rocha, P. K. (2025). Implementation of the I-DECIDED® tool for PIVC assessment and decision making: Discussion paper. *British Journal of Nursing, 34*(2), S12–S20. https://www.semanticscholar.org/paper/a215cb6dbeb7f19f33b8270f4bafc44a8c531c90 (accessed on 30th June 2025).

48. Rhodes, A., Evans, L., Alhazzani, W., Levy, M. M., Antonelli, M., Ferrer, R., Kumar, A., *et al.* (2017). Surviving Sepsis Campaign: International guidelines for management of sepsis and septic shock: 2016. *Critical Care Medicine, 45*, 486–552. https://doi.org/10.1097/ccm.0000000000002255 (accessed on 30th June 2025).

49. Rice, A., Noseworthy, C., Ashraf, K., Seferian, E., & Nawathe, P. (2022). 1053: Improving PICU patient safety by implementing a robust supply chain management process. *Critical Care Medicine*. https://www.semanticscholar.org/paper/b036d5a310fde0061eed9c5c6c4420e852e7b641 (accessed on 30th June 2025).

50. Sarin, S. K., Kumar, M., Lau, G., Abbas, Z., Chan, H. L. Y., Chen, C. J., Chen, D. S., *et al.* (2015). Asian-Pacific clinical practice guidelines on the management of hepatitis B: A 2015 update. *Hepatology International, 10*, 1–98. https://doi.org/10.1007/s12072-015-9675-4 (accessed on 30th June 2025).

51. Schwartz, D. M. (2020). Implementation and evaluation of a compassion satisfaction program for healthcare providers of children with medical complexity. https://core.ac.uk/download/322851769.pdf (accessed on 30th June 2025).

52. Simpson, L., & Struchen-Shellhorn, W. (2008). The promise of health information technology: Ensuring that Florida's children benefit. https://core.ac.uk/download/71342408.pdf (accessed on 30th June 2025).

53. Slawomirski, L., Auraaen, A., & Klazinga, N. S. (2017). The economics of patient safety. *OECD Health Working Papers*. https://doi.org/10.1787/5a9858cd-en (accessed on 30th June 2025).

54. Stout, K., Daniels, C. J., Aboulhosn, J., Bozkurt, B., Broberg, C. S., Colman, J. M., Crumb, S. R., *et al.* (2018). 2018 AHA/ACC guideline for the management of adults with congenital heart disease: A report of the American College of Cardiology/American Heart Association task force on clinical practice guidelines. *Circulation, 139*. https://doi.org/10.1161/cir.0000000000000603 (accessed on 30th June 2025).

55. Thabet, F., Zayani, S., Daya, A., Chouchane, C., & Chouchane, S. (2025). Enhancing safety in mechanical ventilation: A quality improvement initiative targeting unplanned estuations in a Tunisian PICU. *Pediatric Quality & Safety, 10*. https://www.semanticscholar.org/paper/6788911bbf3a0f08ac8a94a386fba6aee23ec138 (accessed on 30th June 2025).

56. Trivedi, K. K., Schaffzin, J. K., Deloney, V. M., Aureden, K., Carrico, R., Garcia-Houchins, S., Garrett, J. H., *et al.* (2023). Implementing strategies to prevent infections in acute-care settings. *Infection Control and Hospital Epidemiology, 44*, 1232–1246. https://doi.org/10.1017/ice.2023.103 (accessed on 30th June 2025).

57. Vega, L. M. (2024). The implementation of an educational program to improve registered nurses' knowledge levels and reduce delays to admission to the operating room–A quality improvement project. https://core.ac.uk/download/643773280.pdf (accessed on 30th June 2025).

58. Whelton, P. K., Carey, R. M., Aronow, W. S., Casey, D. E., Collins, K. J., Dennison Himmelfarb, C., DePalma, S. M., *et al.* (2017). 2017 ACC/AHA/AAPA/ABC/ACPM/AGS/APhA/ASH/ASPC/NMA/PCNA guideline for the prevention, detection, evaluation, and management of high blood pressure in adults: A report of the American College of Cardiology/American Heart Association Task Force on Clinical Practice Guidelines. *Hypertension, 71*. https://doi.org/10.1161/hyp.0000000000000065 (accessed on 30th June 2025).

INDEX

G

H

I

K

L

M